Decision Making in Otolaryngology

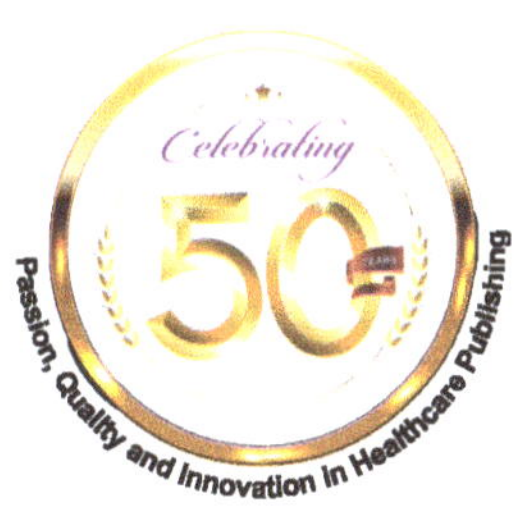

Decision Making in Otolaryngology

Second Edition

Editors

Cuneyt M Alper MD
Professor of Otolaryngology and Clinical and Translational Science
University of Pittsburgh School of Medicine
Vice-Chair of Research, Division of Pediatric Otolaryngology
Children's Hospital of Pittsburgh
University of Pittsburgh Medical Center
Pittsburgh, Pennsylvania, USA

Eugene N Myers MD FACS FRCS Edin (Hon)
Distinguished Professor and Emeritus Chair
Department of Otolaryngology
University of Pittsburgh School of Medicine
Professor
Department of Oral Maxillofacial Surgery
University of Pittsburgh School of Dental Medicine
Pittsburgh, Pennsylvania, USA

David E Eibling MD FACS
Professor of Otolaryngology
University of Pittsburgh School of Medicine
Vice-Chair for Education
Department of Otolaryngology
Assistant Chief of Surgery
VA Pittsburgh
Co-Director VA Pittsburgh Inter-professional Fellowship in Patient Safety
Pittsburgh, Pennsylvania, USA

Foreword

Michael M Paparella MD

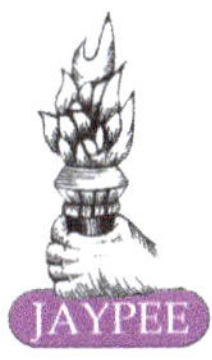

JAYPEE BROTHERS MEDICAL PUBLISHERS
The Health Sciences Publisher
New Delhi | London | Panama

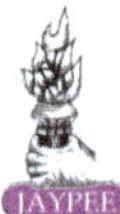 **Jaypee Brothers Medical Publishers (P) Ltd**

Headquarters

Jaypee Brothers Medical Publishers (P) Ltd
4838/24, Ansari Road, Daryaganj
New Delhi 110 002, India
Phone: +91-11-43574357
Fax: +91-11-43574314
Email: jaypee@jaypeebrothers.com

Overseas Offices

J.P. Medical Ltd
83 Victoria Street, London
SW1H 0HW (UK)
Phone: +44 20 3170 8910
Fax: +44 (0)20 3008 6180
Email: info@jpmedpub.com

Jaypee-Highlights Medical Publishers Inc
City of Knowledge, Bld. 235, 2nd Floor, Clayton
Panama City, Panama
Phone: +1 507-301-0496
Fax: +1 507-301-0499
Email: cservice@jphmedical.com

Jaypee Brothers Medical Publishers (P) Ltd
Bhotahity, Kathmandu, Nepal
Phone +977-9741283608
Email: kathmandu@jaypeebrothers.com

Website: www.jaypeebrothers.com
Website: www.jaypeedigital.com

Decision Making in Otolaryngology

First Edition: 2001 (Saunders)

Second Edition: **2019**

ISBN: 978-93-8605-608-5

Dedication

I dedicate our book *Decision Making in Otolaryngology 2nd Edition*
to my mother Meral, my father Zeki,
my sister Sule Nesrin, my son Berk and all my teachers.

Cuneyt M Alper

I dedicate our book *Decision Making in Otolaryngology 2nd Edition*
to my wife Barbara, our daughter Marjorie Fulbright, her husband Cary,
and their sons Alex and Chip, our son Jeffrey N Myers, MD, PhD, his wife Lisa,
and their sons Keith, Brett, and Blake. The book is also dedicated to my parents Dr David
and Rosalind N Myers for their lifetime commitment to the specialty of Otolaryngology
and the legacy they left.

Eugene N Myers

This book is dedicated to the residents I have worked with for the past 47 years who have taught me so much.
As I have aged I realize now that I have learned much more from them than they have learned from me.
I also dedicate it to my wife Carol who (more or less) tolerated the piles of draft chapters, edited chapters, and proofs generated
by the development of this book that nearly covered our dining room table for the past year and a half!

David E Eibling

Shelly Abramowicz DMD MPH
Assistant Professor
Oral and Maxillofacial Surgery and
Pediatrics
Emory University
Children's Healthcare of Atlanta
Atlanta, Georgia, USA

William G Albergotti MD
Clinical Instructor
Medical University of South Carolina
Charleston, South Carolina, USA

Gregory C Allen MD FASC FAAP
Associate Professor
Department of Otolaryngology—
Head and Neck Surgery
University of Colorado School of Medicine
Children's Hospital Colorado
Aurora, Colorado, USA

Cuneyt M Alper MD
Professor of Otolaryngology and
Clinical and Translational Science
University of Pittsburgh School of Medicine
Vice-Chair of Research
Division of Pediatric Otolaryngology
Children's Hospital of Pittsburgh of UPMC
University of Pittsburgh Medical Center
Pittsburgh, Pennsylvania, USA

Samantha Anne MD MS
Assistant Professor
Pediatric Otolaryngology
Head and Neck Institute
Cleveland Clinic
Cleveland, Ohio, USA

Stephanie Moody Antonio MD FACS
Associate Professor
Eastern Virginia Medical School
Children's Hospital of the King's
Daughters
Norfolk, Virginia, USA

Swathi Appachi MD
Resident Physician
Head and Neck Institute
Cleveland Clinic
Cleveland, Ohio, USA

Ellis M Arjmand MD MMM PhD
Chief of Service
Pediatric Otolaryngology
Texas Children's Hospital
Bobby Alford Endowed Chair in
Pediatric Otolaryngology
Professor of Otolaryngology and
Pediatrics, Baylor College of Medicine
Texas Children's Hospital and Baylor
College of Medicine
Houston, Texas, USA

Moisés A Arriaga MD MBA FACS
Clinical Professor of Otolaryngology and
Neurosurgery
Director of Otology and Neurotology
Louisiana State University Medical School
Director, Hearing and Balance Center
Our Lady of the Lake Regional Medical
Center, Baton Rouge, USA
Director, CNC Hearing and Balance
Center, New Orleans, USA
Director, Childrens Hospital Cochlear
Implant Program, New Orleans
New Orleans and Baton Rouge
Louisiana, USA

Elton Ashe-Lambert MD
Assistant Professor
Baylor College of Medicine
Texas Children's Hospital
Houston, Texas, USA

Yehia M Ashry MSc
Research Fellow
Department of Otolaryngology
Boston Children's Hospital
Boston, Massachusetts, USA
Lecturer, Department of Ear
Nose and Throat
Suez Canal University
Ismailia, Egypt

Henry P Barham MD
Otolaryngologist
Sinus and Nasal Specialists of
Louisiana, LLC
Baton Rouge, Lousiana, USA

Julie E Bauman MD MPH
Professor of Medicine
Chief, Division of Hematology/Oncology
University of Arizona Cancer Center
Tucson, Arizona, USA

Sebastian M Brooke MD
Plastic Surgeon/Craniofacial Surgeon
Baylor Scott and White
Temple, Texas, USA

Farrel J Buchinsky MBChB
BSc(Hons)(Med) FACS
Director
Respiratory Papillomatosis Program
Allegheny-Singer Research Institute
Allegheny Health Network
Pittsburgh, Pennsylvania, USA

Craig A Buchman MD FACS
Lindburg Professor and Head
Department of Otolaryngology—
Head and Neck Surgery
Washington University School of Medicine
St Louis, Missouri, USA

Jeffrey M Bumpous MD
J Samuel Bimgardner
Professor and Chairman
Otolaryngology Head and Neck Surgery
and Communicative Disorders
University of Louisville
Louisville, Kentucky, USA

John M Burnheimer DMD MS
Assistant Professor
Department of Otolaryngology
University of Pittsburgh
Pittsburgh, Pennsylvania, USA

Susan E Calderbank DMD
Assistant Professor
Oral Medicine Department
University of Pittsburgh School of
Dental Medicine
Attending Dentist
University of Pittsburgh Medical Center
(UPMC)
Presbyterian Shadyside Dental Center
Pittsburgh, Pennsylvania, USA

Ricardo L Carrau MD FACS
Professor and Lynne Shepard Jones
Chair in Head and Neck Oncology
Department of Otolaryngology—
Head and Neck Surgery
Director of the Comprehensive Skull
Base Surgery Program
The Ohio State University Wexner
Medical Center
Co-Director
Anatomy Laboratory Toward
Visuospatial Surgical Innovations in
Otolaryngology and Neurosurgery
(ALT-VISION)
Columbus, Ohio, USA

Stephen P Cass MD
Professor
Department of Otolaryngology
University of Colorado School of Medicine
Aurora, Colorado, USA

Margaretha L Casselbrant MD PhD
Professor
Department of Otolaryngology
University of Pittsburgh School of
Medicine
Pittsburgh, Pennsylvania, USA

CY Joseph Chang MD
Director
Texas Ear Center
Clinical Professor
Division of Surgery
Department of Otorhinolaryngology
Head and Neck Surgery
University of Texas – McGovern Medical
School
University of Texas MD Anderson
Cancer Center
Houston, Texas, USA

Douglas A Chen MD
Director
Division of Neurotology
Department of Neurosurgery
Allegheny General Hospital
Pittsburgh Ear Associates
Pittsburgh, Pennsylvania, USA

David H Chi MD
Associate Professor of Otolaryngology
University of Pittsburgh School of Medicine
Chief, Division of Pediatric Otolaryngology
Children's Hospital of Pittsburgh
University of Pittsburgh Medical Center
Pittsburgh, Pennsylvania, USA

Adrienne L Childers MD
Assistant Professor
Department of Otolaryngology
Saint Louis University
Saint Louis, Missouri, USA

Sukgi S Choi MD MBA
Lecturer in Otolaryngology
Harvard Medical School
Otolaryngologist
Boston Children's Hospital
Boston, Massachusetts, USA

David A Clump MD PhD
Assistant Professor
Department of Radiation Oncology
University of Pittsburgh School of
Medicine
Pittsburgh, Pennsylvania, USA

David M Cognetti MD FACS
Associate Professor
Department of Otolaryngology—
Head and Neck Surgery
Sidney Kimmel Cancer Center
Thomas Jefferson University
Philadelphia, Pennsylvania, USA

Michael S Cohen MD
Assistant Professor
Department of Otolaryngology
Harvard Medical School
Massachusetts Eye and Ear Infirmary
Boston, Massachusetts, USA

Bernard J Costello DMD MD FACS
Dean
University of Pittsburgh School of
Dental Medicine
Chief
Pediatric Oral and Maxillofacial Surgery
Children's Hospital of Pittsburgh
Professor and Fellowship Program
Director
Department of Oral and Maxillofacial
Surgery
University of Pittsburgh Medical Center
Pittsburgh, Pennsylvania, USA

Joseph M Curry MD FACS
Associate Professor
Sidney Kimmel Cancer Center
Thomas Jefferson University
Philadelphia, Pennsylvania, USA

Sam J Daniel MDCM FRCSC
Professor
Pediatric Surgery and Otolaryngology
Hugh Hallward Chair Pediatric Surgery
McGill University
Montreal, Quebec, Canada

Kavita Dedhia MD
Assistant Professor
Department of Otolaryngology—
Head and Neck Surgery
Emory University
Atlanta, Georgia, USA

Peter N Demas DMD MD
Associate Professor
Department of Oral and Maxillofacial
Surgery
University of Pittsburgh
School of Dental Medicine
Pittsburgh, Pennsylvania, USA

Craig S Derkay MD FACS
Professor and Vice Chairman
Director of Pediatric Otolaryngology
Eastern Virginia Medical School
Norfolk, Virginia, USA

Dipan D Desai MD
Resident Physician
University of Texas Southwestern
Dallas, Texas, USA

Mark A Dettelbach MD
Senior Attending
Georgetown University
Washington DC, USA

Matilda Dhima DMD MS
Assistant Professor
Department of Prosthodontics
University of Pittsburgh School of
Dental Medicine
Pittsburgh, Pennsylvania, USA

Joseph E Dohar MD MS FAAP FACS
Professor of Otolaryngology
University of Pittsburgh School of
Medicine
Pittsburgh, Pennsylvania, USA

Michael Dohopolski BS
Medical Student
University of Pittsburgh School of
Medicine
Pittsburgh, Pennsylvania, USA

Umamaheswar Duvvuri MD PhD
Assistant Professor of Otolaryngology
University of Pittsburgh School of Medicine
Director of Robotic Surgery
Division of Head and Neck Surgery
Director, Center of Advanced Robotics
Training (CART)
Pittsburgh, Pennsylvania, USA

David E Eibling MD FACS
Professor of Otolaryngology
University of Pittsburgh School of Medicine
Vice-Chair for Education
Department of Otolaryngology
Assistant Chief of Surgery
VA Pittsburgh
Co-Director, VA Pittsburgh
Interprofessional Fellowship in
Patient Safety
Pittsburgh, Pennsylvania, USA

Johannes J Fagan MBCHB MMed FCS (ORL)
Professor and Chair
Division of Otolaryngology
University of Cape Town
Cape Town, South Africa

Berrylin J Ferguson MD*
Professor
Department of Otolaryngology
University of Pittsburgh School of Medicine
Pittsburgh, Pennsylvania, USA
*Deceased

Robert L Ferris MD PhD
Hillman Professor of Oncology and
Director
UPMC Hillman Cancer Center
Associate Vice-Chancellor for
Cancer Research
Co-Director
Tumor Microenvironment Center
Professor of Otolaryngology,
Immunology, and Radiation Oncology
Pittsburgh, Pennsylvania, USA

Peter F Ferson MD
Charles G Watson Professor of
Surgical Education
Professor of Cardiothoracic Surgery
University of Pittsburgh School of
Medicine
Pittsburgh, Pennsylvania, USA

Rebecca E Fraioli MD
Assistant Professor
Department of Otolaryngology—
Head and Neck Surgery
Albert Einstein College of Medicine
Montefiore Medical Center
Bronx, New York, USA

Shannon Fraser MD
Otolaryngologist
Alaska Native Medical Center
Anchorage, Alaska, USA

Zachary C Fridirici MD
Chief Resident, PGY-5
Loyola Department of Otolaryngology—
Head and Neck Surgery
Maywood, Illinois, USA

Jenifer Fruit AuD*
Audiologist
University of Pittsburgh Medical Center
Pittsburgh, Pennsylvania, USA
*Deceased

Joseph M Furman MD PhD
Professor
Department of Otolaryngology and
Neurology
University of Pittsburgh School of Medicine
Pittsburgh, Pennsylvania, USA

Joseph C Fusco MD
Pediatric Surgery Research Fellow
Children's Hospital of Pittsburgh of
University of Pittsburgh Medical Center
Pittsburgh, Pennsylvania, USA

Jackie L Gartner-Schmidt PhD CCC-SLP
Speech-Language Pathologist
Department of Otolaryngology
University of Pittsburgh Medical Center
Pittsburgh, Pennsylvania, USA

Jessica L Geiger MD
Associate Staff and
Clinical Assistant Professor
Cleveland Clinic Taussig Cancer
Institute and Lerner College of Medicine
of Case Western Reserve University
Cleveland, Ohio, USA

Mathew Geltzeiler MD
Assistant Professor
Otolaryngology—Head and Neck Surgery
Oregon Health and Science University
Portland, Oregon, USA

Grant S Gillman MD FRCS(C)
Associate Professor
Department of Otolaryngology
University of Pittsburgh School of
Medicine
Director, Division of Facial Plastic and
Reconstructive Surgery
Pittsburgh, Pennsylvania, USA

George K Gittes MD
Benjamin R Fisher Chair of Pediatric
Surgery and Surgeon-in-Chief
Children's Hospital of Pittsburgh of UPMC
Professor, Department of Surgery and
Professor of Pediatrics
University of Pittsburgh School of Medicine
Pittsburgh, Pennsylvania, USA

Andrew N Goldberg MD MSCE FACS
Boles Professor and Vice Chair
Director, Division of Rhinology and
Sinus Surgery
Department of Otolaryngology—
Head and Neck Surgery
University of California, San Francisco
San Francisco, California, USA

Jesse Goldstein MD FAAP FACS
Assistant Professor
Department of Plastic Surgery
Children's Hospital of Pittsburgh of
University of Pittsburgh Medical Center
Pittsburgh, Pennsylvania, USA

Nira A Goldstein MD MPH
Professor of Clinical Otolaryngology
State University of New York Downstate
Medical Center
Brooklyn, New York, USA

Nandini Govil MD MPH
Resident Physician
Department of Otolaryngology
University of Pittsburgh Medical Center
Pittsburgh, Pennsylvania, USA

Kenneth M Grundfast MD FACS
Professor
Department of Otolaryngology—
Head and Neck Surgery
Boston University School of Medicine
Boston, Massachusetts, USA

Lorelei J Grunwaldt MD FACS FAAP
Associate Professor of Surgery
Division of Pediatric Plastic Surgery
Cleft-Craniofacial Center
Director of Brachial Plexus Clinic and
Vascular Anomalies Clinic
Children's Hospital of Pittsburgh
University of Pittsburgh Medical Center
Pittsburgh, Pennsylvania, USA

Trevor Hackman MD
Associate Professor
Department of Otolaryngology—
Head and Neck Surgery
University of North Carolina
Chapel Hill, North Carolina, USA

Sheng-Po Hao MD
Professor and Chairman
Department of Otolaryngology
Shin Kong Wu Ho-Su Memorial Hospital
Fu Jen Catholic University Hospital
Taipei, Taiwan

Bridget Hathaway MD
Assistant Professor
Department of Otolaryngology
University of Pittsburgh School of
Medicine
Pittsburgh, Pennsylvania, USA

Larry D Hartzell MD FAAP
Associate Professor of Otolaryngology—
Head and Neck Surgery
The University of Arkansas for
Medical Sciences
Arkansas Children's Hospital
Little Rock, Arkansas, USA

Andrea M Hebert MD MPH
Assistant Professor
Department of Otorhinolaryngology—
Head and Neck Surgery
University of Maryland School of
Medicine
Baltimore, Maryland, USA

Andrew Herlich DMD MD FAAP FASA
Professor and Special Assistant to the Chair
Academic and Faculty Affairs
Department of Anesthesiology
University of Pittsburgh School of
Medicine
Pittsburgh, Pennsylvania, USA

Jacques Herzog MD
Associate Professor
Department of Otolaryngology—
Head and Neck Surgery
Washington University School of Medicine
St. Louis, Missouri, USA

Douglas M Hildrew MD
Assistant Professor
Yale School of Medicine
Department of Surgery
Section of Otolaryngology —
Head and Neck Surgery
Otology, Neurotology and
Skull Base Surgery
New Haven, Connecticut, USA

Barry E Hirsch MD
Professor, Departments of Otolaryngology
Communication Science and Disorders
and Neurological Surgery
University of Pittsburgh School of Medicine
Director, Division of Otology, Neurotology
University of Pittsburgh Medical Center
Pittsburgh, Pennsylvania, USA

David L Horn MD MS
Associate Professor
Department of Otolaryngology—
Head and Neck Surgery
University of Washington
Co-director Cochlear Implant Program
Seattle Children's Hospital
Seattle, Washington DC, USA

Andrew J Hotaling MD
Professor
Department of Otolaryngology—
Head and Neck Surgery and Pediatrics
Loyola University Medical Center
Maywood, Illinois, USA

Sean D Houston MD
Private Practitioner
General Otolaryngology
Neptune, New Jersey, USA

Winslo K Idicula MD
Assistant Professor of Otolaryngology
Texas Tech Health Science Center
School of Medicine
Pediatric Otolaryngologist
Children's Hospital of Colorado
Lubbock, Texas, USA

Glenn Isaacson MD
Professor of Otolaryngology
Head and Neck Surgery and Pediatrics
Lewis Katz School of Medicine at
Temple University
Philadelphia, Pennsylvania, USA

Noel Jabbour MD MS FACS
Assistant Professor
Department of Otolaryngology
University of Pittsburgh School of Medicine
Pittsburgh, Pennsylvania, USA

Minyoung Jang MD
Pediatric Otolaryngology Fellow
Children's Hospital of Wisconsin
Milwaukee, Wisconsin, USA

Niall D Jefferson MBBCh BAO FRACS (OHNS)
Director
Department Otolaryngology
Head and Neck Surgery
John Hunter Adults and Childrens
Hospitals
Newcastle, New South Wales, Australia

David M Johnson MD
Chief Resident
Department of Otolaryngology
University of Pittsburgh Medical Center
Pittsburgh, Pennsylvania, USA

Patricia G Johnson MD
Resident Physician
Temple University Hospital
Head and Neck Institute
Philadelphia, Pennsylvania, USA

Robert G Kaniecki MD
Assistant Professor
Department of Neurology
University of Pittsburgh School of Medicine
Pittsburgh, Pennsylvania, USA

Jason I Kass MD PhD
Instructor
Harvard Medical School
Associate Surgeon
Brigham and Women's Hospital
Boston, Massachusetts, USA

Margaret A Kenna MD MPH
Professor of Otolaryngology
Harvard Medical School
Sarah Fuller Chair for Hearing Loss and
Hearing Restoration
Director of Clinical Research
Department of Otolaryngology and
Communication Enhancement
Boston Children's Hospital
Boston, Massachusetts, USA

David T Kent MD
Assistant Professor
Department of Otolaryngology
Vanderbilt University Medical Center
Nashville, Tennessee, USA

Seungwon Kim MD
Associate Professor
Department of Otolaryngology
University of Pittsburgh School of
Medicine
Pittsburgh, Pennsylvania, USA

Dennis J Kitsko DO
Assistant Professor
Department of Otolaryngology
University of Pittsburgh School of
Medicine
Division of Pediatric Otolaryngology
Children's Hospital of Pittsburgh of
University of Pittsburgh Medical Center
Pittsburgh, Pennsylvania, USA

Cristine Klatt-Cromwell MD
Assistant Professor
Department of Otolaryngology—
Head and Neck
Washington University School of Medicine
Rhinology and Skull Base Surgery
St Louis, Missouri, USA

Karen M Kost MDCM FRCSC
Professor
Otolaryngology Head and Neck Surgery
McGill University Health Center
Director
Voice and Dysphagia Laboratory
McGill University
Montreal, Quebec, Canada

Jamie Ahn Ku MD
Clinical Assistant Professor of Surgery
Cleveland Clinic Lerner
College of Medicine
Case Western Reserve, University Staff
Head and Neck Oncology Surgery
and Facial Plastics
Reconstructive Surgery
Head and Neck Institute
Cleveland Clinic Foundation
Cleveland, Ohio, USA

Efthymios E Kyrodimos MD PhD
Assistant Professor of Otolaryngology
National and Kapodistrian
First Department of Otolaryngology
"Hippocratio" Hospital
University of Athens
Athens, Greece

Miriam N Lango MD
Associate Professor
Department of Otolaryngology
Temple University School of Medicine
Temple University Health System
Department of Surgical Oncology
Head and Neck Surgery Section
Fox Chase Cancer Center
Philadelphia, Pennsylvania, USA

Lorenz Frederick Lassen MD FACS
Neurotologist
Lakeview Medical Center
Bayview Physicians Group
Suffolk, Virginia, USA

Stella E Lee MD
Assistant Professor of Otolaryngology
University of Pittsburgh
School of Medicine
Pittsburgh, Pennsylvania, USA

Paul Leong MD FACS
Director
Sistine Plastic Surgery PC
Pittsburgh, Pennsylvania, USA

Ali Lewandowski MA CCC-SLP
Speech-Language Pathologist
University of Pittsburgh Medical Center
Department of Otolaryngology
Pittsburgh, Pennsylvania, USA

Bryan J Liming MD
Otolaryngologist
Tripler Army Medical Center
Honolulu, Hawaii, USA

Joseph E Losee MD FACS FAAP
Ross H Musgrave Professor and
Executive Vice Chair
Department of Plastic Surgery
University of Pittsburgh School of
Medicine
Division Chief, Pediatric Plastic Surgery
Children's Hospital of Pittsburgh
University of Pittsburgh Medical Center
Pittsburgh, Pennsylvania, USA

Lyndsay L Madden DO
Assistant Professor of Otolaryngology
Department of Otolaryngology—
Head and Neck Surgery
Wake Forest University
Winston-Salem, North Carolina, USA

Raymond Maguire DO
Assistant Professor
Department of Otolaryngology
University of Pittsburgh School of Medicine
Pittsburgh, Pennsylvania, USA

Ellen M Mandel MD
Associate Professor
Department of Otolaryngology
University of Pittsburgh School of
Medicine
Research Pediatrician
Division of Pediatric Otolaryngology
Children's Hospital of Pittsburgh
University of Pittsburgh Medical Center
Pittsburgh, Pennsylvania, USA

David L Mandell MD
Affiliate Associate Professor
Charles E Schmidt College of Medicine
Florida Atlantic University
Boca Raton, Florida, USA
Clinical Associate Professor
Division of Otolaryngology
NOVA Southeastern University College
of Osteopathic Medicine
Fort Lauderdale, Florida, USA
Voluntary Associate Professor
Department of Otolaryngology
Miller School of Medicine
University of Miami
Miami, Florida, USA
Center for Pediatric Otolaryngology-
Head and Neck Surgery
Boynton Beach, Florida, USA

Mark Mandell-Brown MD
Director
The Plastic Surgery Experts
Mandell-Brown Plastic Surgery Center
Volunteer Instructor
Department of Otolaryngology
University of Cincinnati College of Medicine
Cincinnati, Ohio, USA

Scott C Manning MD
Professor
Department of Otolaryngology
University of Washington
Seattle, Washington, USA

Gerardo Marrazzo MD
Mohs Surgeon
The Skin Surgery Center
Hickory, North Carolina, USA

Jameson K Mattingly MD
Neurotology Fellow
Department of Otolaryngology—
Head and Neck Surgery
The Ohio State University
Columbus, Ohio, USA

Andrew A McCall MD
Assistant Professor
Department of Otolaryngology
University of Pittsburgh School of Medicine
Pittsburgh, Pennsylvania, USA

Wade McClain DO
Assistant Professor of Otolaryngology/
Head and Neck Surgery
The University of North Carolina at
Chapel Hill
Chapel Hill, North Carolina, USA

Andrew A McCormick MD
Assistant Professor of Pediatrics
Vascular Anomaly Center of Pittsburgh
University of Pittsburgh School of Medicine
Children's Hospital of Pittsburgh
University of Pittsburgh Medical Center
Pittsburgh, Pennsylvania, USA

Mariann C McElwain MD PhD
Assistant Professor
Department of Otolaryngology
University of Pittsburgh School of Medicine
Pittsburgh, Pennsylvania, USA

Gregory L McHugh MD
Clinical Assistant Professor
University of Pittsburgh School of Medicine
Department of Anesthesiology
Children's Hospital of Pittsburgh of
University of Pittsburgh Medical Center
Pittsburgh, Pennsylvania, USA

Brian J McKinnon MD
Associate Professor
Department of Otolaryngology—
Head and Neck Surgery
University of Tennessee Health Science
Center
Memphis, Tennessee, USA

Deepak Mehta MD
Associate Professor
Baylor College of Medicine
Texas Children's Hospital
Houston, Texas, USA

Chelsea R Metzger BS
Medical Student
Mercer University School of Medicine
Savannah, Georgia, USA

Justine S Moe DDS MD
Surgery Resident
Department of Oral and Maxillofacial
Surgery
Emory University
Atlanta, Georgia, USA

Erica Montgomery MD PhD
Professor
Department of Otolaryngology—
Head and Neck Surgery
Temple University School of Medicine
Director
Division of Otology and Neurotology
Philadelphia, Pennsylvania, USA

Charles M Myer III MD
Professor
Division of Pediatric Otolaryngology
Cincinnati Children's Hospital Medical
Center
Cincinnati, Ohio, USA

Jeffrey N Myers MD PhD FACS
Alando J Ballantyne
Distinguished Professor and Chairman
Department of Head and Neck Surgery
MD Anderson Cancer Center
Houston, Texas, USA

Jayakar V Nayak MD PhD
Assistant Professor
Co-Director, Rhinology Fellowship Program
Division of Rhinology and Endoscopic
Skull Base Surgery
Department of Otolaryngology—
Head and Neck Surgery
Stanford University School of Medicine
Stanford, California, USA

Vu T Nguyen MD
Assistant Professor
University of Pittsburgh School of Medicine
Residency Program Director
Department of Plastic Surgery
University of Pittsburgh Medical Center
Pittsburgh, Pennsylvania, USA

Julia E Noel MD
Resident Physician
Stanford University
Stanford, California, USA

Daniel W Nuss MD FACS
Professor and Chairman
Department of Otolaryngology
Head and Neck Surgery
Louisiana State University
New Orleans, Louisiana, USA

Todd D Otteson MD MPH FAAP FACS
Associate Professor, Department of
Pediatric Otolaryngology/Head and
Neck Surgery
Assistant Dean, Office of Student Affairs
Case Western Reserve University School
of Medicine
Chief, Pediatric Otolaryngology
The James Arnold MD, Tom and Nancy
Seitz Chair in Pediatric Otolaryngology
Department of Otolaryngology—
Head and Neck Surgery
University Hospitals Cleveland
Medical Center
Rainbow Babies and Children's Hospital
Cleveland, Ohio, USA

Jonathan B Overdevest MD PhD
Clinical Instructor
Department of Otolaryngology—
Head and Neck Surgery
Stanford University
Stanford, California, USA

Catherine V Palmer PhD
Associate Professor
Departments of Otolaryngology and
Communication Science and Disorders
University of Pittsburgh School of Medicine
Director of Audiology
University of Pittsburgh
Medical Center
Pittsburgh, Pennsylvania, USA

Renee E Park MD MPH
Assistant Professor of Pediatric
Otolaryngology
Loma Linda University Children's
Hospital
Loma Linda, California, USA

Guy J Petruzzelli MD PhD MBA FACS
Physician-in-Chief and Vice President
for Oncology Programs
Curtis and Elizabeth Anderson Cancer
Institute and Memorial University
Medical Center
Professor of Surgery—
Head, Neck and Endocrine Surgery
Savannah, Georgia, USA

Karen T Pitman MD
Professor
Department of Otolaryngology
The Johns Hopkins School of Medicine
Medical Director
The Milton J Dance Jr Head and Neck
Center at GBMC
Baltimore, Maryland, USA

Dennis S Poe MD PhD
Professor
Department of Otolaryngology
Harvard Medical School
Boston Children's Hospital
Boston, Massachusetts, USA

Aron Z Pollack MD
Assistant Professor
Department of Otolaryngology—
Head and Neck Surgery
Hofstra-Northwell School of Medicine
Lenox Hill Hospital and Manhattan Eye,
Ear and Throat Hospital
New York City, New York, USA

Anna M Pou MD FACS
Professor
Administrative Vice Chair
Louisiana State University Health
Sciences Center, New Orleans
Our Lady of the Lake Regional
Medical Center
Baton Rouge, Louisiana, USA

Sheila R Pratt PhD
Professor
University of Pittsburgh and the
Geriatric Research Education and
Clinical Center
VA Pittsburgh Healthcare System
Pittsburgh, Pennsylvania, USA

Emmanuel P Prokopakis MD PhD
Assistant Professor
Department of Otorhinolaryngology—
Head and Neck Surgery
University of Crete School of Medicine
Heraklion, Crete, Greece

Christopher H Rassekh MD FACS
Associate Professor
Department of Otorhinolaryngology—
Head and Neck Surgery
University of Pittsburgh School of Medicine
Director, Penn Medicine Sialendoscopy
Program
Co-Chair, Hospital University of
Pennsylvania Airway Safety Committee
Director of Risk Reduction and Director
of Professional Practice
Department of Otorhinolaryngology—
Head and Neck Surgery
University of Pennsylvania
Philadelphia, Pennsylvania, USA

Brian K Reilly MD FACS
Associate Professor
Department of Otolaryngology and
Pediatrics
George Washington University
Washington DC, USA

James S Reilly MD FACS
Professor
Department of Otolaryngology and
Pediatrics
Thomas Jefferson University
Philadelphia, Pennsylvania, USA

Gresham T Richter MD FACS
Professor and Chief Pediatric
Otolaryngology
The University of Arkansas for Medical
Sciences
Arkansas Children's Hospital
Little Rock, Arkansas, USA

Pamela C Roehm MD PhD
Professor
Department of Otolaryngology—
Head and Neck Surgery
Temple University School of Medicine
Director
Division of Otology and Neurotology
Philadelphia, Pennsylvania, USA

Clark A Rosen MD
Professor and Morrison Chair of
Laryngology
University of California—San Francisco
San Francisco, California, USA

Richard M Rosenfeld MD MPH
Distinguished Professor and Chairman
of Otolaryngology
SUNY Downstate Medical Center
Brooklyn, New York, USA

Noémie Rouillard-Bazinet
MD MSc FRCSC
Pediatric Otolaryngologist
Centre Hospitalier Universitaire
Sainte-Justine
Department of Otolaryngology
Université de Montréal
Montréal, Canada

Nicholas R Rowan MD
Fellow in Head and Neck Surgery
Department of Otolaryngology
Medical University of South Carolina
Charleston, South Carolina, USA

Benjamin J Rubinstein MD
Resident
Eastern Virginia Medical School
Norfolk, Virginia, USA

Nivedita Sahu MD
Resident
Department of Otolaryngology
University of Pittsburgh School of
Medicine
Pittsburgh, Pennsylvania, USA

Barry M Schaitkin MD
Professor
Department of Otolaryngology
University of Pittsburgh School of
Medicine
Pittsburgh, Pennsylvania, USA

Nicole C Schmitt MD
Associate Professor
Department of Otolaryngology
University of Pittsburgh School of
Medicine
Pittsburgh, Pennsylvania, USA

John V Segas MD PhD
Professor of Otolaryngology
National and Kapodistrian
University of Athens
Chairman of the 1st Department of
Otolaryngology
"Hippocratio" Hospital
Athens, Greece

Joshua B Silverman MD PhD
Associate Professor
Department of Otolaryngology
Hofstra Northwell School of Medicine
Long Island Jewish Medical Center—
Cohen Children's Medical Center
New Hyde Park, New York, USA

Alfred A Simental Jr MD FACS
Professor and Chairman
Department Otolaryngology—
Head and Neck Surgery
Loma Linda University School of Medicine
Loma Linda, California, USA

Jeffrey P Simons MD
Associate Professor
Department of Otolaryngology
University of Pittsburgh School of Medicine
Division of Pediatric Otolaryngology
Children's Hospital of Pittsburgh of
University of Pittsburgh Medical Center
Pittsburgh, Pennsylvania, USA

Demetrios G Skedros MD
Adjunct Assistant Professor
Division of Otolaryngology
University of Utah
Salt Lake City, Utah, USA

Libby J Smith DO
Associate Professor
Department of Otolaryngology
University of Pittsburgh School of Medicine
Pittsburgh, Pennsylvania, USA

Richard JH Smith MD
Sterba Hearing Research Professor and
Vice-Chair
Department of Otolaryngology
University of Iowa
Carver College of Medicine
Director
Molecular Otolaryngology and Renal
Research Laboratories
Iowa City, Iowa, USA

Carl H Snyderman MD MBA
Professor
Departments of Otolaryngology and
Neurological Surgery
University of Pittsburgh School of Medicine
Pittsburgh, Pennsylvania, USA

Mario G Solari MD
Assistant Professor
Plastic Surgery and Otolaryngology
Department of Plastic Surgery
University of Pittsburgh School of Medicine
Pittsburgh, Pennsylvania, USA

John I Song MD
Associate Professor
Department of Otolaryngology
University of Colorado School of Medicine
Aurora, Colorado, USA

Ryan J Soose MD
Associate Professor
Department of Otolaryngology
University of Pittsburgh School of
Medicine
Pittsburgh, Pennsylvania, USA

Shaum S Sridharan MD
Assistant Professor
Georgetown University Hospital
Georgetown, Washington DC, USA

Amanda L Stapleton MD
Assistant Professor
Department of Otolaryngology
University of Pittsburgh School of
Medicine
Pittsburgh, Pennsylvania, USA

Susan Tonya Stefko MD FACS
Associate Professor
Department of Ophthalmology
University of Pittsburgh School of Medicine
Pittsburgh, Pennsylvania, USA

Allison Tobey MD
Assistant Professor of Otolaryngology
University of Pittsburgh School of Medicine
Division of Pediatric Otolaryngology
Children's Hospital of Pittsburgh
University of Pittsburgh Medical Center
Pittsburgh, Pennsylvania, USA

Elizabeth Toh MD MBA
Vice Chairman
Department of Otolaryngology
Director, Balance and
Hearing Implant Center
Co-Director, Center for
Cranial Base Surgery
Lahey Hospital and Medical Center
Burlington, Massachusetts, USA

Jason Trahan MD
Resident
Department of Otolaryngology—
Head and Neck Surgery
Louisiana State University Health
Sciences Center
New Orleans, Louisiana, USA

Meghan T Turner MD
Assistant Professor
Department of Otolaryngology/Head
and Neck Surgery
West Virginia University Medical Center
Morgantown, West Verginia, USA

Andrew C Urquhart MD FACS
Attending Otolaryngologist
Department of Otolaryngology—
Head and Neck Surgery
Marshfield Clinic
Marshfield, Wisconsin, USA

Alec Vaezi MD PhD
Assistant Professor
Department of Otolaryngology—
Head and Neck Surgery
Department of Radiation Oncology
Department of Neurosurgery
University of Massachusetts Memorial
Medical Center
Worcester, Massachusetts, USA

Ryan D Walker MD
Pediatric Otolaryngologist
Advanced ENT
Voorhees, New Jersey, USA

Rohan R Walvekar MD
Associate Professor
Mervin L. Trail Endowed Chair in Head
and Neck Oncology
Director, Salivary Endoscopy Service
Department of Otolaryngology—
Head and Neck Surgery
Louisiana State University Health
Sciences Center
New Orleans, Louisiana, USA

Eric W Wang MD
Associate Professor
Departments of Otolaryngology
Neurological Surgery and
Ophthalmology
University of Pittsburgh
School of Medicine
Pittsburgh, Pennsylvania, USA

Hailun Wang MD
Chief Resident
Department of Otolaryngology
Mount Sinai Hospital
New York City, New York, USA

Peter C Weber MD MBA
Professor
Department of Otolaryngology
Boston University Medical School
Boston, Massachusetts, USA

Jay Werkhaven MD
Associate Professor
Vanderbilt University
School of Medicine
Nashville, Tennessee, USA

Susan L Whitney DPT PhD
Professor in Physical Therapy
University of Pittsburgh School of
Medicine
Pittsburgh, Pennsylvania, USA

Robert A Williamson MD
Clinical Assistant Professor
Department of Surgery and
Perioperative Care
Dell Medical School at the University of
Texas
Department of Otolaryngology/ENT
Austin Regional Clinic
Austin, Texas, USA

Todd M Wine MD
Assistant Professor of Pediatric
Otolaryngology
Department of Otolaryngology
University of Colorado
School of Medicine
Children's Hospital of Colorado
Aurora, Colorado, USA

Robert F Yellon MD
Instructor
Lake Erie College of Osteopathic
Medicine
Bradenton, Florida, USA

VyVy N Young MD
Associate Professor
Department of Otolaryngology—
Head and Neck Surgery
University of California
San Francisco, California, USA

Sancak Yuksel MD
Assistant Professor
Department of Otorhinolaryngology
McGovern Medical School
University of Texas Health Science Center
Houston, Texas, USA

Adam M Zanation MD FACS
Associate Professor
Department of Otolaryngology—
Head and Neck Surgery
University of North Carolina
Chapel Hill, North Carolina, USA

Carlton J Zdanski MD FACS
Associate Professor of Otolaryngology/
Head and Neck Surgery and Pediatrics
The University of North Carolina at
Chapel Hill
Chief, Division of Pediatric
Otolaryngology/Head and Neck Surgery
Surgical Director, The North Carolina
Children's Airway Center
Chapel Hill, North Carolina, USA

Larry A Zieske MD FACS
Adjunct Clinical Associate Professor
Uniformed Services University of the
Health Sciences
Minneapolis, Minnesota, USA

John A Zitelli MD
Adjunct Clinical Associate Professor
Dermatology
Otolaryngology, Plastic Surgery
University of Pittsburgh School of
Medicine
Pittsburgh, Pennsylvania, USA

Foreword

The Department of Otolaryngology—Head and Neck Surgery at the University of Pittsburgh has a long-standing history of being one of the best academic departments in the United States and elsewhere. Their faculties proven expertise encompasses all aspects of otology, otolaryngology and head and neck surgery. Their many graduate students, residents and fellows have come from the United States and many corners of the earth and further have made significant contributions to patient care, education and research worldwide.

For this and other reasons I am pleased and privileged to add a foreword to this, the second edition of *Decision Making in Otolaryngology*. The editors, Drs Cuneyt M Alper, Eugene N Myers and David E Eibling are to be congratulated for educating us all regarding the importance of decision making which helps us make a correct diagnosis and provide appropriate treatment to our patients.

An analogy, perhaps. The IBM company, a long-standing technology company whose net worth is approximately 85 billion dollars has recently emphasized artificial intelligence (AI) as its major emphasis for research and business for the future. It created Watson, a product whose purpose is to produce Cognitive Computing under the aegis of AI. including its ability to diagnose diseases. This approach will clearly grow and become more important in all aspects of life, however, the human factor will continue to be essential in *Decision Making in Otolaryngology*.

We are all taught differential diagnosis in our first year of medical school and when possible, a specific diagnosis of a disease is critical to the treatment of that disease. While many diseases in Otolaryngology are clear cut, either black or white, many can and do occur in the gray zone. While technology will continue to develop to become more useful in decision making, the human brain will continue to be paramount. Amongst other examples of the brains cognitive and memory capabilities, intrinsic and experience abilities will continue to be critical in the diagnosis and treatment of otolaryngological diseases.

The editors of *Decision Making in Otolaryngology* include all appropriate aspects of the human factor and available technology in the diagnosis and treatment of otological and otolaryngological and head and neck diseases. They also provide us a road map with graphics to assist us in our journey to help our patients in the best way possible.

Michael M Paparella MD
Director, Otology/Neurotology Fellowship
Paparella Ear, Head and Neck Institute
Director, Otopathology Laboratory
Clinical Professor and Chairman Emeritus
Department of Otolaryngology
University of Minnesota
Founder, International Hearing Foundation
Minneapolis, Minnesota, USA

The passage of 17 years since the First Edition of our book *Decision Making in Otolaryngology* has put us in sync with the current era of the "Millennials" in which as much information as possible is relayed to the reader within a minimal amount of time. We have accomplished this task by incorporating as much detail as possible into the algorithms. We believe that we have met this goal and that the reader will be able to easily grasp these concepts, as well as the critical details of the management of the basic problems encountered in our specialty.

Most of the chapters in our book have been written by current and former members of the faculty of the Department of Otolaryngology in the University of Pittsburgh School of Medicine and the University of Pittsburgh Medical Center. To these friends and colleagues, we owe our sincere thanks.

Cuneyt M Alper
Eugene N Myers
David E Eibling

Acknowledgments

It has been an honor and a privilege to work with Dr Eugene N Myers and Dr David E Eibling on the 2nd Edition of our book *Decision Making in Otolaryngology*. When Dr Myers invited me to discuss production of a potential book on decision algorithms in 1999, I had little idea what I was getting into. The following month, I did a Grand Rounds presentation to our Department on decision trees in Otolaryngology. With the guidance and leadership of Dr Myers, with me as the Senior Editor, we published the 1st Edition of Decision-Making in the Ear, Nose and Throat Disorders, in 2001.

Joe Rusko from Jaypee Brothers Medical Publishers approached me almost 15 years after, with their interest in publishing the 2nd Edition, as part of their Decision Making series. Special thanks to the Development Editor Bridget H Meyer, who assisted the initial phase of development, later taken over by the Development Editor Ms Nedup Denka, who worked tirelessly to make certain of the success of this project. I would like to acknowledge the great help and support of Ms Chetna Malhotra Vohra (Associate Director-Content Strategy) of M/s Jaypee Brothers Medical Publishers, New Delhi, India.

Editors acknowledge the contributions of authors in the 1st Edition of this book, "Decision Making in Ear, Nose and Throat Disorders". As per Editors' advice, authors in the 2nd Edition used the content in the former Edition, when applicable.

Cuneyt M Alper

Contents

Section 4: Larynx, Trachea and Bronchi

Section 5: Neck

SECTION

1

Ear and Temporal Bone

CHAPTER 1

Clinical Examination of the Ear in Children

Cuneyt M Alper

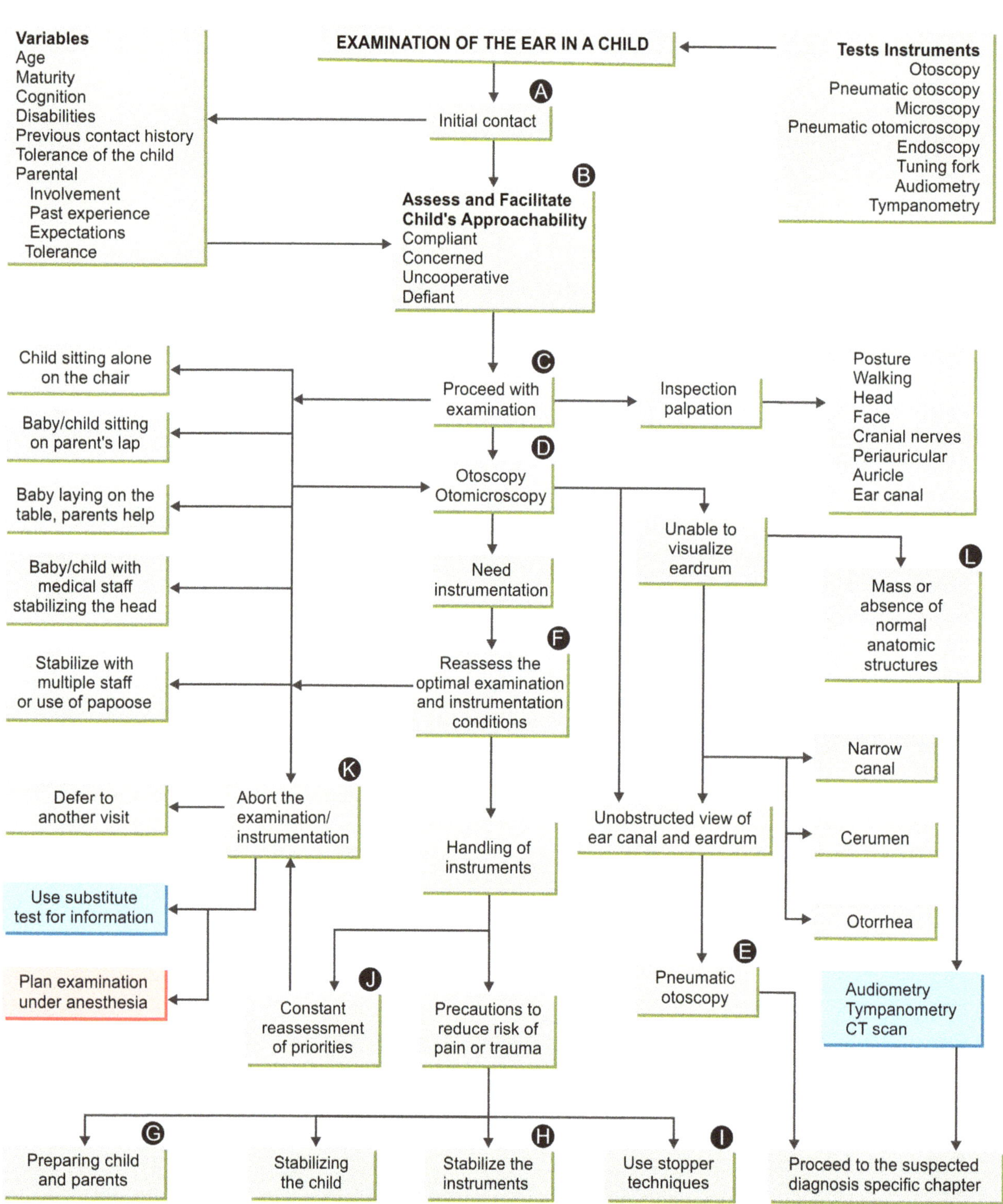

Clinical examination of the ear in children may be challenging, especially in infants and young children. Description of symptoms is often limited and inaccurate, reflecting parents' perception. High volume clinician practice limits time spent with the patients, enhancing the importance of focused and efficient history taking, examination and decision making.

A Initial contact and interaction is very important to realize the full potential of the patient-clinician encounter. Attention should immediately be directed to the child with a display of smile as a universal sign of friendliness. The clinician's attention to the child's toy's, clothes or hair as the lead to the conversation may soften the initial fear, distance, or reactive attitude.

B The child's response to the clinician's attempt to establish contact will provide insight about the child's character, cognitive and maturity level, past experience with other clinicians, and the mood that he/she is in at the time of the examination.

C The examination is performed with the least possible restraint. Early and escalated restraint may break the bond and bring the need for more restraint. It is important to make the child feel that he is making the decisions. Asking permission to start, explaining the next step, promising to stop if painful, and keeping the promise, may lead to unexpected compliance from a child even below age 2 and pleasantly surprise parents.

D Holding the pinna to pull back as the initial physical contact with the child should be avoided. Instead, laying ones hand over the head and face may comfort and distract the child and facilitate a more seamless transition to the insertion of the speculum in the external auditory canal (EAC).

E Pneumatic otoscopy is the standard of care in pediatric otoscopy. Ignoring the need, not having a proper otoscope, and failure to achieve a seal in the EAC may lead to misdiagnosis. The seal of the otoscope head should be tested each time, after inserting the speculum, by closing the tip and squeezing the bulb. Squeezing the bulb before getting an external ear canal (EEC) seal facilitates bidirectional pressure change with minimal change in bulb volume. Otomicroscopy is not needed routinely. Otoendoscopy may not be safe in children.

F The clinician should balance the need for a complete unobstructed view of the EEC and tympanic membrane (TM) with the risk of causing pain and reverse any gain in interaction achieved until that time.

G Preparing the child and parents for necessary and acceptable modes of restraint and instrumentation is essential.

H The use of multipoint holding (usually the 3rd finger on the shaft) and anchoring (4th and/or 5th finger on the speculum edge), and head, and shaft is needed for stable instrumentation. The chosen stabilizing method should be enhanced to reduce the risk of pain or injury with movement by visual and tactile feedback methods (palm on the head while fingers gently pull the pinna).

I The clinician should anticipate and be prepared for sudden movements in every child and should use the "stopper or anchor techniques" by placing the instrument holding hand or fingers on the patient's head, edge of the speculum, or on the speculum holding hand. Therefore, the distance between the tip of the instrument and the TM or middle ear structures is not affected by the movement of the head, as any movement will push the instrument with the holding hand, maintaining a safe distance and angle.

J As the assessment and manipulations proceed, priorities and goals should be constantly reassessed based on the compliance of the child and the reactions of the parents.

K When it is not likely that the tasks will be finalized, information from tympanometry and/or audiometry may reset the priorities, with the option of not proceeding, deferring the tasks until a later time, changing restraint method, examination under anesthesia or imaging.

L Suspicion of a mass or abnormal anatomic structures should prompt audiometric and tympanometric testing, and possibly imaging.

SUGGESTED READING

Alper CM, Cohen MS. Clinical examination of the ear. In: Sataloff RT, Hartnick SJ (Eds). Sataloff's Comprehensive Textbook of Otolaryngology—Head and Neck Surgery, 1st edition, Vol 6. Daryaganj, New Delhi: Jaypee Brothers; 2015. pp. 119-142.

Bluestone CD, Klein JO. Diagnosis. In: Bluestone CD, Klein JO (Eds). Otitis Media in Infants and Children, 3rd edition. Philadelphia, PA: WB Saunders; 2001. pp. 120-179.

Bluestone CD, Klein JO. Methods of examination: clinical examination. In: Bluestone CD, Stool SE, Alper CM (Eds). Pediatric Otolaryngology, 4th edition. Philadelphia: WB Saunders; 2003. pp. 172-186.

Carlson LH, Carlson RD. Diagnosis. In: Rosenfeld RM, Bluestone CD (Eds). Evidence-Based Otitis Media, 2nd edition. Hamilton, London: BD Decker, Inc.; 2003. pp. 136-146.

Isaacson GC. Examination of the tympanic membrane for otitis media. In: Alper CM, Bluestone CD, Casselbrant ML, et al. (Eds). Advanced Therapy of Otitis Media. Hamilton, London: BC Decker, Inc.; 2004. pp. 14-20.

Failed Newborn Hearing Screening

Dennis J Kitsko

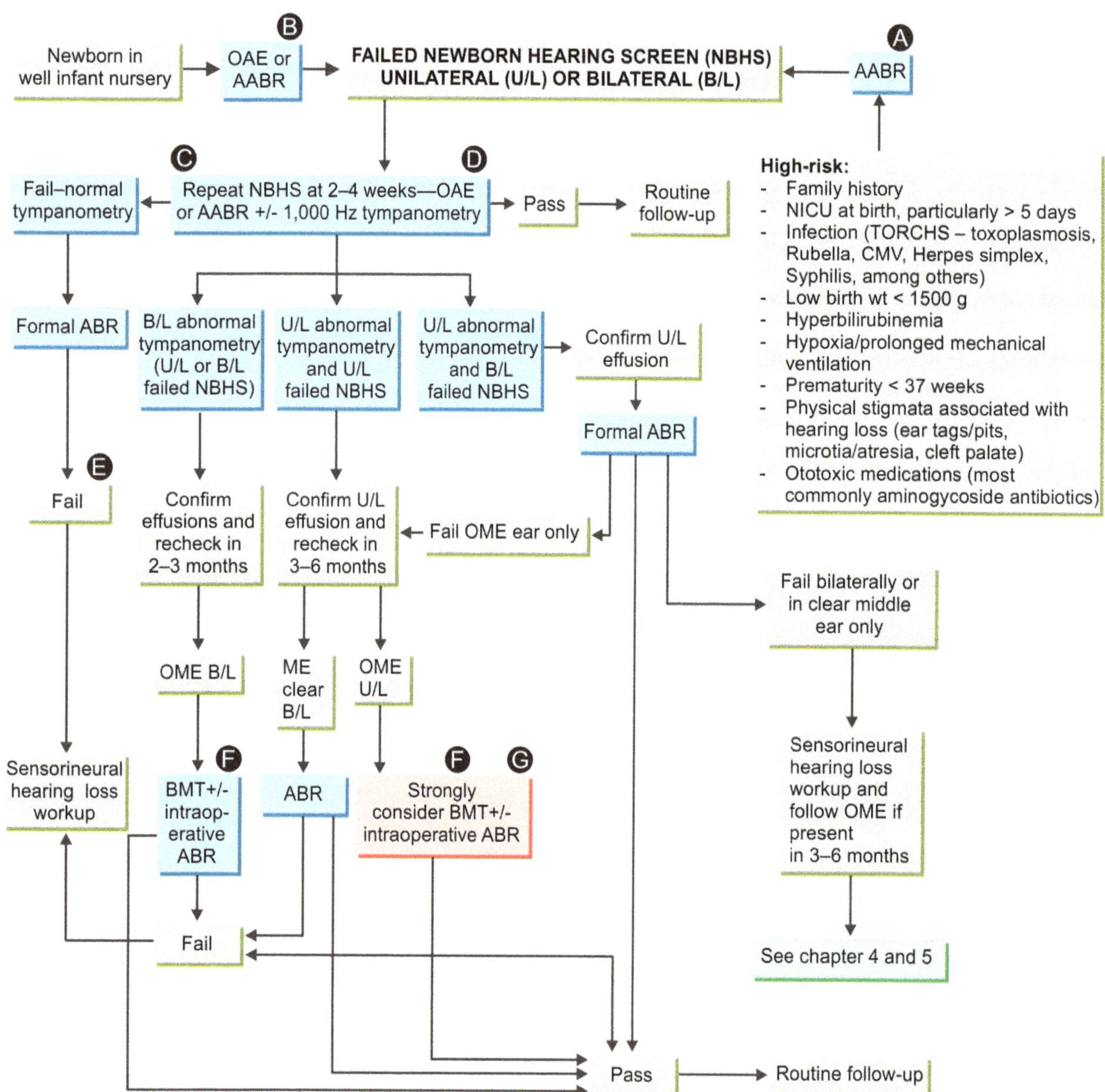

As of 2015, legislation mandating universal newborn hearing screening has been passed in 43 states and in the District of Columbia. In the other states, screening is offered but can be refused by parents. Currently, >95% of all infants born in the United States have a newborn hearing screening. This is noteworthy because prior to a 1993 National Institutes of Health conference on the early identification of hearing loss, only 11 hospitals nationwide screened >90% of their newborns.

A Auditory brainstem response (ABR) testing is recommended in these infants given the higher prevalence of auditory neuropathy spectrum disorder (ANSD) in neonatal intensive care unit (NICU) graduates. The rationale for this is that children with ANSD will often have otoacoustic emissions (OAEs) present.

B The Joint Commission on Infant Hearing position statement in 2007 recommended a "1-3-6" rule. This states that all children should be appropriately screened (OAEs or ABR testing) by 1 month of age. Those who do not pass screening should have a comprehensive audiological evaluation by 3 months of age, and if hearing loss is confirmed, appropriate intervention with healthcare and educational professionals should occur by 6 months of age.

C It has been reported that up to 30% of newborns will fail an initial OAE screening, most commonly thought to be due to vernix in the ear canal or transient middle ear effusion after birth. Rescreening has been shown to decrease the referral rate to a much more reasonable 5% rate. Controversy exists about whether OAE or automated ABR (AABR) is the ideal screen in well-infants. Automated ABR is more specific and can identify ANSD, but is also more expensive. Many institutions have instituted a "two-step" technique that initially screens with OAEs, followed by AABR for those who fail initial screening.

D Tympanometry is an easy and effective means of identifying potential middle ear disease in infants. Typically, tympanometry is performed at a 226-Hz frequency. However, studies have shown that in the newborn ear, it is less reliable, possibly due to the increased compliance of the ear canal. To that end, high-frequency 1,000-Hz tympanometry is recommended in infants of <4 months of age.

E Repeat ABR testing can be considered to confirm a failed test, particularly if the testing was difficult to perform (i.e. the newborn aroused/awakened during testing). If repeat testing is desired, however, it should be performed as soon as possible after the initial ABR and before 6 months of age. After 6 months of age, most infants will require sedation for ABR testing—obviously this sedation should be avoided if possible.

F As previously mentioned, ABR testing without sedation after 6 months of age is often not possible. By the time that bilateral otitis media with effusion is diagnosed, followed for 2–3 months, and the decision for surgery is made, most infants will be approaching, if not, already 6 months of age. Therefore, it is prudent to consider ABR testing intraoperatively after tympanostomy tube insertion. Care should be taken to be as gentle as possible when inserting tympanostomy tubes in this setting, and even minimal bleeding, if encountered, should be completely dried up before ABR testing is started. Even with these precautions, however, ABR testing can still be inaccurate when performed intraoperatively with bilateral myringotomy with tubes (BMT). If this is suspected, a follow-up ABR should be performed when the middle ears have completely cleared.

G Research and national guidelines suggest that unilateral otitis media with effusion can be monitored in many children without significant impairment. However, these guidelines also recommend that when fluid is observed for >3-6 months, both hearing and language should be tested and intervention considered if there is significant hearing loss or language delay. Furthermore, "at-risk" children are excluded from these guidelines, although otherwise healthy infants with otitis media with effusion (OME) are not specifically mentioned within this "at-risk" group. Given that the assessment of language is difficult in very young children and hearing has not been accurately assessed at baseline, it is more than reasonable to consider tympanostomy tube insertion after 3–6 months of observation. An argument could also be made that the inability to accurately assess language milestones in these young infants automatically makes them "at risk."

SUGGESTED READING

American Academy of Pediatrics, Joint Commission on Infant Hearing. Year 2007 position statement: principles and guidelines for early hearing detection and intervention programs. Pediatrics. 2007;120:159-163.

Berg AL, Spitzer JB, Towers HM, et al. Newborn hearing screening in the NICU: profile of failed auditory brainstem response/passed otoacoustic emission. Pediatrics. 2005;116:933-938.

Dedhia K, Kitsko D, Sabo D, et al. Children with sensorineural hearing loss after passing the newborn hearing screen. JAMA Otolaryngol Head Neck Surg. 2013;139:119-123.

Rosenfeld RM, Culpepper L, Doyle KJ, et al. Clinical practice guideline: otitis media with effusion. Otolaryngol Head Neck Surg. 2004;130:S95-118.

Rosenfeld RM, Schwartz SR, Pynnonen MA, et al. Clinical practice guideline: tympanostomy tubes in children. Otolaryngol Head Neck Surg. 2013;149:S1-35.

Stewart DL, Mehl A, Hall JW III, et al. Universal newborn hearing screening with automated auditory brainstem response: a multisite investigation. J Perinatol. 2000;20:S128-131.

CHAPTER 3

Conductive Hearing Loss

Barry E Hirsch

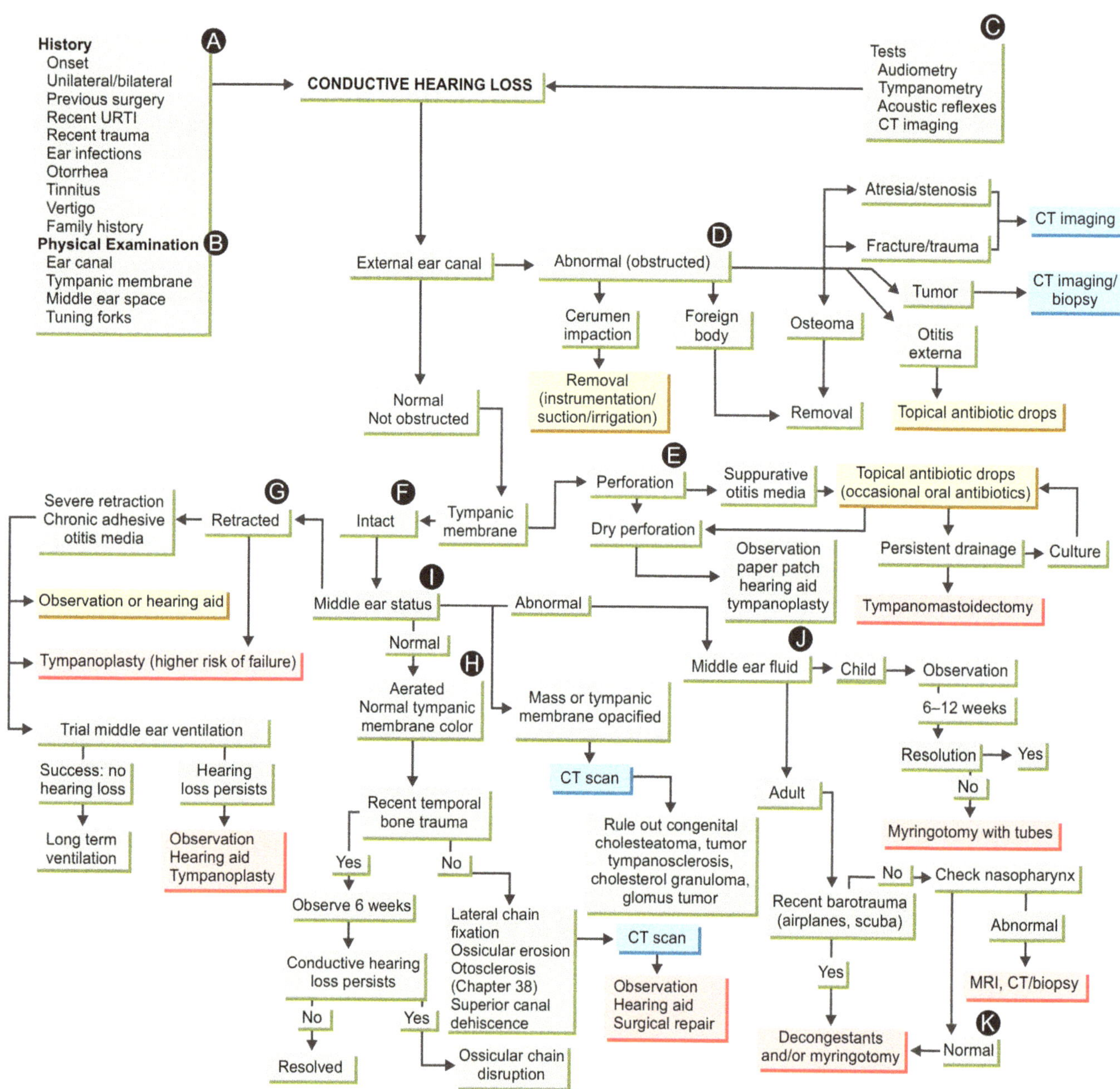

Conductive hearing loss is due to failure of sound energy to reach hair cells of the cochlea as a result of obstruction or incomplete transmission from problems of the tympanic membrane, middle ear space, ossicular chain, or rarely, the inner ear.

A The history identifies whether the hearing loss is sudden in onset, long-standing, or progressive. Associated symptoms of otorrhea, trauma, tinnitus, or vertigo should be elicited. A family history of hearing loss treated with surgery provides useful information. Autophony (hearing one's voice, breathing, or other bodily sounds) should raise suspicion for superior canal dehiscence.

B Physical examination of the ear includes the pinna and external auditory canal. An abnormal or obstructed canal can be the result of processes listed in Step D. Tuning-fork testing is important in the verification of the presence of a conductive hearing loss and in estimating its magnitude.

C An audiogram is necessary to determine the type and degree of hearing loss. Speech discrimination testing is important, especially if surgical instrumentation or intervention is to be undertaken. Physical examination with pneumatic otoscopy typically precludes the need for tympanometry unless visualization of the tympanic membrane is inconclusive. Acoustic reflexes are absent in most sources of conductive hearing loss. Acoustic reflexes remain present in superior canal dehiscence.

Computed tomography (CT) can be helpful in providing information in conductive hearing loss following trauma or in the presence of a normal middle ear (see Step K).

Computed tomography imaging is mandatory is cases of congenital atresia, obstructing polyps, or tumors of the external or middle ear, and the clinician should suspect complications of acute or chronic otitis media.

D Osteoma of the ear canal can completely occlude the ear canal causing conductive hearing loss.

Congenital atresia can be managed with a bone conduction hearing aid or bone-anchored device or by surgical correction of the atretic canal and tympanoplasty.

E A perforation of the tympanic membrane can be dry or associated with otorrhea. If the ear does not respond to topical and systemic antibiotics culture-specific therapy should be given. Failure to achieve a dry ear may warrant surgical intervention. A small dry perforation with conductive hearing loss can be electively repaired with a paper patch if cholesteatoma or ossicular chain involvement is not suspected or by tympanoplasty for larger defects. Amplification with a hearing aid is also an option, but has the potential to promote further otorrhea.

F The presence of an intact tympanic membrane and a conductive hearing loss requires further evaluation of the position of the tympanic membrane and status of the middle ear space.

G A conductive hearing loss and retracted tympanic membrane may be reversed with middle ear ventilation. If this is successful, repeated placement of myringotomy tubes can be offered. Prolonged ventilation with a Per-Lee or T tube provides a longer term solution. On rare occasion, middle ear ventilation can increase the conductive hearing loss if the tympanic membrane is lateralized from a natural type III tympanoplasty (stapediopexy) in the presence of erosion of the incudostapedial joint. Patients with persistent conductive hearing loss despite ventilation may be offered hearing aid amplification or exploratory tympanotomy and ossicular reconstruction.

An intact tympanic membrane that is severely adherent to the ossicular chain and promontory implies possible irreversible eustachian tube (ET) dysfunction. Middle ear ventilation at the time of surgery or in the immediate postoperative period may increase the success of tympanoplasty.

H The history of hearing loss should be confirmed when a patient with conductive hearing loss has a tympanic membrane that is intact, not retracted and there is normal middle ear ventilation. Patients with recent temporal bone trauma should be observed for 4–6 weeks to monitor for resolution. Patients with persistent conductive hearing loss can be offered surgical exploration or hearing aid amplification.

Patients with long-standing conductive hearing loss since childhood should be suspected of having congenital fixation of the lateral chain or stapedial footplate.

This can be either unilateral or bilateral. Computed tomography imaging is warranted. Slowly progressive conductive hearing loss without evidence of middle ear disease suggests otosclerosis. Similar to other situations having conductive hearing loss without significant middle ear disease, treatment options include observation, hearing aid amplification, and surgical correction. Otosclerosis is further discussed in Chapter 38.

Superior semicircular canal dehiscence (SSCD) may present with conductive hearing loss, vestibular symptoms, or both. Acoustic reflexes remain present in SSCD and thus are important to establish. Coronal CT imaging can identify this finding. Intervention is based on the severity of symptoms via the middle fossa or transmastoid approaches.

I It may be difficult to determine the status of the middle ear in the presence of an opacified tympanic membrane. Dense myringosclerosis can appear similar to a congenital cholesteatoma. A pulsatile mass within the middle ear could be an encephalocele or glomus tumor. A discolored middle ear mass that is blue or violaceous red could represent a cholesterol granuloma, aberrant carotid artery, or dehiscent jugular bulb. The diagnosis in all of these situations can usually be ascertained with CT imaging.

J Middle ear effusion is more common in children than in adults. A middle ear effusion can be seen in adults after acute otitis media, temporal bone trauma, or barotrauma. Unilateral effusion is usually self-limited and resolves within a few weeks. It is reasonable to offer myringotomy without a tube for patients desiring more immediate intervention. Adult patients with idiopathic effusion should be further evaluated. The nasopharynx should be carefully examined for obstructing pathology. An abnormal mass identified on endoscopy warrants imaging and biopsy. Children with recurrent otitis media or persistent effusion are managed based on the presence of hearing loss or speech delay. Myringotomy with tube placement is warranted in the patients in whom medical management fails (see Chapter 25).

K There is preliminary evidence that procedures directed at the ET may restore function. These include cartilage framework surgery, laser tuboplasty, and dilation with balloons (see Chapter 22).

SUGGESTED READING

Dougherty W, Kessler BW. Management of conductive hearing loss in children. Otolaryngol Clin N Am. 2015;48:955-974.

Fetterman BL, Luxford WM. The rehabilitation of conductive hearing impairment. Otolaryngol Clin N Am. 1997;30(5):783-801.

Kim SH, Cho YS, Chu HS, et al. Open-type congenital cholesteatoma: differential diagnosis for conductive hearing loss with a normal tympanic membrane. Acta Otolaryngol. 2012;132(6):618-623.

Kim SC, Lee WS, Kim M, et al. Third windows as a cause of failure in hearing gain after exploratory tympanotomy. Otolaryngol Head Neck Surg. 2011;145(2):303-308.

Rosenfeld RM, Schwartz SR, Pynnonen MA, et al. Clinical Practice Guideline: Tympanostomy tubes in children. Otolaryngol Head Neck Surg. 2013;149(1):A1-35.

Rosenfeld RM, Shin JJ, Schwartz SR, et al. Clinical Practice Guideline: Otitis media with effusion executive summary (update). Otolaryngol Head Neck Surg. 2016;154(2):201-214.

Sensorineural Hearing Loss

Robert A Williamson, Ellis M Arjmand

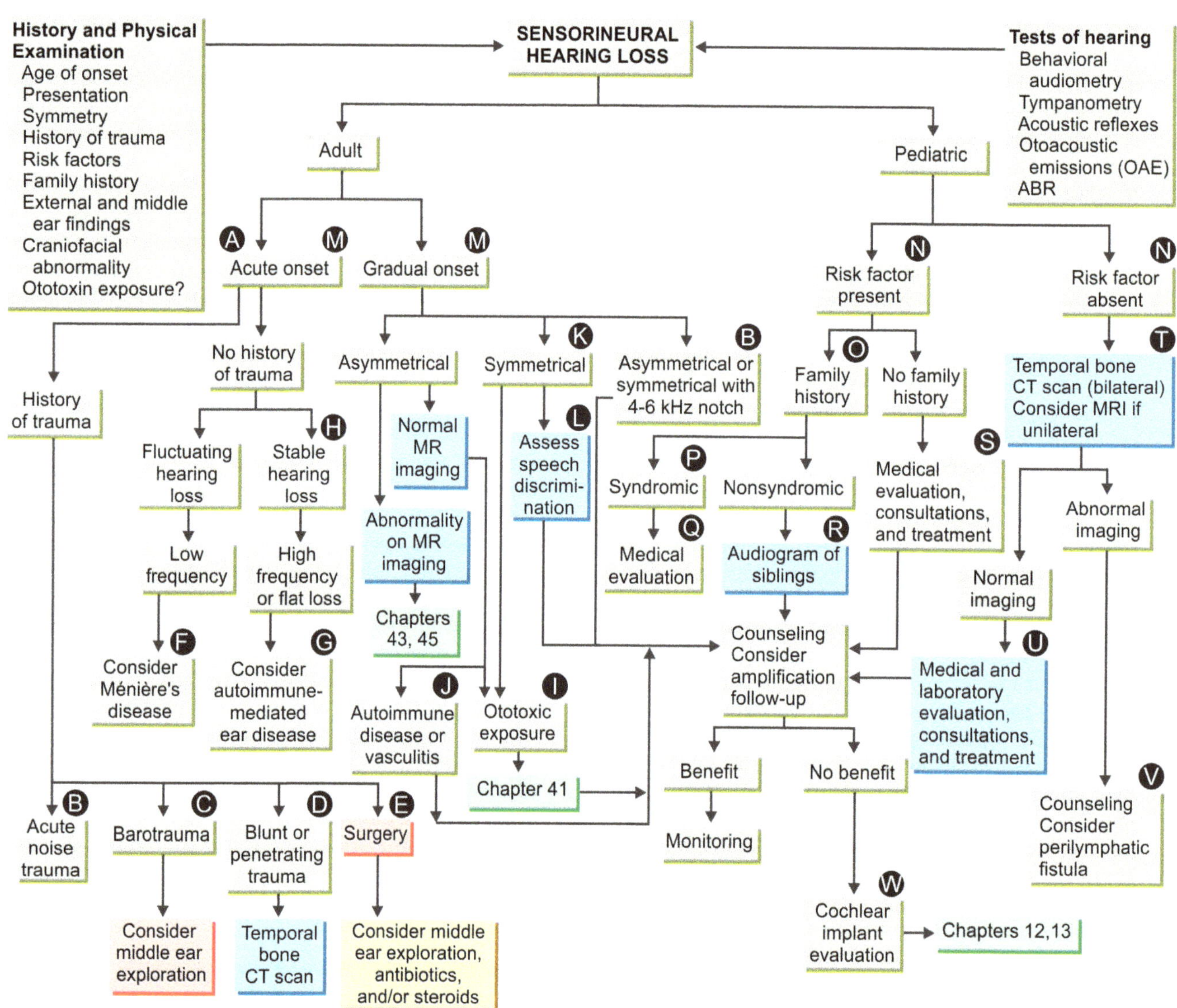

The evaluation and treatment of sensorineural hearing loss poses many challenges for the physician. The presentation varies and the causes are many. Studies on the utility and cost-effectiveness of diagnostic evaluation and treatment are for the most part not definitive, leaving many important clinical questions unanswered. Consequently, there is considerable variation in physician practice. Our goal in this chapter is provide an overall framework for evaluating patients of all ages who present with hearing loss.

A Sudden hearing loss may occur abruptly (minutes) or develop over several hours and up to 3 days, by definition.

B Acoustic trauma causing acute hearing loss may be unilateral or bilateral. There is typically a discrete history with subsequent hearing loss. Tinnitus often accompanies the hearing loss. A conductive component may be present. The loss may be temporary or permanent. Noise exposure is often associated with a "notch" centered around 4 kHz. Handgun or firearm exposure may also cause asymmetrical hearing loss. Counseling on ear protection from further noise exposure should be provided.

C Barotrauma may result in sensorineural hearing loss (SNHL) by inducing rupture of the membranous labyrinth or the mechanism of perilymphatic fistula.

D Severe trauma may result in SNHL and other acute injuries. After stabilization of other injuries, high-resolution computed tomography (CT) of the temporal bone is indicated to evaluate the otic capsule. Hearing loss may be present even in the absence of a skull base fracture.

Surgical intervention may be required for facial nerve injury and/or persistent cerebrospinal fluid leak.

E Hearing loss may occur after otologic surgery; immediate loss suggests labyrinthine trauma and may occur due to excessively forceful manipulation of the ossicles or dissection in the oval- or round-window niches. Labyrinthine or cochlear fistulae also pose a risk during removal of cholesteatoma or granulation tissue. Delayed loss can occur due to granuloma formation related to a stapes prosthesis.

F Ménière's disease typically is unilateral but may be bilateral. Diagnosis is suggested by fluctuating hearing loss, tinnitus, aural fullness, and episodic vertigo. Audiometry should confirm SNHL. If the patient does not respond to treatment, evaluation for other causes of fluctuating SNHL is indicated. Serologies for fluorescent treponemal antibody absorption test (FTA-ABS), allergy, and autoimmune disease are appropriate. Magnetic resonance imaging (MRI) should also be considered.

G If fluctuating loss is high frequency or flat, immune-mediated ear disease should be considered. Treatment with high-dose corticosteroids is indicated, and serologies for FTA-ABS and immune-mediated diseases are appropriate.

H If the physical examination does not reveal evidence of acute or chronic ear disease or other middle ear pathology then neurologic, vascular, or viral causes (e.g. Ramsay Hunt syndrome with ipsilateral vesicular eruption and facial paralysis) should be considered.

I Ototoxicity typically causes subacute or gradually progressive SNHL. High-frequency loss is often detected first. Systemic exposure to aminoglycosides, loop diuretics, quinine, and platinum-based chemotherapeutic agents results in bilateral loss. Unilateral hearing loss may occur after intratympanic gentamicin treatment for Meniere's disease. Rarely, long-term application of ototoxic drops with either tympanic membrane perforation or ventilation tube may lead to SNHL.

J Immune-mediated diseases and vasculitides can be associated with unilateral or bilateral SNHL. Physical examination and serology aid in the diagnosis of SNHL associated with Cogan's syndrome, periarteritis nodosa, Wegener's disease, sarcoidosis, and systemic lupus erythematosus. Lyme disease is a rare but treatable cause of SNHL and typically associated with other symptoms.

K Adult-onset gradual, progressive SNHL may be the result of syndromic or nonsyndromic hereditary hearing loss. Evaluation for a family history of adult-onset hearing loss is important for genetic screening and counseling.

L Presbycusis results in either a downsloping or flat SNHL, usually with preservation of speech discrimination. If there is no benefit from a trial of amplification, cochlear implantation should be considered.

M Syphilitic labyrinthitis can manifest as almost any pattern of SNHL. Evaluation with FTA-ABS should be performed.

N Risk factors for childhood SNHL have been recognized by the Joint Committee on Infant Hearing. Universal newborn hearing screening has replaced risk-based screening. Protocols typically include either screening-format otoacoustic emissions or automated auditory brainstem response (ABR). As many as 50% of affected children do not have a known risk factor for SNHL.

O Approximately 50% of all cases of childhood SNHL are hereditary. Autosomal recessive inheritance is the most common pattern.

P Hereditary SNHI is syndromic in ~30% of cases and non-syndromic in ~70%. Autosomal recessive nonsyndromic SNHL accounts for ~25% of all pediatric SNHL cases.

Q Consultation with a geneticist should be obtained when a syndrome is present or suspected.

R Family history of SNHL is an indication to test a child's hearing; thus, siblings of children with SNHL should have audiometric testing (either behavioral or ABR-based if indicated by age).

S Medical evaluation must be determined on the basis of which risk factors have been identified and tailored specifically for each child. An ophthalmologic consultation should be considered in each case to be certain that the child is not affected by additional sensory deficits.

T CT scan of the temporal bones should be obtained when the etiology of SNHL is unknown. Inner ear anomalies are seen in up to 25% of children with SNHL. In cases of unilateral SNHL, MRI should also be considered to evaluate possible retrocochlear etiologies.

U Medical evaluation of children with SNHL of unknown cause is an area of controversy. An ophthalmology consult should be obtained. In addition, the following are of use in confirming and excluding certain disorders: TORCH syndrome titers, FTA-ABS, urinalysis, thyroid function tests, complete blood count, chemistry panel, rheumatoid factor, antinuclear antibody assay, and electrocardiogram. Electrocardiogram should be obtained to rule out Jervell and Lange–Nielsen (QT prolongation), which is untreated.

V Certain inner ear malformations (e.g. enlarged vestibular aqueduct and associated cochlear dysplasia) may place the child at risk for progressive SNHL after head trauma or barotrauma; the patient and family should be counseled appropriately. Contact sports should be avoided, and long-term serial audiometry is advised.

W Cochlear implantation may be performed in children young as 12 months of age and should be considered when limited or no benefit is obtained from amplification.

SUGGESTED READING

American Academy of Pediatrics Joint Committee on Infant Hearing: 2007 Position Statement (update). Pediatrics. 2007;120(4):898-921.

DeMarcantonio M, Choo DI. Radiographic evaluation of children with hearing loss. Otol Clin North Am. 2015;48(6):913-932.

Foteff C, Kennedy S, Milton AH, et al. Economic evaluation of treatments for pediatric bilateral severe to profound sensorineural hearing loss: an Australian perspective. Otol Neurotol. 2016;37(5):462-469.

Jayawardena ADL, Shearer AE, Smith RJH. Sensorineural hearing loss: a changing paradigm for its evaluation. Otolaryngol Head Neck Surg. 2015;153(5):843-850.

Park AH, Duval M, McVicar S, et al. A diagnostic paradigm including cytomegalovirus testing for idiopathic pediatric sensorineural hearing loss. Laryngoscope. 2014;124(11):2624-2629.

Prosser JD, Cohen AP, Greinwald JH. Diagnostic evaluation of children with sensorineural hearing loss. Otol Clin North Am. 2015;48(6):975-982.

CHAPTER 5

Congenital Hearing Loss

Bryan J Liming, Richard JH Smith

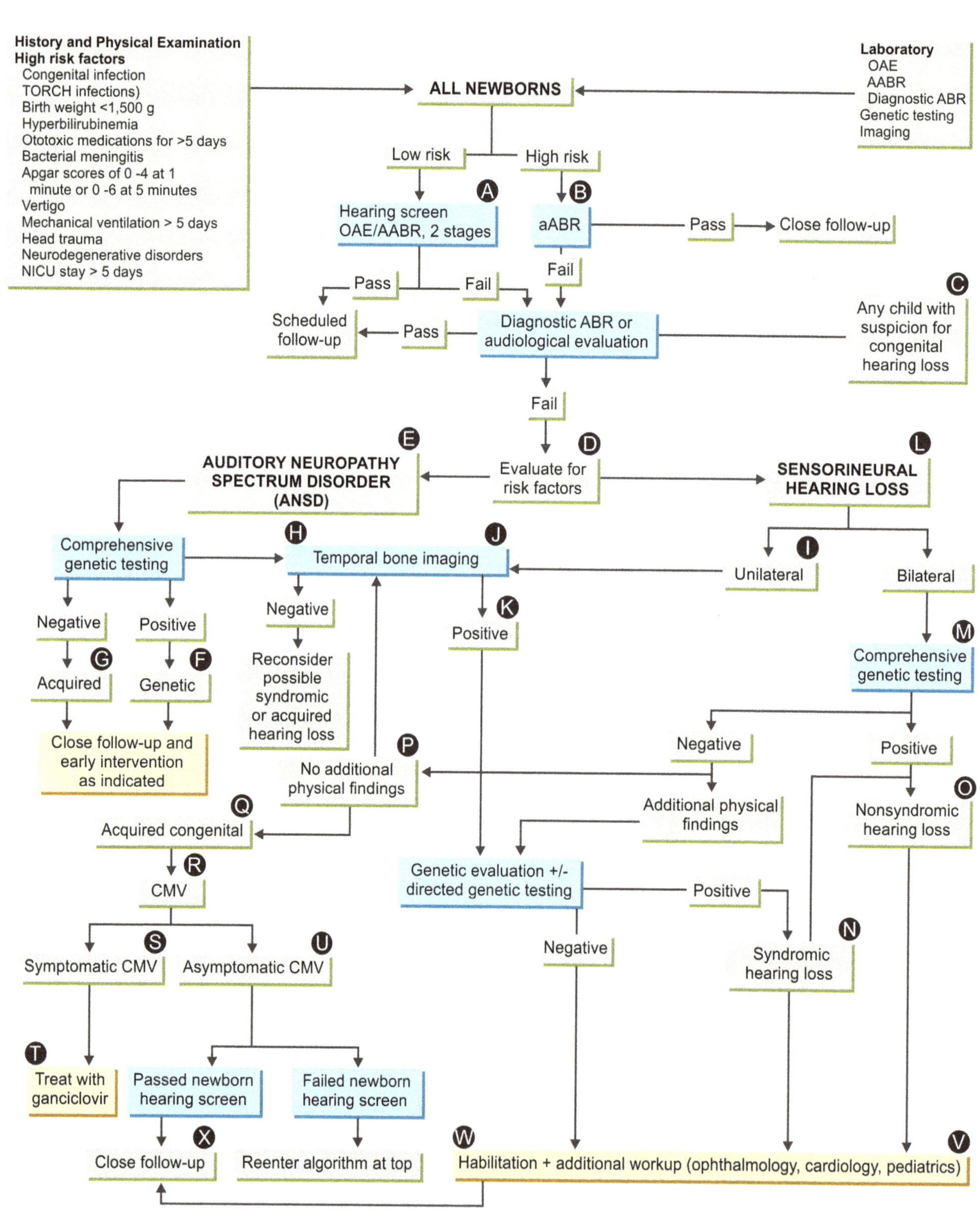

Congenital hearing loss affects 2–3 out of 1,000 children born in the United States. By definition, congenital hearing loss is present at birth and affected children are deaf or have a hearing loss great enough to affect speech and language development. The understanding of the genetic causes of hearing loss has rapidly expanded and dramatically altered the Evaluation of children with hearing loss.

A Universal screening of all infants has been recommended by the American Academy of Pediatrics, the American Academy of Otolaryngology—Head and Neck Surgery, and the National Institutes of Health Consensus Group with the goal of identifying and habilitating children with hearing loss before 6 months of age. Early intervention is associated with improved language development, educational achievement, and speech skills. All states have established early detection and intervention programs, and screening is mandated in 43 states. If screening were performed only in high-risk infants, 50% of infants with congenital hearing loss would go undetected. In the child without risk factors, screening can be accomplished by either otoacoustic emissions (OAEs) or automated auditory brainstem response (AABR). A two-stage approach is often used where children who fail OAEs will have a follow-up AABR as a screen.

B In the high-risk child, an AABR is the initial screening test of choice to avoid missing a diagnosis of auditory neuropathy spectrum disorder (ANSD), which is more prevalent in the high-risk population. High-risk factors include congenital infection or childhood infection known or suspected to be associated with hearing loss (i.e. TORCH infections), birth weight <1,500 g, hyperbilirubinemia exceeding indication for exchange transfusion, ototoxic medications used for >5 days (including antibiotics and loop diuretics), bacterial meningitis, Apgar scores of 0–4 at 1 minute or 0–6 at 5 minutes, prolonged mechanical ventilation > 5 days, head trauma, neurodegenerative disorders, and neonatal intensive care unit (NICU) stay > 5 days. Infants readmitted within the first month of life after a normal hearing screen should also have repeat screening prior to discharge.

C Children in whom hearing loss should be suspected include children with language delay or those with a parental concern. Hearing loss should be confirmed by ABR or behavioral audiometry or both. Other causes of language delay include autism, neurodegenerative diseases, environmental deprivation, attention deficit disorder, specific learning disorders, and mental retardation. Referral to a communication disorders clinic for evaluation may be helpful in children whose hearing is normal.

D Irrespective of the initial reason for referral, all children should be evaluated for developmental milestone achievement, craniofacial abnormalities, middle ear disease, gestational and neonatal risk factors, and other risk factors for hearing loss. A thorough family history, including any family history of hereditary childhood sensorineural hearing loss (SNHL) and/or consanguinity, is imperative for the evaluation of the child with hearing loss. Hearing thresholds of parents and possibly other family members should be determined if inherited hearing loss remains in the differential diagnosis.

E Auditory neuropathy spectrum disorder is diagnosed when OAEs and/or cochlear microphonic are present, but there is an absent or abnormal ABR. The ANSD can manifest as mild-to-profound hearing loss or normal hearing thresholds in the presence of reduced speech discrimination and can be caused by dysfunction at any point along the auditory pathway.

F Approximately 40–50% of ANSD diagnoses have a genetic etiology while the remainder is acquired. The most common genetic cause is mutation of OTOF (DFNB9), which encodes the protein otoferlin. Typically, DFNB9-related hearing loss manifests as profound prelingual deafness. Other genes implicated in ANSD include TIMM8A, AIFM1, PJVK, mtDNA (m.N9ST>C), PMP22, MPZ, TMEM126A. Identifying the specific genetic cause may impact habilitation options. For example, persons with TIMM8A mutations do not do well with cochlear implants, while persons with mutations in A1FM1 can have auditory nerve agenesis and may require brain stem implants.

G Early acquired ANSD is strongly associated with an extended stay in the neonatal intensive care unit and is related to associated hypoxia, prematurity, metabolic toxins, and hyperbilirubinemia. Acquired ANSD can improve with time, and with close surveillance and repeat testing it may be possible to differentiate acquired from genetic ANSD.

H Magnetic resonance imaging (MRI) is an option in ANSD and may reveal abnormalities in the inner ear, cochlear nerve, brain, or posterior cranial fossa in up to 60% of cases.

I Temporal bone imaging can be considered with the discovery of unilateral hearing loss. Twenty-five to 64% of these children will be found to have an abnormality on temporal bone imaging.

J Temporal bone imaging should not be reflexively ordered in most children with congenital hearing loss, although it is indicated in children who are cochlear implant candidates. However, in the presence of unilateral hearing loss, especially at the severe-to-profound range, either computed tomography (CT) or high-resolution T2-weighted MRI can resolve abnormalities of the cochlear and labyrinth as well as the VIIIth cranial nerve complex. The most commonly discovered abnormalities are dilated vestibular aqueduct (DVA) and cochlear nerve deficiency, each which occurs at a rate of ~20% of children with unilateral SNHL.

K Cochlear nerve deficiency can be associated with ANSD as well as CHARGE and VACTERL syndromes. The DVA is associated with Pendred's syndrome. Genetics consultation should be considered for an individual with complex temporal bone abnormalities.

L The subsequent evaluation of SNHL depends on a thorough history, a comprehensive physical examination, and a focused family history.

M The evaluation of hearing loss in children has substantially improved with the advent of comprehensive genetic testing (CGT). After an audiogram, CGT is the single best test to order in the evaluation of hearing loss and has a diagnostic rate of 40–65%. Establishing a diagnosis facilitates genetic counseling and directs subsequent steps in the management of the individual with hearing loss. In the future, genetic testing will be the foundation for various types of gene therapy to prevent or reverse hearing loss.

N Thirty percent of genetic hearing loss is syndromic. More than 500 types of syndromic deafness have been described, most of which are extremely rare. Relatively common forms include Stickler's syndrome, Pendred's syndrome, Usher's syndrome, branchio-oto-renal syndrome, Alport's syndrome, neurofibromatosis, and Waardenburg syndrome. Confirmatory genetic testing is available.

O When a specific nonsyndromic genetic cause is identified, a thorough search of the literature should be performed to guide subsequent counseling and management.

P Temporal bone imaging can be considered if CGT is negative or inconclusive. The diagnostic rate is relatively low (~30% for CT, ~26% for MRI).

Q About 2 to 5% of neonates with one or more risk factors have a moderate-to-profound hearing loss.

R Cytomegalovirus (CMV) deserves special consideration. Congenital CMV is the most common nongenetic cause of congenital SNHL in the United States. It causes 9–25% of early-onset bilateral SNHL and 9% of early unilateral SNHL. Approximately 0.6–0.7% of newborns in industrialized countries are infected with CMV, most without outward signs of infection. The rates of hearing loss are 7–15% for asymptomatic CMV and 33% for symptomatic CMV. Most children with CMV-associated congenital hearing loss also have vestibular dysfunction (and therefore delayed motor milestones). The hearing loss can be bilateral, fluctuating, and progressive or unilateral. The CMV testing can be performed on banked infant blood spots when available. Currently, the majority of congenital CMV-related SNHL is not identified by newborn hearing screening programs.

S Symptomatic CMV is often associated with a spectrum of symptoms including petechiae, conjugated hyperbilirubinemia, thrombocytopenia, hepatosplenomegaly, seizures, microcephaly, and intracranial calcifications. The diagnosis is confirmed by polymerase chain reaction of urine or saliva within 3 weeks of birth.

T In symptomatic children, intravenous ganciclovir has been shown to improve audiologic outcomes at 6 months of age, but the benefit is less clear at age 2. Oral valganciclovir for 6 months may mitigate long-term hearing and neurodevelopmental morbidity.

U Most children with CMV-related SNHL are asymptomatic and initially pass the newborn hearing screen (NBHS). It is not clear how to adequately identify which children are at risk for SNHL. If CMV status is known to be positive, these children should be monitored closely for the development of hearing loss.

V Rarely, additional diagnostic tests (e.g. urinalysis, ultrasonography of kidneys, electroretinography, electrocardiography, chromosomal testing, and thyroid function tests) may identify the cause of hearing loss and inconspicuous medical comorbidity. This directed investigation is often driven by CGT results. Rare medically treatable causes of hearing loss include congenital syphilis, toxoplasmosis, Lyme disease, tuberculosis, hypercholesterolemia, tumors, and several enzyme abnormalities, such as biotinidase deficiency and Refsum's disease. The most common comorbidities are mental retardation (11%), ophthalmologic (30–40%), and cerebral palsy (3%). Ophthalmologic evaluation may identify syndromic deafness, although in Usher's syndrome, fundoscopy can remain normal during the childhood years.

W Habilitation options include amplification, cochlear implantation, or middle ear reconstruction as indicated. A wide variety of communication modalities exist. The intervention team ideally includes individuals with expertise in deafness and training in otolaryngology, deaf education, speech-language pathology, childhood development, and audiometric testing. The Joint Committee on Infant Hearing position statement states that children should receive appropriate intervention by no later than 3 months of age.

X Periodic follow-up is essential to ensure the efficacy of auditory intervention, monitor for fluctuation and progression of hearing loss, aggressively treat reversible and preventable exacerbations of hearing loss, monitor for emerging comorbidity, and identify syndromic features that may appear over time. Infants who are identified as high risk should be closely followed even in the presence of a normal hearing screen.

SUGGESTED READING

Alford RL, Arnos KS, Fox M, et al. American College of Medical Genetics and Genomics guideline for the clinical evaluation and etiologic diagnosis of hearing loss. Genet Med. 2014;16(4): 347-355.

American Academy of Pediatrics: Year 2007 Position Statement: principles and guidelines for early hearing detection and intervention programs. Pediatrics. 2007;120(4):898-921.

Bernard S, Wiener-Vacher S, Van Den Abbeele T. Disorders in children with congenital cytomegalovirus infection. Pediatrics. 2015;136(4):e887-995.

Dahl JP, Stadler ME, Huang BY. Connexin-Related (DFNB1) hearing loss: is routine computed tomography imaging necessary? Otolaryngol Head Neck Surg. 2015;152(5):889-896.

Deklerck AN, Acke FR, Janssens S, et al. Etiological approach in patients with unidentified hearing loss. Int J Pediatr Otorhinolaryngol. 2015;79(2):216-222.

Goderis J, De Leenheer ED, Smets K. Hearing loss and congenital CMV infection: a systematic review. Pediatrics. 2014;134(5):972-982.

Jayawardena AD, Shearer AE, Smith RJ. Sensorineural hearing loss: a changing paradigm for its evaluation. Otolaryngol Head Neck Surg. 2015;153(5):843-850.

Norrix LW, Velenovsky DS. Auditory neuropathy spectrum disorder: a review. J Speech Lang Hear Res. 2014;57(4):1564-1576.

Shearer AE, Black-Ziegelbein EA, Hildebrand MS, et al. Advancing genetic testing for deafness with genomic technology. J Med Genet. 2013;50(9):627-634.

Shearer AE, Smith RJH. Massively parallel sequencing for genetic diagnosis of hearing loss: the new standard of care. Otolaryngol Head Neck Surg. 2015;153(2):175-182.

Sudden Sensorineural Hearing Loss

Peter C Weber

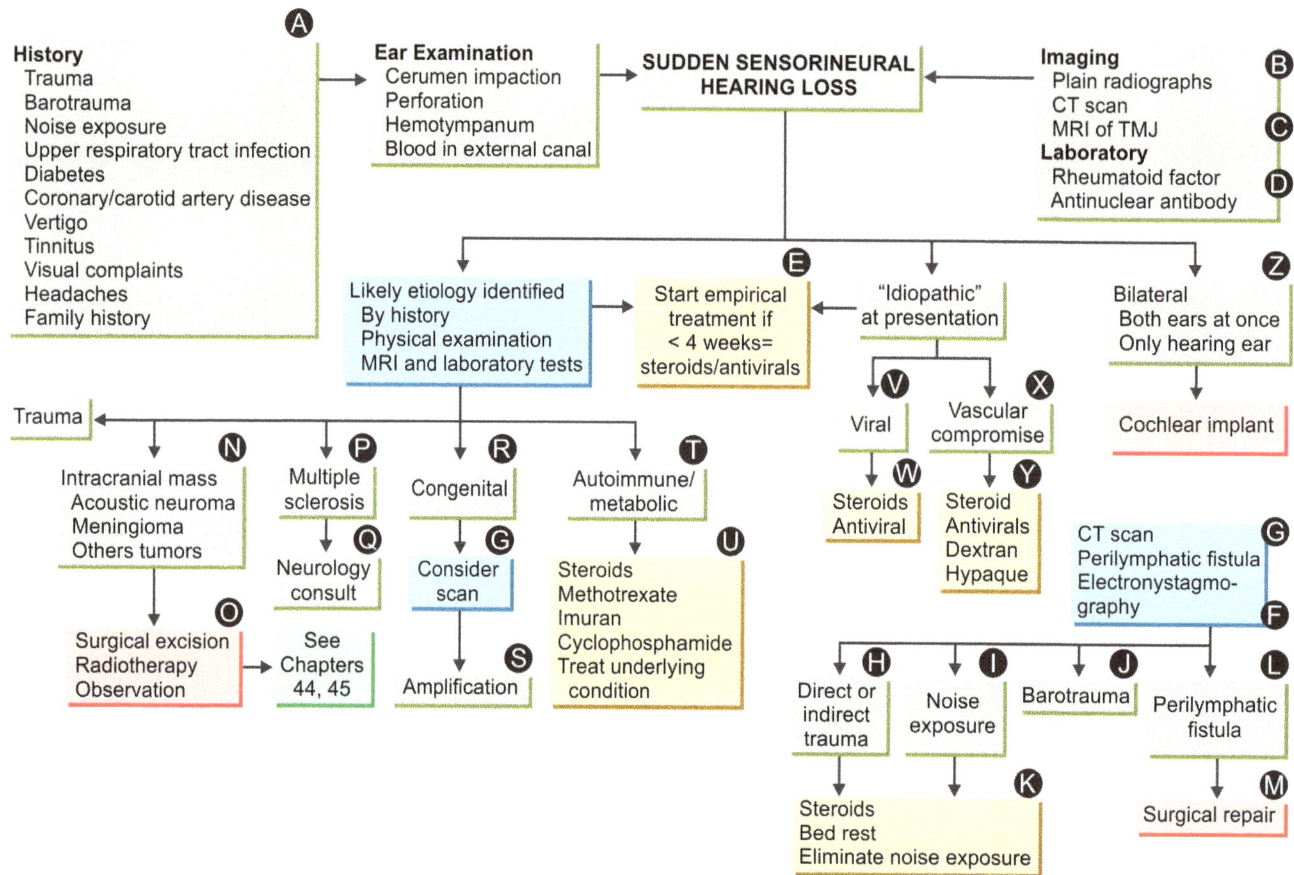

Sudden hearing loss, defined as a >30-dB hearing reduction in at least three continuous frequencies, occurring over a period of ≤72 hours, can be the result of any number of etiologies. The term is usually used for sudden sensorineural loss, although patients may perceive "sudden loss" from other causes such as otitis media with effusion (OME). Early intervention is key, particularly in autoimmune hearing loss; hence, there should be a sense of urgency when addressing this complaint.

A The history will often indicate the actual cause for the sudden sensorineural hearing loss. Examination of the ear and tympanic membrane is important and, although usually normal, it may reveal the presence of hemotympanum, a mass, or a perforation of the tympanic membrane.

B Any patient who complains of hearing loss (with no apparent cause such as otitis media) should undergo audiometric studies at the earliest opportunity.

C Any patient who has a sudden sensorineural hearing loss should have an MRI with gadolinium, regardless of whether or not the hearing returns to normal with or without treatment. Multiple sclerosis, acoustic neuroma, meningioma, or other type of central cause (e.g. cerebrovascular accident) must be ruled out by imaging.

D It is important to ascertain that the patient does not have any type of autoimmune disorder, blood dyscrasias, hypo- or hyperthyroidism, or other abnormalities in the metabolic panel.

E The results of MRI, computed tomography (CT) scan, and laboratory tests are often pending when therapy is initiated. If the onset has been <4 weeks, I recommend starting prednisone [either 60 mg per day (all in the AM) for 10 days; intratympanic injections of dexamethasone (one a week for 3 weeks), or both for adults] and valacyclovir (Valtrex, 1 g three times a day for 10 days for adults) if there are no medical contraindications. The recent American Academy of Otolaryngology—Head and Neck Surgery guidelines question the use of Valtrex if not initiated immediately but with minimal side effects I offer it if the etiology appears to be viral. I also use intratympanic injections after failure of oral medication and for up to 8–12 weeks after the loss of hearing.

F Any patient who has a history of barotrauma, nystagmus with pneumoscopy, or trauma should be evaluated for the possibility of perilymphatic fistula or semicircular canal dehiscence.

G A CT scan is usually indicated in patients who have suffered head trauma and in those for whom there is concern about a congenital abnormality or superior semicircular canal dehiscence. Many congenital abnormalities can be diagnosed with MRI with gadolinium. Computed tomography may also be indicated in the patient with suspected cochlear otosclerosis or some other type of bony lesion.

H Indirect or direct trauma may cause a sudden sensorineural hearing loss as a result of either temporal bone fractures or concussive forces, which cause an increased pressure or shearing force within the cochlear.

I Although prolonged exposure to noise can cause a progressive sensorineural hearing loss, extremely loud sounds can cause a sudden loss. These sounds are usually >160 dB. For some people who are sensitive, the intensity of the sound may be significantly less (≥100 dB).

J Barotrauma is seen most commonly in divers, but it can also be seen in people who fly airplanes. Hearing loss is usually due to a rupture of the cochlear membranes or a perilymphatic fistula.

K Treatment for trauma, whether direct, indirect, noise induced, or barotrauma, includes steroids and rest. If a traumatic perilymphatic fistula is suspected, then exploratory surgery and packing of the oval and round window fistulas are also appropriate. Elimination of exposure to loud noise is also necessary.

L Perilymphatic fistula can cause sudden hearing loss and can result from congenital abnormalities or trauma. Pressure changes, even as simple as increased pressure from nose blowing can cause a fistula.

M Treatment for PLF is surgical repair, packing of the oval and round windows with muscle and fascia or other connective tissue. Alternatively, one can treat as described above with steroids, rest, and noise elimination, and if no response surgery can then be considerd.

N The most common intracranial mass is an acoustic neuroma, which presents with sudden sensorineural hearing loss in 10–15% of cases.

O Treatment for an intracranial mass includes observation if the tumor is very small and confined to the internal auditory canal and the patient has no other symptoms. More symptomatic masses are managed with surgical excision or stereotactic radiation therapy.

P Multiple sclerosis can present as a sudden sensorineural hearing loss in up to 10% of cases. An MRI with gadolinium usually discloses a plaque; however, lumbar puncture may be needed for testing cerebrospinal fluid.

Q Multiple sclerosis is usually managed with medications by a neurologist. In the case of sudden loss, high-dose steroids have proven useful.

R This may be due to congenital malformations of the inner ear, such as enlarged vestibular aqueduct, or some type of familial disorders.

S Treatment for congenital sensorineural hearing loss is amplification.

T An autoimmune cause usually results in an asymmetric sudden bilateral hearing loss. The hearing loss typically occurs at different times, and the hearing levels are usually different in each ear. Sedimentation rates may be elevated, unfortunately, 68-KD cochlear autoantigens are not diagnostic. Metabolic causes such as hypo- and hyperthyroidism are identified by laboratory tests.

U Autoimmune inner ear disease is treated with steroids. Once there is a response with high-dose steroids, the steroids are reduced until a very low maintenance dose is found. If the steroids do not help or a low dose cannot be determined to keep the hearing stable, then the use of methotrexate, azathioprine (Imuran), and cyclophosphamide may prove useful.

V Virus will likely remain the most common cause of sudden sensorineural hearing loss. Herpes simplex virus 1 is considered the most common etiology.

W Treatment of a viral cause consists of high-dose prednisone or the weekly intratympanic injections of dexamethasone for 3 weeks, along with antivirals. Typically, there is an 85% chance of return of hearing, and usually hearing will start to improve within the first few weeks to 2 months.

X Vascular compromise is considered in people who have diabetes or coronary/carotid artery disease and in those who are most prone to transient ischemic attacks or strokes, such as the elderly.

Y Treatment for vascular compromise is with steroids, although in those individuals with diabetes, the use of intratympanic steroid injections is preferred. The long term use of aspirin may also be indicated.

Z Occasionally, a patient may lose hearing suddenly bilaterally. Causes can include ototoxicity, noise, and viral. Cochlear implantation should be considered if no improvement is seen after 3–6 months of treatment.

SUGGESTED READING

Awad Z, Huins C, Pothier DD. Antivirals for idiopathic sudden sensorineural hearing loss. Cochrane Database Syst Rev. 2012;15:8.

Grandis JR, Hirsch BE, Wageur MM. Treatment of idiopathic sudden sensorineural hearing loss. Am J Otol. 1993;14:183-185.

Kim SH, Jung SY, Kim MG, et al. Comparison of steroid administration methods in patients with idiopathic sudden sensorineural hearing loss: a retrospective observational study. Clin Otolaryngol. 2015;40:183-190.

Weber PC, Prey BA, Bluestone CD. Middle ear abnormalities associated with congenital perilymphatic fistulas. Laryngoscope. 1993;103:160-164.

Weber PC, Zbar R, Gantz B. Appropriateness of MRI in sudden sensorineural hearing loss. Otolaryngol Head Neck Surg. 1997;116:153-156.

Noise-induced Hearing Loss

Catherine V Palmer, Jenifer Fruit

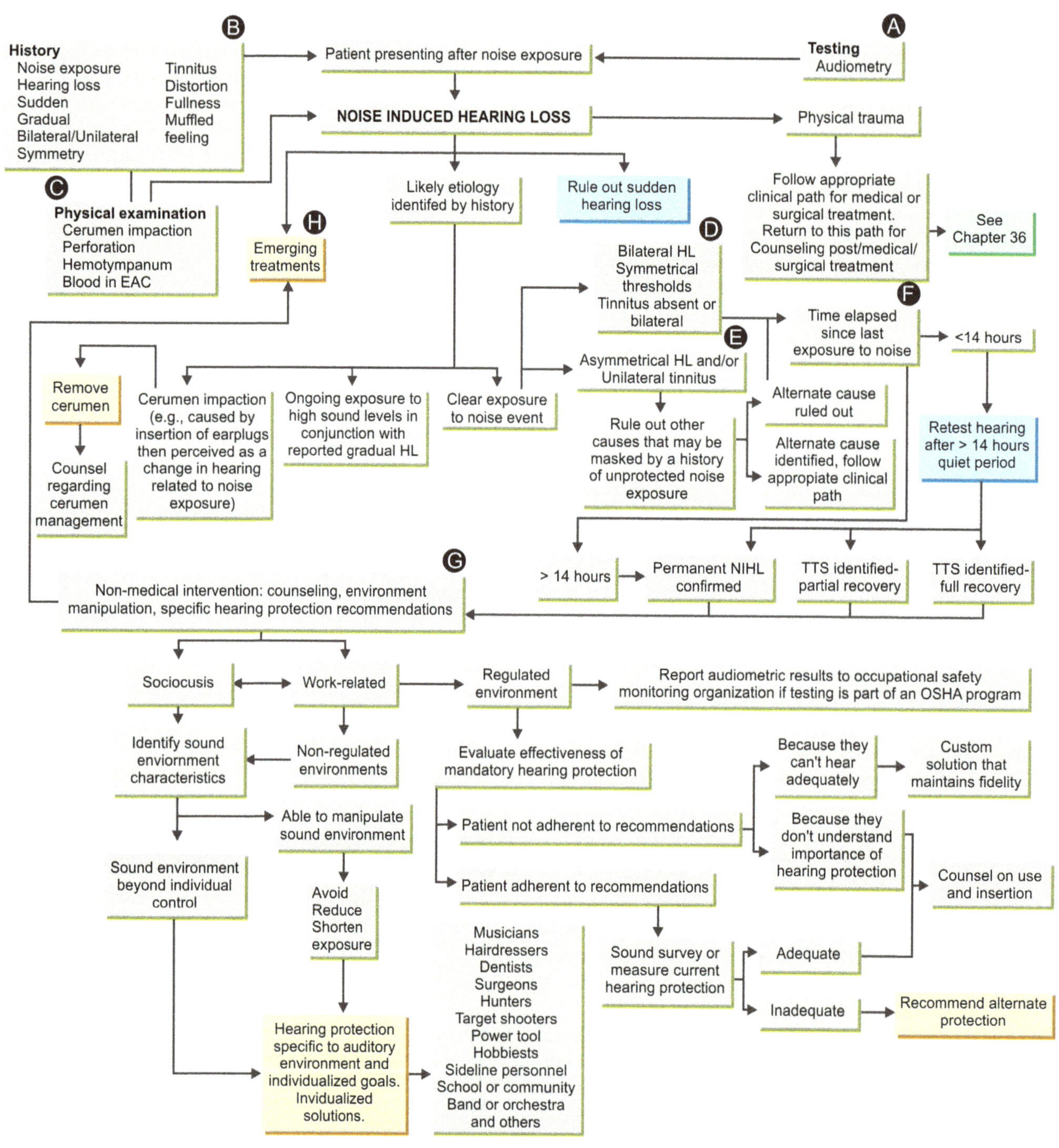

Loud noise exposure is a common, often preventable, cause of temporary or permanent auditory threshold shift. Hearing loss of this type, often referred to as noise-induced hearing loss (NIHL), may result from one exposure to a very loud sound or as a cumulative effect of extended exposure to loud sounds. Hearing loss which is the result of extended exposure to noisy work environments is called occupational noise-induced hearing loss (ONIHL), whereas hearing loss resulting from loud recreational activities is called socioacusis. The term acoustic trauma is often used to refer to NIHL resulting from exposure to one very loud sound, such as an explosion or gun shot, and implies additional physiologic changes such as rupture of the tympanic membrane or damage to physical structures in the inner ear. Tinnitus is frequently associated with NIHL or acoustic trauma.

In the United States, the Occupational Safety and Health Administration (OSHA) regulates the amount of noise to which workers are permitted to be exposed. According to the National Institute for Occupational Safety and Health, 30 million American workers are exposed to potentially damaging amounts of noise each year. With appropriate protections in place, the risk of ONIHL is largely mitigated for employees of companies that fall under OSHA regulations. Loud noise resulting from nonoccupational sources is not regulated and poses a great risk for NIHL. Sources of nonoccupational noise include but are not limited to hobbies such as wood-working, motorcycle riding, car racing, lawn care, hunting and target shooting, performing music, and attending concerts or sporting events. Working-age adults are not the only population at risk for NIHL. An estimated 12.5% of children and adolescents aged 6–19 years (~5.2 million) have hearing loss as a result of exposure to loud noise.

Noise-induced hearing loss is preventable with appropriate hearing protection and other noise mitigation. Pharmaceutical interventions for NIHL are in development. The majority of research in this area is focused on otoprotective use of the amino acid D-methionine (D-met), and research regarding its application is in Phase 3 FDA clinical trials (2015). In addition, there is research underway investigating the use of inner ear-gene therapy administered to the ear as a potential treatment for acquired hearing loss. At this time, there is no accepted medical treatment for NIHL. The proactive clinician may dedicate part of his/her practice to educating the community about NIHL and individualized hearing protection. Most typically, however, the clinician will see the patient after the damage has been done and will be in a position to rule out other causes of hearing loss, manage any permanent hearing loss (typically with the use of amplification), and recommend appropriate hearing protection for future use to avoid further damage.

Ⓐ A comprehensive audiometric evaluation will reveal the type, severity, and configuration of hearing loss and will aid in ruling out other potential causes of hearing loss. A recent study indicated that only 40% of NIHL will present with the typical noise notch (hearing loss at 2,000–6,000 Hz with recovery at 8,000 Hz).

Ⓑ The history will give the clinician a clear indication of a noise event or long-term exposure to noise. Interview the patient regarding work and nonwork exposure.

Ⓒ There are cases of individuals using in-ear hearing protection that results in impacted cerumen. Although the hearing loss is due to the cerumen impaction, they associate it with the noise and use of hearing protection.

Ⓓ Noise exposure most typically causes bilateral damage if both ears are unprotected. If the sound source is clearly located on one side over time, an asymmetrical hearing loss may be revealed. For instance, a drummer who has cymbals on one side may experience more hearing loss in the ear closest to the sound.

Ⓔ Patients with NIHL may describe unilateral tinnitus because of uneven exposure between ears, but the clinician will want to rule out other causes in these cases. The noise exposed individual can have other underlying causes of hearing loss that may be masked by the NIHL overlay.

Ⓕ Occupational Safety and Health Administration suggests a 14-hour quiet period post-noise exposure prior to measuring hearing because of the possibility of temporary threshold shift.

Ⓖ If a diagnosis of NIHL is determined on the basis of audiometric findings and case history while other causes of hearing loss have been ruled out, the clinician will want to enter into nonmedical intervention that will include counseling, environment manipulation, and specific hearing protection recommendations. Individualized hearing protection solutions are available for a variety of noisy activities and are designed to meet specific hearing needs. Most typically, an audiologist will supply this information and will make recommendations related to hearing protection along with acquiring earmold impressions needed to fit custom solutions. Hearing protection can be measured in the clinic to assess the noise reduction provided in the individual ear.

Ⓗ Emerging treatments include pharmacological based therapies that are currently in clinical trials.

ACKNOWLEDGEMENT

Jenifer Fruit passed away at an untimely young age several months after completing work on this chapter. She is sorely missed by her colleagues

SUGGESTED READING

Campbell K, Claussen A, Meech R, et al. D-methionine (D-met) significantly rescues noise-induced hearing loss: timing studies. Hear Res. 2011;282(1):138-144.

Franks JR, Stephenson MR, Merry CJ. Preventing occupational hearing loss—a practical guide. US Department of Health and Human Services Public Health Service Centers for Disease Control and Prevention National Institute for Occupational Safety and Health Division of Biomedical and Behavioral Science Physical Agents Effects Branch June 1996. Revised October 1996. www.cdc.gov/niosh/docs/96-110/pdfs/96-110.pdf.

Kirchner DB, Evenson E, Dobie RA, et al. Occupational noise-induced hearing loss: ACOEM task force on occupational hearing loss. J Occup Environ Med. 2012;54(1):106-108.

Niskar AS, Kieszak SM, Holmes AE, et al. Estimated prevalence of noise induced hearing threshold shifts among children 6 to 19 years of age: The Third National Health and Nutritional Examination Survey, 1988–1994, United States. Pediatrics. 2001;108:40-43.

Occupational Safety Health Administration, Occupational Noise Exposure; Hearing Conservation Amendment 2aCRF1910.95, Federal Register Rules and Regulations. Part II Department of Labor. 12/12/1981. www.osha.gov/pls/oshaweb/owadisp.show_document?p_table=DIRECTIVES&p_id=1865.

Pearlman RC. Presbycusis: the need for a clinical definition. Am J Otol. 1982;3(3):183-186.

Shargorodsky J, Curhan SG, Curhan GC, et al. Change in prevalence of hearing loss in US adolescents. JAMA. 2010;304(7):772-778.

Wilson RH. Some observations on the nature of the audiometric 4000 Hz Notch: data from 3430 Veterans. J Am Acad Audiol. 2011;22(1):23-33.

Unilateral Deafness

Kavita Dedhia

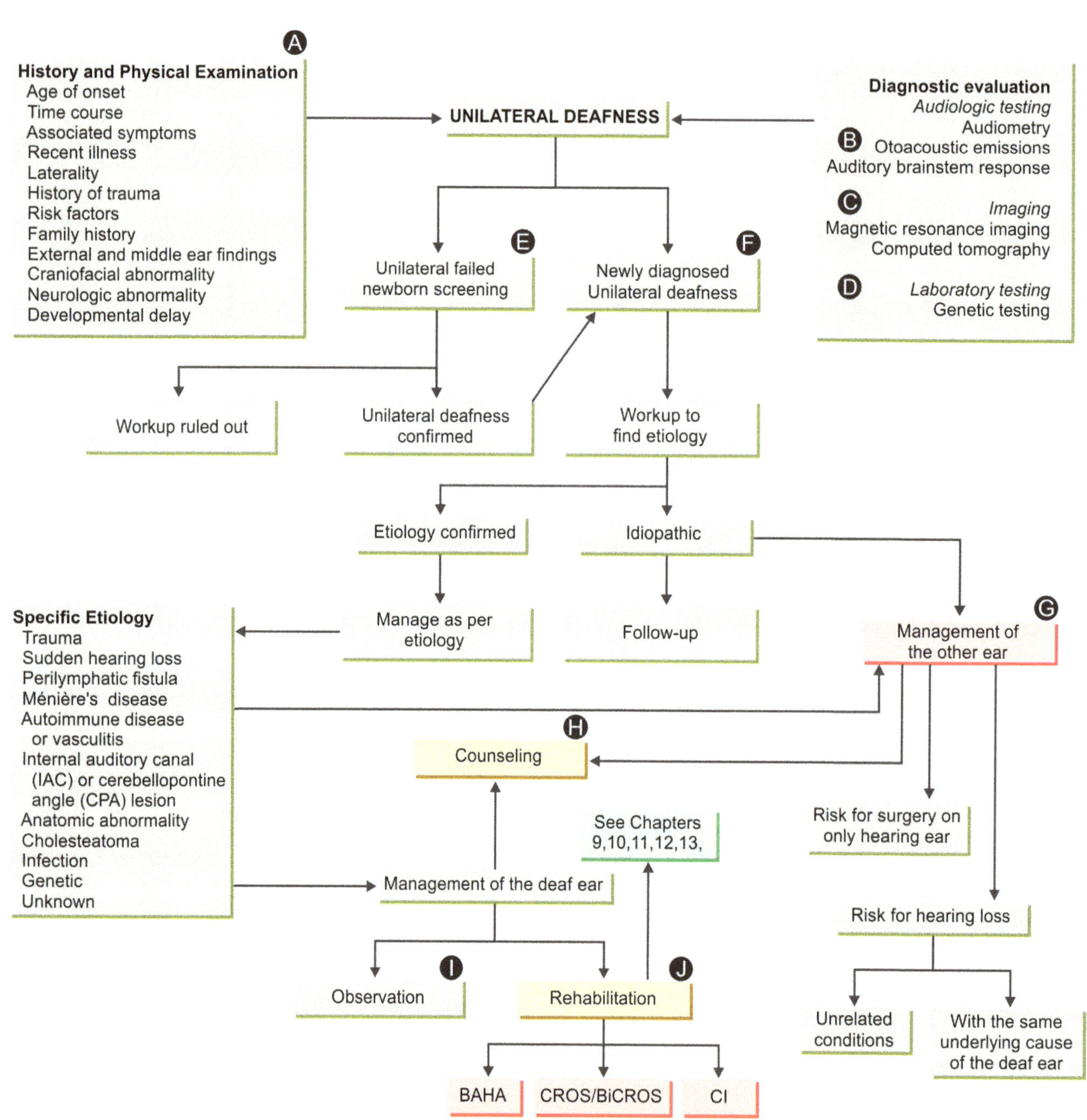

Patients with unilateral deafness have complete hearing loss in one ear and normal hearing or a mild to severe loss on the contralateral side. These patients have often been overlooked with respect to hearing rehabilitation due to the belief that the normal ear will compensate. They experience multiple audiologic difficulties, as they cannot hear anything on the nonhearing side; these difficulties are exacerbated in the presence of competing sounds.

A When evaluating patients with unilateral deafness, it is important to perform a thorough history and physical examination including microscopic examination of the tympanic membrane and pneumatic otoscopy.

B All adult patients should undergo a conventional audiogram. For pediatric patients, the type of audiologic testing depends on the age: 0–6 months behavioral observation, 6 months–2 years visual reinforcement, 2–4 years conditions play, and >4 conventional audiogram. Cases in which the audiogram is not diagnostic, or unable to be performed, evaluation may require otoacoustic emissions testing or an auditory brainstem response (ABR).

C Adult patients with unilateral deafness should undergo magnetic resonance imaging as 0.8–4% of these patients may have lesions in the internal auditory canal or cerebellopontine angle lesions. Young adults and children should also undergo a CT scan, since they are more likely to have an anatomic abnormality such as cochlear dysplasia, Mondini malformation, or enlarged vestibular aqueduct.

D Laboratory testing is not routinely indicated as laboratory evaluation of patients with unilateral hearing loss has a low diagnostic yield. Testing should only be performed when there is specific clinical suspicion. Genetic testing however should be offered to all patients, as 50% of hearing loss is due to a genetic etiology.

E Failed unilateral newborn hearing screen should still follow the 1-3-6 rule. Screening by 1 month, diagnosis by 3 months, and intervention by 6 months. Behavioral testing should be performed after 6 months to confirm the deafness and future audiograms to follow the hearing in the contralateral ear. Audiograms should be performed every 3–4 months the first year, every 6 months the second year and yearly afterward, if the hearing is stable.

F Newly diagnosed deafness should be evaluated with a full history and physical examination, audiologic testing, imaging, genetic testing, and laboratory testing if needed, as discussed above. The management of each individual etiology listed in this algorithm is discussed elsewhere in this book.

G Patients should be advised regarding the management of the contralateral ear. They should be counseled regarding future hearing loss, or progression if there is already hearing loss. If the patient absolutely requires surgery in the only hearing ear, they should be counseled regarding the risk of losing hearing in the only hearing ear after surgery. For the patient with hearing loss in the nondeaf ear amplification is recommended with a bilateral contralateral routing of signal (BiCROS).

H Patients should be counseled regarding the effect of unilateral deafness; developmental, social, educational, and economic effects should be discussed. Aural rehabilitation should be recommended, and adults can also be given the choice of observation. In addition, all patients should have an understanding of what services are available for them with respect to early intervention, school services, and the American Disabilities Act. All school-aged children should have preferential seating at school and the use of an FM system if available.

I If they choose to observe, then they should be followed with subsequent audiograms to evaluate for progression or fluctuation of the hearing loss. This is not the recommended management especially for children given the social and educational implications.

J If they choose aural rehabilitation, then they currently have the option of the bone-anchored hearing aid (BAHA) or a contralateral routing of signals (CROS/BiCROS) hearing aid. The main difference between the two modalities is that the BAHA requires a surgical procedure, and is only worn on the side of the deafness, whereas the CROS requires two hearing aids (one transmitter and one receiver) to be worn but no surgical procedure. They should be counseled that these types of hearing devices would restore sound awareness but do not provide sound localization. Only cochlear implants (CI) can restore both in patients; however, they are not currently approved by the Federal Drug Administration for unilateral deafness. New studies have looked at the benefit of CI in patients with unilateral deafness. Those patients with a shorter period of auditory deprivation showed the best performance with the CI.

SUGGESTED READING

Arndt S, Aschendorff A, Laszig R, et al. Comparison of pseudobinaural hearing to real binaural hearing rehabilitation after cochlear implantation in patients with unilateral deafness and tinnitus. Otol Neurotol. 2011;32:39-47.

Arndt S, Laszig R, Aschendorff A, et al. Unilateral deafness and cochlear implantation: audiological diagnostic evaluation and outcomes. HNO. 2011;59:437-446.

Arndt S, Prosse S, Laszig R, et al. Cochlear implantation in children with single-sided deafness: does aetiology and duration of deafness matter? Audiol Neurootol. 2015;20(Suppl 1):21-30.

Finbow J, Bance M, Aiken S, et al. A comparison between wireless CROS and bone-anchored hearing devices for single-sided deafness: a pilot study. Otol Neurotol. 2015;36:819-825.

Hassepass F, Aschendorff A, Wesarg T, et al. Unilateral deafness in children: audiologic and subjective assessment of hearing ability after cochlear implantation. Otol Neurotol. 2013;34:53-60.

Holstrum JW, Gaffney M, Gravel JS, et al. Early intervention for children with unilateral and mild bilateral degrees of hearing loss. Trends Amplif. 2008;12:35-41.

Leterme G, Bernardeschi D, Bensemman A, et al. Contralateral routing of signal hearing aid versus transcutaneous bone conduction in single-sided deafness. Audiol Neurootol. 2015;20:251-260.

Newman CW, Sandridge SA, Wodzisz LM. Longitudinal benefit from and satisfaction with the BAHA system for patients with acquired unilateral sensorineural hearing loss. Otol Neurotol. 2008;29:1123-1131.

Stachler RJ, Chandrasekhar SS, Archer SM, et al. Clinical practice guideline: sudden hearing loss. Otolaryngol Head Neck Surg. 2012;146:S1-35.

Stewart CM, Clark JH, Niparko JK. Bone-anchored devices in single-sided deafness. Adv Otorhinolaryngol. 2011;71:92-102.

Habilitation and Rehabilitation of Pediatric Hearing Loss

Sheila R Pratt

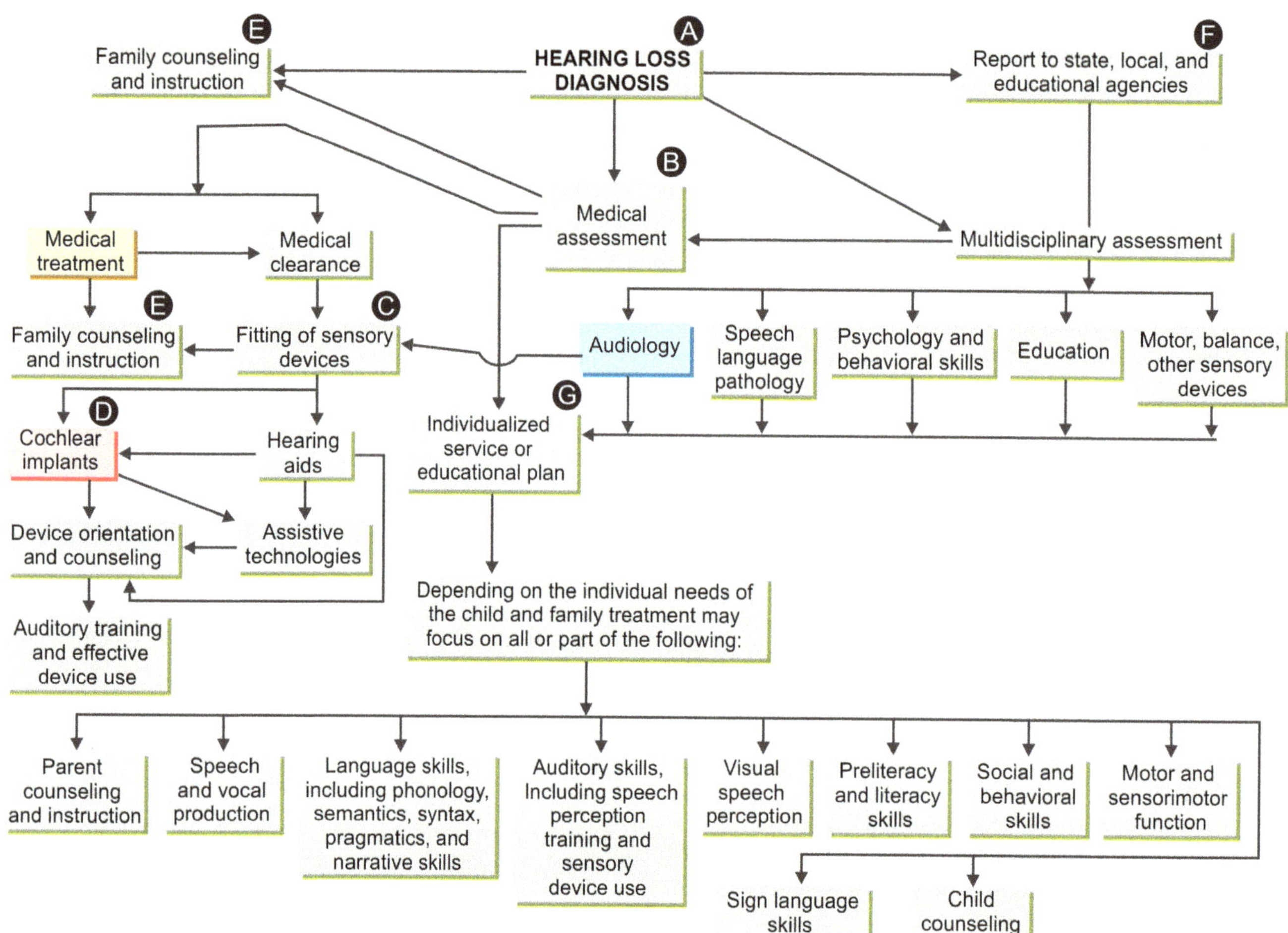

Hearing loss has negative consequences regardless of the age of onset and level of severity. However, congenital and early childhood hearing losses are particularly devastating to children and their families. It impacts speech perception and consequently the acquisition of speech, language, concept development, verbal memory, auditory attention, and literacy skills. Some children also have associated medical issues, as well as cognitive, sensory, and motor deficits that further compromise development. When hearing loss is detected early in infants and young children and their families receive early and high-quality intervention, many of the negative consequences of hearing loss are reduced or alleviated. However, the constellation of problems and needed services vary substantively across children and families, and therefore rehabilitation should be individualized to be effective. Many pediatric patients with hearing loss require some level of services across childhood.

A Hearing loss is a common disorder in infancy and childhood. The most recent data from the Centers for Disease Control-Early Hearing Detection and Intervention Program indicated a prevalence of 1.5 per 1,000 live births in the United States (US) with rates varying from 0.3 to 11.4 across the US states and territories. With age, the rate of hearing loss increases, and it has been shown that about 14.9% of school-aged children have some level of permanent hearing loss. It is recommended that congenital hearing loss and hearing loss occurring in the neonatal period should be identified by 1-month of age, diagnosed by 3 months, and early intervention initiated by 6 months.

B Upon diagnosis of hearing loss, infants and children are referred for a medical evaluation, and subsequent clearance for fitting of sensory devices as deemed appropriate.

C Infants recommended for hearing aids should be fitted by 6 months of age as part of early intervention. For older infants and children, hearing aids should be fitted shortly after diagnosis.

D Currently in the US, infants with a severe-to-profound hearing loss do not receive cochlear implants until they reach 12 months of age. This age requirement can be waived if imaging suggests the onset of cochlear ossification following meningitis. Infants who are cochlear implant candidates typically receive hearing aids shortly after diagnosis and are entered into behavioral rehabilitation for 3–6 months in preparation for implantation.

E Families should receive instruction and counseling throughout the rehabilitation process, but it is critical at diagnosis, and with device fittings and behavioral interventions.

F State and local agencies are responsible for early intervention [covered under Part C of the Individuals with Disabilities Education Act (IDEA), 2004] and should be contacted shortly after diagnosis to initiate services for infants 0 years through 2 years (in some states 0 years through 5 years). Children aged 3–21 years are covered under Part B of IDEA and can receive services through their local school system. As such, it is important that, with parent's permission, a child's school must be informed of a newly diagnosed hearing loss or a substantive change in hearing status.

G Local early intervention agencies and most schools initiate a multidisciplinary assessment shortly after diagnosis and in advance of developing an individualized service or educational plan. Under Part C the plan is referred to as the Individual Family Service Plan (IFSP) but with older children the school-based plan is referred to as the Individualized Education Plan (IEP). It is also common for families to access diagnostic and treatment services through private insurance, Medicaid, or by paying out-of-pocket. Typical professional groups evaluating and making recommendations for these infants and children include audiologists, physicians, speech-language pathologists, educators, psychologists, social workers, physical therapists, and occupational therapists.

SUGGESTED READING

Centers for Disease Control and Prevention. (2016). Summary of 2013 National CDC Early Hearing Detection & Intervention Data [online]. Available from: www.cdc.gov/ncbddd/ehdi/data.htm [Accessed December 2016].

Individuals With Disabilities Education Act, 20 USC. Public law. 2004;108-446.

Joint Committee on Infant Hearing. Year 2007 position statement: principles and guidelines for early hearing detection and intervention programs. Pediatrics. 2007;120:898-921.

Krover AM, Konings S, Dekker FW, et al. Newborn hearing screening vs later hearing screening and developmental outcomes in children with permanent childhood hearing impairment. JAMA. 2010;304:1701-1708.

Niskar AS, Kieszak SM, Holmes A, et al. Prevalence of hearing loss among children 6 to 19 years of age: The Third National Health and Nutrition Examination Survey. J Am Med Asso. 1998;279:1071-1075.

CHAPTER 10

Hearing Aids and Assistive Devices

Catherine V Palmer, Jenifer Fruit

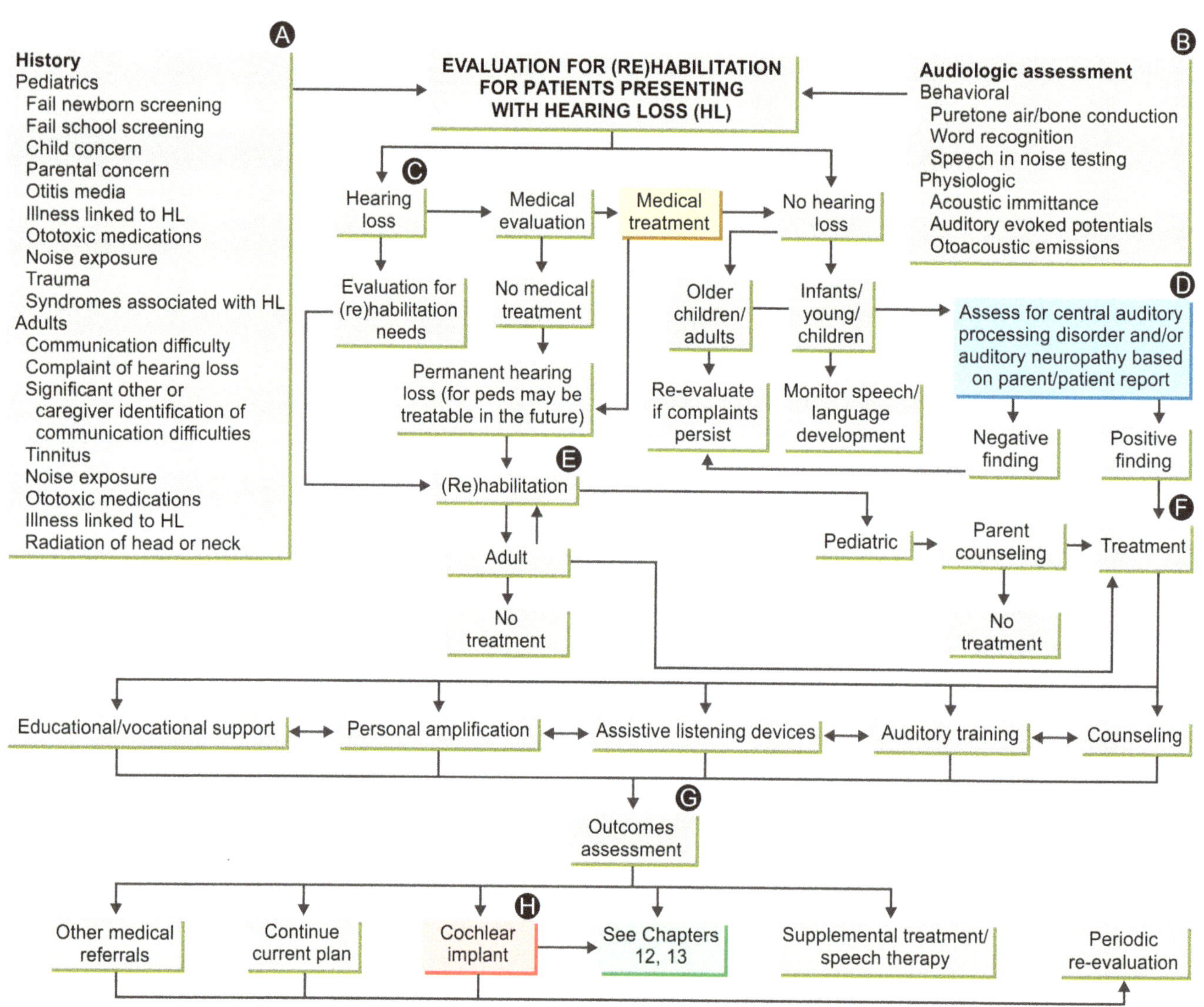

Approximately 30 million Americans aged 12 years and older have bilateral hearing loss with the estimate increasing to 48.1 million when individuals with unilateral hearing loss are included. The prevalence of hearing loss increases with every decade of age. Welcome to Medicare Center for Medicare and medicaid services (CMS) includes the recommendation for a hearing screening for all patients entering Medicare coverage. Increase in social isolation, depression, falls and cognitive decline are related to untreated hearing loss.

Between 1 and 6 infants per 1,000 births are reported as having hearing loss. Most children with congenital hearing loss have hearing loss at birth and are potentially identifiable by newborn hearing screening protocols. The Centers for Disease Control and prevention (CDC) reports that 97% of newborns in the United States are now screened for hearing loss. Some congenital hearing losses will appear later in life and, therefore, require vigilance from the family and the pediatrician. Speech and language development as well as reading proficiency is related to adequate hearing.

Complete hearing health care is provided when the otolaryngologist and audiologist work together. Once a hearing loss is deemed untreatable medically, the audiologist will most often take over the leadership role in nonmedical management. Nonmedical treatments most often include amplification (hearing aids), enhancement of signal-to-noise ratio (assistive listening devices), and environmental manipulation. Management of sensorineural hearing loss or conductive hearing loss that is not responsive to medical treatment is important for both adults and pediatric patients.

A A thorough history elicits information regarding otologic history and symptoms, family history of hearing loss, and other pertinent medical history. The important information to be obtained during an adult or pediatric case history is similar but not identical.

B A comprehensive audiologic assessment helps to determine the type, degree, and configuration of hearing loss. These results will point toward possible medical management and/or nonmedical management of the hearing loss. Behavioral and/or physiologic assessment techniques may be used as appropriate for an individual patient, given their age and developmental status.

C Following the evaluation for patients presenting with complaints of hearing loss or family members reporting hearing loss, possible medical treatments should be completed or ruled out. For hearing losses for which there is no medical treatment, the patient should enter into an evaluation for (re)habilitation needs. The term 'rehabilitation' is used for those with acquired hearing loss, whereas habilitation is used for young children who have not yet acquired speech and language skills.

D If normal peripheral hearing is documented in light of patient or family complaints of hearing problems, an evaluation for auditory processing disorder (older children and adults) or an assessment of auditory neuropathy (any age) may be completed.

E (Re)habilitation will depend on the severity of hearing loss, age of the patient, lifestyle, and communication goals. For young children, habilitation will focus on auditory input for the development of speech and language. For adults, rehabilitation will focus on their listening and communication needs.

F Treatments may include educational and vocational support and modifications. For the school-age child, the audiologist will work closely with the educational audiologist/school to ensure auditory access to the educational environment. This often will include assistive listening devices that enhance the signal-to-noise ratio. Personal amplification is the most common treatment for permanent hearing loss and is custom-fit to the individual's hearing and lifestyle. Specifically, hearing aids are tuned on the basis of frequency-specific threshold data in order to provide audible sound for soft, moderate, and loud inputs without causing discomfort. In order to achieve audibility and comfort, the individual's ear canal size and acoustics must be accounted for via real ear probe microphone measures. For very young children, these real ear measures will be repeated each time they need a new earmold to account for the growth of their outer ear, which will impact the amplification delivered to the eardrum. Conventional amplification delivers an air-conducted signal, but a patient may also be fit with a bone-conducted signal that is either applied to the skull with a tight band

or surgically implanted. Auditory training programs are available to pediatric and adult patients and may improve their ability to use amplified sound. Counseling is an essential part of treatment to assist parents/guardians of children to understand the importance of hearing to their child's normal speech and language development. Adults often benefit from counseling in order to encourage full-time use of amplification.

G As health care continues to evolve, a formal outcome assessment of the treatment of permanent hearing loss will become critical. Traditionally, audiologists have assumed that if a patient purchases amplification and does not return it, then they are successful. This is not an acceptable measure of success and there are numerous valid, reliable outcome assessments targeted at the use of amplification.

H For patients with severe-to-profound hearing loss, a trial with amplification will be completed first to assess whether the individual can benefit from traditional amplification. If not, a cochlear implant assessment will be completed. For infants identified at birth with hearing loss, the guidelines indicate that they should have a diagnostic audiometric evaluation by 3 months and should be fit with amplification no later than 6 months of age. Infants with severe-to-profound permanent hearing loss, may receive a cochlear implant by 12 months of age based on Food and Drug Administration guidelines. For patients who have contracted meningitis and have experienced profound bilateral hearing loss, bilateral implants will be recommended immediately because of the expected ossification of the inner ear eventually preventing insertion of the electrode.

SUGGESTED READING

American Academy of Audiology. Clinical practice algorithms and statements. Audiol Today. (Special Issue) 2000;32-49. Available at: http://audiology-web.s3.amazonaws.com/migrated/Clinical PracticeAlgorithms.pdf_53994878207278.74980219.pdf (accessed on 10/27/2016).

American Academy of Audiology. Guidelines for the audiologic management of adult hearing impairment. Audiol Today. 2006;18(5). Available from: http://audiology-web.s3.amazonaws. com/migrated/haguidelines.pdf_53994876e92e42.70908344.pdf (accessed on 10/27/2016).

American Academy of Audiology. Pediatric amplification practice guidelines. [online] Available from: www.audiology.org/ publications-resources/document-library/pediatric-reha-bilitation-hearing-aids [Accessed June 2013]. Available at http://www.audiology.org/sites/default/files/publications/ PediatricAmplificationGuidelines.pdf (accessed on 10/27/2016).

Lin FR, Yaffe K, Xia J, et al.; Health ABC Study Group. Hearing loss and cognitive decline in older adults. JAMA Intern Med. 2013;173(4):293-299.

Implantable Hearing Aids

Patricia G Johnson, Pamela C Roehm

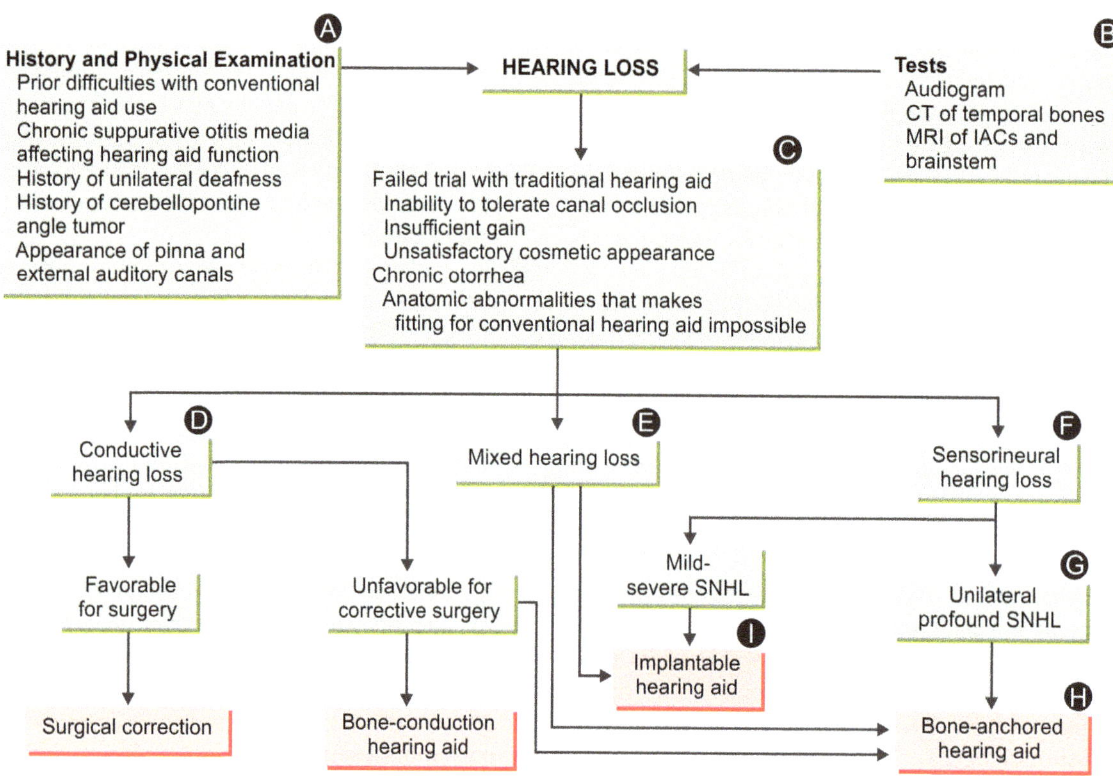

Not all patients can tolerate the use of a conventional hearing aid, and certain types of hearing loss respond better to bone-anchored or implantable hearing aids than conventional hearing aids. The use of these devices can avoid complaints of many hearing aid users, including external auditory canal occlusion and irritation and acoustic feedback. Bone-anchored hearing aids rely on osseointegration for direct bone conduction of sound to both cochleas. This allows sound to completely bypass the conductive hearing portions of the middle ear. Implantable hearing aids convert sound into mechanical energy through either piezoelectric or electromagnetic processors. Sound is received by way of an audio processor, and energy is transferred through the processor and converted into mechanical energy that oscillates the device attached to the ossicles. The choice of bone-anchored or implantable hearing aid is predicated upon a number of factors, including age, amount of hearing loss (HL), type of HL, ear anatomy, and reason(s) for conventional hearing aid failure.

A A full history should be obtained as noted in the previous chapters on HL. In particular, factors regarding implantable hearing prosthesis candidacy should be elicited, including prior difficulties with hearing aid use, chronic suppurative otitis media, history of unilateral deafness, history of cerebellopontine angle or temporal bone tumors, and history of aural atresia/microtia (including plans for surgical correction). A complete physical examination, including pneumatic otoscopy and tuning fork examination, should also be performed.

B Audiometry is essential, as the type and the amount of HL are the most important factors affecting the choice of a bone-anchored or implantable device. High-resolution computed tomography (CT) of the temporal bones should be performed on patients with conductive or mixed hearing losses (MHLs), particularly those involving aural atresia or chronic suppurative otitis media. The CT scan is also required to assess for adequate space to allow successful implantation of the devices. MR imaging of the internal auditory canals and temporal bones is indicated in the evaluation of patients with a history of the cerebellopontine angle tumors or carcinoma of the temporal bone.

C Inability to tolerate canal occlusion, chronic otorrhea, insufficient gain, anatomic abnormalities that make conventional hearing aid fitting impossible, and unsatisfactory cosmetic appearance are contraindications for conventional hearing aids and may lead to lack of patient compliance. These patients should be considered for either bone-anchored or implantable hearing aids.

D Patients with a conductive hearing loss (CHL) may have their HLs remediated by surgery, conventional hearing aids, or bone-anchored hearing aids. However, certain patients may be unlikely to benefit from surgery, and may not be able to wear conventional hearing aids or tolerate bone-conduction aids. One such cause of CHL is aural atresia. Typically, this condition is congenital and results from lack of a bony channel connecting the pinna with the middle ear, although acquired cases resulting from soft-tissue ingrowth following trauma or infection can occur. Patients with aural atresia may have unfavorable middle ear anatomy as defined by the Jahrsdorfer criteria. For these patients, placement of a bone-anchored hearing aid can significantly improve hearing outcomes, compared with relatively poor atresiaplasty results or unsightly and uncomfortable headband bone-conduction aids. Another common cause of CHL that may be best remediated by a bone-anchored hearing aid is chronic suppurative otitis media in the only hearing ear.

E Patients with a mixed conductive and sensorineural hearing loss (SNHL) with mild-to-severe air-conduction levels may benefit from either a bone-anchored or an implantable hearing aid.

F Patients with stable mild-to-severe SNHL may be successfully treated with an implantable hearing aid.

G Patients with unilateral severe-to-profound sensorineural deafness can often be successfully treated with a bone-anchored hearing aid. This can give the wearer the illusion of binaural hearing though patients will still not be able to localize sound normally. For these patients, a percutaneous abutment must be used, because transcutaneous bone-anchored aids lose 15 dB of gain due to the transcutaneous attachment, and so cannot transmit sound energy sufficiently to the contralateral ear.

H There are two types of bone-anchored hearing aids, percutaneous (which have a titanium abutment that projects through the skin, which snaps onto the external components) and transcutaneous (which include a subdermal magnet that attaches to the external components via magnetic attraction). Percutaneous prostheses are approved for unilateral CHL or MHL ≤55-dB HL. Use of a body worn processor increases amplification and allows for fitting of CHL or MHL ≤65-dB HL. While transcutaneous implants are more cosmetically acceptable, they lose 15 dB of gain

and so are not adequate for patients requiring higher gain due to the severity of their ipsilateral CHL or MHL.

I Implantable hearing aids are either fully or semi-implanted, with the difference between the two being the location of the microphone. The semi-implantable devices have an external audio processor held in place by a magnet or a custom audio processor that fits in the external auditory canal. Fully implantable devices include a sound receiver and a processor that are placed under the skin. Fitting curves vary for the different implantable aids on the market, but some brands can amplify up to 65–100 dB HL. Air-conduction levels should be stable for at least 2 years prior to implantation. These implants cannot be placed into an open or draining mastoid cavity and offer no audiologic gain at lower frequencies. Current guidelines for their use include ages ≥18, prior trial of conventional hearing aids, and ample space in the mastoid for device implantation.

SUGGESTED READING

Adunka OF, Buchman CA. Cochlear implants and other implantable auditory prostheses. In: Johnson J, Rosen C (Eds). Bailey's Head and Neck Surgery—Otolaryngology, 5th edition. Philadelphia: Lippincott Williams & Wilkins; 2014. pp. 2624-2653.

Bittencourt AG, Burke PR, Jardim IS, et al. Implantable and semi-implantable hearing aids: a review of history, indications, and surgery. Int Arch Otorhinolaryngol. 2014;18:303-310.

Edmiston RC, Aggarwal R, Green KMJ. Bone conduction implants—a rapidly developing field. J Laryngol Otol. 2015;7:1-5.

Karl A, O'Donoghue GM. Profound deafness in childhood. N Engl J Med. 2010;363:1438-1450.

Lo JF, Tsang WS, Yu JY, et al. Contemporary hearing rehabilitation options in patients with aural atresia. Biomed Res Int. 2014;2014:761579.

Lustig LR, Della Santina CC. Implantable hearing aids. In: Flint P, Haughey B, Lund V, et al. (Eds). Cummings Otolaryngology Head and Neck Surgery, 5th edition. Portland: Elsevier Health Sciences; 2010. pp. 2203-2227.

Schmuzinger N, Schimmann F, Wengen D, et al. Long-term assessment after implantation of the Vibrant Soundbridge device. Otol Neurotol. 2006;27(2):183-188.

Stach BA, Ramachandran V. Hearing aids: Strategies of amplification. In: Flint P, Haughey B, Lund V, et al. (Eds). Cummings Otolaryngology Head and Neck Surgery, 5th edition. Portland: Elsevier Health Sciences; 2010. pp. 2265-2275.

Cochlear Implants in Adults

Barry E Hirsch

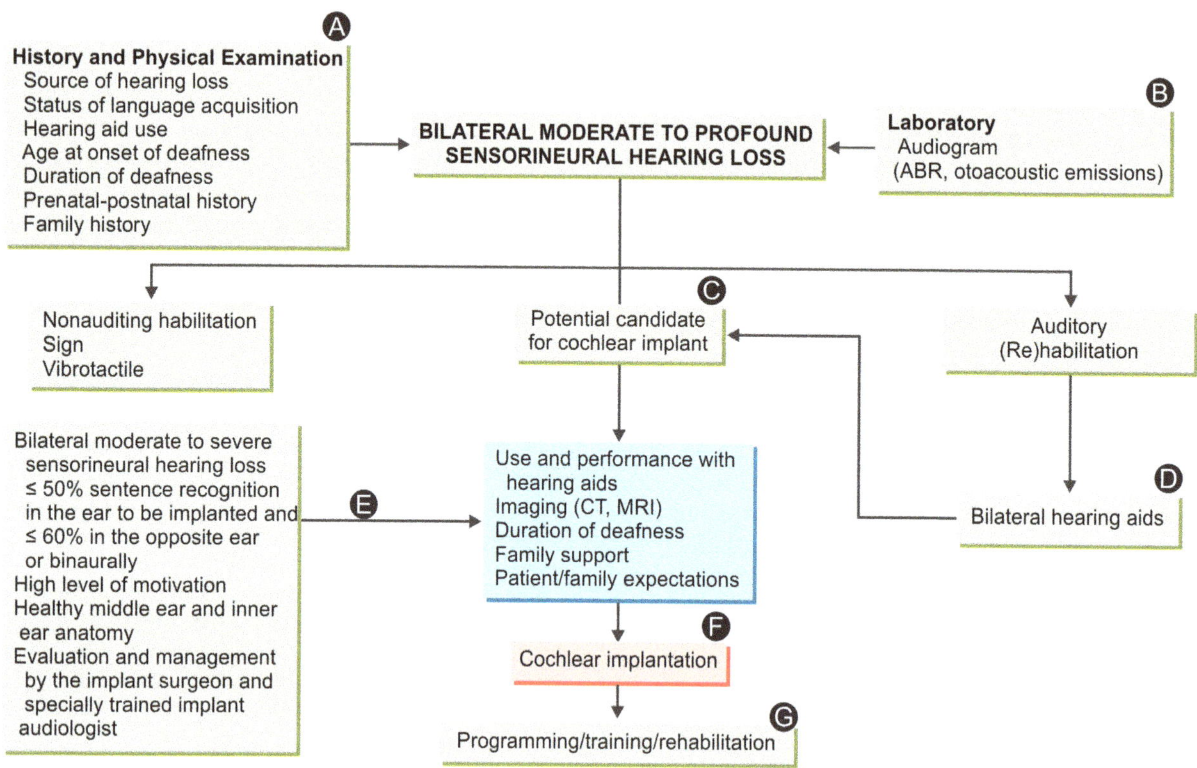

Adult patients with bilateral moderate to profound bilateral hearing loss are potential candidates for a cochlear implant.

A A complete history should review the presumed source of hearing loss, status of language acquisition, and whether hearing aids are being used. Knowledge of age at onset and duration of deafness helps the clinician predict the likely success of the cochlear implant. In young adults, a comprehensive history, including prenatal and post-natal course, any recurrent ear infections or meningitis, and any family history of hearing loss must be obtained. Patients need to be categorized as having prelingual, perilingual, or postlingual deafness. Children born deaf (acquired or hereditary congenital sensorineural hearing loss) are considered to have prelingual deafness. Hearing loss between ages 1 and 3 years is perilingual deafness, and hearing loss after age 3–4 is postlingual deafness. See Chapter 13 for cochlear implantation in children.

The patient's ability to understand spoken language and communicate orally should be estimated. The physician should evaluate the patient's lip-reading or speech-reading skills and whether the patient is wearing hearing aids. Handicaps such as blindness or disturbance of fine hand motor coordination may affect the rehabilitation process. Physical examination of the ears should focus on the postauricular skin, pinna, external auditory canal, tympanic membrane, and the middle ear space.

B Audiometric analysis of the patient's residual hearing abilities is necessary. Patients with postlingual deafness can undergo comprehensive behavioral audiometric testing. Along with pure tones, their ability to understand words (speech or word discrimination) is determined. Auditory neuropathy, auditory dyssynchrony is a condition affecting central neural processing of sound and speech. It is often identified in childhood and characterized by identifying functioning cochlear outer hair cells [otoacoustic emissions (OAE) testing] and absent central transmission [ABR (auditory brainstem response) testing]. The assessment of hearing in children is covered in Chapters 2 and 4.

C A decision must be made by the patient, family, and physician regarding (re)habilitation when the patient is identified as having bilateral moderate-to-profound sensorineural hearing loss. Parents of young patients may choose nonauditory habilitation (sign, total communication) for language acquisition and education. Hearing aids should be strongly encouraged. Despite wishes for obtaining normal hearing, young adults with prelingual deafness are not good candidates for a cochlear implant and should be discouraged and alternative communication reinforced.

D Postlingually deafened adult patients can self-determine the course of rehabilitation that they wish to pursue. Patients who have residual hearing and acquired language may wish to pursue or remain with bilateral hearing aid amplification. If never amplified, a trial of hearing aids is necessary.

Patients with moderate-to-profound sensorineural hearing loss using bilateral hearing aids may be functioning suboptimally because of the limits of amplification. They may seek further evaluation for implant candidacy.

E If never previously amplified, a trial of hearing aids is warranted.

The inclusion criteria for cochlear implant candidacy include:

- *Bilateral moderate-to-severe sensorineural hearing loss*: Useful hearing in one ear precludes candidacy based on current Food and Drug Administration criteria. A hybrid device (electric and acoustic stimulation) was made available in 2014 that allows patients with normal-to-moderate loss in the low frequencies and severe to profound loss in the high frequencies to be a candidate for this specific device.

- Testing for speech understanding is done with power hearing aids in place of using sentence presentations and recording the word recognition. The two common paradigms are HINT and AZBio sentences. These can be delivered in quiet or with competing background sound. The signal-to-noise presentation levels are between +5 and +10 dB. Patients are implant candidates if they have ≤50% sentenced recognition in the ear to be implanted and ≤60% in the opposite ear or binaurally. Again, both ears must qualify in order to be a candidate.

- *High level of motivation*: It is important to be motivated to persevere in the rehabilitation process. Family support is just as important for adults as with children.

- *Healthy middle ear and inner ear anatomy to safely implant the device*: The mastoid anatomy and configuration of the cochlea is ascertained by thin cut bone algorithm computed tomography scanning. Concern for retrocochlear disease and patency of the cochlear turns can be defined by magnetic resonance imaging. High-resolution T2 sequences can identify possible problems of inner ear fibrosis (labyrinthitis ossificans). This can occur following hearing loss from meningitis. Implantation can still be performed but incomplete insertion of the full electrode array may be anticipated.

- Adult patients can be evaluated and managed by the implant surgeon and specially trained implant audiologist.

F *Side of implantation*: The choice of which side to implant is based on a number of factors. The worse hearing ear is usually implanted first. This allows the contralateral ear to have ongoing stimulation through the existing hearing aid. If there is long-standing hearing loss, the ear more recently deafened is likely to better respond to electric stimulation. In situations where both ears have comparable loss, the side with more favorable anatomy based on imaging is chosen. Patient preference is also strongly taken into account when the decision is otherwise equivocal. A cochlear implant is surgically placed under general anesthesia. The procedure takes between 2 and 3 hours depending on the amount of time devoted to intraoperative device testing and imaging. This can be performed on an outpatient basis in adults.

G The postoperative rehabilitation is critical for achieving a successful outcome. This involves not only members of the cochlear implant team but also the encouragement and support of family members and, in the case of children; educators. The device has to be programmed (or mapped) at the initial stimulation (hook-up) and during frequent subsequent visits to ensure optimum performance. Programming, training on its use and rehabilitation is an ongoing process. Implant audiologists develop their preferred protocol for initial and subsequent stimulation. Multiple reprogramming visits are scheduled in the first few months of activation and use. Consideration is given for bilateral implantation, though most of my adult patients are satisfied with one implant and a contralateral hearing aid.

SUGGESTED READING

Hood LJ. Auditory neuropathy/dys-synchrony disorder. Otolaryngol Clin N Am. 2015;48(6):1027-1040.

Niparko JK, Kirk KI, Mellon NK. Cochlear Implants: Principles and Practices. Philadelphia, PA: Lippincott Williams & Wilkins; 2000.

Nikolopoulos TP, O'Donoghue GM, Archbold S. Age at implantation: its importance in pediatric cochlear implantation. Laryngoscope. 1999;109:595-599.

Nucleus Hybrid L24 Cochlear Implant System – P130016. Available from: http://www.fda.gov/MedicalDevices/ProductsandMedical Procedures/DeviceApprovalsandClearances/Recently-Approved Devices/ucm392836.htm. [Accessed February 8, 2016].

CHAPTER 13

Pediatric Cochlear Implants

David H Chi

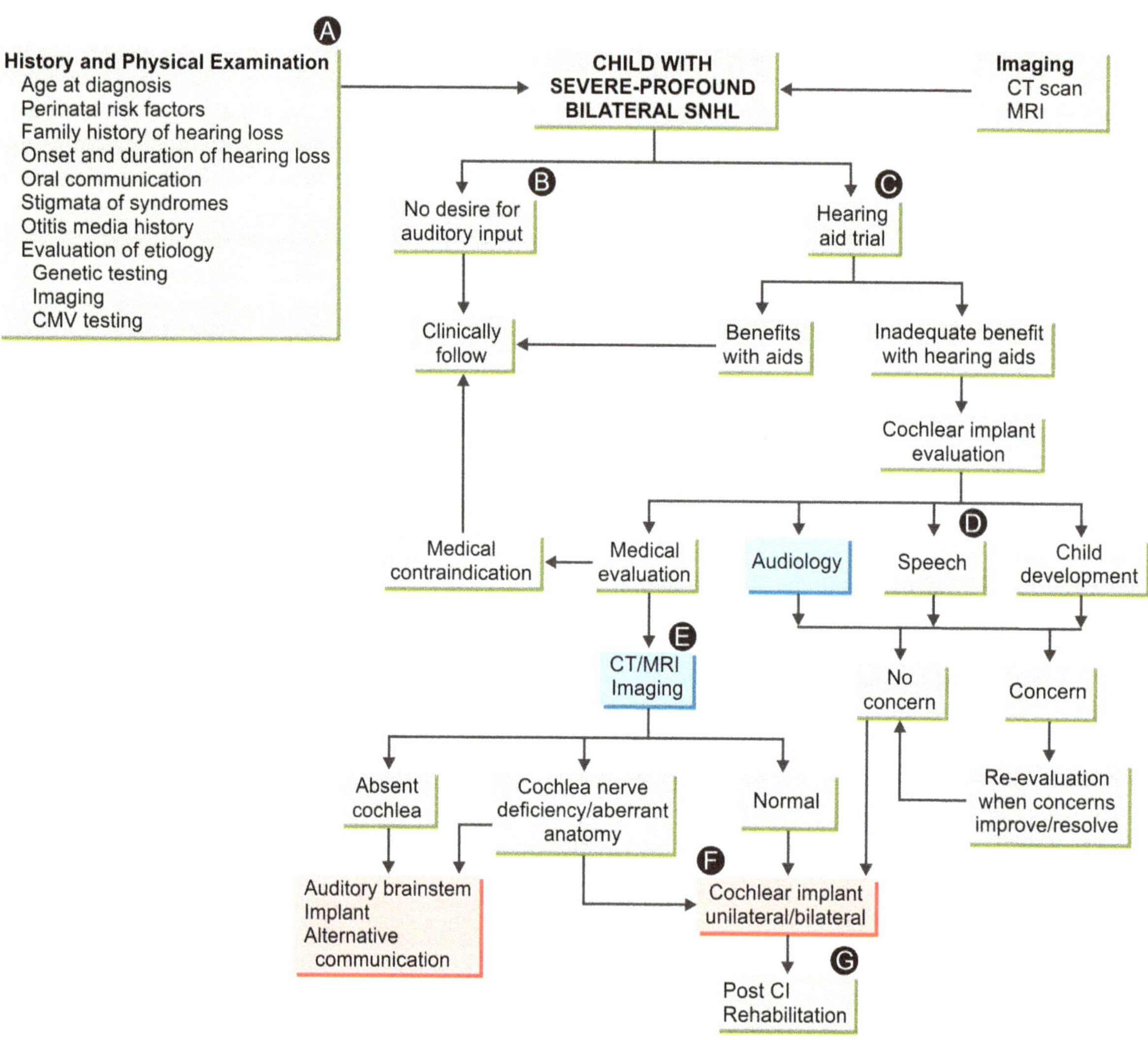

Congenital hearing loss occurs in 1–3 out of 1,000 births. While many children may benefit with hearing aids alone, some have profound hearing loss in which hearing aids are insufficient. For these children, cochlear implants provide the opportunity for appropriate development of speech and language. The indications for pediatric implants continue to evolve.

Current indications are as follows:

- Severe to profound bilateral hearing loss in children between the ages 24 months and 17 years. The hearing loss should be profound in pediatric patients of 12–24 months of age. In select patients, implants may be performed in those less than 12 months of age. With some highly motivated parents, implants may be completed around 6–12 months of age in healthy infants whose hearing can be followed by an audiologist.
- Lack of auditory development and minimal benefit from a hearing aid. A hearing aid trial of approximately 3 months is completed. The infant or child is monitored closely to assess progress with hearing aids. Exception to an extended hearing aid trial will be patients with hearing loss secondary to meningitis. In these individuals, quick progression to cochlear implantation (CI) should occur prior to development of fibrosis or ossification of the perilymphatic space of the cochlea.
- No medical contraindications.
- High motivation and realistic expectations from family and patient. The family has to be active participants in the rehabilitation of the child.

A A pediatric patient may present with severe-to-profound sensorineural hearing loss (SNHL) in two ways. An infant may have congenital hearing loss. The otolaryngologist should assess for perinatal risk factors. The status of the newborn hearing screen and follow-up testing is documented. Genetic evaluation should be obtained. Cytomegalovirus (CMV) testing if performed in the first

2–3 weeks of life may provide opportunities for treatment. Family history of hearing loss is identified. Alternatively, an older child may have developed hearing loss or have progression of known hearing loss. A similar assessment for etiology is obtained, but other important aspects of history are the duration and onset of hearing loss, and past and current ability for oral communication.

Physical examination includes the assessment for stigmata of syndromes. The tympanic membrane should be intact and without evidence of acute otitis media. In a child who is otitis media prone, a tympanostomy tube may be inserted in a separate surgery. The tube may be removed at the time of cochlear implant surgery or left in place, per surgeon preference.

B Parents may decide to pursue manual communication as a choice for their child's habilitation and not pursue implantation. Certain families, such as those in the deaf community, may not want their child to have audiologic input and prefer to communicate via sign language. Physicians need to be sensitive to these wishes and respect them.

C A hearing aid trial is necessary. Hearing aid fitting should be as soon as possible. The infant or child is monitored closely to assess progress with hearing aids. I recommend that every patient, including those with profound hearing loss, undergo a trial as responses are not always predictable and that the child and family get accustomed to having a device worn on the ear.

D A multidisciplinary evaluation is required. Otolaryngologist, audiologist, speech and language pathologist, psychologist, and social workers collaborate to assess infants and children. The speech and language evaluation determines whether developmental language or articulation disorders are present, defines the child's current communication abilities, and develops expectations and plans for speech therapy after implantation. The child development evaluation assesses the intelligence and may identify cognitive disabilities that could affect a child's performance with a cochlear implant. Families are counseled that some conditions such as autism and attention deficit disorders may not be evident until the child reaches 2 years of age. The audiologist assesses for progress with hearing aids. In infants, speech perception tasks are not readily attainable and decisions about implant depend on electrophysiologic measures and detection thresholds. In older children, aided and unaided hearing thresholds are obtained. Additional audiologic testing may identify unique conditions such as auditory neuropathy spectrum disorder. These children may benefit from CI but their outcome can be variable secondary to the heterogeneous causes of the disorder.

E The medical evaluation consists of determining surgical candidacy and identifying medical conditions that preclude anesthesia and surgery. Also, the surgical anatomy is evaluated with radiographic imaging.

Preoperative imaging is necessary for surgical planning. Up to one-third of children may have a cochleovestibular anomaly identified with imaging. A CT scan is helpful to identify bony anomalies, aeration of the temporal bone course of the facial nerve and abnormal vasculature such as an anterior sigmoid sinus or high riding jugular bulb. MRI is useful to assess the internal auditory canal and cochlear nerve anatomy. A child with a history of meningitis should also have an MRI

performed to assess for patency of the cochlea. Cochlear anomalies do not preclude implantation, but identification of anomalies helps the surgeon with electrode selection and prediction of complications such as cerebrospinal fluid leak. The presence of an abnormal cochlea also helps to determine outcomes with CI.

Cochlear implantation for cochlear nerve deficiency (CND) remains controversial. Initially, CND was considered a contraindication for cochlear implants, but children with CND may benefit with CI. However, children with complete absence of a cochlear nerve do poorly with CI and may benefit from an auditory brainstem implant.

If the child had meningitis, and fibrosis or ossification of the cochlea is noted on CT and MRI, the surgeon must be prepared with various electrodes at the time of surgery.

F Prior to surgery, every child should receive pneumococcal vaccine. In infants, care is taken to observe for blood loss, and careful hemostasis is maintained throughout surgery. If an abnormal cochlea is present then intraoperative imaging may be performed to assess electrode position in the cochlea.

The Otolaryngologist also has to determine whether unilateral or bilateral cochlear implants will be considered. Bilateral implants provide the recipient improved hearing in noisy environments. Other benefits include sound localization and assurance of a functional implant whether the internal receiver-stimulator or the external processor malfunctions. The position of the American Academy of Otolaryngology is that bilateral cochlear implants are an accepted medical practice. However, various factors influence the decision of unilateral or bilateral implantation: (1) Family motivation for the child have two implants; (2) Medical considerations, for example, inner ear malformations may create some concern about how a child may respond to a cochlear implant. Prior to proceeding with bilateral implants, the performance with the first implant is assessed; (3) The cost of surgery and surgical and anesthesia risks.

G Postoperative habilitation is essential for speech and language outcomes with cochlear implants. Initial activation occurs approximately 3–4 weeks after surgery. Frequent programming of the device may be necessary. Speech therapists and educators of the deaf contribute to maximizing performance of cochlear implants. Children who are prelingually deaf will take additional time to demonstrate improvement compared to those who are post-lingually deaf.

SUGGESTED READING

Basura GJ, Eapen R, Buchman CA. Bilateral cochlear implantation: current concepts, indications, and results. Laryngoscope. 2009; 119(12):2395-2401.

Buchman CA, Teagle HF, Roush PA, et al. Cochlear implantation in children with labyrinthine anomalies and cochlear nerve deficiency: implications for auditory brainstem implantation. Laryngoscope. 2011;121(9):1979-1988.

Lammers MJ, van der Heijden GJ, Pourier VE, et al. Bilateral cochlear implantation in children: a systematic review and best-evidence synthesis. Laryngoscope. 2014;124(7):1694-1699.

Noij KS, Kozin ED, Sethi R, et al. Systematic review of nontumor pediatric auditory brainstem implant outcomes. Otolaryngol Head Neck Surg. 2015;153(5):739-750.

Vlastarakos PV, Nikolopoulos TP, Pappas S, et al. Cochlear implantation update: contemporary preoperative imaging and future prospects - the dual modality approach as a standard of care. Expert Rev Med Devices. 2010;7(4):555-567.

Tinnitus

David E Eibling

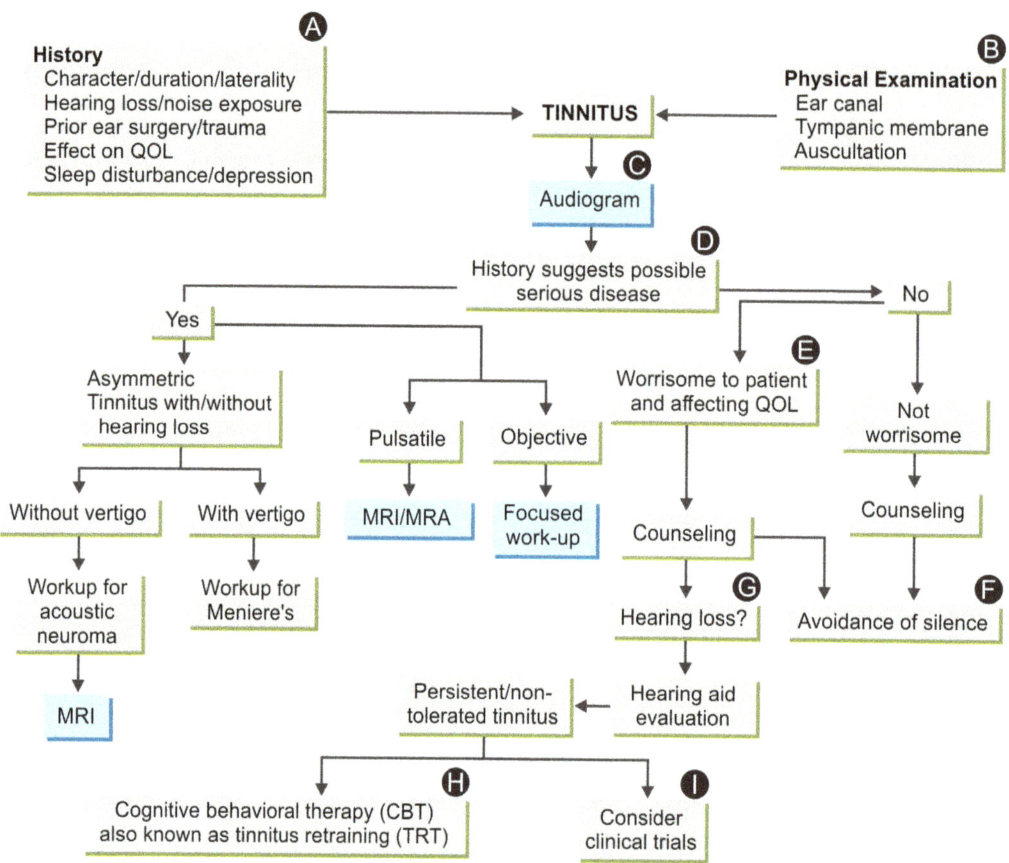

Tinnitus is a common complaint, affecting ~10–15% of the population, with wide variability in its effect on different individuals. The economic cost is high, with ~1 million US veterans receiving disability compensation for tinnitus as of 2012. An authoritative Clinical Practice Guideline (CPG) addressing tinnitus was recently published by the American Academy of Otolaryngology, and the reader is referred to this document for more detailed discussion.

Recent studies identify the dorsal cochlear nucleus as the origin of the perceived sound, which originates from a maladaptive response to reduced input. The correlation between the degree of hearing loss and the intensity of tinnitus is inconsistent, as some of the most severely affected patients have minimal hearing loss. There is strong correlation between the effect of tinnitus on quality of life and underlying mood disorders, a correlation which must be considered when evaluating affected patients.

A The character, duration, and laterality should be elicited. The 2014 CPG suggests a threshold of 6 months' duration; however, any patient concerned about tinnitus will benefit from evaluation and counseling. A history of pre-existent hearing loss suggests causation, as does a history of prior ear surgery or trauma, head injury, or noise exposure. Tinnitus may be associated with a single event, such as noise trauma, or develop over a period of years. Pulsatile tinnitus suggests a vascular cause, and associated vertigo suggests Meniere's disease. A medication history should include any prior administration of ototoxic drugs or current use of aspirin (ASA). Patients should be questioned as to whether the tinnitus has resulted in sleep disturbance. Depression, as well as other neuropsychiatric diseases, is a common associated diagnosis; hence, treatment of antidepressant may be of benefit.

B Physical examination of the ear canal and tympanic membrane is essential. All patients with tinnitus, especially those with pulsatile tinnitus, should undergo auscultation over and around the ear canal. Venous hums may be heard commonly and typically are of low pitch, whereas higher pitched pulsatile bruits suggest arterial disease or arteriovenous malformation. Examination of the oropharynx for palatal myoclonus may be revealing in patients with symptoms suggestive of this disorder.

C Although not mandated by the 2014 CPG, pure tone audiometry as well as speech discrimination should probably be obtained on all patients with complaints of tinnitus. Vascular malformations with loud bruits may mask sound and lead to inaccurate assessment of hearing function. Cerumen impaction may result in a spurious conductive loss. Imaging is reserved only for those patients with pulsatile tinnitus and those with asymmetrical hearing loss in whom a cerebellopontine angle tumor is suspected.

D Although uncommon, tinnitus may be indicative of serious disease, a suspicion of which is typically suggested by history. Unilateral tinnitus with asymmetric hearing loss could be due to a cerebellopontine tumor; so magnetic resonance imaging is indicated. Pulsatile tinnitus may be an indication of a vascular abnormality; so appropriate imaging required. Most affected patients with symptomatic tinnitus do not have an identifiable cause. Patients with possible depression or other neuropsychiatric disease should be referred for further evaluation and management.

E The 2014 CPG emphasizes the importance of eliciting from the patient the degree to which the tinnitus is bothersome. Only about 10% of patients with tinnitus are impacted sufficiently to require treatment, but all can benefit from counseling with a discussion of the etiology and management.

F Regardless of the symptoms, essentially all patients benefit from avoidance of silence. If the tinnitus is symptomatic at night and when the patient is in quiet surroundings, the routine use of background noise-generating devices such as a fan or music from a bedside radio may alleviate the symptoms.

G Amplification often results in reduction of symptoms in patients with hearing loss.

H If bothersome symptoms persist despite these interventions, the patients can be offered formal cognitive behavioral therapy, often termed Tinnitus Retraining.

I Highly motivated patients should be considered for innovative clinical trials. The 2014 CPG recommends against the routine use of transcranial magnetic stimulation as several clinical trials have failed to demonstrate improvement.

SUGGESTED READING

Davis A, El Refaie A. Epidemiology of tinnitus. In: Tyler R (Ed). Tinnitus Handbook. San Diego, CA: Singular; 2000.

Jastreboff PJ, Jastreboff MM. Tinnitus retraining therapy (TRT) as a method for treatment of tinnitus and hyperacousis patients. J Am Acad Audiol. 2000;11:162-177.

McKenna L, Handscomb L, Hoare DJ, et al. A scientific cognitive-behavioral model of tinnitus: novel conceptualizations of tinnitus distress. Front Neurol. 2014;5:196-221.

Middleton JQ, Kiritani T, Pedersen C, et al. Mice with behavioral evidence of tinnitus exhibit dorsal cochlear nucleus hyperactivity because of decreased GABAergic inhibition. Proc Natl Acad Sci USA. 2011;108:7601-7606.

Tunkel DE, Bauer CA, Sun GH, et al. Clinical practice guideline: tinnitus. Otolaryngol—Head Neck Surg. 2014;15:S1-S40.

Dizziness

Joseph M Furman, Susan L Whitney

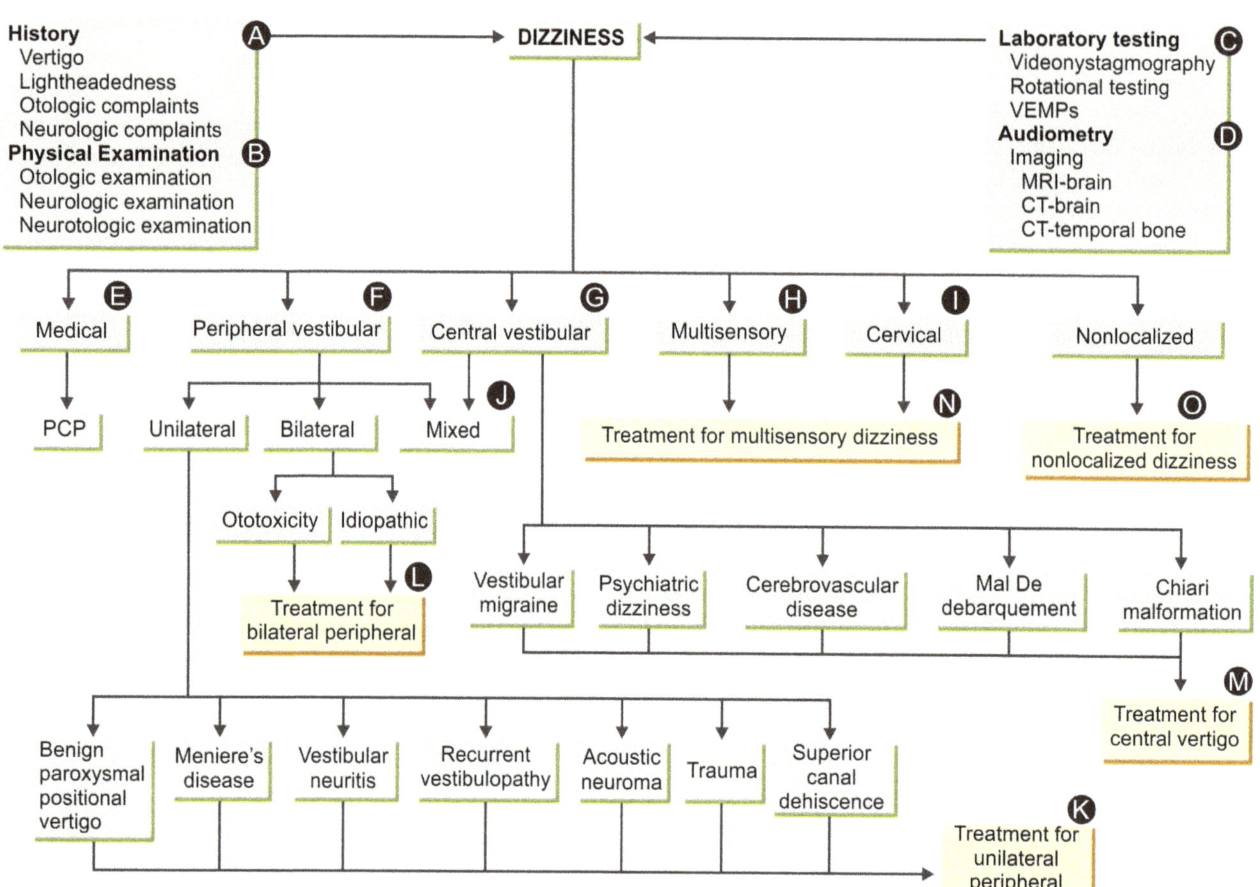

Dizziness, a nonspecific complaint, can be a manifestation of both vestibular and nonvestibular abnormalities. Vestibular abnormalities can be peripheral, central, or mixed. Also, dizziness may be based on sensory changes either in addition to or other than vestibular. Choice of treatment often depends upon the specific diagnosis.

A Whereas a complaint of dizziness may not suggest a vestibular abnormality, vertigo suggests involvement of peripheral or central vestibular structures. The presence of hearing loss, tinnitus, and a feeling of fullness in the ear suggests an otologic diagnosis, whereas complaints of altered vision, weakness, and numbness suggest neurologic ailments. The time course and pattern of a patient's dizziness assist in assigning a diagnostic category.

B The neurotologic examination includes some specialized techniques, among them assessment of nystagmus using infrared video goggles, both seated and during the Dix-Hallpike maneuver, the Romberg test on a firm surface and on a compliant foam pad, and assessment of the vestibulo-ocular reflex using the head impulse test.

C Laboratory testing of the dizzy patient should be ordered selectively. Videonystagmography includes a search for positional nystagmus and recording responses to thermal (caloric) stimulation. Rotational testing is particularly helpful in assessing the status of compensation. Vestibular evoked myogenic potential (VEMPs) assessing otolith organ function may also be of value.

D Brain imaging may be useful in patients with history or physical examination findings suggestive of an abnormality of the central nervous system. A computed tomography (CT) scan of the temporal bones should be used to search for superior canal dehiscence.

E It is critical to rule out medical disorders before embarking on an evaluation of vestibular abnormalities. Orthostatic hypotension, cardiac disease, and side effects of medications are particularly common causes of dizziness which is best managed by the patient's primary care physician (PCP).

F A peripheral vestibular disorder is suggested by vertigo, vestibular nystagmus, a normal neurologic examination, reduced caloric responses, and normal brain imaging.

Acute peripheral vestibular disorders cause vertigo, nausea, and vomiting, and usually manifest vestibular nystagmus and gait ataxia. Unilateral peripheral vestibular loss of gradual onset does not usually cause dizziness because the central nervous system compensates. Bilateral peripheral vestibular loss, regardless of cause, manifests as Dandy's syndrome, i.e. oscillopsia and gait ataxia.

G A central vestibular disorder is suggested by symptoms referable to the central nervous system, an abnormal neurologic examination, abnormal eye movement testing in the laboratory, and abnormal brain imaging.

H Multisensory dysequilibrium occurs in patients who have an impairment of all three sensory inputs important for balance (i.e. vision, somatosensation, and vestibular sensation). Patients with diabetes mellitus are particularly prone to this disorder.

I Individuals who have suffered from flexion-extension injuries (whiplash) and those with severe cervical degenerative joint disease may suffer from dizziness on the basis of impaired afferent information from the neck to central vestibular structures.

J Patients with dizziness may suffer from a mixed peripheral and central vestibular disorder on the basis of either a single diagnosis or multiple, possibly unrelated, diagnoses. Mixed peripheral and central vestibular disorders may be particularly symptomatic, because central compensatory processes may be impaired.

K Treatment for unilateral peripheral disorders may consist of pharmacotherapy, physical therapy, and rarely surgical intervention. Patients with benign paroxysmal positional vertigo usually respond to a particle repositioning maneuver. Patients with Ménière's disease are treated with a diuretic and sodium restriction. Patients with vestibular neuritis may be treated with corticosteroids briefly along with a short course of vestibular suppressants and physical therapy. Patients with recurrent vestibulopathy are treated symptomatically. Patients with an acoustic neuroma require an evaluation by a neurotologic surgeon. Patients with labyrinthine trauma may respond to a combination of pharmacotherapy and physical therapy. Patients with a superior canal dehiscence require a surgical opinion.

L Treatment of patients with bilateral peripheral vestibular disease usually includes physical therapy and the use of assistive devices such as a cane. Vestibular suppressant medications should be avoided.

M Treatment of patients with central vestibular disorders is complex and depends upon the specific diagnosis. Patients with vestibular migraine may be treated with migraine prophylaxis agents, migraine abortive agents, and symptomatic pharmacotherapy. Vestibular rehabilitation therapy may also be beneficial. Patients with psychiatric dizziness should be treated by addressing the underlying psychiatric disorder. Patients with vascular causes of dizziness should be evaluated by an expert in cerebrovascular disease and treatment. Patients with mal de debarquement syndrome usually respond to pharmacotherapy. Patients with Chiari malformation should be evaluated by a neurosurgeon.

N Treatment of patients with multisensory disequilibrium usually includes vestibular rehabilitation therapy and may include other sensory aids. Treatment of patients with cervicogenic dizziness includes a combination of physical therapy for the neck and a muscle relaxant.

O Treatment of patients with nonlocalized dizziness typically includes symptomatic pharmacotherapy including a combination of vestibular suppressants, antinausea agents, and antianxiety agents. Vestibular rehabilitation may also be helpful.

SUGGESTED READING

Baloh RW, Halmagyi GM. Disorders of the Vestibular System. New York: Oxford University Press; 1996.

Brandt T. Vertigo, Its Multisensory Syndromes, 2nd edition. London: Springer-Verlag; 2003.

Eggers SD, Zee D. Vertigo and Imbalance: Clinical Neurophysiology of the Vestibular System. Amsterdam: Elsevier; 2010.

Furman JM, Cass SP, Whitney SL. Vestibular Disorders: A Case Study Approach, 3rd edition. New York: Oxford University Press; 2010.

Furman JM, Jacob R. Psychiatric dizziness. Neurology. 1997;48: 1161.

Herdman SJ, Clendaniel R. Vestibular Rehabilitation (Contemporary Perspectives in Rehabilitation), 4th edition. Philadelphia, PA: FA Davis; 2014.

Vestibular Rehabilitation

Susan L Whitney, Joseph M Furman

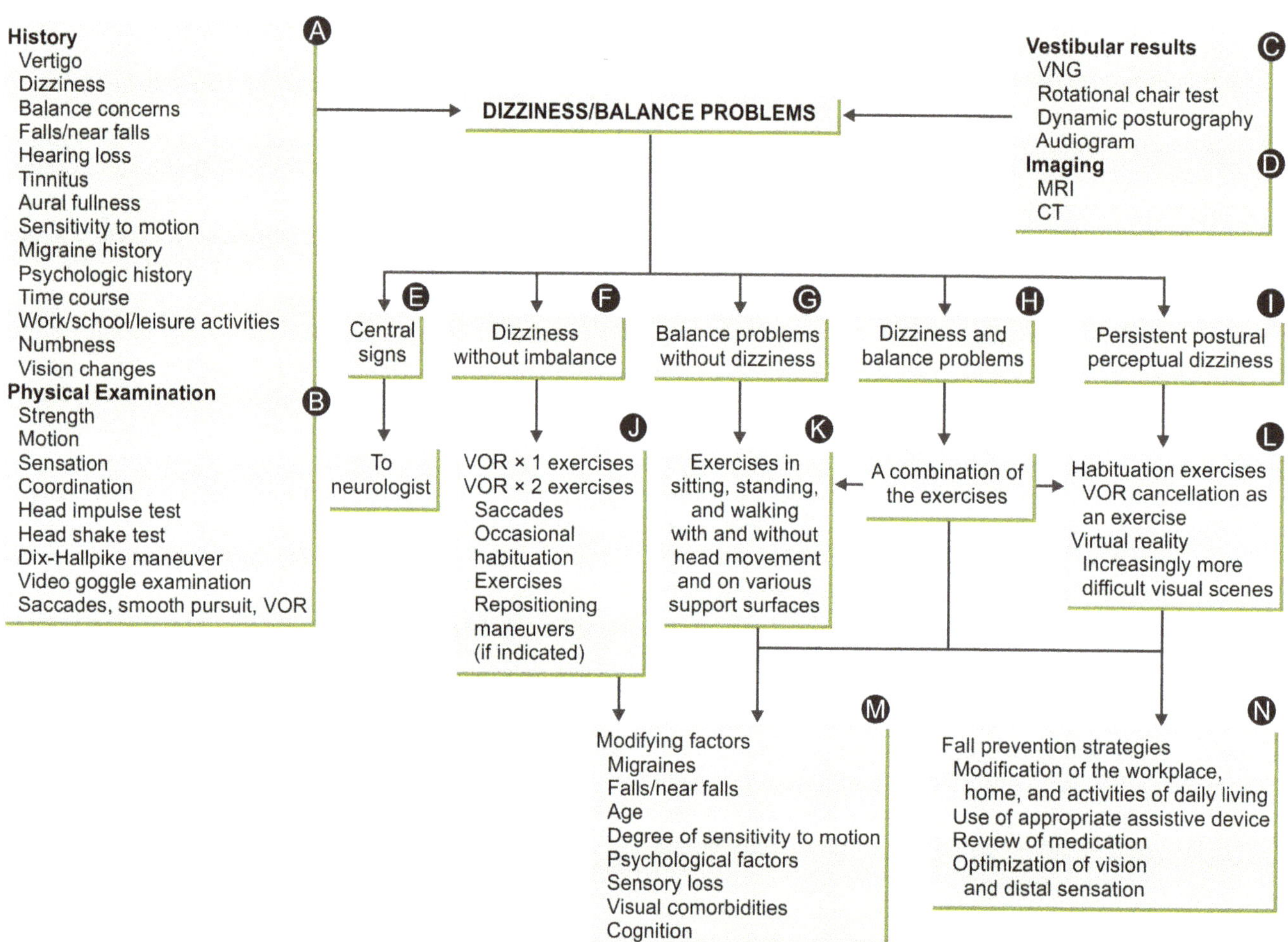

Vestibular disorders are common in both adults and children. In a recent publication, the authors have suggested that the population prevalence of balance and vestibular disorders is >5% in children between the ages of 3 and 17 in the United States. Getting people moving after a vestibular disorder in order to recalibrate the gain of the VOR, desensitizing them to movement, increasing their activity level, and teaching them to live with their condition are all components of a vestibular rehabilitation program. There is ample evidence that vestibular rehabilitation is effective in the management of balance and dizziness problems. A common complaint of a person with a vestibular disorder is vertigo. Vertigo is often considered the sensation of spinning. Dizziness is a word that is often used but can have many different meanings to patients such as the feeling of sensation of lightheadedness and that they might faint (never vestibular) or a sensation of floating.

A Patient reports of dizziness, vertigo, balance, or sensitivity to motion of self or surroundings suggest that physical therapy may be indicated. When tinnitus, aural fullness, or hearing loss is noted, referral to an Otolaryngologist is indicated. History of migraine, sensitivity to motion, and psychological comorbidity will complicate the rehabilitation process.

B The physical therapy examination includes assessing impairments and functional testing of the VOR. Video examination of extraocular eye movements and performance of the Dix-Hallpike maneuver (to examine posterior and anterior canal BPPV) and roll test (to examine horizontal canal BPPV in supine with the head rotated to the right and then left to determine, if they demonstrate horizontal direction changing nystagmus) are key components of the physical therapist examination. Determining, if the person is presenting with central or peripheral vestibular findings will assist with determining their functional prognosis.

C Vestibular test result findings will provide information about whether certain exercises should be performed. For persons with bilateral loss, if no vestibular function is noted, VOR exercises will most likely have little value. Computerized dynamic posturography results can assist in quantifying balance loss and selecting key exercises for intervention.

D CT and MRI are recommended for consideration in persons with suspected superior canal dehiscence, or central pathology and to rule out other diagnoses when migraine is suspected.

E When central findings are noted (and not otherwise identified by the patient's physician), immediate referral back to the physician is indicated. A neurologic or neurotologic referral should be considered.

F Dizziness is a common complaint and it may be the patients only complaint. Other causes of dizziness such as medication induced dizziness or postural hypotension need to be ruled out before proceeding with an exercise program.

G Balance complaints may have a vestibular component or may be related to other functional impairments such as sensory loss, visual loss, fear of falling, or psychiatric comorbidities.

H Dizziness and balance problems in combination are common and require interventions to remediate both conditions. It may take longer for patients to improve than if they had either an isolated dizziness or balance complaint.

I Persistent postural perceptual dizziness has been described in the literature as phobic postural vertigo, visual vertigo, space and motion discomfort, or chronic subjective dizziness. Persons who have visual sensitivity are more difficult to treat and may need both physical therapy, pharmacologic, and behavioral interventions.

J Exercises to increase the gain of the vestibulo-ocular reflex (VOR) are helpful for persons with a low VOR gain. Repositioning maneuvers are indicated for persons with BPPV. It is common to also have balance deficits especially in older adults with BPPV, so a balance examination is indicated after addressing the positional dizziness with the repositioning maneuvers.

K Balance exercises are indicated, if the person has complaints of unsteadiness during upright stance or gait instability during ambulation. Balance activities are progressed based on stance position, head position, eye movements, speed, and support surface.

L Persistent postural perceptual dizziness is a complex phenomenon that is most likely caused by multiple factors functionally the person has difficulty in complex visual environments. Virtual reality scenes, disco ball simulations, and viewing visually complex visual scenes on a computer may assist in recovery.

M Modifying factors may affect response to physical therapy. These include active or a history of migraine, falls/near falls, age, motion sensitivity, psychological factors, sensory loss, visual comorbidities, and cognition. Medication can be either a facilitator or an inhibitor of functional recovery.

N Preventing falls at home, work, and during leisure activities is essential. Teaching persons how to fall and get up from the floor, a home assessment, use of an assistive device, and optimizing the use of vision, and proprioception can assist in decreasing the risk of falling.

SUGGESTED READING

Agrawal Y, Carey JP, Della Santina CC, et al. Disorders of balance and vestibular function in US adults: data from the National Health and Nutrition Examination Survey, 2001–2004. Arch Intern Med. 2009;169(10):938-944.

Bhattacharyya N, Baugh RF, Orvidas L, et al. Clinical practice guideline: benign paroxysmal positional vertigo. Otolaryngol Head Neck Surg. 2008;139(5 Suppl 4):S47-S81.

Herdman SJ, Clendaniel RA. Vestibular Rehabilitation, 2nd edition. Philadelphia, PA: FA Davis Company; 2014.

Li CM, Hoffman HJ, Ward BK, et al. Epidemiology of dizziness and balance problems in children in the united states" a population-based study. J Pediatr. 2016;171:240-247.

Klatt BN, Carender WJ, Lin CC, et al. A conceptual framework for the progression of balance exercises in persons with balance and vestibular disorders. Phys Med Rehabil Int. 2015;2(4):1-8.

Whitney SL, Alghwiri A, Alghadir A. Physical therapy for persons with vestibular disorders. Curr Opin Neurol. 2015;28(1):61-68.

Otalgia

Andrew A McCall

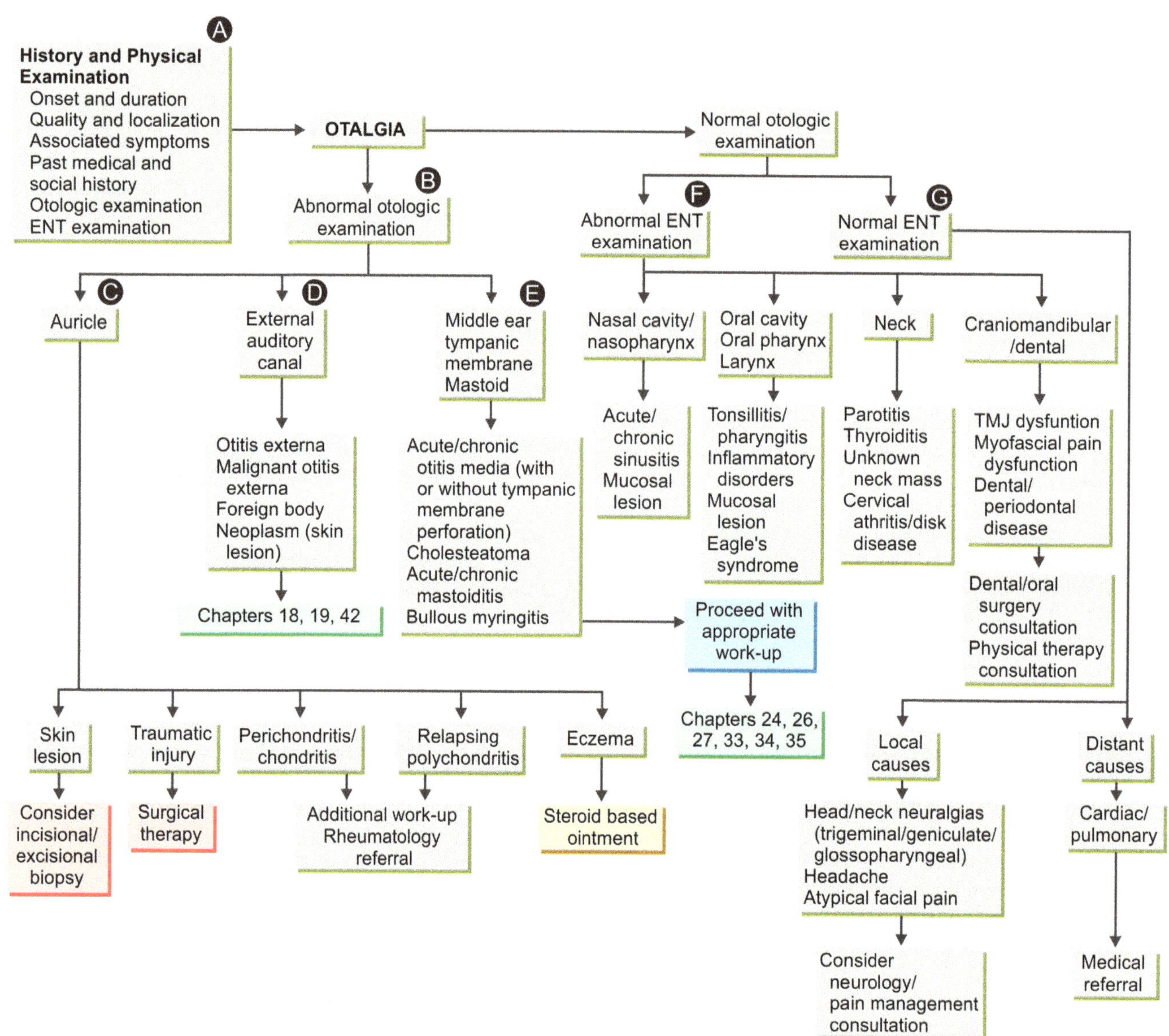

Otalgia is the sensation of pain perceived to be emanating from the ear. It can occur as the result of a diverse array of diagnoses: the clinician must remain aware that otalgia may be the result of primary otologic pathology or the result of referred pain from disease involving adjacent or distant structures. The underlying etiology for otalgia dictates management.

A A detailed history and physical examination is typically sufficient to narrow the differential diagnosis for otalgia. Otalgia onset, duration, location, and quality of pain are important to elicit. Associated symptoms including otorrhea, hearing changes, pruritus of the ear, skin changes or swelling, or the perception of a mass in the ear suggest an otologic source. The physical examination is especially helpful in determining the source of otalgia. An abnormal otologic examination suggests a primary otologic problem causing otalgia keeping in mind that other disorders could be causing the otalgia, and that the findings on abnormal otologic examination may not be the source of pain. When the otologic examination is normal, the otalgia usually results from abnormalities of adjacent or distant structures. A full examination of the head and neck, including assessment of the cranial nerves and particular attention to the temporomandibular joint (TMJ) and surrounding musculature, is warranted to evaluate for a source of otalgia. Upper airway endoscopic examination and/or head and neck imaging should also be considered, especially in cases where the remainder of the examination fails to reveal a source or if a patient fails to respond appropriately to therapy.

B The otologic examination will reveal pathology in cases with an otogenic source for otalgia. The examination of the pinna, external auditory canal, or tympanic membrane/middle ear may reveal a source.

C A variety of disease processes can affect the pinna and result in otalgia. Primary skin lesions occur in this location with frequency because the pinna often sustains significant sun exposure. If a skin lesion is present, and in particular if it is associated with pain, biopsy is warranted. Traumatic lesions, such as a laceration or hematoma, are usually obvious and dealt with surgically. The skin of the pinna, at the meatus especially, can be affected by eczema. Pruritus is a common co-occurring symptom of this disorder. Steroid-based ointments are used to control the disease. Cartilagenous disorders, chondritis/perichondritis and relapsing polychondritis, can be painful and typically require systemic therapy with antibiotics and steroids, respectively. Furthermore, if relapsing polychondritis is suspected, additional head and neck manifestations should be sought, and rheumatologic consultation is warranted.

D Disorders of the external auditory canal are common sources of otalgia. Evaluation and treatment of otitis externa and malignant otitis externa will be discussed in Chapters 18 and 19. Foreign bodies or firm cerumen impactions can cause pain and should be removed. Neoplasms can also occur in the external auditory canal; they can be of cutaneous origin, cerumen gland tumors, or salivary gland tumors. Workup and treatment of these lesions is described in Chapter 42.

E Disorders of the tympanic membrane, middle ear, and mastoid can lead to otalgia. Acute or chronic otitis media and their sequelae are discussed in Chapters 24, 26, 27, and 33–35.

F In cases where the otologic examination is unremarkable, in cases in which the otologic findings do not appear to explain the otalgia, or in cases where a patient's otalgia does not respond to appropriate management, other sources for the otalgia should be sought. A thorough head and neck examination is often revealing. Referred pain from upper aerodigestive sources is a common source of otalgia. Causative disorders include infectious etiologies (such as referred pain from upper respiratory tract infection) and neoplastic etiologies (such as upper respiratory tract squamous cell carcinoma) among others (see flow chart). Treatment is directed at the underlying etiology. Particular attention should be given to the TMJ and associated musculature because disorders in this area are amongst the most common causes of otalgia. Tenderness in the area of or clicking and popping of the TMJ may suggest TMJ arthralgia or myofascial pain (Chapter 90). Referral to a dental or physical therapy professional who specialized in treatment of these disorders is appropriate.

G Some patients presenting with otalgia have normal otologic, head and neck, and neurologic physical examinations. Local or distant pathology may be responsible for the otalgia. If the presenting otalgia is characterized by sharp shooting pain, cranial neuralgias should be considered in the differential diagnosis. Palpation of areas innervated by the affected nerve may elicit the otalgia. Neurologic consultation should be obtained. Cardiac and pulmonary disorders can result in referred pain to the auricle by stimulation of the vagus nerve; medical referral is warranted when such an etiology is suspected.

SUGGESTED READING

Charlett SD, Coatesworth AP. Referred otalgia: a structured approach to diagnosis and treatment. Int J Clin Pract. 2007;61(6):1015-1021.

Neilan RE, Roland PS. Otalgia. Med Clin North Am. 2010;94(5):961-971.

Shah RK, Blevins NH. Otalgia. Otolaryngol Clin North Am. 2003;36(6):1137-1151.

CHAPTER 18

Otorrhea

Joseph E Dohar

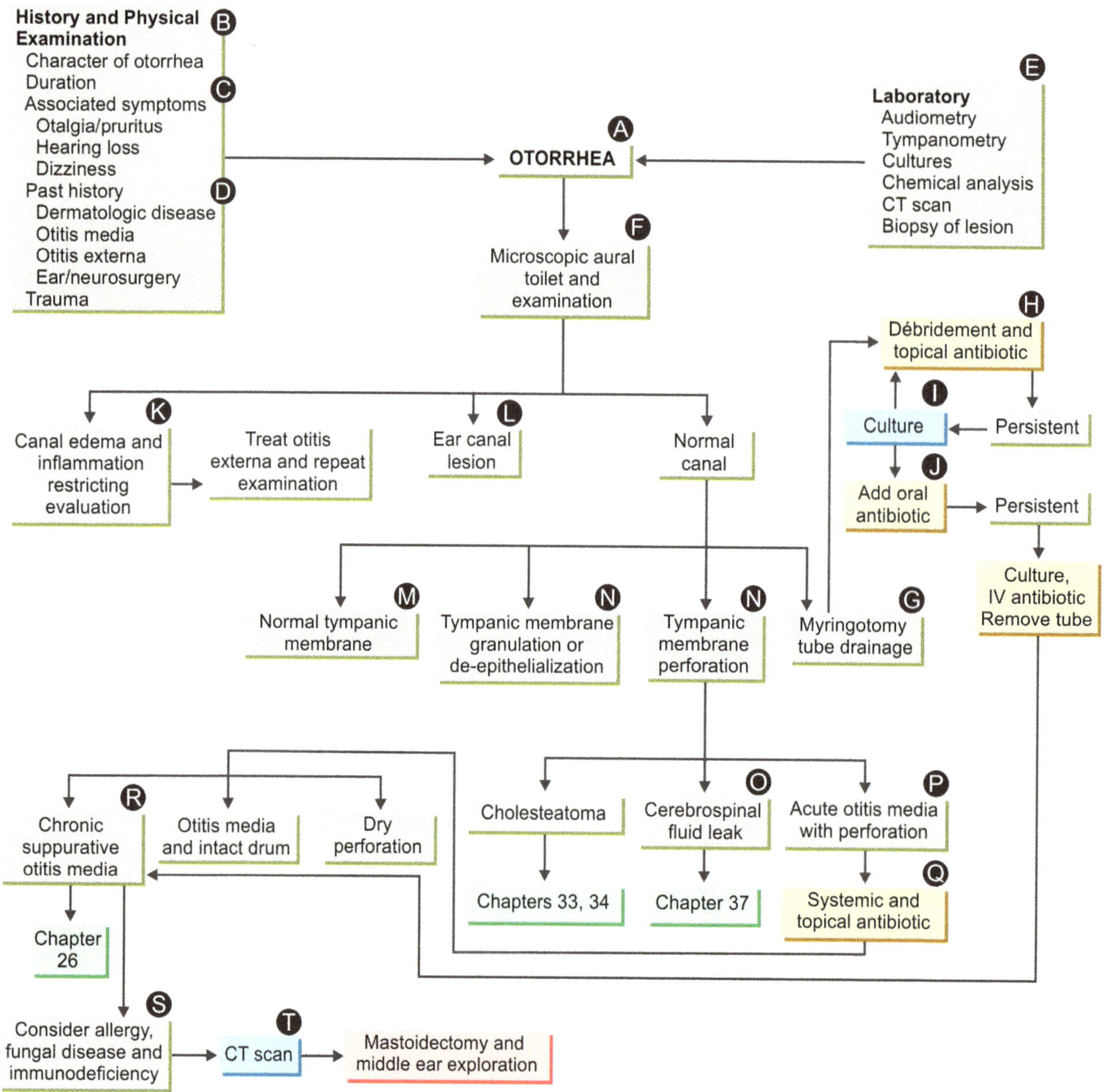

Otorrhea is one of the most frequent chief complaints prompting consultation with an Otolaryngologist. Although often oversimplified, the evaluation and management of otorrhea may be quite complex. Determining the source of the drainage is complicated by edema and debris, which obscures pneumatic otoscopy. Interpreting microbiology data is not trivial and assuming infectious etiology often delays the diagnosis of noninfectious causes of the illness, which can be life-threatening and even fatal.

A Not unlike most algorithms, a detailed history and physical examination are paramount in evaluating otorrhea with an emphasis on establishing associated otalgia, high fever (>102°F), antecedent trauma, respiratory tract infection, water exposure, otologic surgery, and onset.

B Clear, watery otorrhea must be analyzed for the possibility of cerebrospinal fluid (CSF). The diagnosis of CSF otorrhea (leakage of CSF into the ear canal) is usually a result of head trauma, tumor, congenital malformation, or surgery but may also occur spontaneously. Confirmation of the presence of CSF in drainage is also challenging. Traditional chemical analyses (e.g. glucose, protein, and specific gravity) are unreliable tests for CSF. Radiographic studies, especially those involving the injection of dyes or radiographic compounds, are costly and may introduce additional risks to the patient. β-2 transferrin is a CSF-specific variant of transferrin and is often used as an endogenous marker of CSF leakage.

C Bloody otorrhea is most commonly due to granulation tissue associated with a retained tympanostomy tube or from a robust host inflammatory response. However, it is potentially indicative of a serious condition. In the absence of a history of trauma or prior surgery, bloody otorrhea must be investigated with temporal bone imaging and tissue biopsy to rule out malignancy.

D Dermatologic disease such as eczema or psoriasis may involve the skin of the ear canal, predisposing to recurrent otitis externa. Past surgery for otitis media or cholesteatoma suggests recurrence of middle ear or mastoid disease. Neurosurgical procedures involving or adjacent to the temporal bone may be followed by immediate or delayed CSF otorrhea.

E Audiometry is best deferred if the ear canal is obstructed unless tuning fork tests or vestibular symptoms suggest sensorineural hearing loss. Tympanometry is painful in otitis externa and is contraindicated in suspected CSF otorrhea, because pneumocephalus could result. Topical antibiotics will interfere with culture growth and should not be started until after cultures are obtained. An aspirate from deep in the canal or from a perforation will be the most representative. Cultures should include aerobes, anaerobes, and fungi.

F Examination of the ear under the microscope with debridement is the key to diagnosis. Otitis externa may be secondary to otitis media and yet may prevent middle ear examination. Antibiotic, topical steroid, and repeated debridement may be required. An unsuspected foreign body may be encountered.

G Purulent otorrhea is the most commonly encountered situation. In the presence of a tympanostomy tube and associated with an acute upper respiratory tract infection, standard ototopical therapy with aural toilet should suffice. Otorrhea is common after myringotomy tube insertion. Avoiding water exposure with suitable ear plugs is an important preventive measure.

H A short course of a topical antibiotic will be sufficient in most cases. Ototoxicity from topical aminoglycosides is a concern. A partially obstructed tube should be debrided.

I When treating with ototopical antibiotics, culture is relevant only in terms of confirming bacterial pathogenicity versus other possibilities such as fungal infection. When bacterial pathogens are isolated, in vitro susceptibility results should be disregarded as the break points are established for systemic antibiotic administration and are not adjusted for much higher concentrations delivered topically.

J Culture and susceptibility data may inform systemic antibiotic selection, particularly when delivery of topical therapy is compromised or with suppurative complications. Microbiologic identification also carries significant clues to pathophysiology as certain pathogens are more likely to derive from the external auditory canal (i.e. Staphylococcus aureus) versus the nasopharynx (*Streptococcus pneumoniae*), while other pathogens may suggest chronicity (*Pseudomonas aeruginosa*) over more acute infections. These clues are particularly helpful in cases where the otorrhea is recurrent and/or chronic.

K In refractory otitis externa, canal stenosis may be present. Congenital and traumatic types of stenosis have a high incidence of cholesteatoma. Computed tomography is important before surgery. In a very edematous external auditory canal, otowick placement has traditionally been recommended with re-evaluation as soon as the edema has resolved to the point where the tympanic membrane can be visualized. High-level evidence supports otowick placement even in external auditory canals of adequate size.

L Various lesions of the ear canal may present with secondary otitis externa: osteoma, exostoses, ear canal cholesteatoma, and canal dehiscence into the mastoid or glenoid fossa, skin lesions, and neoplasm. Generally, these conditions are managed surgically. A CT scan and a biopsy may be required for surgical planning.

Ⓜ Occasionally, a patient may complain of frequent scant otorrhea but has a normal examination. This may represent moisture trapping after washing or may be related to the use of a hearing aid or ear plugs. Several drops of topical isopropyl alcohol can be used to dry the ear as needed.

Ⓝ Granular myringitis will, usually, slowly respond to topical steroid or 5-fluorouracil. Debridement of the granulation can often be done without violating the tympanic membrane. An intact but de-epithelialized tympanic membrane after infection or tympanoplasty may respond to drying agents such as Burow's solution. A split-thickness skin graft may be required.

Ⓞ Copious watery otorrhea through a perforation suggests CSF otorrhea; however, the leak may be subtle or intermittent. On closure of the perforation, CSF will drain through the Eustachian tube (*see* Chapter 37).

Ⓟ A tympanic membrane perforation with otorrhea will generally respond to topical and systemic antibiotics. Culture is performed in refractory cases. An uninfected ear with a "dry perforation" or functioning myringotomy tube may be seen in a patient with intermittent otorrhea. Episodes may follow contamination with water or upper respiratory tract infections (*see* Chapters 24, 26, and 30).

Ⓠ Otorrhea from acute otitis media with perforation is frequently bloody, causing the patient to be alarmed. The perforation seldom provides free drainage. Systemic antibiotic is indicated; however, topical antibiotic may enter the middle ear and will prevent secondary otitis externa. In refractory cases, it is wise to perform cultures before changing antibiotics. A pinpoint perforation should be enlarged to achieve adequate drainage.

Ⓡ Persistent otorrhea from a myringotomy tube requires cultures and adequate systemic antibiotic. Removal of the tube and repeated debridement may be necessary for adequate drainage. Methicillin-resistant *S. aureus* (MRSA) otorrhea has become increasingly more common and, although once considered an iatrogenic infection, is now commonly contracted in the community. Chasing this infection with systemic antibiotics identified in vitro to be active against MRSA is doomed to failure. Identifying the reservoir, avoiding systemic antibiotics active against *S. aureus,* and topical therapy with time directed at eradication of the carriage state have proven to be effective strategies for long-term success.

Ⓢ Although traditionally listed as an indication for tympanomastoidectomy surgery, chronic suppurative otitis media without cholesteatoma is rarely, if ever, best treated by

this approach. Identifying underlying immunodeficiency or allergy will enable specific medical interventions to augment antimicrobials. This should be considered before surgery. When considering possible allergic etiologies, one must not only consider inhalant or food triggers but also household triggers such as shampoos and even medication reactions. Of the ototopical options used, neomycin is purported to most often induce an allergic response while even topical steroids may induce such a response. The latter is somewhat counterintuitive since steroids are often used to treat allergic skin reactions but must be kept in mind since several combination ototopical agents include a steroid component. Arguably, the most challenging culture result to interpret is isolation of a fungal organism. One must beware of the perfunctory assignment of a pathologic role to fungal isolates as not unlike in paranasal sinuses, fungus in the ear may be an invasive fulminant pathogen in immunocompromised hosts, an invasive nonfulminant pathogen in immunocompetent hosts, a focal mycetoma without any invasive potential, an allergen-triggering allergic fungal otomastoiditis (which has been reported), or a simple saprophyte opportunistically growing in an environment that is dark, moist, and warm without any other pathophysiologic role. Distinguishing these scenarios is not trivial or simply an academic exercise and demands far more consideration than is typically appreciated. Furthermore, treatment is vastly different for each individual case rendering the importance of this differential diagnosis critical in achieving a cure.

Ⓣ Computed tomography imaging and surgery are final steps in this algorithm. Surgery is designed to remove irreversible mucosal disease in the middle ear and mastoid. In the event of chronic or recurrent cases of otorrhea, other surgical interventions such as removal/replacement of the tympanostomy tubes, adenoidectomy, or excision/debridement of aural granulomas must be considered and can be effective in properly selected patients.

SUGGESTED READING

Dohar JE. All that drains is not infectious otorrhea. Int J Pediatr Otorhinolaryngol. 2003;67(4):417-420.

Dohar JE. Evolution of management approaches for otitis externa. Pediatr Infect Dis J. 2003;22(4):299-305; quiz 306-308.

Dohar JE. Otitis externa. In: Rakel RE. Conn's Current Therapy. Philadelphia: WB Saunders; 2002; pp. 114-117.

Dohar JE. Topical quinolones in the treatment of chronic suppurative otitis media and recurrent otorrhea. Ear Nose Throat J. 2002;81(8 Suppl 1):20.

Dohar JE, Antonelli PJ, Poole MD. Tympanostomy tube otorrhea: treating the first infection. Highlights of a roundtable discussion sponsored by Alcon Laboratories, Inc; October 16, 2004; Fort Worth, Texas. Ear Nose Throat J. 2005;84(2 Suppl 1):5-15.

Inglis AF Jr. Tympanostomy tubes. In: Cummings CW, Fredrickson JM, Harker LA, et al. (Eds). Otolaryngology Head and Neck Surgery, vol 5, 3rd edition. St Louis, MO: CV Mosby; 1998. p. 478.

Parisier SC, Kimmelman CP, Hanson MB. Diseases of the external auditory canal. In: Hughes GB, Pensak ML (Eds). Clinical Otology. New York: Thieme; 1997. p. 191.

Roland PS, Antonelli PJ, Dohar JE, et al. Managing acute otitis media in children with tympanostomy tubes. Panel discussion. Ear Nose Throat J. 2005;8(4 Suppl 2):7-15.

Otitis Externa

Brian J McKinnon

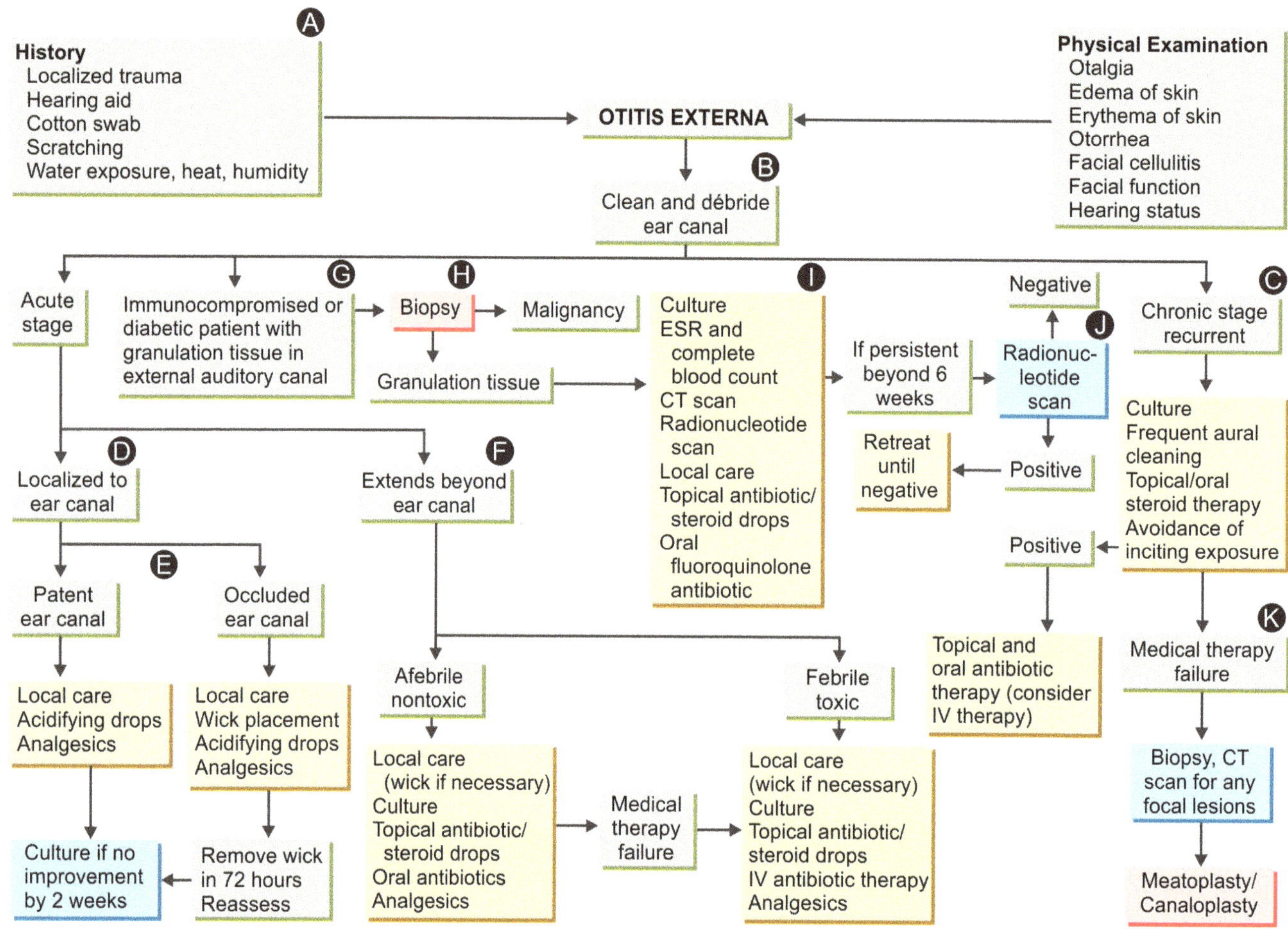

Otitis externa, a common clinical complaint, is a diffuse inflammation of the skin of the external auditory canal (EAC), which may extend to the tympanic membrane and auricle. Acute otitis externa is a cellulitis of the external ear, with a common feature of pain on manipulation of external ear or auricle that seems greater than what would be expected on the basis of the examination. Chronic otitis externa may not be painful, and etiology can be infection, allergic, or autoimmune.

A While the EAC is normally protected by a mildly acidic pH of 4–5 and a lipid film from the skin/cerumen barrier, an accumulation of moisture (i.e. frequent water exposure) and the frequent removal or absence of cerumen can lead to the development of a more alkaline pH. Trauma to the EAC epithelium permits local invasion of bacteria, with resultant inflammation of the underlying soft tissues.

B Gentle cleaning and debridement of the desquamated epithelium and debris with evaluation of the tympanic

membrane and middle ear space are important first steps in management. The examination is frequently quite uncomfortable and must be done with care.

C Localized painful inflammation of the lateral one-third of the EAC with a history of frequent swimming or trauma is typical of acute otitis externa. Chronic otitis externa typically presents with mild discomfort, intense itching, and excoriated skin; on examination, hypertrophic EAC skin and absent cerumen reflect the persistent low-grade inflammatory and/or infectious process. Recurrent otitis externa may be due to repeated water exposure without dry ear precautions, or routine daily hearing aid use.

D Inspection of the auricle, pre- and postauricular skin, and upper cervical lymph node chain assesses for extension of the infectious process. Significant erythema of the auricle, edema or tenderness of the periauricular skin, or fullness and pain in the upper neck indicates infection beyond the confines of the EAC.

E Edema of the lateral EAC skin will trap moisture and debris, abet the inflammatory cycle, and prevent topical acidifying otic drops from reaching the inflamed epithelium. Placement of a wick (cotton wick, porous cellulose, or nonadherent gauze strips) will facilitate contact of the otic drops with the inflamed epithelium. Frequency of follow-up visits is dictated by the degree of inflammation and amount of debris present.

F Extension of the infectious process beyond the EAC warrants more intensive therapy. The addition of topical antibiotic otic/ophthalmologic drops (with steroid) and systemic antibiotics may be necessary. Culture of the EAC may direct medical therapy provided the patient has not been previously treated with antibiotic medication. Antibiotic coverage should be directed against the most common pathogens of Pseudomonas aeruginosa and Staphylococcus aureus. Intravenous antibiotic therapy is indicated with systemic involvement (fever, chills, generalized malaise). If infection progresses, the involvement of less common pathogens (gram-negative bacteria, fungi) should be investigated, for example, using culture samples in Amies transport medium with charcoal.

G The immunocompromised or diabetic patient requires careful initial evaluation and vigorous therapy as they are extremely susceptible to rapid spread of soft-tissue infection, with progression to osteomyelitis of the EAC bone and surrounding skull base (malignant or necrotizing otitis externa). Clinical signs of skull base progression include severe trismus (glenoid fossa), facial nerve paresis/paralysis (stylomastoid foramen), and paresis/paralysis of cranial nerves IX, X, and XI (jugular foramen). As P. aeruginosa is the most common pathogen, initial topical and systemic therapy should be directed at this organism. Classically, granulation is present on the floor of the EAC at the bony-cartilaginous junction, and otalgia is disproportionate to the physical findings. Malignant or necrotizing otitis externa can progress rapidly despite appropriate therapy and can be lethal.

H Biopsy of EAC granulation tissue assesses for occult malignancy as presenting symptoms can be identical.

I Oral fluoroquinolone antibiotic therapy is extremely effective in the treatment of malignant otitis externa.

If the patient does not respond rapidly, consideration should be given to converting therapy to intravenous aminoglycoside administration. Radiologic imaging is necessary for the diagnosis of osteomyelitis of the skull base and is useful in determining the extent of the infection. Limited radionucleotide imaging (technetium-99m scan) confirms the diagnosis, and temporal bone computed tomography (CT) assesses the extent of involvement. While white blood cell count is frequently normal, erythrocyte sedimentation rate is usually quite elevated.

J Prolonged antibiotic therapy is necessary to treat the bony involvement adequately, despite the EAC appearing normal within several weeks. As Technetium-99m scanning will remain positive despite resolution of the infection, Gallium radionucleotide scanning is used to determine the end point for antibiotic therapy. Premature termination of antibiotic therapy may lead to recurrence and/or progression.

K Chronic otitis externa can be refractory to intensive and prolonged medical therapy. While rarely indicated, surgical procedures are directed at enlarging the EAC, removing the hypertrophic, scarred subcutaneous tissue, and resurfacing the EAC. The CT imaging should be obtained before any definitive surgical procedures, and any focal changes within the EAC should undergo biopsy to assess for occult malignancy.

SUGGESTED READING

Carfrae MJ, Kesser BW. Malignant otitis externa. Otolaryngol Clin North Am. 2008;41:537-549.

Kesser BW. Assessment and management of chronic otitis externa. Curr Opin Otolaryngol Head Neck Surg. 2011;19(5):341-347.

Llor C, McNulty CA, Butler CC. Ordering and interpreting ear swabs in otitis externa. BMJ. 2014;349:5259-5263.

Rosenfeld RM, Schwartz SR, Cannon CR, et al. Clinical practice guideline: acute otitis externa. Otolaryngol Head Neck Surg. 2014;150(1 Suppl):S1-S24.

Thompson SW. Otitis externa. In: Alper CM, Myers EN, Eibling DE (Eds). Decision Making in Ear Nose and Throat Disorders, 1st edition. St Louis, MO: Saunders; 2001.

Deformities of the Auricle

Noel Jabbour

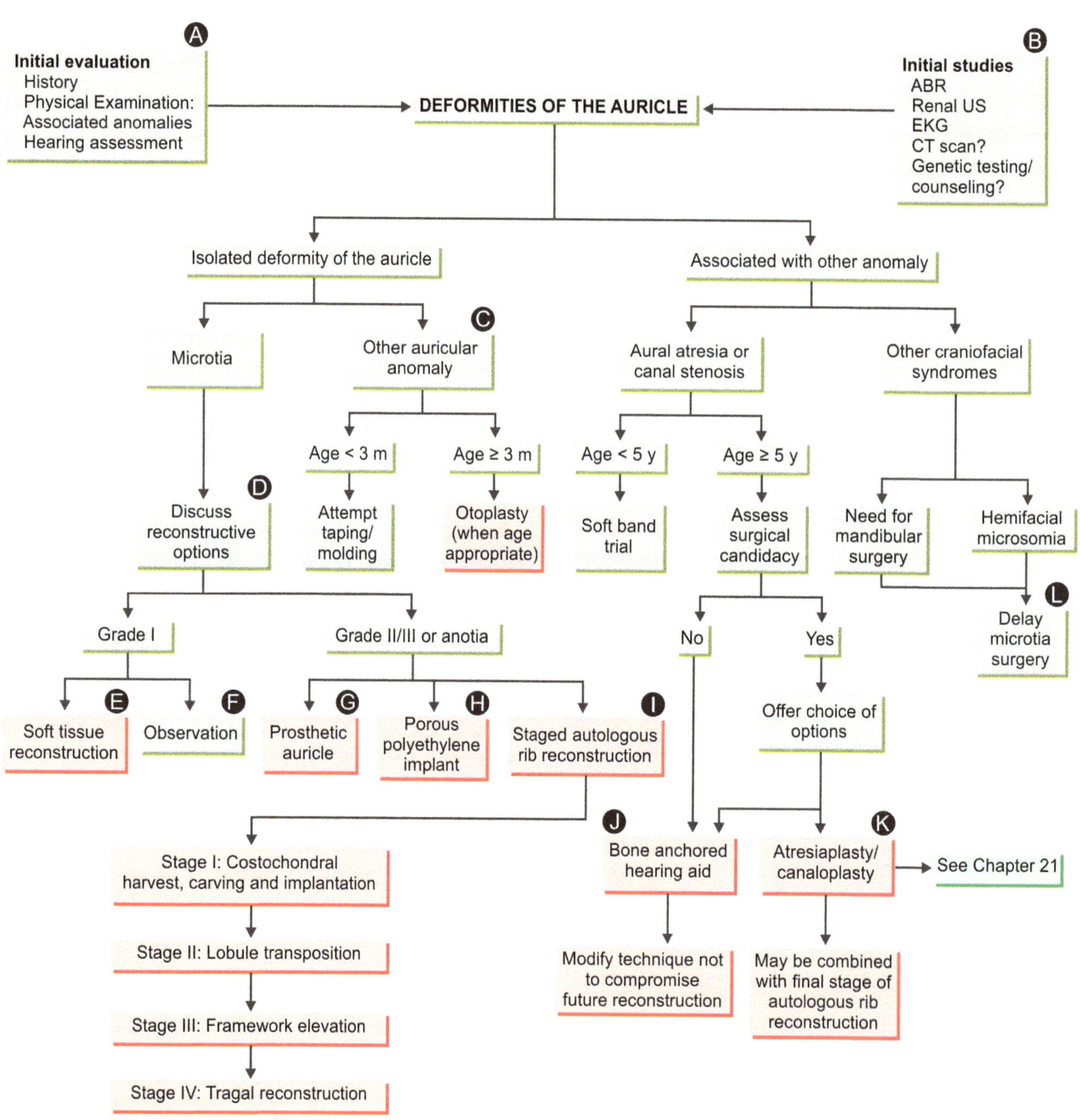

Microtia and aural atresia occur from 0.83 to 17.4 per 10,000 live births and may be unilateral or bilateral. These anomalies are found in association with other congenital anomalies and in up to 10% as part of known syndromes, such as Goldenhar, CHARGE, or Treacher Collins syndrome. However, more subtle auricular and ear canal anomalies are even more common.

A Initial evaluation should include a careful family history, birth history including potential teratogenic exposures, and medical history including other known anomalies. In the vast majority of cases, no specific cause is identified. Physical examination should include grading the severity of the ear abnormalities as well as a careful search for other commonly associated anomalies including choanal atresia/stenosis, hemifacial microsomia, cleft palate, hemipalatal paresis, and other craniofacial anomalies, as well as initial hearing assessment to confirm the hearing status in the affected and unaffected ear(s).

B Since development of the auricle occurs at the same gestational time-period as development of the heart and kidney renal ultrasound and EKG may serve as baseline screening tests for associated renal or cardiac anomalies. If there is a question regarding the hearing, auditory brainstem response testing should be performed to evaluate conductive versus sensorineural hearing loss. Some centers perform a CT scan of the internal auditory canal at the time of initial evaluation, though it may be more prudent to wait until a later age, when considering surgical options, in order to reduce the patients exposure to the radiation.

C Other of the auricular anomalies that are not microtia should be identified, such as macrotia, lop ear deformity, Stahl's deformity, prominauris, or cryptotia. There is evidence that children under the age of 3 months may benefit from nonsurgical splinting with either tape or ear molding. After 3 months of age, the circulating maternal estrogen decreases and the cartilage stiffens and these techniques may be less likely to be successful; otoplasty may be considered when the ear is approaching its adult size at 5–6 years of age. Otoplasty is most commonly performed from a post-auricular approach. Incisionless techniques have been described. If the auricle is deficient in cartilage, grafting from the contralateral auricle may be required.

D Treatment options for microtia are dependent on severity. Microtia is graded as follows: Grade I—nearly normal ear with deficiency in at least one dimension; Grade II—ear with structural deficiencies but recognizable anatomy; Grade III—rudimentary soft tissue with "peanut" remnant; Grade IV— anotia (absent external ear).

E Soft tissue reconstructive techniques may be used to address Grade I microtia. These may involve local rotation or advancement flaps as well as cartilage grafts or composite grafts from the contralateral ear.

F Many patients and families express a preference not to proceed with reconstructive options or to wait until the patient is old enough to choose for himself or herself.

G Prosthetic auricles may be constructed by an anaplastologist as a mirror image of the unaffected ear or a chosen model ear in bilateral cases. In the near future,

3-D printing may reduce the cost and improve availability of prosthetic ears. These may be affixed temporarily by tape or glue or more permanently by osseointegrated abutments or magnets.

H MEDPOR auricular reconstruction involves a one- to two-stage surgical reconstruction in which a porous, high-density polyethylene auricular implant is covered by a vascularized temporoparietal fascia flap and skin grafts. The aesthetic results can be excellent, though there are reports of extrusion of the implants. The age at time of reconstruction has been reported as early as 3 years of age.

I Staged-autologous rib reconstruction has been described in two to four stages. Traditionally, the four-stage approach involves rib cartilage framework implantation carved from the contralateral costochondral cartilage. Subsequent stages involve lobule rotation, auricle elevation, and touch-up of the tragus and conchal bowl.

J For transcutaneous abutments, a small, stab incision may be used to minimize any compromise to the blood supply for future microtia reconstruction. For magnetic implants, the location of the incision should be chosen to not preclude the use of a temporoparietal flap in future repair.

K Management of anomalies of the ear canal is dependent upon severity (*see* Chapter 21). Timing of repair, if indicated, may be combined with subsequent stages of microtia repair, most commonly, for formation of the tragus.

L If mandibular surgery is indicated, especially in hemifacial microsomia, microtia surgery may be delayed to ensure proper placement of the reconstructed auricle.

SUGGESTED READING

Brent B. Microtia repair with rib cartilage grafts: a review of personal experience with 1000 cases. Clin Plastic Surg. 2002;29:257-271.

Guilfoyle R, Wilkes GH, Wong J. Microtia reconstruction. Plast Reconstr Surg. 2014;134(3):464e-479e.

Nagata S. A new method of total reconstruction of the auricle for microtia. Plast Reconstr Surg. 1993;92:187-201.

Reinisch JF, Lewin S. Ear reconstruction using a porous polyethylene framework and temporoparietal fasca flap. Facial Plast Surg. 2009;25(3):181-189.

Ullmann Y, Blazer S, Ramon Y, et al. Early nonsurgical correction of congenital auricular deformities. Plast Reconstr Surg. 2002;109:907-913.

Congenital Aural Atresia and Congenital External Auditory Canal Stenosis

Robert F Yellon

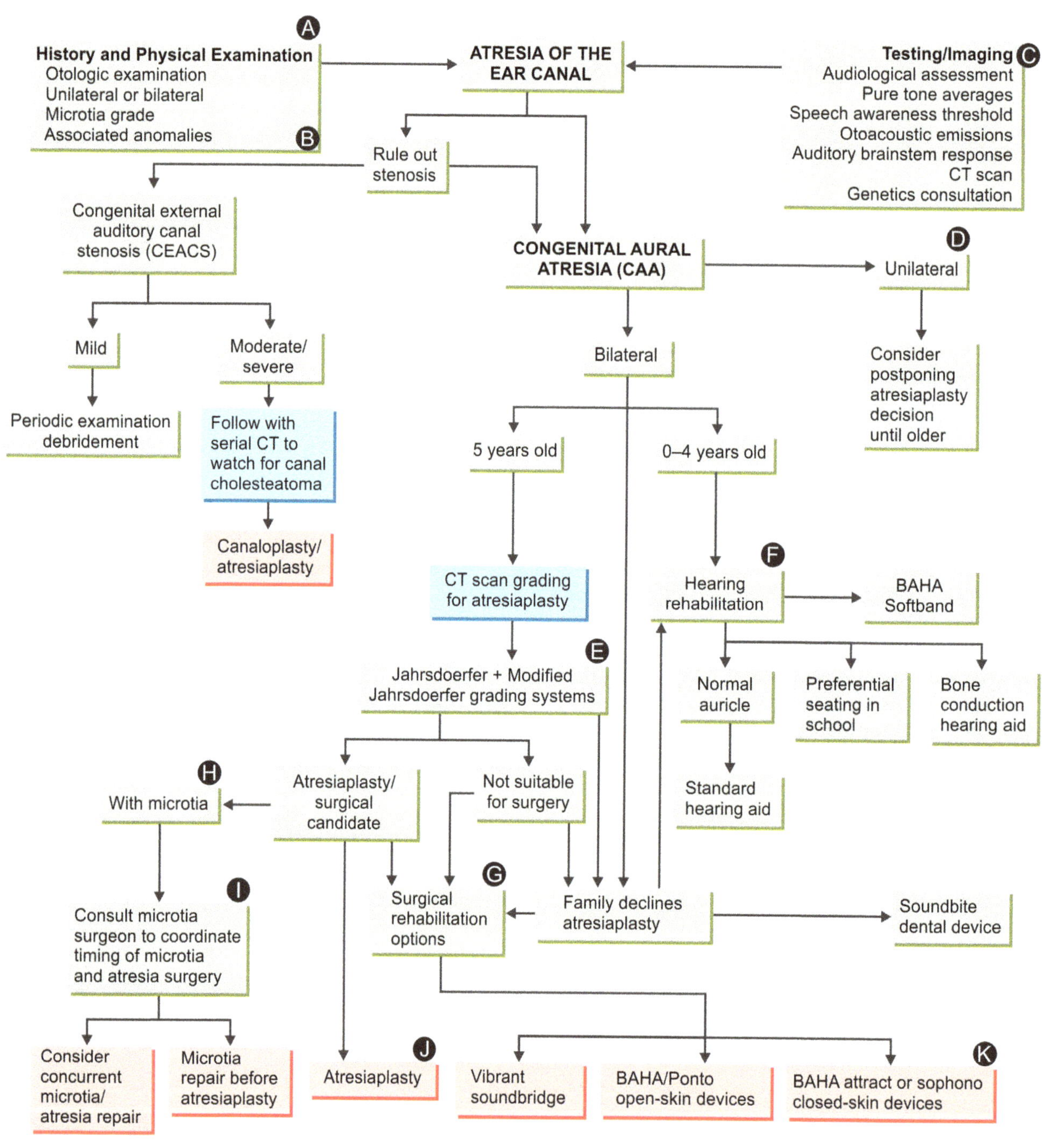

Surgical management of microtia and congenital aural atresia (CAA) and congenital external auditory canal stenosis (CEACS) continues to be one of the most exciting, challenging, and rewarding areas of reconstructive and otologic surgery. The decision for surgery and the type of surgery depends upon the child's age, hearing, thickness of the cortical bone, severity of the middle ear malformation, the surgeon's experience, and the choice of the patient/family.

A Congenital anomalies of the auricle are graded as follows:
Grade 1: nearly normal ear, abnormal in some dimension;
Grade 2: an ear with moderate structural deficiencies;

Grade 3: classic severe "peanut deformity;" and Grade 4: anotia or no auricle and earlobe.

B Microtia/CAA/CEACS may occur with ocular, cervical, cardiac, airway, and feeding issues that must be treated. Genetics and Craniofacial Team consults may be required.

C The great majority of children with CAA and CEACS have conductive hearing loss (CHL) and normal sensorineural hearing. Auditory brainstem response testing may be required to evaluate the sensorineural component. For unilateral CAA, CHL is more frequent in the "normal" ear, so bilateral testing is required.

D Unilateral hearing loss is not associated with speech and learning problems.

E Jahrsdoerfer and modified Jahrsdoerfer systems for grading CT scans of the temporal bone help to identify patients who are favorable candidates for atresiaplasty. See Yeakley, et al., and Dedhia, et al. in Suggested Reading.

F For patients who are younger than 5 years, hearing rehabilitation options include bone-conduction metal headband hearing aid, Bone Anchored Hearing Aid (BAHA) Softband, and if an adequate auricle is present a standard hearing aid.

G For patients who are not atresiaplasty candidates or for those who decline atresiaplasty, surgical implant options include BAHA and Ponto open-skin implants, closed-skin bone magnetic conduction devices (Sophono Alpha, BAHA Attract), Vibrant Soundbridge active middle ear implant, and Bonebridge. Minimum age is 5 years in the United States for all except Vibrant Soundbridge, which has >18 year limit. Bonebridge is not yet approved by the US Food and Drug Administration. Patients >18 years can use the Soundbite dental device.

H Some surgeons advocate for early microtia and CAA/CEACS reconstruction, whereas others recommend that the patient understands risk when they are older and makes their own decision.

I Education of the family about all options for microtia reconstruction is important including: no surgery, glueon prosthetic ears, prosthetic ears attached to bone anchors, autologous costal cartilage graft auricle reconstruction, and Medpor polyethylene implants.

J Atresiaplasty can be performed successfully with both canal-wall-up and canal-wall-down techniques. Canal-wall-up technique is preferred to avoid mastoid bowl problems. Complications of atresiaplasty surgery include postsurgical stenosis of the external auditory canal stenosis, infections, lateralization of the tympanic membrane, persistent or progressive CHL, and rarely, injury to the facial nerve or sensorineural hearing loss. The best possible outcome is uncomplicated atresiaplasty with excellent hearing. Atresiaplasty is a long procedure with more risk. However, the average hearing result of atresiaplasty is not as good as the average hearing result with the implants (*see* G).

K Implants, however, are not without complications and are less cosmetically acceptable. Complications of open-skin BAHAs include site infections, scalp thickening requiring revision surgery, and loss of the implant.

SUGGESTED READING

Byun H, Moon IJ, Woo S-Y, et al. Objective and subjective improvement of hearing in noise after surgical correction of unilateral aural atresia in pediatric patients: a prospective study using the hearing in noise test, the sound-spatial-quality questionnaire, and the glasgow benefit inventory. Ear Hear. 2015;36;e183-189.

Dedhia K, Yellon RF, Branstetter BF, et al. Anatomic variants on computed tomography in congenital aural atresia. Otolaryngol Head Neck Surg. 2012;147(2):323-328.

Denoyelle F, Coudert C, Thierry B, et al. Hearing rehabilitation with the closed skin bone-anchored implant Sophono Alpha 1: results of a prospective study in 15 children with ear atresia. Int J Pediatr Otorhinolaryngol. 2015;79:382-387.

Fan Y, Zhang Y, Wang S, et al. Auditory development after placement of bone-anchored hearing aids Softband among Chinese Mandarin-speaking children with bilateral aural atresia. Int J Pediatr Otorhinolaryngol. 2014;78(1):60-64.

Frenzel H, Sprinzl G, Streitberger C, et al. The Vibrant Soundbridge in children and adolescents: preliminary European multicenter results. Otol Neurotol. 2015;36:1216-1222.

Jensen DR, Grames LM, Lieu JEC. Effects of aural atresia on speech development and learning. Retrospective analysis from a multidisciplinary craniofacial clinic. JAMA Otolaryngol Head Neck Surg. 2013;139(8):797-802.

Nadaraja GS, Gurgel RK, Kim J, et al. Hearing outcomes of atresia surgery versus osseointegrated bone conduction device in patients with congenital aural atresia: a systematic review. Otol Neurotol. 2013;34:1394-1399.

Sprinzl GM, Wolf-Magele A. The Bonebridge bone conduction hearing implant: indication criteria, surgery and a systematic review of the literature. Clin. Otolaryngol. 2016;41(2):131-143.

Yeakley J, Jahrsdoerfer RA. CT evaluation of congenital aural atresia: what the radiologist and surgeon need to know. J Comput Assist Tomogr. 1996;20:724-731.

Yellon RF, Denoyelle F. Evaluation and management of congenital aural atresia. In: Cummings Otolaryngology Head and Neck Surgery, 6th edition. Philadelphia, PA: Saunders Elsevier; 2015. pp. 3006-3018.

CHAPTER 22

Eustachian Tube Dysfunction

Cuneyt M Alper

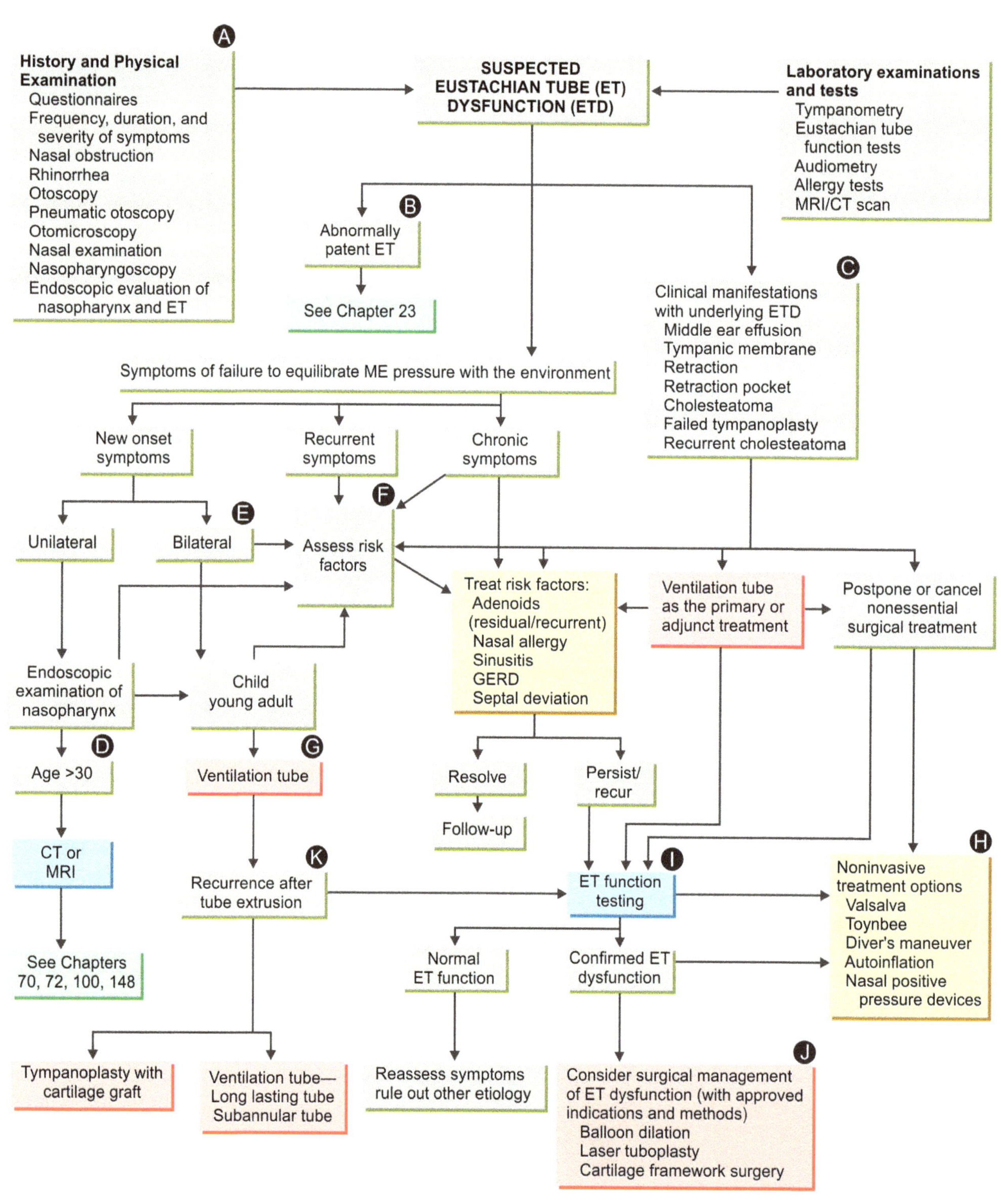

Eustachian tube (ET) dysfunction (ETD) is defined as the inability for ET to maintain middle ear (ME) pressure close to the pressure in the environment. Gases in the ME are constantly exchanging through the mucosa toward equilibrating the partial pressures with the blood. The ultimate result of complete equilibration, if the absorbed gases are not replaced, is approximately –600 mm of H_2O, at which level aerated ME with normal tympanic membrane position and/or structure is not possible and could lead to ME effusion due to transudation and exudation, tympanic membrane retraction (TMR), retraction pocket (RP), or cholesteatoma. Although marginal ET function can maintain ME pressure under normal conditions, it may fail to keep up with the increased demand with the rapid changes in the environmental pressure or worsened equilibrating ability with upper respiratory tract infections.

A Obstructed ET may present with symptoms of otalgia, popping, snapping, mild hearing loss, tinnitus, disequilibrium, and even vertigo. Signs of obstruction, commonly diagnosed by otoscopy, otomicroscopy, or tympanometry, include the presence of middle-ear negative pressure, retraction of the tympanic membrane, and diffuse erythema of the tympanic membrane when caused by barotrauma.

B Abnormally patent ET, termed as patulous ET, not only have similar symptoms but also have autophony (hearing one's own voice/breathing in the ear). A patulous ET may be associated with movement of the tympanic membrane synchronous with breathing and phonation, failure to get a full tympanometry curve and/or recording of synchronous pressure changes.

C A number of clinical manifestations may have presumed underlying ETD; however, the pathogenesis of ME effusion, TMR, RP, and cholesteatoma are multifactorial, and although these may have been the primary cause in the pathogenesis, it does not necessarily indicate a current ETD.

D New onset unilateral ETD in adults should prompt an endoscopic evaluation of the nasopharynx and imaging to rule out a neoplastic process.

E New onset ETD is usually associated with upper respiratory tract infection, allergy, or barotrauma.

F Recurrent acute or chronic obstruction can have the same causes as acute obstruction but can also be secondary to hypertrophy of the adenoids, residual or recurrent adenoids, peritubal lymphoid tissue, exacerbation of nasal allergy, paranasal sinusitis, gastroesophageal reflux disease, intranasal diseases/disorders (e.g. deviated septum, polyps), or craniofacial disorders, such as cleft palate.

G Insertion of a ventilation tube (VT) is the least invasive and most commonly used treatment method; although it does not cure ETD, it may resolve the symptoms while VT is in and functioning. Symptoms that persist after VT are not related to ET obstruction.

H If ongoing ETD is suspected when there is an indication for ME surgery, concurrent VT insertion, postponing nonessential surgery until ETD is assessed and managed, and/or trial of noninvasive treatment methods may be considered.

I To evaluate ETD, a number of methods including the ability to increase ME pressure with Valsalva, ability to correct positive and negative ME pressures created with tympanometer, nine-step test, sonotubometry, inflation–deflation test, tubomanometry, forced response test, and pressure chamber tests. While most of these methods are used only in selected centers, tests with widely available tympanometers can provide information on ET function.

J Newly developed specific treatment methods targeting ETD, such as laser tuboplasty, cartilage framework surgery, or balloon dilation of ET, may be considered.

K Currently, significantly symptomatic ears or findings of persistent, recurrent, or progressive ETD manifestations have limited treatment options other than replacement of VTs, insertion of long-lasting VTs, subannular tubes, and/or cartilage tympanoplasty.

SUGGESTED READING

Alper CM. Autoinflation for the treatment of otitis media with effusion. In: Alper CM, Bluestone CD, Casselbrant M, et al. (Eds). Advanced Therapy in Otitis Media. Hamilton, Ontario: BC Decker; 2004. pp. 189-193.

Alper CM, Swarts JD, Singla A, et al. Relationship between the electromyographic activity of the paratubal muscles and Eustachian tube opening assessed by sonotubometry and videoendoscopy. Arch Otolaryngol Head Neck Surg. 2012; 138(8):741-746.

Alper CM, Teixeira MS, Swarts JD. Correlations between videoendoscopy and sonotubometry of Eustachian tube opening during a swallow. Laryngoscope. 2016;126(12):2778-2784.

Alper CM, Teixeira MS, Swarts JD, et al. Quantitative description of Eustachian tube movements during swallowing as visualized by transnasal videoendoscopy. JAMA Otolaryngol Head Neck Surg. 2015;141(2):160-168.

Bluestone CD. Eustachian Tube. Structure, Function, Role in Otitis Media. Hamilton, London: BC Decker Inc; 2005.

Bluestone CD, Cantekin EI, Douglas GS. Eustachian tube function related to the results of tympanoplasty in children. Laryngoscope. 1979;89(3):450-458.

Doyle WJ, Swarts JD, Banks J, et al. Sensitivity and specificity of Eustachian tube function tests in adults. Otolaryngol Head Neck Surg. 2013;139(7):719-727.

Piltcher OB, Alper CM. Persistent and recurrent negative middle ear pressure. In: Alper CM, Bluestone CD, Casselbrant M, et al. (Eds). Advanced Therapy in Otitis Media. Hamilton, Ontario: BC Decker; 2004. pp. 501-507.

Takahashi H, Hasebe S, Sudo M. State of Eustachian tube function in tympanoplasty. In: Alper CM, Bluestone CD, Casselbrant M, et al. (Eds). Advanced Therapy in Otitis Media. Hamilton, Ontario: BC Decker; 2004: pp. 436-439.

Patulous Eustachian Tube Dysfunction

Yehia M Ashry, Dennis S Poe

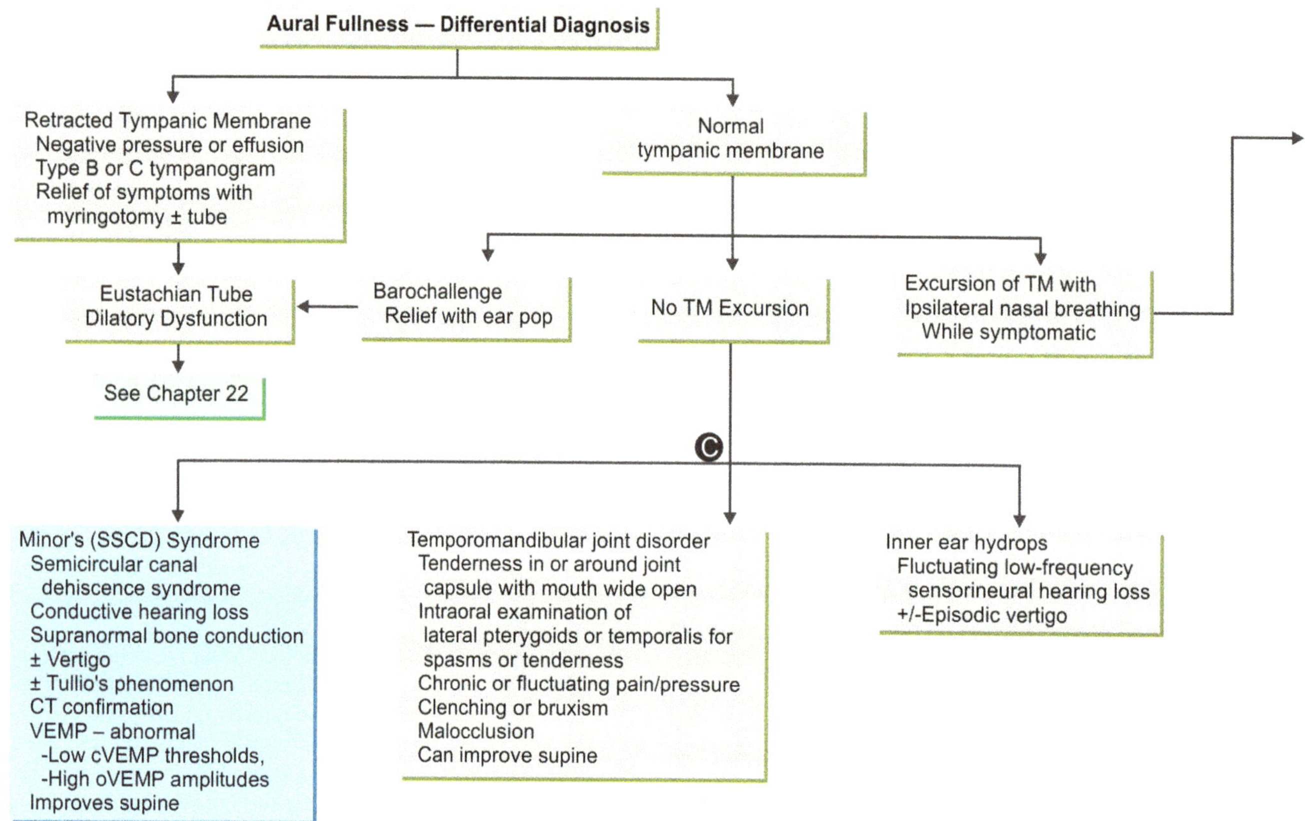

Contd...

Contd...

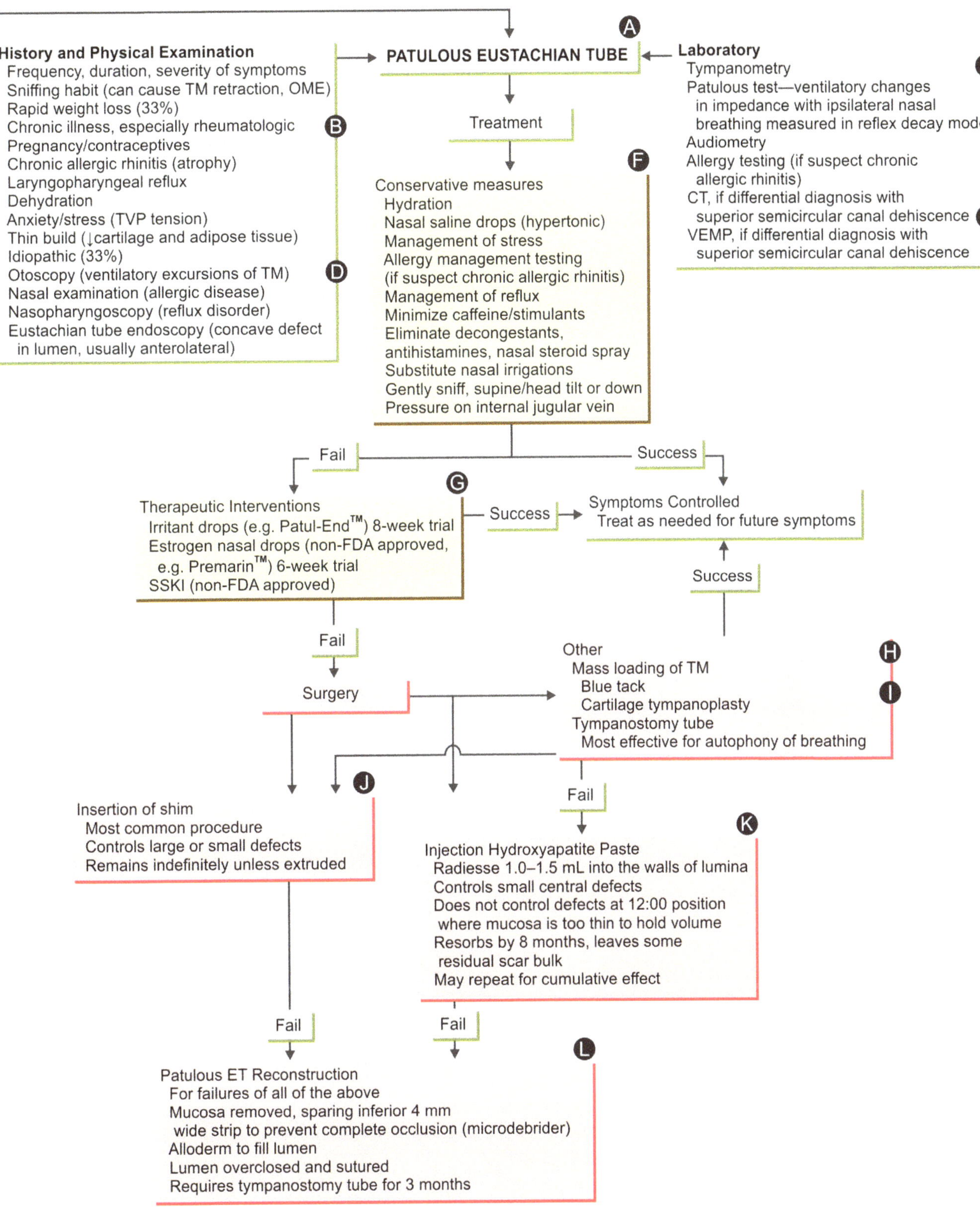

History and Physical Examination
Frequency, duration, severity of symptoms
Sniffing habit (can cause TM retraction, OME)
Rapid weight loss (33%)
Chronic illness, especially rheumatologic
Pregnancy/contraceptives
Chronic allergic rhinitis (atrophy)
Laryngopharyngeal reflux
Dehydration
Anxiety/stress (TVP tension)
Thin build (↓cartilage and adipose tissue)
Idiopathic (33%)
Otoscopy (ventilatory excursions of TM)
Nasal examination (allergic disease)
Nasopharyngoscopy (reflux disorder)
Eustachian tube endoscopy (concave defect
in lumen, usually anterolateral)
B
D
PATULOUS EUSTACHIAN TUBE
A
Treatment
F
Conservative measures
Hydration
Nasal saline drops (hypertonic)
Management of stress
Allergy management testing
(if suspect chronic allergic rhinitis)
Management of reflux
Minimize caffeine/stimulants
Eliminate decongestants,
antihistamines, nasal steroid spray
Substitute nasal irrigations
Gently sniff, supine/head tilt or down
Pressure on internal jugular vein
Laboratory
Tympanometry
Patulous test—ventilatory changes
in impedance with ipsilateral nasal
breathing measured in reflex decay mode
Audiometry
Allergy testing (if suspect chronic
allergic rhinitis)
CT, if differential diagnosis with
superior semicircular canal dehiscence
VEMP, if differential diagnosis with
superior semicircular canal dehiscence
E
C
Fail
Success
G
Therapeutic Interventions
Irritant drops (e.g. Patul-End™) 8-week trial
Estrogen nasal drops (non-FDA approved,
e.g. Premarin™) 6-week trial
SSKI (non-FDA approved)
Success
Symptoms Controlled
Treat as needed for future symptoms
Success
Fail
Surgery
Other
Mass loading of TM
Blue tack
Cartilage tympanoplasty
Tympanostomy tube
Most effective for autophony of breathing
H
I
J
Fail
Insertion of shim
Most common procedure
Controls large or small defects
Remains indefinitely unless extruded
Injection Hydroxyapatite Paste
Radiesse 1.0–1.5 mL into the walls of lumina
Controls small central defects
Does not control defects at 12:00 position
where mucosa is too thin to hold volume
Resorbs by 8 months, leaves some
residual scar bulk
May repeat for cumulative effect
K
Fail
Fail
L
Patulous ET Reconstruction
For failures of all of the above
Mucosa removed, sparing inferior 4 mm
wide strip to prevent complete occlusion (microdebrider)
Alloderm to fill lumen
Lumen overclosed and sutured
Requires tympanostomy tube for 3 months

The Eustachian tube (ET) connects the middle ear (ME) with the nasopharynx and normally remains closed, opening intermittently with swallowing, yawning or passively with pressure differences between the ME and ambient. Patulous ET is defined as the lumen of ET remaining open continuously or for extended periods of time. Differential diagnosis should start with ruling out the other causes of the most common presenting symptom; aural fullness.

A Patulous ET is due to incomplete closure of the cartilaginous segment of the ET secondary to loss of tissue volume in the anterolateral wall of the ET's functional valve.

B Patients with patulous ET may complain of aural fullness, autophony, and habitual sniffing. Temporary relief of autophony may occur during an upper respiratory infection, supine position, head down, or by applying pressure to the neck veins.

C The diagnosis must be differentiated from superior semicircular canal dehiscence (Minor's syndrome), temporomandibular joint disorders, ET dilatory dysfunction, and endolymphatic hydrops.

D Otoscopy during active patulous ET symptoms may confirm the diagnosis if tympanic membrane movements are seen in synchrony with ipsilateral nasal breathing. Endoscopic examination of a patulous ET will reveal a longitudinal concave defect in the anterolateral wall of the ET valve.

E Impedance tympanometry is the most sensitive test to corroborate the diagnosis of patulous ET. Tympanometry, performed in reflex decay mode to have a 10–15 seconds window, usually demonstrates sawtooth tracings coinciding with irregular deep breaths.

F The frequent passage of air through the lumen of the ET contributes to desiccation and atrophy of the mucosa. Measures should be taken to rehydrate and thicken the mucosa and increase its secretions. Nasal drops with isotonic saline may be sufficient, but for an additional irritant effect, hypertonic saline drops can be used.

G Measures can be taken to thicken the mucosa or secretions by irritation or hormonal effect. A topical irritant (e.g. Patul-End™) administered two or three times daily for 2 months can provide lasting benefit. Estrogen nasal drops (off-label use) can also provide lasting benefit using Premarin™ 25 mg IV Secule in 30 mL NS 3 drops tid or Depo-Estradiol™ drops 5 mg IV solution in 30 mL NS 3 drops tid. Less commonly, saturated solution of potassium iodide (SSKI) may be used, 1 g/mL 10 gtt in cup of fruit juice, tid.

H Surgical management should be sought only after conservative measures have failed. Numerous surgical options have been described including tympanostomy tube, mass loading of the tympanic membrane, aug-mentation procedures including local injection of various materials, curvature inversion of ET cartilage using laser, insertion of a shim, or partial or total occlusion of ET.

I Tympanostomy tube is most beneficial in patients complaining mainly of aural fullness, tympanic membrane excursions with autophony of breathing, but it is not usually as effective for treating autophony of voice.

J Endonasal endoscopic insertion of a shim (IV catheter) filled with bone wax and introduced through the full length of the cartilaginous ET is very effective. The shim is wedged into the bony-cartilaginous isthmus and being flexible, will fit into the anterolateral wall concave defect. It fills the defect, but generally does not obstruct the ET. If the shim remains in position for a sufficient amount of time to rehabilitate the mucosa, symptoms may remain relieved.

K Endoscopic augmentation of the ET using calcium hydroxyapatite injection (off-label) could be used initially in mild or intermittent symptoms with small defects in the midportion of the anterolateral wall. Symptoms may recur as the material is absorbed over ~8 months, but if effective for a sufficiently long period, repeat injection can be administered to try to achieve a cumulative benefit.

L Reconstruction of the patulous ET can be done by subtotal occlusion of the cartilaginous ET. The mucosa of the ET is removed circumferentially, except for a 4 mm-wide strip along the floor, to prevent complete occlusion. A graft material such as Alloderm (also adipose tissue, fascia) is used to completely occlude the lumen as high as can be practically inserted. The lumen and orifice are then oversewn with absorbable sutures with endoscopic techniques. Complete, permanent occlusion may cause mucoid otitis media that can repeatedly occlude tympanostomy tubes, creating a difficult management situation and is performed electively only as a last resort.

ACKNOWLEDGMENT

Authors are grateful to Carleton Eduardo Corrales, MD for his editing contributions.

SUGGESTED READING

Adil E, Poe D. What is the full range of medical and surgical treatments available for patients with Eustachian tube dysfunction? Curr Opin Otolaryngol Head Neck Surg. 2014;22:8-15.

Brace MD, Horwich P, Kirkpatrick D, et al. Tympanic membrane manipulation to treat symptoms of patulous Eustachian tube. Otol Neurotol. 2014;35:1201-1206.

Chen D, Luxford W. Myringotomy and tube for relief of patulous Eustachian-tube symptoms. Am J Otology. 1990;11:272-273.

Doherty J, Slattery W. Autologous fat grafting for the refractory patulous Eustachian tube. Otolaryngol Head Neck Surg. 2003; 128:88-91.

McGrath AP, Michaelides EM. Use of middle ear immittance testing in the evaluation of patulous Eustachian tube (Report). J Am Acad Audiol. 2011;22:201-207.

Oshima T, Kikuchi T, Kawase T, et al. Nasal instillation of physiological saline for patulous Eustachian tube. Acta Otolaryngol. 2010;130:550-553.

Poe DS. Diagnosis and management of the patulous Eustachian tube. Otol Neurotol. 2007;28:668-677.

Poe DS, Abou-Halawa A, Abdel-Razek O. Analysis of the dysfunctional Eustachian tube by video endoscopy. Otol Neurotol. 2001;22:590-595.

Rotenberg B, Davidson B. Endoscopic transnasal shim technique for treatment of patulous Eustachian tube. Laryngoscope. 2014; 124:2466-2469.

Schroder S, Lehmann M, Sudhoff H, et al. The patulous Eustachian tube-novel surgical approaches. HNO. 2013;61:1017-1025.

Acute Otitis Media

Ellen M Mandel, Margaretha L Casselbrant

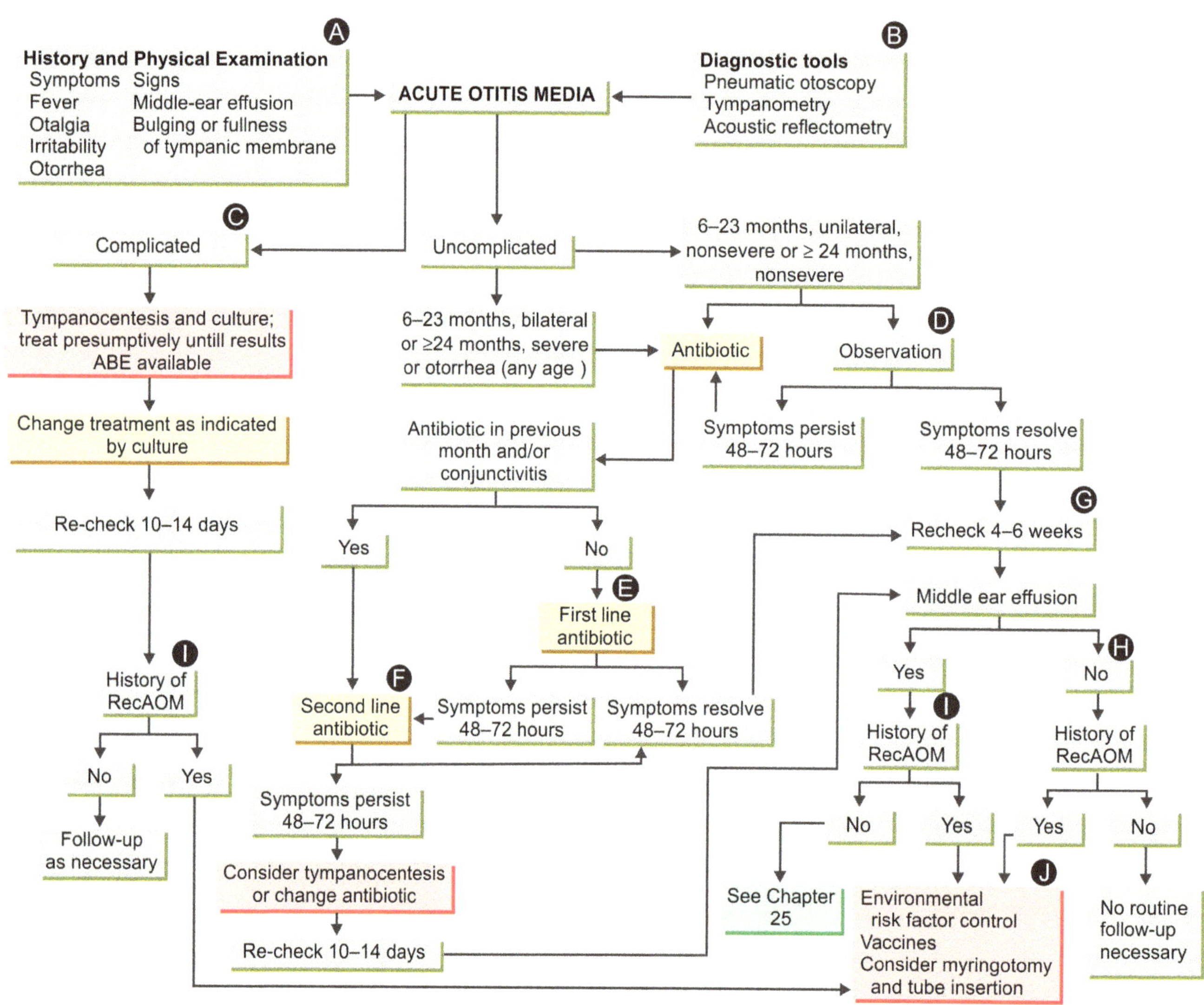

Acute otitis media (AOM) is one of the most common diseases in children and a significant indication for antibiotic and surgical treatment. It has many causes, including microbiologic, anatomic, and immunologic factors, and its treatment has been the object of intense study. As AOM is often self-limiting, treatment of AOM walks a fine line between risks and benefits.

A The definition of AOM is not uniform in the literature. Some authors require both signs and symptoms, whereas others require signs or symptoms. We define AOM by the presence of one or more symptoms and one or more signs. AOM should be distinguished from otitis media with effusion (OME) (Chapter 25).

B These tests, if abnormal, may support a finding of middle ear effusion (MEE), but they cannot distinguish between AOM and OME.

C Patients considered "complicated" include those who have persistent symptoms while on a second-line antibiotic, immune-suppressed patients, newborns, and patients who have suspected extracranial or intracranial complications. Extracranial complications include mastoiditis, petrositis, labyrinthitis, and facial paresis. Intracranial complications include meningitis, extradural abscess, subdural empyema, brain abscess, and lateral sinus thrombosis (see Chapters 27 and 35). Tympanocentesis should be considered before initiation of medical therapy to establish with certainty the diagnosis of AOM and the precise bacteriologic diagnosis. Treatment may be started based on Gram stain results until definitive information from culture and antimicrobial sensitivity is available.

D As initial management, observation may be offered to selected patients with nonsevere disease, but a mechanism must be in place for follow-up and treatment with an appropriate antibiotic if the child's condition worsens or fails to improve in 48–72 hours after onset of symptoms.

E The "first-line" antibiotic for uncomplicated AOM in a child not treated in the previous month and who does not have conjunctivitis is usually amoxicillin ("high dose," 90 mg/kg/day). If the patient is penicillin allergic but does not have a history of anaphylaxis, cefdinir (14 mg/kg/day), or cefuroxime (30 mg/kg/day) can be used. Macrolides have less efficacy against *Streptococcus pneumoniae* and *Haemophilus influenzae.*

F Second-line antibiotics include amoxicillin clavulanate (90 mg/kg/day of amoxicillin with 6.4 mg/kg/day of clavulanate) and ceftriaxone (50 mg IM or IV for 3 days).

G Even if symptoms resolve, a follow-up examination may be helpful in determining whether MEE found at a later time is residual effusion from this episode of AOM or a new effusion.

H If no MEE is present, further scheduled follow-up may not be necessary. If effusion persists, see recommendations in Chapter 25.

I Recurrent AOM (RecAOM) is usually considered to be three episodes of AOM in 6 months or four episodes in 12 months.

J Remediable environmental risk factors, such as day care attendance and exposure to tobacco smoke should be sought and discussed with the patient's parents. Pneumococcal and influenza vaccines may prevent some episodes of AOM. Myringotomy with tube insertion has been shown to be helpful in managing recurrent AOM, but adenoidectomy, with greater risks and costs, has been shown to have limited short-term efficacy and is not recommended as the first-line surgical treatment for recurrent AOM. Antimicrobial prophylaxis has demonstrated efficacy but is not recommended because of increasing bacterial resistance and is reserved for selected rare cases.

SUGGESTED READING

Bluestone CD, Klein JO. Otitis Media in Infants and Children, 4th edition. Hamilton, Ontario: BC Decker, Inc; 2007.

Hoberman A, Paradise JL, Rockette HE, et al. Treatment of acute otitis media in children under 2 years of age. N Engl J Med. 2011;364:105-115.

Lieberthal AS, Carroll AE, Chonmaitree T, et al. The diagnosis and management of acute otitis media. Pediatrics. 2013;131:e964-966.

Paradise JL, Bluestone CD, Colborn DK, et al. Adenoidectomy and adenotonsillectomy for recurrent acute otitis media. JAMA. 1999;282:945-953.

Pichichero ME. Use of selected cephalosporins in penicillin-allergic patients: a paradigm shift. Diagn Microbiol Infect Dis. 2007;57(Suppl 3):13S-18S.

Rosenfeld RM, Schwartz SR, Pynnonen MA, et al. Clinical practice guideline: Tympanostomy tubes in children. Otolaryngol Head Neck Surg. 2013;149(1 Suppl):S1-35.

Tahtinen PA, Laine MK, Huovinen P, et al. A placebo-controlled trial of antimicrobial treatment for acute otitis media. N Engl J Med. 2011;364:116-126.

Otitis Media with Effusion

Margaretha L Casselbrant, Ellen M Mandel

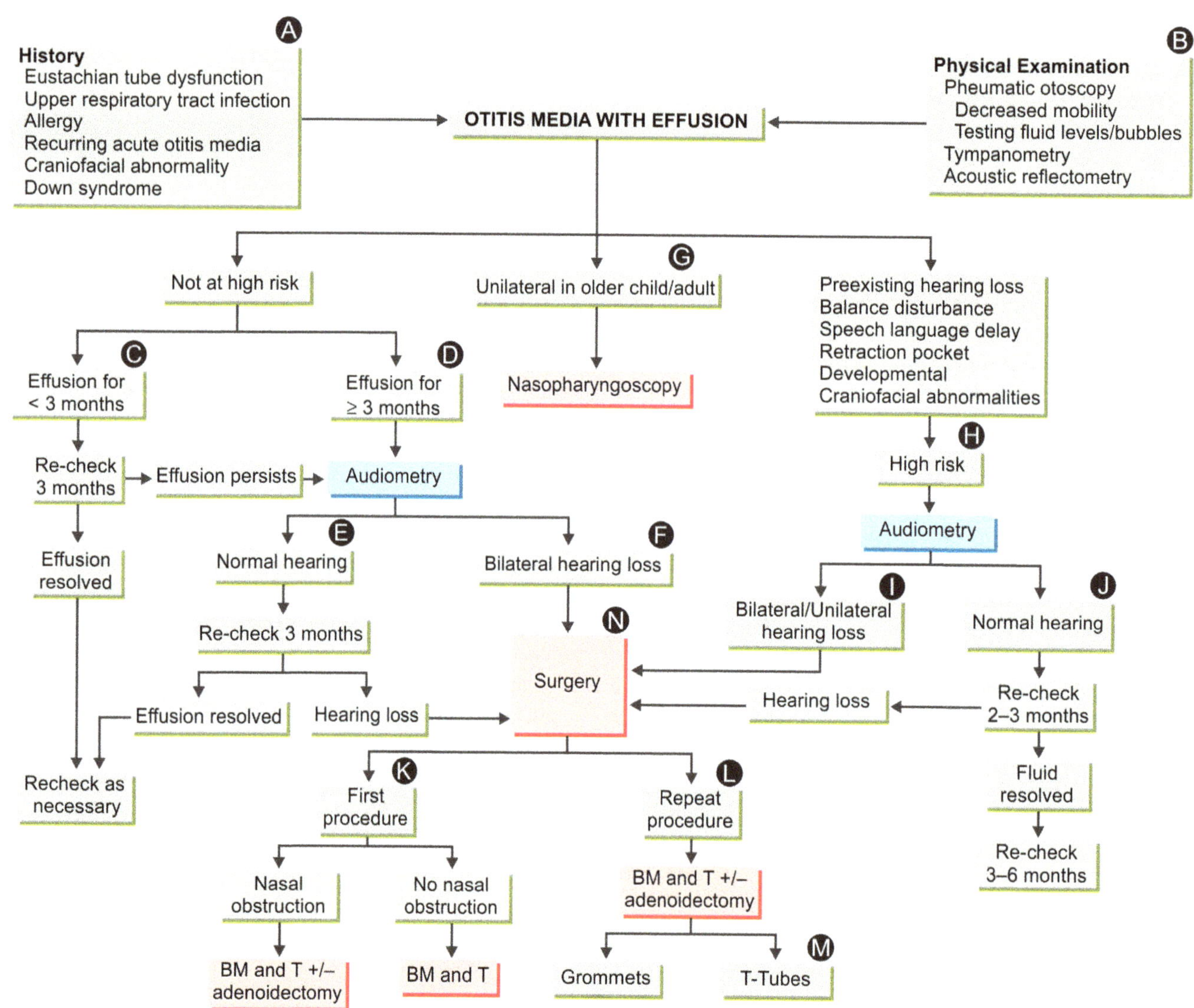

Otitis media with effusion (OME) is middle ear effusion (MEE) without signs and symptoms of infection. Its "true" incidence is difficult to determine, as it is by definition "asymptomatic" but may cause hearing loss, speech-language delay, poor school performance, balance disturbance and may affect the child's quality of life.

A The pathophysiology of OME is multifactorial with overlapping factors such as anatomical/physiological, infectious, and environmental and host-related factors. Risk factors, such as day-care attendance, absence of breastfeeding, and exposure to tobacco smoke should be discussed with the parents at the initial visit. Antibiotics, steroids, antihistamine, and/or decongestant are not indicated for the management of OME.

B Pneumatic otoscopy is the primary diagnostic method for OME, as it will allow for assessment of tympanic membrane mobility, fluid levels, and/or bubbles. Additional diagnostic tools are tympanometry and acoustic reflectometry. Audiometry may guide management but is not routine at the initial diagnosis.

C Children "not at high risk" with <3 months of MEE and no hearing loss, speech-language and balance concerns should be rechecked every 3 months until fluid resolves; if MEE persist and hearing loss and/or speech-language problems develop, audiometry is recommended.

D For children "not at high risk" with MEE for ≥3 months audiometry is recommended.

E If normal hearing is present in at least one ear and there are no speech-language problems, watchful waiting is recommended with recheck every 3 months until the fluid resolves. If at any time symptoms that are likely attributable to MEE (such as hearing loss, speech-language problems, balance difficulties, behavioral problems, poor school performance, or reduced quality of life) or structural abnormalities of the tympanic membrane or middle ear are suspected, reassessment and consideration for bilateral myringotomy and tube insertion (BM&T) with or without adenoidectomy are recommended.

F If fluid is present with documented bilateral hearing loss and/or speech-language problems are identified reassessment and consideration for surgery is indicated.

G If an older child or adult has persistent unilateral OME without a prior history of OME, it is important to exclude a nasopharyngeal tumor. Endoscopy and possibly imaging should be performed. If the work-up for tumor is negative re-enter the algorithm.

H Children at "high risk" for speech-language or learning problems caused by sensory, physical, cognitive, or behavioral factors should be promptly evaluated with audiometry, speech language evaluation, and assessed for need for intervention.

I Surgery should be recommended for "high-risk" children with bilateral/unilateral hearing loss.

J If hearing is normal and there are no speech-language or learning problems, watchful waiting with recheck every 2–3 months until fluid resolves; if hearing loss and/or speech-language problems develop, surgery is recommended.

K BM&T is recommended as a first-line procedure. Adenoidectomy should be considered only for relief of nasal obstruction resulting from adenoid hypertrophy.

L For repeat BM&T, adenoidectomy may be considered regardless of nasal symptoms. The child should be re-evaluated for risk factors and underlying comorbid conditions and need for treatment.

M Grommet-type tubes are the most commonly used type of tubes, while T-tubes may be considered if the tube is needed for a prolonged period of time or the tympanic membrane is very atrophic.

N Parents should be counseled regarding expected duration of tube function, follow-up schedule including audiometry at the first visit, as well as treatment of episodes of otorrhea and detection of complications and sequelae. Water precaution is no longer recommended except for children with recurrent episodes of otorrhea.

SUGGESTED READING

Bluestone CD, Klein JO. Otitis media and Eustachian tube dysfunction. In: Bluestone CD, Simons JP, Healey GB (Eds). Bluestone and Stool's Pediatric Otolaryngology, 5th edition. Shelton, CT: People's Medical Publishing House; 2014. pp. 633-759.

Browning GG, Rovers MM, Williamson I, et al. Grommets (ventilation tubes) for hearing loss associated with otitis media with effusion in children (review). The Cochrane Database Syst Rev. 2010;(10):1-38.

Hellström S, Groth A, Jorgensen F, et al. Ventilation tube treatment: a systematic review of the literature. Otolaryngol Head Neck Surg. 2011;145(3):383-395.

Rosenfeld RM, Schwartz SR, Pynnonen MA, et al. Clinical practice guideline: tympanostomy tubes in children. Otolaryngol Head Neck Surg. 2013;149(1 Suppl):S1-S35.

Rosenfeld RM, Shin JJ, Schwartz SR, et al. Clinical practice guideline: otitis media with effusion. Otolaryngol Head Neck Surg 2016;154(1 Suppl):S1-S41.

Ryan D Walker, Margaret A Kenna

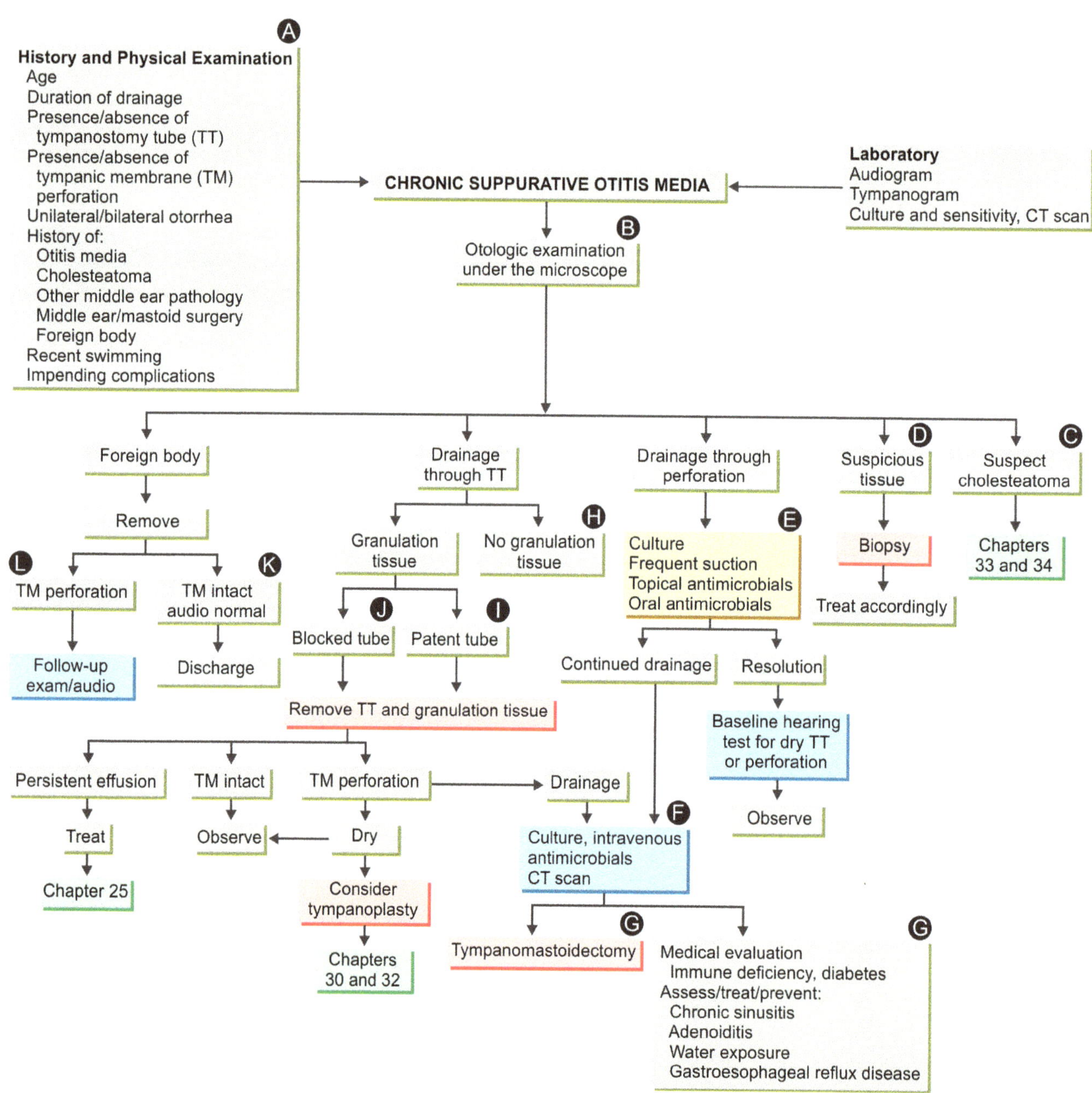

Chronic suppurative otitis media (CSOM) may occur in both children and adults. By definition, CSOM involves drainage through a non-intact tympanic membrane (TM) [tympanostomy tube (TT) or perforation]. Although the World Health Organization definition requires only 2 weeks of otorrhea, most Otolaryngologists and publications discussing about CSOM use a definition of at least 6 weeks of otorrhea unresponsive to medical therapy. Although the treatment algorithm is approximately the same for both children and adults, duration of treatment and consideration of alternative diagnoses other than straightforward CSOM may vary with age.

A Historical elements that should specifically be elicited include otologic history, particularly a history of TTs or other ear surgery, and signs or symptoms of intracranial complications such as severe headache, fever, visual changes, mental status changes, or abnormal neurologic examination. If there is any concern about an impending intracranial complication of otitis media (OM), please refer to Chapter 35.

B Otologic microscopic examination is indicated to evaluate for a foreign body (FB), cholesteatoma, abnormal tissue, and the presence or absence of a TT. Abnormal tissue, including granulation tissue, polyps, or any other abnormal appearing tissue arising from the TM, middle ear, or the external auditory canal (EAC), may suggest the presence of a retraction pocket, cholesteatoma, or FB.

C If cholesteatoma is suspected by the degree of hearing loss or the physical presence of squamous debris involving the middle ear or external auditory meatus, see the discussion of cholesteatoma in Chapters 33 and 34. Cholesteatoma, either acquired or congenital, should always be considered, especially in the absence of a recent history of OM and when the drainage is unilateral. Computed tomography (CT) scan of the temporal bones, assessing for bone erosion, may help determine whether cholesteatoma is present. In cases of diagnostic uncertainty, particularly in the postoperative ear, magnetic resonance imaging (MRI) with diffusion-weighted imaging can be useful to differentiate cholesteatoma from postsurgical changes or other soft tissue.

D Neoplasms of the middle ear and EAC such as Langerhans cell histiocytosis, rhabdomyosarcoma, leukemia, squamous cell carcinoma, and salivary gland tumors—though uncommon—should be considered when there is minimal or no history of OM before the onset of drainage and the drainage does not respond promptly to standard therapy (ototopical drops or culture guided systemic or topical therapy). Older age and a normal contralateral ear examination should raise added concern for a neoplastic process. If OM seems less likely based on history, physical examination, and/or audiogram, a CT or MRI of the temporal bone is indicated. Biopsy should be performed if there is suspicion for a neoplastic process.

E Middle ear drainage often persists because the antimicrobial (topical or systemic) initially chosen was not effective for the bacteria or fungus present. Common causes of intractable otorrhea include *Pseudomonas, Staphylococcus aureus,* and fungal species. Frequent suctioning of the EAC and TT provides mechanical removal of otorrhea, allowing topical antimicrobials access to the EAC and middle ear. Culture-directed therapy or empiric therapy covering these organisms will typically provide adequate treatment.

F If the middle ear continues to drain after appropriate topical and oral antimicrobials, repeat culture of the otorrhea and intravenous antimicrobials should be considered. If a CT scan of the temporal bone has not been obtained, it should be at this point to look for bone erosion or other abnormalities. Removal of a TT (if present) at this point may be effective in stopping the drainage, although this is less likely if the drainage is coming mainly from the middle ear, is constant, and is not associated with granulation tissue attached to the TT.

G If drainage persists after appropriate intravenous and topical antimicrobials then tympanomastoidectomy should be considered. Local causes of continued drainage include occult cholesteatoma, aditus block, fungal or other less common infectious organisms, and neoplasm. Systemic medical problems that may contribute to ongoing CSOM include immune deficiency, diabetes, and immotile cilia. Other potential aggravating factors—especially in children—include chronic sinusitis, adenoiditis, water exposure, and nasopharyngeal reflux of gastric contents with gastroesophageal reflux disorder.

H In a child with a TT/perforation and a strong history of OM, otorrhea for several weeks is not rare. Topical fluoroquinolone antibiotics should be used as the first-line therapy to avoid ototoxicity.

I Granulation tissue is not an uncommon reaction to the presence of a TT (similar to a FB reaction). If the TT is not functional, it should be removed, along with any associated granulation tissue. If, after the TT is removed, the TM is intact, then further management depends on whether there is OM with effusion or not. If the TM is not intact but dry, observation is appropriate. In older children with a dry perforation and no evidence of ongoing Eustachian tube dysfunction, tympanoplasty could be considered.

J Granulation tissue associated with a TT will often resolve if appropriate topical antimicrobials, or antimicrobial/steroid combination, are used. If this is not successful, removal of the TT often results in cessation of otorrhea (especially, if the otorrhea was coming mainly from the TT and not from the middle ear).

K A FB, if found, should be removed. If the TM and EAC are normal and intact and hearing is normal, follow-up can be as needed.

L If a FB is removed but there is a residual TM perforation, laceration of the EAC, or both, then the patient should be followed to resolution of their injury. Some practitioners may consider the use of steroid-containing topical antibiotic drops to treat significant swelling or epithelial injury. The hearing should be checked once healing is complete to confirm that there has been no ossicular disruption or other change in hearing.

SUGGESTED READING

Acuin J. (2004). Chronic Suppurative Otitis media: Burden of Illness and Management Options. World Health Organization. [online] Available from: http://www.who.int/pbd/publications/chronic-suppurativeotitis_media.pdf

Bluestone CD, Chi DH, Klein JO. Complications and sequelae of otitis media. In: Bluestone CD, Simons JP, Healy GB (Eds). Pediatric Otolaryngology, 5th edition. Shelton CT: People's Medical Publishing House; 2014; pp. 761-847.

Bluestone CD, Klein JO. Otitis media and eustachian tube dysfunction. In: Bluestone CD, Simons JP, Healy GB (Eds). Pediatric Otolaryngology, 5th edition. Shelton CT: People's Medical Publishing House; 2014; pp. 633-759.

Daniel SJ, Kozak FK, Fabian MC, et al. Guidelines for the treatment of tympanostomy tube otorrhea. J Otolaryngol. 2005;34(Suppl 2):S60-63.

Kenna MA. Otitis media and the new guidelines. J Otolaryngol. 2005;34(Suppl 1):S24-32.

Kenna MA, Rosane B, Bluestone CD. Update on medical management of chronic suppurative otitis media. Am J Otol. 1993;14:469-473.

Rosenfeld RM, Culpepper L, Doyle KJ, et al. Clinical practice guideline: otitis media with effusion. Otolaryngol Head Neck Surg. 2004;130(5 Suppl):S95-118.

van der Veen EL, Schilder AG, van Heerbeek N, et al. Predictors of chronic suppurative otitis media in children. Arch Otolaryngol Head Neck Surg. 2006;132(10):1115-1118.

van Egmond SL, Stegeman I, Grolman W, et al. A systematic review of non-echo planar diffusion-weighted magnetic resonance imaging for detection of primary and postoperative cholesteatoma. Otorhinolaryng Head Neck Surg. 2016;154(2):233-240.

Wasson JD, Yung MW. Evidence-based management of otitis media: a 5S model approach. J Laryngol Otol. 2015;129(2):112-119.

Extracranial Complications of Otitis Media

Sancak Yuksel

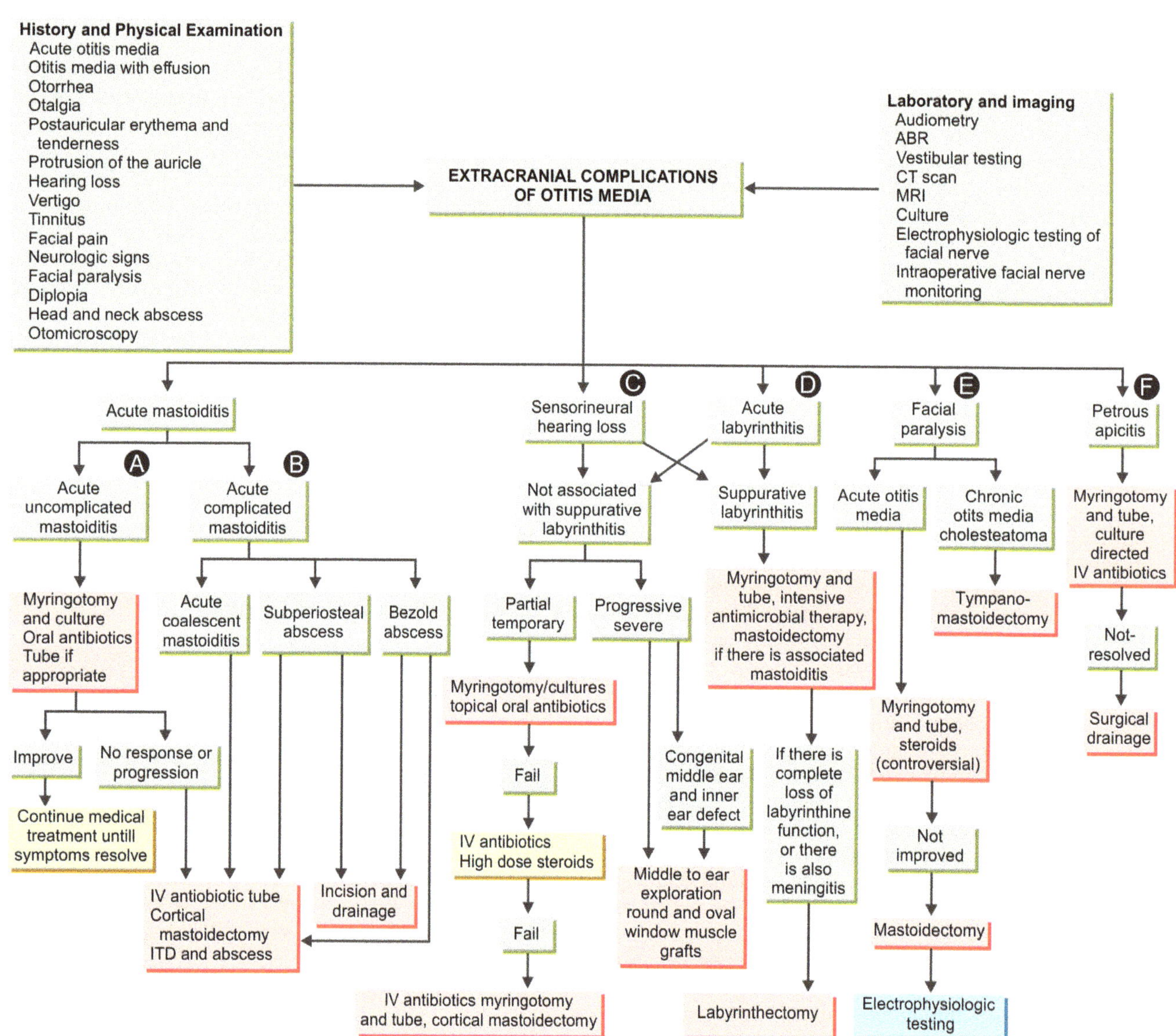

Acute otitis media (AOM) remains one of the most frequent diseases of early infancy and childhood. Despite the widespread use of antibiotics, complications and sequelae of otitis media (OM) are still prevalent and remain potentially life-threatening and morbid. There are intracranial and extracranial complications of OM. This chapter focuses on the extracranial complications of AOM. Chronic conditions such as cholesteatoma or chronic OM and sequelae such as conductive hearing loss, adhesive OM or fixation or disarticulation of the ossicles are emphasized elsewhere in this book. Extracranial complications of AOM include mastoiditis, subperiosteal abscess, Bezold's abscess, acute sensorineural hearing loss (ASNHL), acute labyrinthitis, acute facial paralysis, and petrous apicitis.

A Acute uncomplicated mastoiditis (mastoiditis without periostitis/osteitis) is an extension of effusion or purulent exudate due to OM into the mastoid air cells and it is not strictly a complication. Management is identical to standard treatment options when AOM or OM with effusion is present and the status of the mastoid is unknown. If there are signs of progression such as postauricular swelling, erythema, tenderness, and protrusion of the auricle, it should be treated as a complicated mastoiditis. If an acute complicated mastoiditis is suspected, a computed tomography (CT) scan should be obtained.

B Acute complicated mastoiditis, termed acute coalescent mastoiditis, is a progression of AOM with osteitis. Classic signs and symptoms such as fever, otalgia, protrusion of the pinna, postauricular erythema, and tenderness are present in this stage. A subperiosteal abscess is present if purulent exudate accumulates under the mastoid periosteum. If the infection extends into the neck along with the sternocleidomastoid muscle, it indicates the presence of a Bezold's abscess that usually presents with neck pain and fluctuant neck mass along the anterior and posterior boundary of the muscle. Management in this stage consists of intravenous antibiotic therapy, insertion of a tympanostomy tube, and cortical mastoidectomy. The abscess requires incision and drainage. Some authors suggest that incision and drainage without a mastoidectomy may also be sufficient.

C Identification of ASNHL is important in AOM as many patients will already have conductive hearing loss due to purulent secretions in the middle ear and thickening of the tympanic membrane due to inflammation. A tuning fork should be used in the acute setting until a formal audiogram is obtained. Once ASNHL is diagnosed a CT scan should be done. It could be due to either serous or suppurative labyrinthitis. Dysequilibrium or vertigo may or may not be present. If hearing loss is temporary or partial, myringotomy with cultures is performed and the patient is treated with topical and oral antibiotic. If hearing loss is progressive and/or there is a congenital cochleolabyrinthine defect, an exploration of oval and round windows and repair with muscle grafts should be performed.

D Acute labyrinthitis should be suspected if a patient with AOM develops vertigo and SNHL. It could be either serous or suppurative labyrinthitis. In serous labyrinthitis, endotoxins and by-products of infection enter the inner ear and symptoms are partial and often reversible. It could be managed as described in Step D when SNHL is mild or not progressive. Suppurative labyrinthitis occurs if bacteria also invade the inner ear and it requires an aggressive approach. An audiogram and auditory brainstem response will be performed, CT of the temporal bone and brain are important to determine whether there is another suppurative complication or congenital cochlear anomaly. Intensive antimicrobial therapy is initiated and a tympanostomy tube is placed. If acute mastoiditis is present, a cortical mastoidectomy should also be performed. In the antibiotic era, indications for opening the labyrinth for drainage are very few. Labyrinthectomy should be performed only if there is complete loss of labyrinthine function or if the infection has spread to the meninges despite antibiotic therapy.

E Acute facial paralysis may develop during/after an AOM likely due to infection entering the Fallopian canal and causing edema and pressure injury to the nerve. An immediate tympanocentesis is required for cultures and a tympanostomy tube is placed. Steroids are initiated even though it is controversial. Computed tomography of the temporal bone and brain are usually obtained. If there is no improvement, mastoidectomy is indicated to drain the mastoid infection. Facial nerve decompression in this setting is controversial and usually not recommended.

F If a patient with AOM develops retro-orbital pain, otorrhea and esotropia due to abducens palsy, an acute petrositis or petrous apicitis is suspected. This is termed Gradenigo's syndrome. The pain is in the distribution of the ophthalmic division of cranial nerve V. A CT scan of the temporal bone should be obtained, systemic antibiotics should be initiated, and myringotomy with placement of a pressure equalizing tube should be performed. If the patient fails to improve, surgical drainage via either transmastoid or middle fossa approach should be performed.

SUGGESTED READING

Bluestone CD. Clinical course, complications and sequelae of acute otitis media. Pediatr Infect Dis J. 2000;19:S37-46.

Bluestone CD. Suppurative complications. In: Rosenfeld RM, Bluestone CD (Eds). Evidence Based Otitis Media, 2nd edition. Hamilton, Ontario: BC Decker Inc; 2003. p. 494.

Bluestone CD, Klein JO. Definitions, terminology and classification. In: Bluestone CD, Klein JO (Eds). Otitis Media in Infants and Children, 4th edition. Hamilton, Ontario: BC Decker Inc; 2007. pp. 6-10.

Hellstrom S. Tympanic membrane perforation. In: Alper CM, Bluestone CD, Casselbrant ML, et al. (Eds). Advanced Therapy of Otitis Media. Hamilton, Ontario: BC Decker Inc; 2004. pp. 382-385.

Kumar A, Wiet R. Aural complications of otitis media. In: Gulya AJ, Minor LB, Poe DS (Eds). Glasscock-Shambaugh Surgery of the Ear, 6th edition. Shelton, CT: People's Medical Publishing House—USA; 2010. pp. 437-440.

Pang LHY, Barakete MS, Havas TE. Mastoiditis in a pediatric population: a review of 11 years' experience in management. Int J Pediatr Otolaryngol. 2009;73:1520-1524.

Quinton G. Middle ear and mastoid. In: Gopen G (Ed). Fundamental Otology, Pediatric and Adult Practice. Philadelphia, PA: JP Brothers; 2013. pp. 105-108.

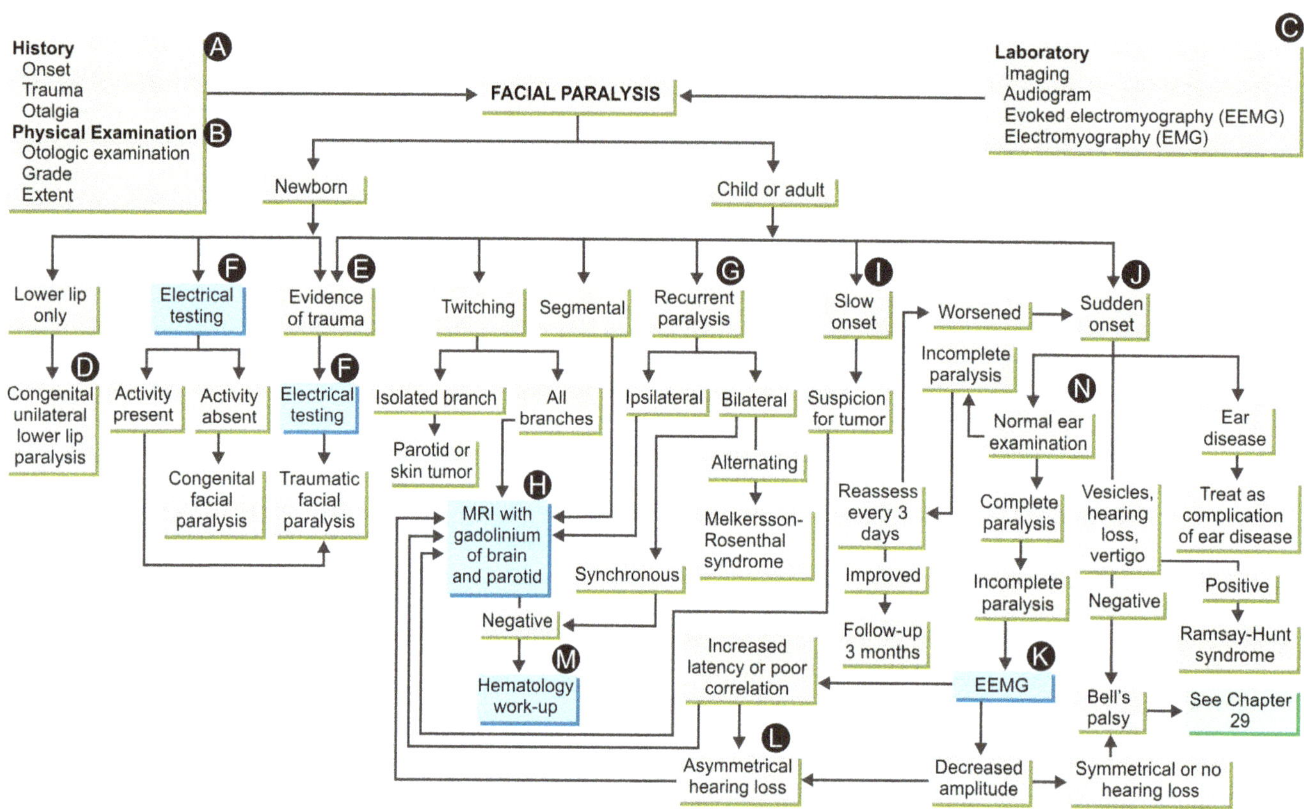

Peripheral facial paralysis (FP) remains a diagnostic challenge. This algorithm cannot be all-inclusive but is a reminder of Terence Cawthorne's epigram "All that palsies is not Bell's." The tortuous course of the facial nerve gives rise to a wide variety of disorders that can lead to paresis or paralysis.

A The most important features of the history are the timing of the paralysis, presence of recurrent paralysis, and a history of malignancy. In the latter case, early imaging is essential with preference for magnetic resonance imaging (MRI) of the brain and parotid gland. Bilateral FP has its own short diagnostic list. May's' Table 4-1 in The Facial Nerve offers a more complete differential diagnosis.

B On physical examination, the finding of vesicles, facial twitching, or a palpable mass near the extratemporal facial nerve is most critical. All patients with FP should be given topical eye care to avoid exposure keratitis.

C The use of appropriate testing is logically driven by the history.

D Congenital unilateral paralysis of the lip is sometimes associated with other congenital malformations (e.g. 22q11 syndromes).

E Battle's sign, hemotympanum, and computed tomography (CT) evidence of temporal bone fracture are keys to making the diagnosis. Treatment decisions often depend upon whether the onset of paralysis was immediate or delayed.

F In patients with a traumatic FP, responses on needle electromyography (EMG) will be present initially if the nerve is intact but may be lost over the first 3 days due to Wallerian degeneration. Similarly, the amplitude of the evoked EEG (EEMG, also called electroneurography or ENoG) may start at a high level and then be lost over the first 3–5 days with traumatic FP. Congenital FP will have no decay of the initial electrical response over time.

G In patients with recurrent ipsilateral paralysis, investigation should always be undertaken for the possibility of a tumor of the facial nerve, most commonly schwannoma or osseous hemangioma. However, the vast majority of patients actually have a recurrent Bell's palsy. One in 10 patients with Bell's palsy will have recurrence, although two-thirds of these will be on the contralateral side.

H The MRI with contrast must include the brain stem and the parotid gland to rule out neoplasm. If an intraparotid lesion is identified or suspected, ultrasonography with fine-needle aspiration biopsy is an alternative diagnostic modality. The MRI of the brain may demonstrate T2 hyperintensities, a finding with its own broad differential diagnosis including multiple sclerosis.

I The time course of FP, although helpful, is not always able to differentiate tumor from other causes, although the algorithm does display it that way. Slow progression is usually defined as patients who continue to lose function beyond 3 weeks. Bell's palsy, blunt trauma, and even surgical trauma can progress over 10 days, which is not considered slow progression. Only 60% of patients with Bell's palsy present with a sudden complete paralysis. Slowly progressive FP has been seen in 60% of 197 patients with tumors. One-third of patients with acoustic neuroma and 17% of patients with cancer of the head and neck who had FP before treatment reported sudden onset.

J Examination of the ear will direct the algorithm to other chapters dealing specifically with the management of these conditions simultaneous with FP. A red chorda tympani, although not diagnostic, when seen suggests a viral cause, either Bell's palsy or herpes zoster oticus (Ramsay-Hunt syndrome).

K Patients with complete paralysis should undergo an evoked EMG (EEMG), which helps to assess the likelihood of recovery based on the amplitude of the responses. Preservation of 10–25% amplitude on the involved side, compared to the normal side, gives a 70% chance of a good outcome (House-Brackmann III or better). Less than 10% of the normal-side response carries a poor prognosis for good recovery. Standard EMG can provide diagnostic information: increased response latency suggests neoplasm, and further work-up should be directed toward this differential.

L Patients who have a mass in the cerebellopontine angle frequently present with an asymmetrical hearing loss in addition to facial nerve symptoms. Herpes zoster oticus not infrequently affects hearing and may present with vestibular symptoms as well.

M Hematologic evaluation should include CRP (C-reactive protein)/ESR (erythrocyte sedimentation rate), ANCA (antineutrophil cytoplasmic antibodies), ACE (angiotensin converting enzyme), RF (rheumatoid factor), ANA (antinuclear antibodies), SSA (anti-Sjögren's-syndrome-related antigen A)/SSB, FTA-ABS (fluorescent treponemal antibody-absorption)/VDRL (venereal disease research laboratory test), TSH (thyroid stimulating hormone), glucose, CBC (complete blood count), antiphospholipid antibodies, and porphyrobilinogen. Negative serologies, if accompanied by negative MRI and low likelihood of malignancy by history, warrant serial clinical follow-up every 6 months, with contrast-enhanced CT of the temporal bone and parotid gland if facial function continues to worsen. However, patients at high risk for malignancy should undergo positron emission tomography (PET)/CT and consideration of facial nerve biopsy.

N Lyme titer and empiric treatment may be prudent based on history for those living in an endemic location.

SUGGESTED READING

Guntinas-Lichius O, Schaitkin BM. Facial Nerve Disorders and Diseases: Diagnosis and Management. New York: Thieme; 2015.

Hohman MH, Hadlock TA. Etiology, diagnosis, and management of facial palsy: 2000 patients at a facial nerve center. Laryngoscope. 2014;124:E283-293.

Rioja-Mazza D, Lieber E, Kamath V, et al. Asymmetric crying facies: a possible marker for congenital malformations. J Matern Fetal Neonatal Med. 2005;18(4):275-277.

Schaitkin BM, May M. The Facial Nerve. New York: Thieme; 1999.

Facial Paralysis—Bell's Palsy

Elizabeth Toh

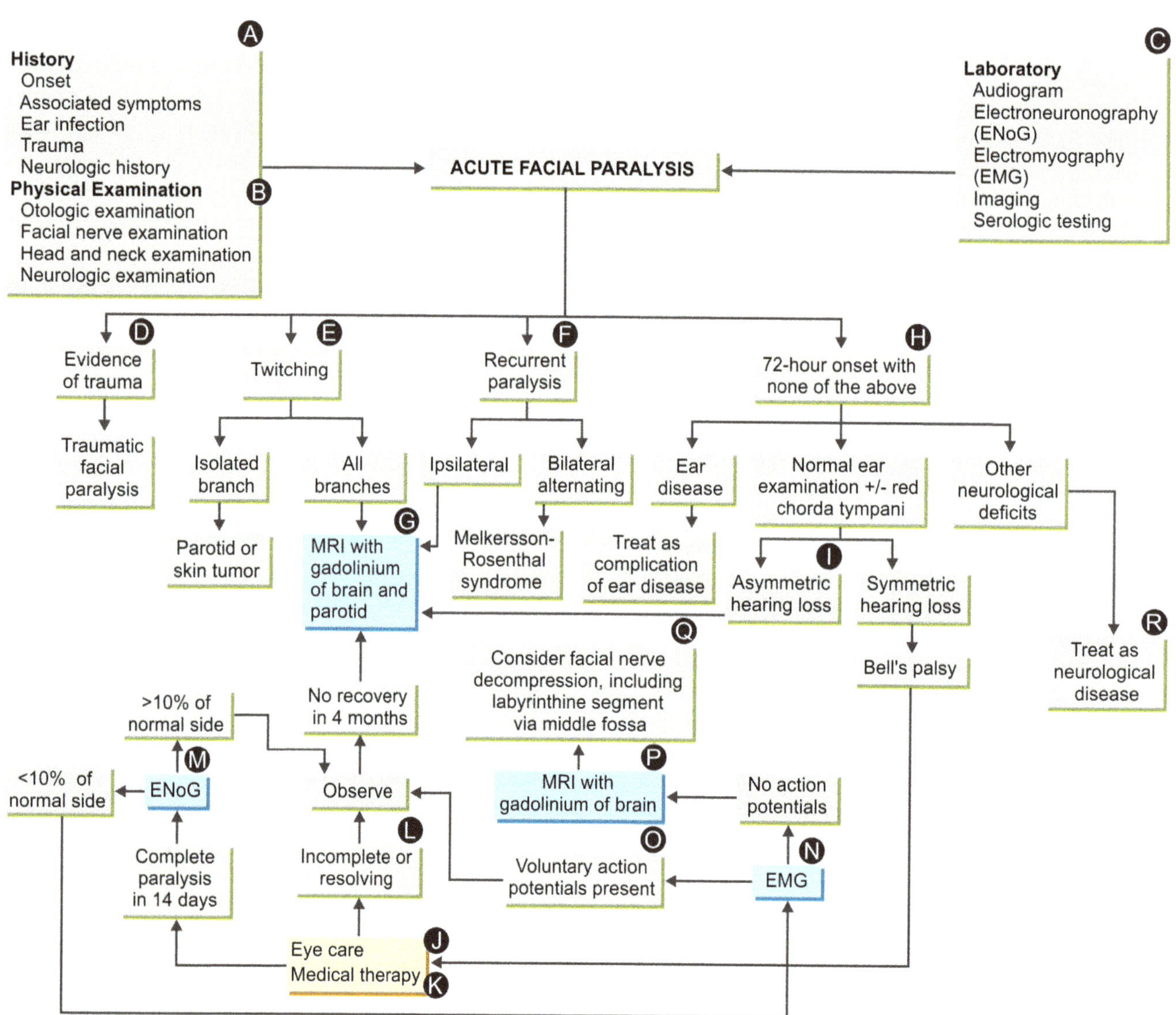

Bell's palsy is a diagnosis of exclusion and remains the most common cause of acute facial paralysis. Current literature suggests the role of herpes simplex virus reactivation as the etiology for what was historically considered an idiopathic disease. A thorough history, physical examination, and testing are necessary in order to exclude other causes. This algorithm focuses on acute onset facial paralysis.

A Key features in the history are onset, progression, extent, recurrence, and associated symptoms. Onset in Bell's palsy occurs within 72 hours and does not progress beyond 2 weeks. Otalgia or retroauricular pain is experienced in over 50% of Bell's palsy patients and may precede the onset of paralysis. Other associated symptoms may include hyperacusis and dysgeusia. Hearing loss, dizziness, and otorrhea are not usually reported.

B On physical examination, unilateral involvement of all branches of the facial nerve should be evident in Bell's palsy. Facial function should be graded and tracked over the course of time to help prognosticate recovery and guide management. The ear should be examined to exclude vesicular lesions, otitis media, cholesteatoma, and tumors of the temporal bone. The remainder of the physical examination should focus on excluding any masses along the extratemporal course of the facial nerve or accompanying neurological deficits.

C An audiogram should be obtained on all patients with acute onset facial palsy. Additional testing is logically driven by the patient's history.

D Clinical signs of temporal bone trauma including hemotympanum, laceration of the ear canal, and Battle's sign associated with a history of trauma and computed tomography evidence of temporal bone fracture support a traumatic etiology.

E Suspect underlying tumor of the facial nerves, when hyperkinesis is associated with facial weakness.

F In patients with recurrent ipsilateral paralysis, investigation should always be undertaken to exclude the possibility of a tumor of the facial nerve, most commonly schwannoma or osseous hemangioma. However, the vast majority of patients actually have recurrent Bell's palsy. Bell's palsy may recur in up to 15% of patients although contralateral recurrence is more common (two-thirds of recurrences).

G A gadolinium-enhanced magnetic resonance imaging (MRI) of the brain and parotid is the imaging study of choice for evaluating the facial nerve in the absence of trauma or abnormal ear examination. Routine MRI is not recommended for Bell's palsy unless no functional recovery is noted 4 months after onset of paralysis. Segmental enhancement of the perigeniculate facial nerve is seen on MRI in Bell's palsy.

H In the majority of patients with Bell's palsy facial weakness peaks within 72 hours but may sometimes continue to progress over 10–14 days. Approximately 70% of patients with Bell's palsy present with a sudden complete paralysis. Physical examination readily differentiates Bell's palsy from other causes of acute paralysis with a similar time course. The algorithm for management of other conditions causing acute facial paralysis is discussed in Chapter 28. A red chorda tympani, while not diagnostic, is suggestive of a viral etiology such as Bell's palsy or herpes zoster oticus.

I Hearing asymmetry correlating to the affected side of the face is suspicious for a retrocochlear tumor. A gadolinium-enhanced MRI of the brain is indicated when asymmetric sensorineural hearing loss is detected. Herpes zoster oticus may also cause sensorineural hearing loss.

J Eye care is critical to prevent exposure keratitis and corneal ulceration. This can be accomplished with natural tear drops during the day and combining an ocular lubricant ointment at night with a moisture chamber. Taping of the eyelids should be avoided due to the risk of corneal abrasion. If the paralysis is determined to be long term then an upper eyelid weight may be indicated. Alternatively, if dry eye symptoms are bothersome, temporary upper eyelid weights may be applied externally. Complaints of eye discomfort or visual signs of eye irritation should prompt an ophthalmology consultation for inspection of the cornea.

K Medical therapy for Bell's palsy consists of systemic steroids administered over 7–10 days. Oral antiviral therapy in combination with steroids is controversial but may offer improved outcomes if administered within 72 hours after onset.

L Patients with incomplete facial paralysis have a 98% likelihood of a good outcome in Bell's palsy.

M Electrical testing is indicated only if paralysis is complete since all incomplete paralysis will recover well. Electroneurography (ENoG) is performed within the first 2 weeks after onset of complete paralysis. Patients who have over 10% preservation of the action potential amplitude on ENoG on the affected side will have a 70% likelihood of a good outcome (House–Brackmann grades I–II). Patients with a <10% ENoG response compared to the normal side have a poor prognosis for functional recovery and may be considered potential candidates for facial nerve decompression.

N Due to loss of neural synchrony during neural regeneration, ENoG alone may overestimate the extent of injury. The absence of motor unit action potentials (MUAPs) within the first 2 weeks confirms absence of neural regeneration and poor prognosis. After 2 weeks, EMG (electromyography) testing is valuable for prognosticating recovery. Spontaneous fibrillation potentials indicate severe muscle denervation and is prognostic for incomplete recovery. Polyphasic action potentials with voluntary facial contraction signal muscle reinnervation and favor functional recovery.

O The presence of voluntary MUAPs indicates neural regeneration that favors spontaneous recovery of function. Surgical decompression is not indicated in these patients.

P Gadolinium-enhanced MRI of the brain with attention to the internal auditory canals is used to guide possible surgical decompression of the facial nerve.

Q Surgical decompression of the facial nerve for Bell's palsy remains controversial. There is limited medical evidence to support decompression of the meatal foramen and labyrinthine segment using a middle fossa craniotomy approach when electrodiagnostic criteria are met within the first 14 days after onset of complete paralysis (ENoG < 10% normal side and absence of voluntary MUAPs). If hearing is poor on the affected side, a translabyrinthine approach may be used.

R Consider serologic testing (angiotensin converting enzyme test lyme titers, syphilis titers) in recurrent ipsilateral palsy, bilateral palsy, contralateral paralysis and multiple cranial neuropathies.

SUGGESTED READING

Axelsson S, Berg T, Jonsson L, et al. Bell's palsy-the effect of prednisolone and/or valacyclovir versus placebo in relation to baseline severity in a randomized controlled trial. Clin Otolaryngol. 2012;37:283-290.

Berg T, Bylund N, Marsk E, et al. The effect of prednisolone on sequelae in Bell's palsy. Arch Otolaryngol Head Neck Surg. 2012;138(5):445-449.

Engstrom M, Berg T, Stjernquist-Desatnik A, et al. Prednisolone and valaciclovir in Bell's palsy: a randomized, double-blind, placebo-controlled, multicenter trial. Lancet Neurol. 2008;7:993-1000.

Gantz BJ, Rubenstein JT, Gidley P, et al. Surgical management of Bell's palsy. Laryngoscope. 1999;109(8):1177-1188.

Gronseth GS, Paduga R. Evidence-based guideline update: steroids and antivirals for Bell's palsy: report of the Guideline Development Subcommittee of the American Academy of Neurology. Neurology. 2012;79:2209-2213.

Murakami S, Mizobuchi M, Nakashiro Y, et al. Bell's palsy and herpes simplex virus: identification of viral DNA in endoneurial fluid and muscle. Ann Intern Med. 1996;127:27-30.

Peitersen E. Bell's palsy: the spontaneous course of 2,500 peripheral facial nerve palsies of different etiologies. Acta Otolaryngol Suppl. 2002;549:4-30.

Sullivan FM, Swan IRC, Donnan PT, et al. Early treatment with prednisolone or acyclovir in Bell's palsy. N Engl J Med. 2007;357:1598-1607.

Sequelae of Chronic Otitis Media

Douglas A Chen

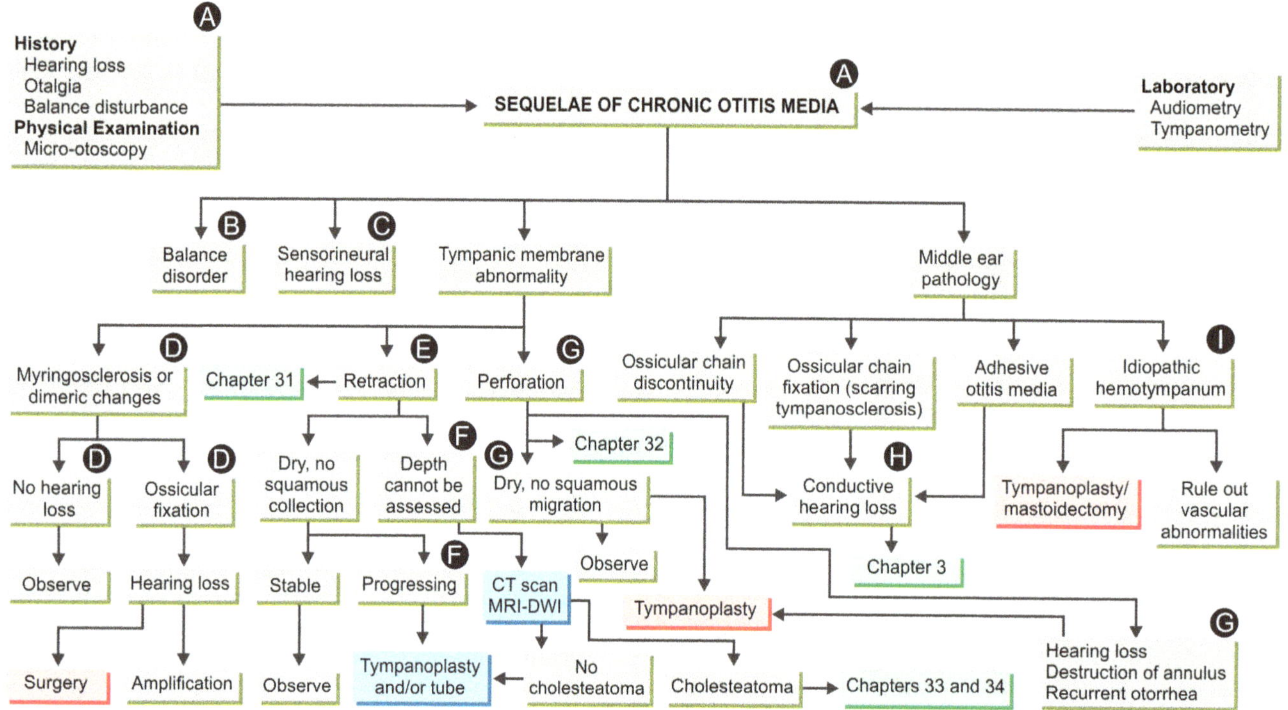

Categorization of long-standing inflammatory changes of the middle ear, mastoid and Eustachian tubes can be helpful. "Active" chronic otitis media implies that there is an ongoing process, the most common being purulent discharge. This is also known as chronic "suppurative" otitis media. The term "inactive" implies that a previously active process has resolved and probably will not recur. The resultant damage to the ear in the inactive state is also known as "sequelae" of chronic otitis media. A "quiescent" state implies that there is a recurrent nature to the inflammatory process, with possible progression of the sequelae.

A The sequelae typically are the symptoms about which the patient complains. Physical examination requires otomicroscopy with suction and palpation.

B Sequelae of chronic otitis media related to the inner ear are rare, but do exist. Balance disorders can occur, especially if chronic otitis media is active. Fistula formation, labyrinthitis, and ototoxicity from topical antibiotics are all possible causes.

C Sensorineural hearing loss has been related to chronic otitis media. The pathogenesis is thought to be related to the spread of inflammation through the round window membrane.

D Changes in the tympanic membrane are the most common sequelae of chronic otitis media. Myringosclerosis and dimeric changes of the tympanic membrane rarely produce symptoms such as hearing loss. Most of these changes do not require treatment. Rarely dense myringosclerosis can fix the malleus and produce conductive hearing loss, which is treatable with surgery or amplification.

E Retraction pockets of the tympanic membrane can occur in the pars tensa or flaccida. Varying degrees of retraction exist from very shallow pockets in which the limits can be seen, to deep pockets in which there is bone erosion and collection of squamous debris. A grading system for pars flaccida retraction has been described by Sade: grade I, shallow pocket; grade II, pocket that is adherent to the neck of the malleus; grade III, adhesion to the neck of the malleus with some erosion of the scutum; grade IV, adhesion to the neck of the malleus, erosion of the scutum, and collection of keratin.

F In general, as long as the pocket is dry and not collecting squamous debris, and the limits can be seen on otomicroscopy, periodic observation is appropriate. Retraction pockets in which the limits cannot be visualized may require further evaluation with computed tomography. Magnetic resonance imaging (MRI) with diffusion-weighted imaging (MRI–DWI) technique has recently been shown to be helpful for the evaluation of cholesteatoma. Many a dry, clean retraction pocket will progress and begin collecting squamous debris, and will ultimately become a cholesteatoma. These enlarging shallow pockets should be prophylactically treated with tympanoplasty or myringotomy with tube insertion to prevent cholesteatoma formation or ossicular chain damage, even in the absence of symptoms such as drainage or hearing loss.

G Perforations of the tympanic membrane are generally classified as total, inferior, anterior, or posterior. They can also be described as either central (with preservation of the annulus and without migration of epithelium through the perforation) or marginal (with destruction of the annulus and potential for ingrowth of keratinizing epithelium). Dry perforations in which there is no evidence of squamous migration into the middle ear can be managed conservatively without surgery. Alternatively, perforations can be treated surgically to prevent reinfection or to eliminate conductive hearing loss even if relatively asymptomatic. Those patients who decline surgery should observe water precautions or use ear plugs.

H Most disease of the ossicular chain or middle ear occurs in conjunction with abnormalities of the tympanic membrane. However, in many cases, conductive hearing loss may occur in the absence of either significant history or changes in the tympanic membrane. Consequently, the true nature of the ossicular chain problem, either erosion or fixation, may not be known until surgery. Consequently, otosclerosis must be considered in the differential diagnosis in this setting.

I Idiopathic hemotympanum is also known as cholesterol granuloma. Clinically, the tympanic membrane has a blue appearance. The condition must be differentiated from vascular abnormalities of the middle ear such as a dehiscent jugular bulb and glomus tumor. Cholesterol granuloma is composed of chronic granulation with foreign body giant cells in the middle ear and mastoid. Clinically, the fluid is thick and brown like motor oil. Treatment is tympanoplasty and mastoidectomy.

SUGGESTED READING

Paparella MM, Oda M, Hiraide F, et al. Pathology of sensorineural hearing loss in otitis media. Ann Otol Rhinol Laryngol. 1972;81:632-647.

Sade J, Fuchs C, Kuntz M. Shrapnell's membrane and mastoid pneumatization. Arch Otolaryngol Head Neck Surg. 1997;123:584-588.

Schwartz KM, Lane N, Bolster BD, et al. The utility of diffusion weighted imaging for cholesteatoma evaluation. Am J Neuroradiol. 2011;32:430-436.

Sheehy JL, Linthicum FH, Greenfield EC. Chronic serous mastoiditis, idiopathic hemotympanum and cholesterol granuloma of the mastoid. Laryngoscope. 1969;79:1189-1217.

Tympanic Membrane Retraction and Retraction Pockets

Cuneyt M Alper

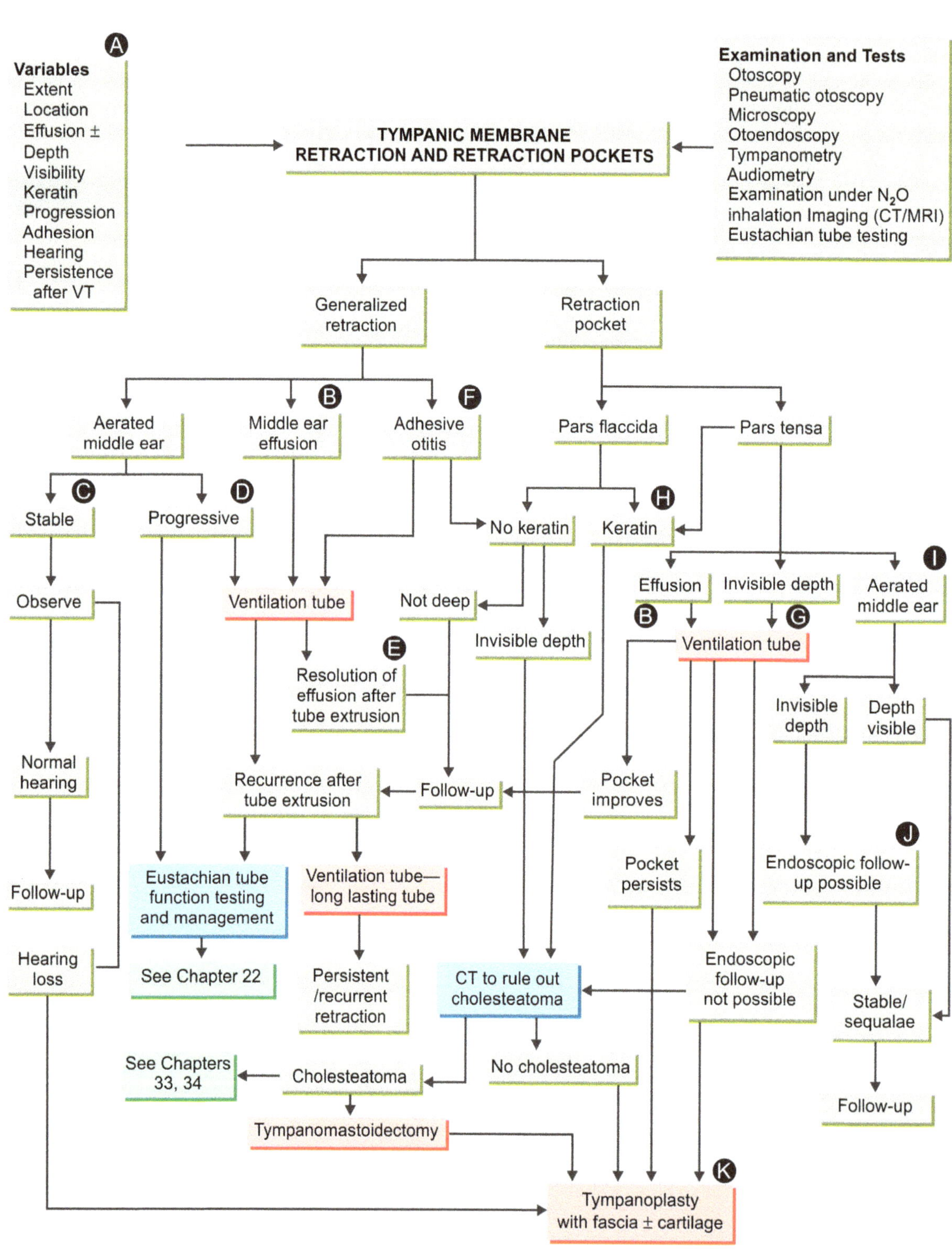

Tympanic membrane (TM) retraction (TMR) and retraction pockets (RPs) are considered as sequelae of otitis media (OM) and/or Eustachian tube dysfunction (ETD); however, the term sequelae should not imply a stable abnormal end point. Often, especially in children, the condition is variable depending upon risk factors and progressive, potentially with the risk of development of cholesteatoma, requiring close follow-up and further surgeries for treatment or prevention.

(A) The most common classification is from Sade, grading the TMR based on the degree of retraction and how much the TM reaches the middle ear (ME) structures, as Sade had suggested. Other classifications focus on location, degree of bone erosion at the scutum as per the classification suggested by Tos, mobility of TM, fixation, whether or not the TMR is controllable according to Charachon, and visibility of the depth as Dornhoffer thought more critical factor for the classification. These classifications differ by focusing on a specific feature of the TMR and RP and may be helpful in decision making.

(B) In an ear with TMR or RP, presence of OM with effusion (OME) and/or frequent episodes of OM should lead to ventilation tube (VT) insertion as the first-line treatment.

(C) A stable TMR or RP without hearing loss that is not showing signs of progression or keratin formation and with the visible full depth with the microscope and/or endoscope can be followed without intervention.

(D) A progressive TMR or RP should initially receive a VT to stop the progression.

(E) Recurrence of TMR with effusion requires repeat VT, possible long-lasting VT. If there is VT or no effusion, ETD can be tested.

(F) Nonprogressive, nonkeratinizing, adhesive OM, without OME, or hearing loss may be stable and followed. If any of these are present, it is best to try to find an ME space for VT insertion. Often, advanced TMR and adhesive OM have extremely thin and atrophic TM that will not hold a regular tube, requiring a long-lasting VT.

(G) An RP with OME should also initially receive a VT, irrespective of the full visibility of its depth. An RP whose depth is invisible may resume its normal anatomical position after the VT and may become safe.

(H) The presence of keratin within an RP will most likely require surgery for removal of cholesteatoma after the imaging. However, if there is OME and presence of advanced bone erosion is not likely, it is better to initially place a VT before the CT scan to better differentiate cholesteatoma from effusion.

(I) The patient with an RP with dry ME and visibility of the full depth with an otoscope, microscope, or an endoscope can be followed.

(J) Endoscopic visualization and follow-up may not be possible in children. Also, if the close follow-up is not feasible or desirable by the patient or parents of a child, it is better to pursue a method that will more likely keep the ear safe, such as VT insertion or tympanoplasty.

(K) In patients who no longer have a risk for progression, a tympanoplasty with fascia graft that restores the original thickness of the TM may be sufficient. However, if there are ongoing risk factors, and if a VT is not going to be inserted, a cartilage graft will be more suitable. If there is ongoing ETD, unless the entire TM is supported with cartilage, a new RP can develop in an area without cartilage support. Therefore, a VT insertion with a fascia graft is more suitable. If there is persistent ETD with likely OME, a VT insertion should be planned upfront.

SUGGESTED READING

Charachon R, Barthez M, LeJeune JM. Spontaneous retraction pockets in chronic otitis media: medical and surgical therapy. Ear Nose Throat J. 1992;71:578-583.

Dornhoffer JL. Surgical management of the atelectatic ear. Am J Otol. 2000;21:315-321.

Neumann C, Yung M. Management of retraction pockets of pars tensa and pars flaccida: a systematic review of literature. Int Adv Otol. 2012;8:360-365.

Sade J. Treatment of retraction pockets and cholesteatoma. Eur Arch Otorhinolaryngol. 1993;250:193-199.

Tos M, Poulsen G. Attic retractions following secretory otitis. Acta Otolaryngol. 1980;89:479-486.

CHAPTER 32

Tympanic Membrane Perforation

Stephanie Moody Antonio

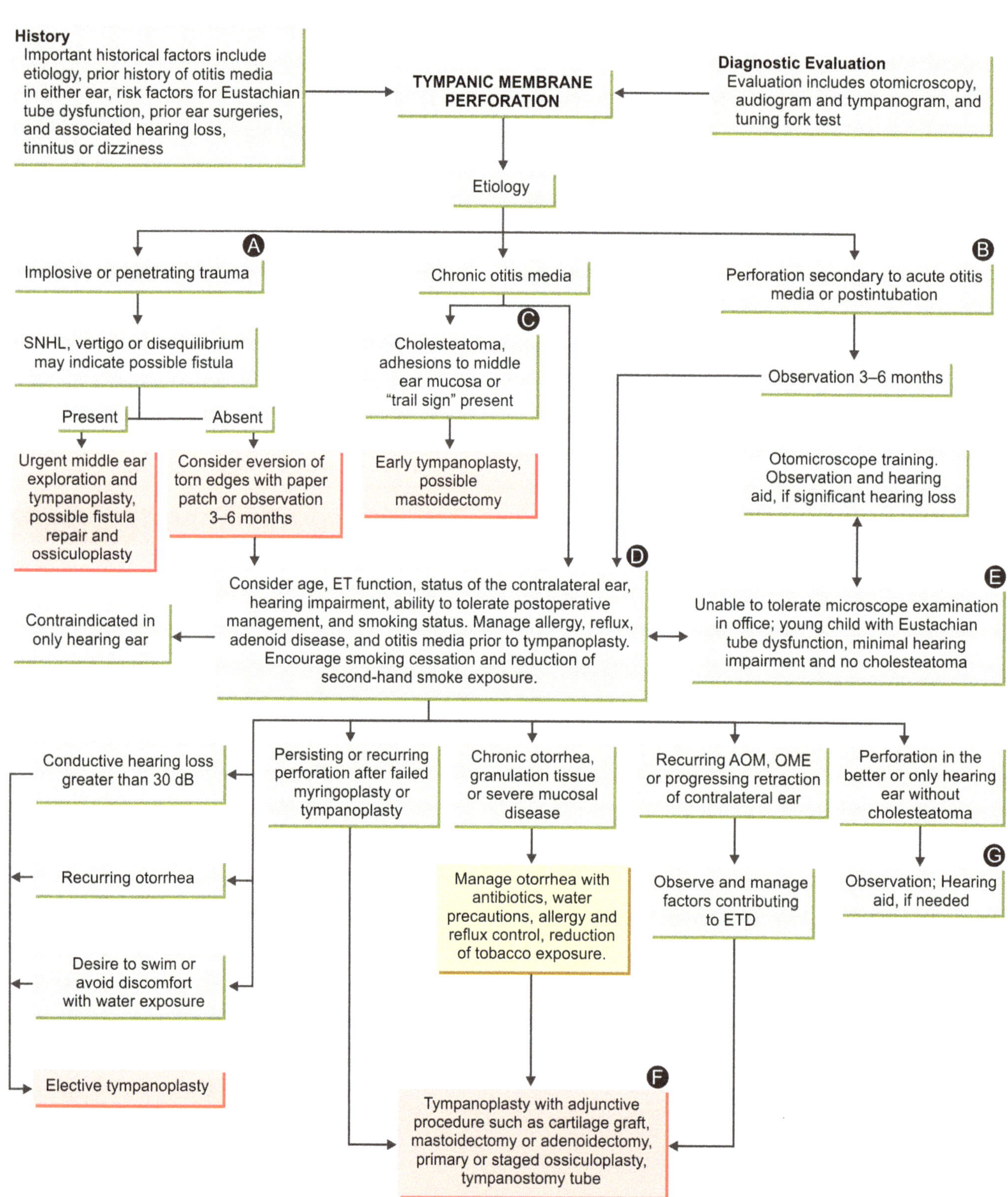

The etiology of tympanic membrane (TM) perforation includes infection, trauma, Eustachian tube (ET) dysfunction (ETD), intubation, and surgical manipulation. Small perforations may be entirely asymptomatic, but larger perforations may result in hearing loss due to the loss of ossicular coupling and reduction in air pressure differential between the middle ear and ear canal. Hearing loss ranges from 0 to 40 dB, directly proportional to the size of the perforation and indirectly proportional to middle ear (ME) volume, with the largest air-bone gap in the lower frequencies. The location of the perforation is not predictive of the degree of hearing loss. The loss of protection, affords the ME exposure to water, cold air, irritants, or pathogens through the external canal or reflux from the nasopharynx may cause discomfort and/or infection. Consider repair of perforation for one of three primary indications: hearing improvement, reduction of risk of contamination, or management or prevention of associated complications such as otorrhea and cholesteatoma. Near absolute contraindication for tympanoplasty would include an only hearing ear or medical risks for anesthesia.

A Eighty percent or more of uncomplicated traumatic perforations close spontaneously within 90 days. Caution must be exercised in cases of implosive or penetrating trauma, since inverted edges, keratin debris, foreign bodies, and burns significantly increase the risk of cholesteatoma, infection, and nonhealing perforations. The rate of spontaneous healing after a blast injury is reported to be between 38% and 82% and is at the lowest end of the spectrum for larger perforations. Perforations that result from exposure to hot slag have a low rate of spontaneous closure due to devascularization. Dizziness, vertigo, disequilibrium, tinnitus, and sensorineural hearing loss could indicate the possibility of a traumatic subluxation of the stapes, and urgent surgical exploration and repair of the perforation should be considered.

B The rate of spontaneous closure after tube extrusion is more than 95%, and after tube removal is about 90%; therefore, it is reasonable to observe postintubation perforations for at least 3–6 months.

C Careful examination by otomicroscopy is critical to detect subclinical cholesteatoma. A "trail sign" or thin line of migrating keratin extending from a posterior marginal perforation or anterior perforation abutting the malleus may indicate involution of squamous epithelium and a risk for developing cholesteatoma.

D Several factors should be considered and managed prior to embarking on tympanoplasty. ETD is not a contraindication for tympanoplasty, but it certainly will have a detrimental effect on healing and long-term outcome. From a practical standpoint, the status of the opposite ear is a good indicator of ET status. Delay tympanoplasty for young children with otitis media or progressive retraction in the opposite ear as they are likely to outgrow ETD. When delayed tympanoplasty is not an option, control all factors contributing to ETD such as allergy, reflux, and exposure to tobacco. Control infection and granulation with antibiotic drops and oral antibiotic if needed, avoiding potentially ototoxic drugs to the ME as much as possible. Otorrhea persisting despite ototopical drops should be cultured. Methicillin-resistant Staphylococcus aureus, if present should be managed aggressively with aural (MRSA) cleansing, and systemic antibiotics drops and, eradication of carrier state.

E Age alone has no significant effect on the rate of closure after tympanoplasty. However, age should be considered, as it relates to several factors that may impact the clinical setting such as status of ET function (ETF), exposure to water, risk for otitis media, postoperative office management, detrimental effects of hearing impairment, and risk of anesthesia.

F The role of mastoidectomy in the management of TM perforations is controversial. In general, mastoidectomy with tympanoplasty does not offer an improved rate of closure compared to tympanoplasty alone and is not necessary for simple perforations. However, some patients, such as those with poor ETF or chronic suppurative otitis media, may benefit from a concurrent mastoidectomy. The volume of the mastoid appears to be inversely related to ME disease. The mechanisms for this relationship are not clear but are hypothesized to be related to a theoretical pressure-buffering and/or ventilatory function of the mastoid. One school of thought suggests that a well-aerated large volume mastoid allows for optimal pressure buffering, reducing the negative effects of inadequate ETF. Alternatively, some surgeons employ mastoidectomy with obliteration or isolation of the mastoid from the ME to reduce the negative effects of a large surface area of nitrogen-absorbing mucosa, which may predispose to negative ME pressure. Whether mastoidectomy reduces the long-term risk of persisting or recurrent perforation, atelectasis, retraction pockets, and cholesteatoma is unclear.

G Surgery on the better or only hearing ear should be avoided, given the small risk of sensorineural hearing loss with tympanoplasty and myringoplasty. Similarly, in most cases, it is unwise to perform bilateral simultaneous tympanoplasty. If both ears have a perforation, repair the worst hearing ear first. Surgical intervention must be considered in a better hearing ear in the case of cholesteatoma or chronic otitis media.

SUGGESTED READING

Ars B, Dirckx J, Ars-Piret N, et al. Insights in the physiology of the human mastoid: message to the surgeon. Int Adv Otol. 2012;8(2):296-310.

Eliades SJ, Limb CJ. The role of mastoidectomy in outcomes following tympanic membrane repair: a review. Laryngoscope. 2013;123(7):1787-1802.

Jellinge ME, Kristensen S, Larsen K. Spontaneous closure of traumatic tympanic membrane perforations: observational study. J Laryngol Otol. 2015;129(10):950-954.

McGrew BM, Jackson CG, Glasscock ME, 3rd. Impact of mastoidectomy on simple tympanic membrane perforation repair. Laryngoscope. 2004;114(3):506-511.

Mehta RP, Rosowski JJ, Voss SE, et al. Determinants of hearing loss in perforations of the tympanic membrane. Otol Neurotol. 2006;27(2):136-143.

Park H, Hong SN, Kim HS, et al. Determinants of conductive hearing loss in tympanic membrane perforation. Clin Exp Otorhinolaryngol. 2015;8(2):92-96.

Remenschneider AK, Lookabaugh S, Aliphas A, et al. Otologic outcomes after blast injury: the Boston Marathon experience. Otol Neurotol. 2014;35(10):1825-1834.

Vercillo NC, Xie L, Agrawal N, et al. Pediatric tympanostomy tube removal technique and effect on rate of persistent tympanic membrane perforation. JAMA Otolaryngol Head Neck Surg. 2015;141(7):614-619.

Cholesteatoma

Moisés A Arriaga

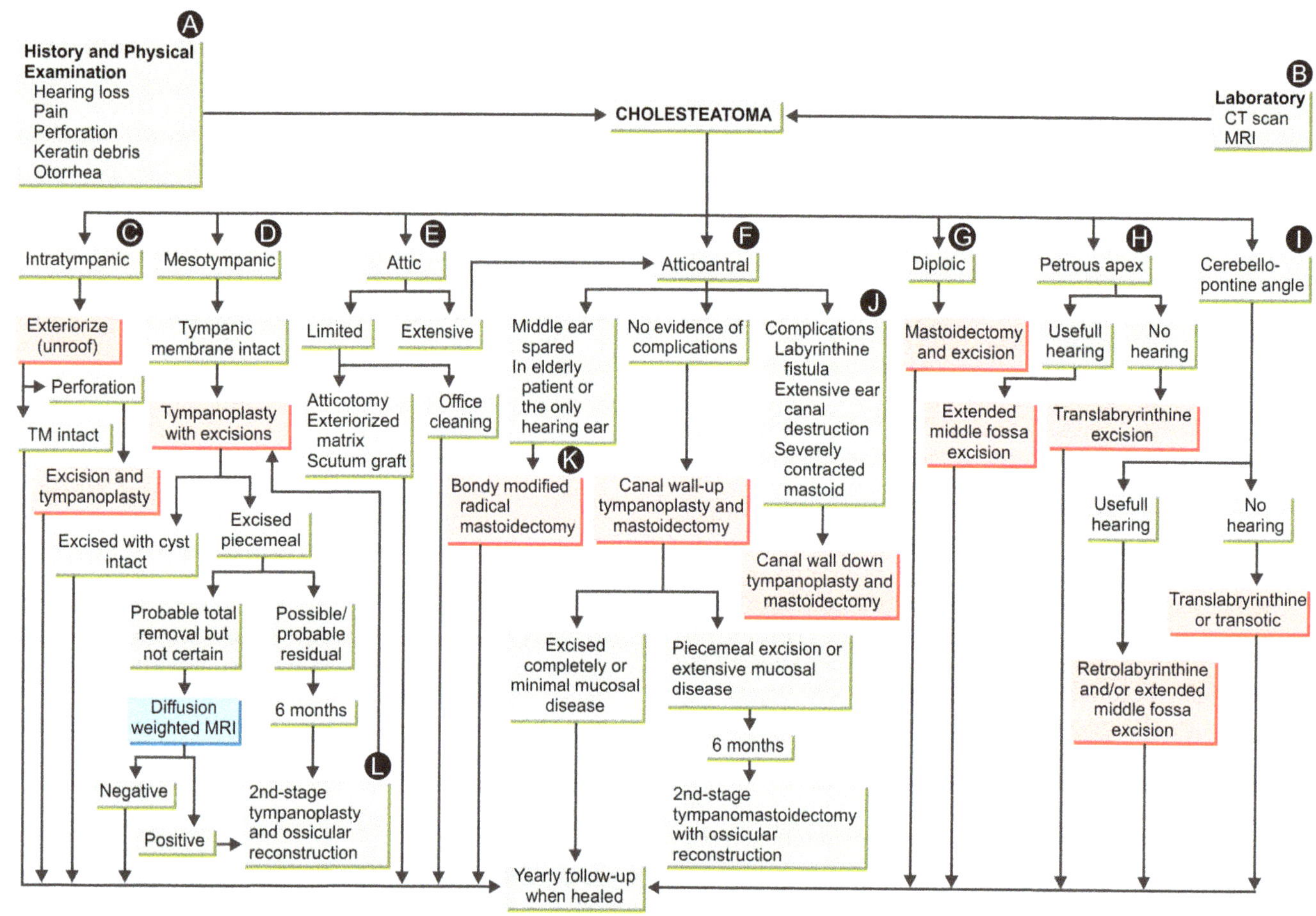

Cholesteatoma is a pathologic accumulation of keratinizing epithelium in the mucosal-lined spaces of the middle ear and mastoid. While they can be congenital or acquired, their damage results from mass effect, erosion, and ongoing infections. The potential damage to the middle ear ossicular system, labyrinth, facial nerve, dura, and intracranial structures makes surgical management of these lesions a priority to avoid further damage.

A Previous ear infections with episodic drainage, pain, and hearing loss are characteristics of cholesteatoma. Although keratin accumulation is typical, narrow-necked cholesteatoma sacs may conceal debris accumulating medially. Right-angled picks or endoscopes are useful to fully visualize small pockets to rule out cholesteatoma. Imaging is useful if uncertainty remains.

B Computed tomography (CT) without contrast reveals bone destruction and soft-tissue accumulation, which can confirm the diagnosis of cholesteatoma, erosion of the semicircular canals, erosion of the tegmen tympani, or the Fallopian canal. Non-echoplanar diffusion-weighted imaging (magnetic resonance imaging, MRI) (DWI) can confirm a cholesteatoma as small as 3 mm. The MRI + contrast can confirm intracranial involvement. While CT is not necessary to diagnose an uncomplicated case, it is helpful in the selection of the surgical technique. Lesions limited to the attic and epitympanum may be appropriate for endoscopic minimally invasive techniques. If complications are suspected, preoperative imaging is necessary for preoperative planning and patient counseling.

C Intratympanic cholesteatomas result from aberrant healing of the tympanic membrane from trauma such as a perforation or a myringotomy. Limited lesions are adequately managed by exteriorization. Deeper lesions require excision and repair.

D Mesotympanic cholesteatoma may be congenital (*see* Chapter 34) or acquired. Progressive conductive hearing loss with a retrotympanic mass is typical in a mesotympanic cholesteatoma.

E Attic cholesteatomas begin as a retraction of the pars flaccida that deepens, accumulates debris, and erodes surrounding bone. Early cholesteatomas may be exteriorized, and the scutum repaired. In patients who are poor surgical risks, frequent cleaning in the office is an appropriate treatment as long as complete cleaning is possible.

F Extensive atticoantral cholesteatoma requires tympanoplasty and mastoidectomy.

G Diploic cholesteatomas are epidermoid cysts of the diploic bone surrounding the temporal bone. Developmental rests of epithelium continue to grow during later life and produce local bone obstruction, pain, and infection. Complete excision is necessary for cure.

H Petrous apex cholesteatoma can be extensive. The progressive bone destruction often involves the Fallopian canal and produces a characteristic facial twitch.

I Cerebellopontine angle cholesteatoma (epidermoid) produces symptoms through mass effect in the posterior fossa. Surgical resection can produce aggressive aseptic meningitis from keratin debris in the cerebrospinal fluid. The signs and symptoms are typical of a posterior fossa tumor (i.e. hearing loss, tinnitus, and vertigo).

J Labyrinthine fistula from cholesteatoma is best managed by leaving the matrix over the fistula and performing a canal wall down mastoidectomy if the fistula is extensive. A small fistula (3 mm) can be managed by careful removal of the matrix and repair with soft tissue, cartilage, or bone. Inadvertent opening of a fistula should be repaired with autologous tissue.

K The Bondy modified radical mastoidectomy is the classic canal wall down procedure for attic cholesteatoma that has not involved the middle ear. A complete canal wall down procedure is accomplished while keeping the tympanic membrane and middle ear undisturbed.

L Staging is appropriate if the matrix is removed piecemeal, and there is question about complete removal. Similarly, if total removal requires extensive resection of middle ear mucosa, staging minimizes adhesions. Silastic sheeting, 0.020 or 0.040 inches thick, is left in the middle ear. Six months to 1 year later, the Silastic sheeting is removed, and the ossicular chain reconstructed. The DWI MRI can be offered to avoid a second stage if the surgeon is confident of complete cholesteatoma removal and ossicular reconstruction was accomplished.

SUGGESTED READING

Arriaga MA. Cholesteatoma in children. Otolaryngol Clin North Am. 1994;27:573-591.

Brackmann D, Shelton C, Arriaga M (Eds). Otologic Surgery, 3rd edition. Philadelphia, PA: Elsevier; 2015.

DeFoer B, Vercruysse JP, Berhaerts A, et al. Detection of postoperative residual cholesteatoma with non-echo-planar diffusion weighted magnetic resonance imaging. Otol Neurotol. 2008;29:513-517.

Sheehy JL. Surgery of chronic otitis media. In: English GM (Ed). Otolaryngology, Vol 1. Philadelphia, PA: JB Lippincott; 1984. pp. 1-87.

CHAPTER 34

Cholesteatoma in the Pediatric Age Group

Cuneyt M Alper

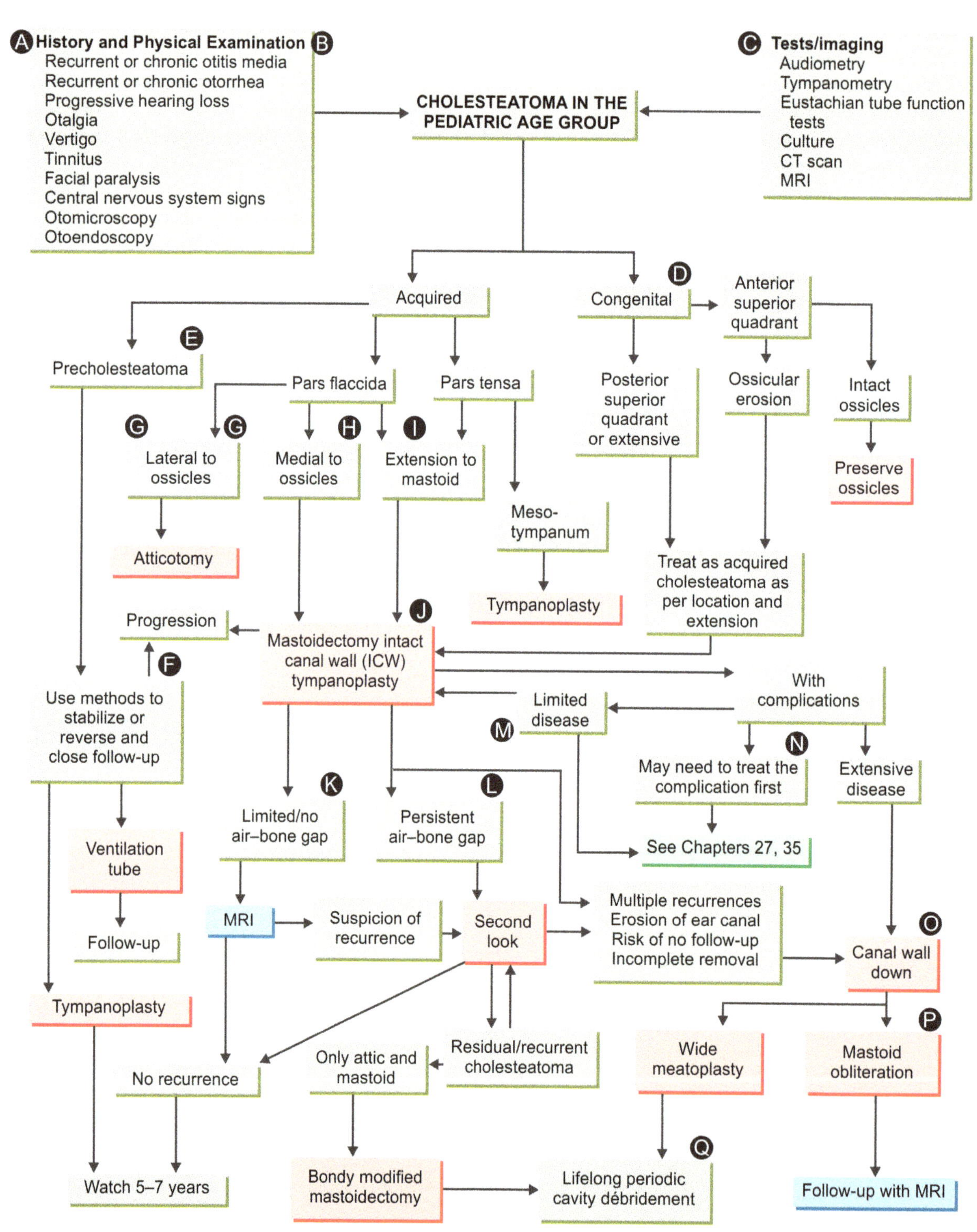

Cholesteatoma in the pediatric population may present as the unique form of congenital cholesteatoma (CC) or as early stages of acquired cholesteatoma, such as the transitional form of precholesteatoma retraction pocket or cholesteatoma with limited extension and minimal or no bone erosion, but at the same time a high rate of residual and recurrent disease, creating diagnostic and treatment challenges. However, a late diagnosed CC may present as quite advanced, having already spread into a previously well-pneumatized temporal bone.

Ⓐ Cholesteatoma in the pediatric age group frequently develops in the absence of signs or symptoms. However, when symptomatic, the child may have recurrent/chronic otitis media (with or without otorrhea) or progressive conductive hearing loss. Recurrent or chronic otalgia is uncommon; when otalgia or headache is associated with cholesteatoma, the clinician should search for a possible complication.

Ⓑ When otorrhea is present, culture-directed therapy may improve the inflammation, surgery conditions, and outcome.

Ⓒ Evaluation should include audiometry. Computed tomography scan of the temporal bone is essential prior to the surgery. Magnetic resonance imaging (MRI) is increasingly used for follow-up of residual disease, but may require sedation or general anesthesia in young children.

Ⓓ Most CC present at the anterosuperior quadrant and are amenable to removal via transmeatal or endaural approach with ossicular preservation. If there is no ossicular erosion, preserving the ossicles should be the goal. If CC presents at the posterosuperior quadrant, the ossicles are eroded or cannot be preserved. Unlike most acquired cholesteatoma CC may present with extensive spread into a well-pneumatized temporal bone, if diagnosed late.

Ⓔ The vast majority of pediatric cholesteatoma evolves from retraction pockets. The transition is not instant or categorical.

Ⓕ Affected with the risk factors, including Eustachian tube dysfunction that varies with viral and bacterial infections, this transition may be halted spontaneously or with intervention such as ventilation tube insertion or cartilage tympanoplasty (*see* Chapter 31).

Ⓖ Small pars flaccida cholesteatoma not extending medial to the ossicles or into the mastoid may be removed through the ear canal, and recurrence prevented with a cartilage graft.

Ⓗ If it extends medial to the ossicles, removal of cholesteatoma requires good visualization of the attic with mastoidectomy, and often removal of the ossicles.

Ⓘ Preserving the posterior canal wall should be aimed at insuring the child's life-long quality of life.

Ⓙ The intact canal wall (ICW) technique increases the risk of residual and recurrent cholesteatoma, resulting in multiple surgeries until the disease is completely eradicated. However, maintenance of anatomy should still be prioritized due to very long life expectancy. Advancements in intraoperative visualization with endoscopes and surveillance with MRI enhances successful outcome with ICW.

Ⓚ If the ossicles have been intact and postoperative air-bone gap is minimal, MRI may be preferred instead of a second look.

Ⓛ A second look operation is often preferred due to higher risk for recurrence in children and if clear for ossicular chain reconstruction.

Ⓜ Although less common in the pediatric population, all extracranial and intracranial complications like extradural abscess, sigmoid sinus thrombosis, and otitis hydrocephalus require tympanomastoidectomy. However, they do not always require a canal wall down (CWD) approach.

Ⓝ Management of subdural abscess, meningitis, and symptomatic brain abscess is prioritized before the surgical management of the middle ear and mastoid, until the patients conditions is stabilized.

Ⓞ Extensive, recurrent, residual cholesteatomas of concern on follow-up may require the CWD approach.

Ⓟ Mastoid obliteration after removal of cholesteatoma may obscure residual cholesteatoma for many years, and needs an MRI to rule it out.

Ⓠ Open mastoid cavity should be avoided in children if possible due to often challenging periodic cavity debridement. Moreover, with normal growth there is often a need to revise the cavity to enhance cleaning and manage recurrent cavity drainage.

SUGGESTED READING

Bennett M, Warren F, Jackson GC, et al. Congenital cholesteatoma: theories, facts, and 53 patients. Otolaryngol Clin North Am. 2006;39(6):1081-1094.

Dornhoffer JL, Friedman AB, Gluth MB. Management of acquired cholesteatoma in the pediatric population. Curr Opin Otolaryngol Head Neck Surg. 2013;21(5):440-445.

Isaacson G. Diagnosis of pediatric cholesteatoma. Pediatrics. 2007;120(3):603-608.

Koitschev A, Behringer P, Bögner D, et al. Does diffusion-weighted MRI (DW-MRI) change treatment strategy in pediatric cholesteatoma? Acta Otolaryngol. 2013;133(5):443-448.

Morita Y, Yamamoto Y, Oshima S, et al. Acquired cholesteatoma in children: clinical features and surgical outcome. Auris Nasus Larynx. 2014;41(5):417-421.

Nevoux J, Lenoir M, Roger G, et al. Childhood cholesteatoma. Eur Ann Otorhinolaryngol Head Neck Dis. 2010;127(4):143-150.

Roger G, Denoyelle F, Chauvin P, et al. Predictive risk factors of residual cholesteatoma in children: a study of 256 cases. Am J Otol. 1997;18:550-558.

Schraff SA, Strasnick B. Pediatric cholesteatoma: a retrospective review. Int J Pediatr Otorhinolaryngol. 2006;70(3):385-393.

Stangerup SE, Drozdziewicz D, Tos M, et al. Surgery for acquired cholesteatoma in children: long-term results and recurrence of cholesteatoma. J Laryngol Otol. 1998;112:742-749.

Yamatodani T, Mizuta K, Hosokawa K, et al. Congenital middle ear cholesteatoma: experience from 26 surgical cases. Ann Otol Rhinol Laryngol. 2013;122(5):316-321.

Intracranial Complications of Otitis Media

Michael S Cohen, Cuneyt M Alper

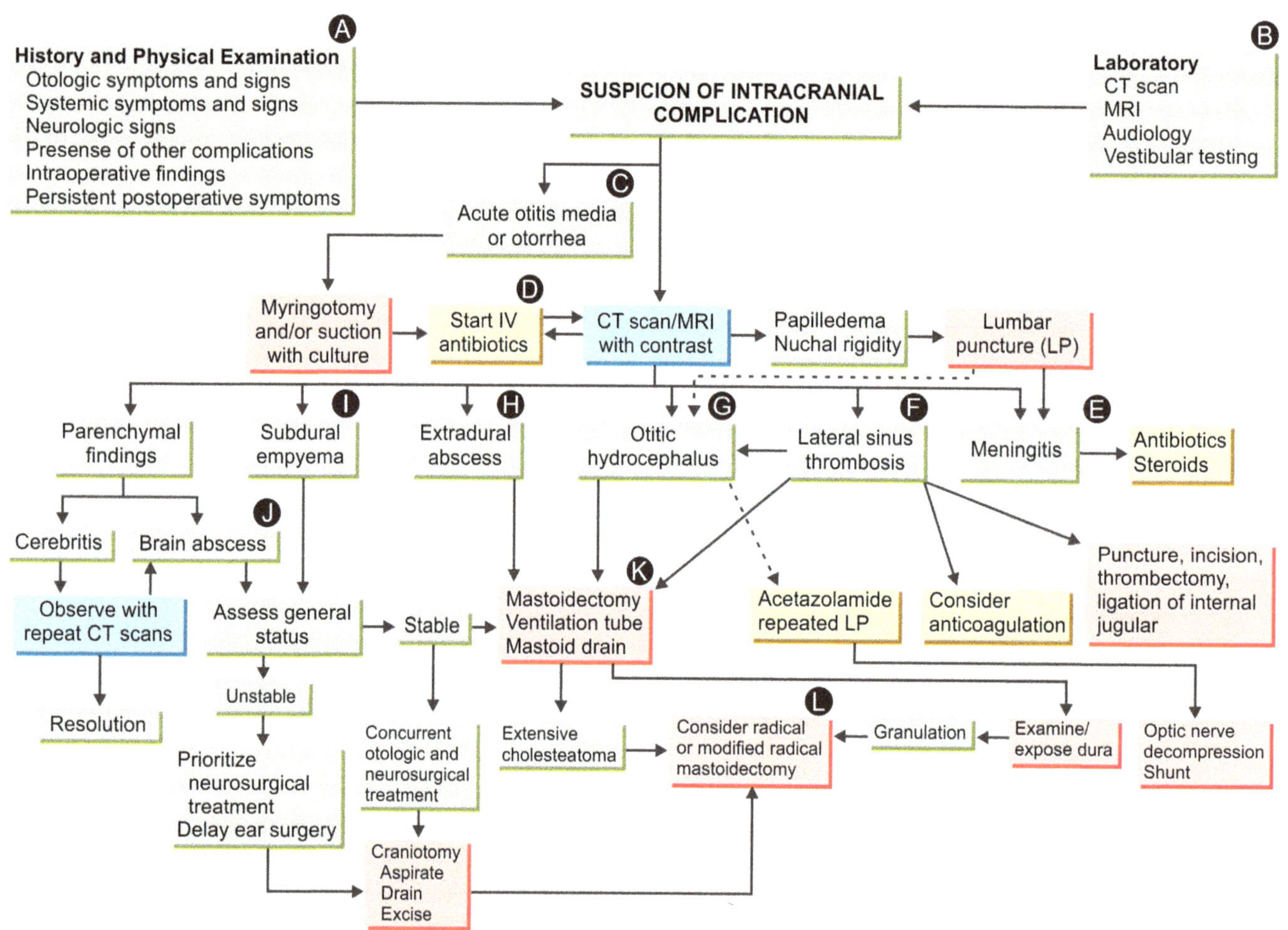

Complications of otitis media (OM) may be secondary to acute or chronic OM with or without cholesteatoma, and may be divided by site into intratemporal complication (ITC) or intracranial complication (ICC). Intracranial complication may occur secondary to, or concurrently with, ITC, and successful treatment of ICC depends upon adequate treatment of all underlying disease. In some cases, ICC may develop after initiation of treatment of either OM or ITC. Awareness of the signs and symptoms of ICC is critical to the early detection and treatment of these conditions in patients with otologic disease.

A Persistent symptoms despite medical or surgical treatment may suggest an ICC. The presence of persistent, severe, and generalized headache, persistent or intermittent fever, nausea, and vomiting, irritability, and lethargy should raise the suspicion for an ICC. Profuse or pulsatile drainage may be consistent with exposed dura. Neurologic symptoms and signs such as mental status change, seizure, nuchal rigidity, ataxia, and visual changes strongly suggest an ICC. Two or more complications may coexist; hence, evidence of any complication requires ruling out others. Persistent otalgia, headache, or fever, despite adequate drainage through a myringotomy, tube, or mastoid drain, suggests ICC.

B Computed tomography (CT) or magnetic resonance imaging (MRI) with contrast should be performed urgently. In the presence of chronic OM with or without cholesteatoma, or with an extracranial complication, the first choice should be a CT scan of the temporal bone and brain with contrast. Thin axial and coronal cuts through the temporal bone are required to provide adequate detail to assess bony destruction of preformed pathways as well as soft tissue changes. In the presence of neurologic symptoms and signs, an MRI with contrast should be obtained in addition to CT. Hearing should be assessed prior to surgery. Vestibular testing may be performed in stable patients with vestibular symptoms.

C When an ICC is suspected in the presence of acute OM, material for culture and Gram stain should be obtained as soon as possible, with adequate drainage through a wide myringotomy or a ventilation tube. If otorrhea is present, the ear canal should first be suctioned and then cultured close to the source of otorrhea.

D Gram-positive organisms are common in acute OM, whereas gram-negative and anaerobic organisms are more prevalent in chronic OM. Intravenous antibiotics with cerebrospinal fluid penetration should be administered to cover Gram-positive, Gram-negative, and anaerobic pathogens pending results of Gram stain or culture results. Antibiotics are continued for 2–6 weeks.

E Meningitis is the most common ICC and presents with severe and generalized headache, vomiting, nuchal rigidity, and Kernig's and Brudzinski's signs. A lumbar puncture (LP), performed after imaging to reduce the risk of brain herniation, classically reveals elevated opening pressure, with decreased glucose, elevated protein, white blood cells, and microorganisms on Gram stain of the cerebrospinal fluid. Management includes stabilization of the patient, radiologic evaluation to rule out other ICC, LP, and antibiotics. Otologic surgery may need to be postponed until the patient is stable. Intravenous dexamethasone, 0.15 mg/kg per dose every 6 hours for 2 days, reduces the morbidity and complications in acute bacterial meningitis especially for *Haemophilus influenzae* type b.

F Lateral sinus thrombosis lacks specific symptoms. In the early (perisinus abscess) stage, only headache and malaise may be present. If the thrombus then becomes infected, septicemia and the classic "picket-fence" pattern of spiking fevers may develop. Progression may result in increased intracranial pressure, papilledema, and postauricular tenderness (Griesinger's sign). Failure of jugular vein compression to cause higher cerebrospinal fluid pressure may be observed on LP (the Tobey-Ayer test or the Queckenstedt sign). This diagnosis requires prompt mastoid surgery with exposure of the lateral sinus. Although controversial, needle aspiration, if confirmed, incision, and thrombectomy are considered. Anticoagulation, also controversial, is considered in cases of progressive dural sinus thrombosis or increasing intracranial pressure.

G Otitic hydrocephalus presents with lethargy, headache, and papilledema. Management consists of acetazolamide, repeated LP, and, if optic nerve complications develop, nerve decompression or shunt.

H Extradural abscess occurs most commonly secondary to bone destruction from coalescent mastoiditis or cholesteatoma. Otorrhea may be creamy and pulsatile and may increase with pressure on the internal jugular vein on the same side.

I Subdural empyema may present with rapidly progressive focal neurologic deficits, seizures, and loss of consciousness.

J Brain abscess may develop in the temporal lobe or cerebellum with associated neurologic symptoms. The initial (cerebritis) stage is reversible with aggressive antimicrobial therapy. Subtle symptoms and signs in the latent phase lasting days to weeks are followed by the expansion stage with severe and progressive symptoms. Initial management is the stabilization followed by surgery for both intratemporal and intracranial foci. Mastoid surgery may be postponed if the patient is neurologically unstable.

K A complete mastoidectomy should be performed in the presence of coalescent mastoiditis. A ventilation tube and a mastoid drain will facilitate adequate drainage. Diseased areas should be monitored to evaluate the dura. When granulation tissue or purulent exudate is present the dura should widely be exposed.

L In the presence of extensive cholesteatoma or widely diseased dura, a modified radical or radical mastoidectomy should be considered.

SUGGESTED READING

Bluestone CD, Chi DH, Klein JO. Complications and sequelae of otitis media. In: Bluestone CD, Simons JP, Healy GB (Eds). Bluestone and Stool's Pediatric Otolaryngology, 5th edition. Shelton, CT: People's Medical Publishing House; 2014. p. 761.

Cass SP. Intracranial complications of otitis media. In: Myers EN (Ed). Operative Otolaryngology Head and Neck Surgery, 1st edition. Philadelphia: WB Saunders; 1997. p. 1343.

Jung TT, Alper CM, Hellstrom SO, et al. Panel 8: Complications and sequelae. Otolaryngol Head Neck Surg. 2013;148(4 Suppl): E122-143.

Kuczkowski J, Tretiakow D, Brzoznowski W. Can we avoid intracranial complications of chronic otitis media? Eur Arch Otorhinolaryngol. 2015;272(9):2581-2582.

Lavin JM, Rusher T, Shah RK. Complications of pediatric otitis media. Otolaryngol Head Neck Surg. 2016;154(2):366-370.

Mattos JL, Colman KL, Casselbrant ML, et al. Intratemporal and intracranial complications of acute otitis media in a pediatric population. Int J Pediatr Otorhinolaryngol. 2014;78(12): 2161-2164.

Sun J, Sun J. Intracranial complications of chronic otitis media. Eur Arch Otorhinolaryngol. 2014;271(11):2923-2926.

CHAPTER 36

Auricular Trauma

Lorenz Frederick Lassen

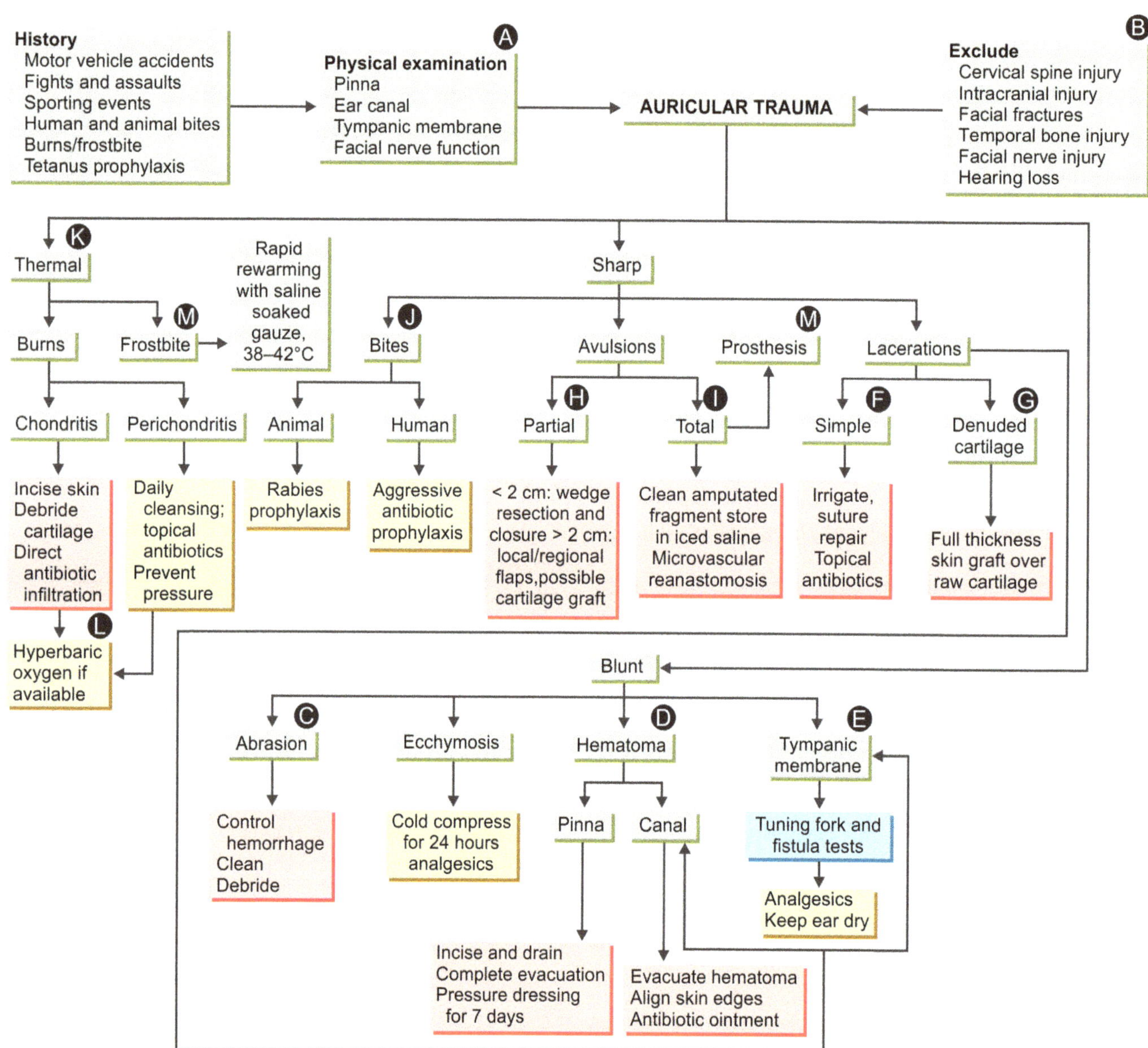

The external ear is very susceptible to trauma because it protrudes from the head and is surrounded by air. Additionally, humans will turn their heads in order to avoid direct facial trauma, thus exposing the ear to the full force of injury. Injuries to the auricle are best categorized by the mechanism of trauma: blunt, sharp, and thermal.

A Examine the external ear by direct inspection and palpation; otoscopic examination must be performed to evaluate the ear canal and tympanic membrane. Snapping the fingers can test hearing in the emergency room setting. The facial nerve traverses the temporal bone and middle ear, facial nerve function should be evaluated and documented.

B Injuries of the auricle may be associated with other life-threatening injuries that should be ruled out before proceeding with evaluation of the auricle. Fractures of the temporal bone may follow a forceful blow to the ear. Fractures of the temporal bone should be suspected if there is cerebrospinal fluid otorrhea, hearing loss, vertigo, laceration of the tympanic membrane, or facial nerve paralysis.

C Abrasions are usually seen in children and should be thoroughly cleaned and debrided in order to avoid infection and tattooing. Abrasions can be dressed with topical bacitracin and a nonstick dressing such as Xeroform.

D Hematoma of the auricle separates the perichondrium from its underlying cartilage. Because the cartilage receives its nutrition from the overlying perichondrium, the cartilage becomes necrotic and is replaced by scar tissue, producing the deformity known as "cauliflower ear." A hematoma of the auricle must be completely evacuated and a pressure dressing applied in order to prevent reaccumulation of blood. Either Telfa gauze or a tie-over, through-and-through bolster of rolled gauze over dental rolls secured with 4-0 nylon suture provide excellent obliteration of any potential dead space and should be left in place for at least 5 days. Systemic antibiotics are not necessary.

E Most tympanic membrane perforations heal spontaneously. Some tympanic membrane perforations can be associated with middle ear and labyrinthine injury causing hearing loss, vertigo, and tinnitus. Weber and Rinne tuning fork tests can help to determine the conductive hearing loss and associated ossicular injury. Pushing the tragus onto the ear canal can perform a bedside fistula test.

F Simple lacerations can be repaired after irrigation and debridement to freshen the raw edges. It is best to use as few sutures as possible. Systemic antibiotics are not necessary. Lacerations of the earlobe usually result from pulling an earring; after excising the epithelial cleft, lacerations of the earlobe may be repaired.

G Loss of skin requires full-thickness skin grafting. If the perichondrium is intact, the skin graft may be done immediately. If there is bare cartilage without perichondrium, then grafting must be delayed until a bed of granulation tissue develops. An excellent donor site is the skin behind the postauricular sulcus.

H A wedge resection can close small (<2 cm) avulsions without significant cosmetic deformity. Larger defects require cartilage grafting. It is most important to preserve or reconstruct the superior ear root. Large partial avulsions, even with tenuous skin paddles, may be reapproximated with a high rate of success.

I Traumatic auricular amputation is very uncommon. The best results for total auricular amputation require microvascular reanastomosis. Most microsurgical techniques are complex and must be performed in specialized centers. For those centers without a microvascular team, various nonmicrovascular techniques have been described for auricular implantation. The amputated fragment should be transported in iced saline with a first-generation cephalosporin. Ancillary treatment includes medical leeches, heparin anticoagulation, and hyperbaric oxygen. Osseointegrated implantation offers an outstanding alternative for reconstructing these defects.

J Bites may be repaired if these are <12 hours old; otherwise, these should be allowed to heal by secondary intention. Human bites require aggressive antibiotic prophylaxis (intravenous (IV), ticarcillin/clavulanate; postoperative, amoxicillin/clavulanate).

K Frostbite should be treated with prompt rewarming with saline soaks. About 50% of head and neck burns involve the auricle. Perichondritis implies contamination with *Pseudomonas* and *Staphylococcus aureus*. Perichondritis should be treated with topical antibiotics (Sulfamylon Burn Cream), oral ciprofloxacin, daily cleaning, and prevention of pressure, or a "lop ear" deformity may develop. Chondritis of the auricle is a true emergency involving incision, drainage, debridement of cartilage, and direct antibiotic infiltration using an IV catheter.

L Hyperbaric oxygen therapy may offer enhanced survival and wound healing for auricular injuries and can be considered where available.

M Affordable three-dimensional printing technologies now make it possible for surgeons to create highly customizable patient-tailored products. This process provides the potential to produce individualized artificial and biologic implants, cell-specific replacement tissue, and regenerative scaffolds. This technology will have an immense impact on the reconstruction of traumatic facial, particularly ear injuries in the near future.

SUGGESTED READING

Abd-Almoktader MA. Nonmicrosurgical single-stage auricular replantation of amputated ear. Ann Plast Surg. 2011;67(1):40-43.

Bauermeister AJ, Zuriarrain A, Newman MI. Three-dimensional printing in plastic and reconstructive surgery: a systematic review. Ann Plast Surg. 2016;77(5):569-576.

Greywoode JD, Pribitkin EA, Krein H. Management of auricular hematoma and the cauliflower ear. Facial Plast Surg. 2010; 26(6):451-455.

Lavasani L, Leventhal D, Constantinides M, et al. Management of acute soft tissue injury to the auricle. Facial Plast Surg. 2010; 26(6):445-450.

Norman ZI, Cracchiolo JR, Allen SH, et al. Auricular reconstruction after human bite amputation using the Baudet technique. Ann Otol Rhinol Laryngol. 2015;124(1):45-48.

Reinisch J. Ear reconstruction in young children. Facial Plast Surg. 2015;31(6):600-603.

Renner G, McClane SD, Early E, et al. Enhancement of auricular composite graft survival with hyperbaric oxygen therapy. Arch Facial Plast Surg. 2002;4(2):102-104.

Rocke DJ, Tucci DL, Marcus J, et al. Osseointegrated implants for auricular defects: operative techniques and complication management. Otol Neurotol. 2014;35(9):1609-1614.

Turpin IM. Microsurgical replantation of the external ear. Clin Plast Surg. 1990;17:397-404.

Yamada A, Ueda K. Total auricular reconstruction after traumatic total amputation of the auricle. J Craniofac Surg. 2012;23(3): e241-246.

Cerebrospinal Fluid Otorrhea

Erica Montgomery, Pamela C Roehm

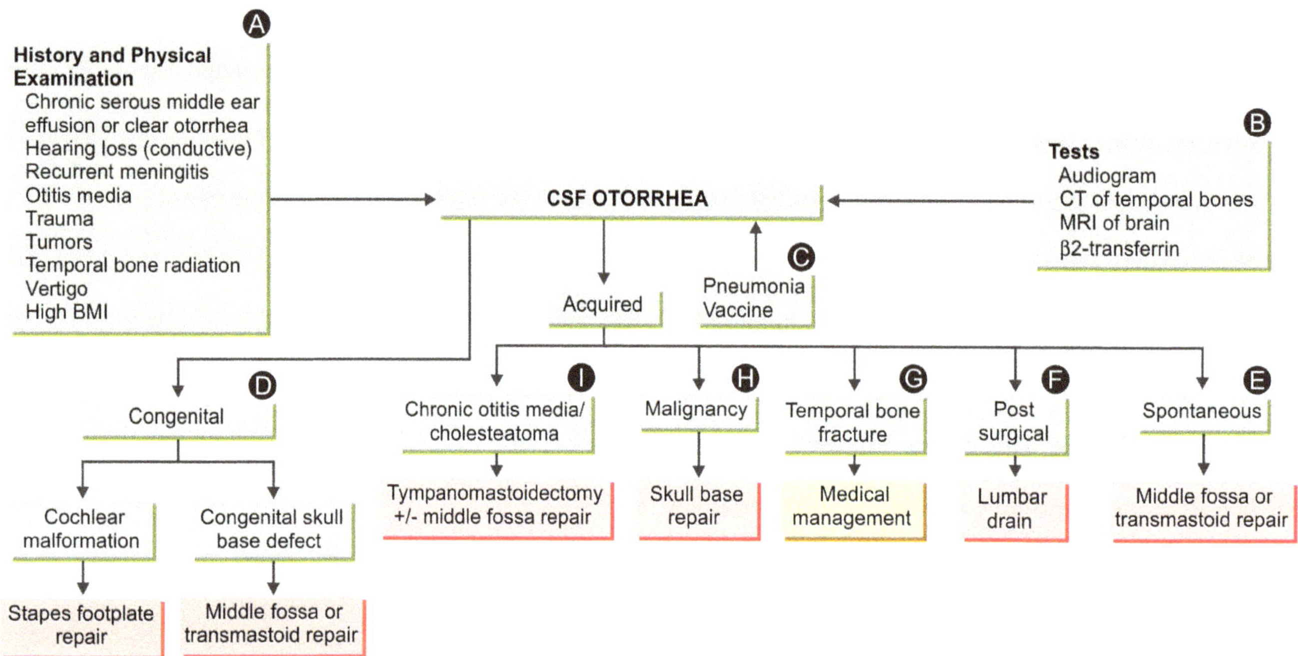

Cerebrospinal fluid (CSF) otorrhea is the pathological condition of CSF within the middle ear and mastoid. A number of conditions can lead to CSF otorrhea, including trauma, tumors, and radiation. Spontaneous CSF otorrhea can also occur, particularly in patients with a high body mass index (BMI) using continuous positive airway pressure for obstructive sleep apnea (OSA). The presence of CSF otorrhea indicates a patent connection between the ear and the CSF space, which if untreated may lead to meningitis or brain abscess due to bacterial seeding from the middle ear.

A Patients with CSF otorrhea may present with chronic serous otitis media or long-standing serous drainage from the ear and/or nose, conductive hearing loss, meningitis, or vertigo. Drainage from the ear only occurs if there is a tympanic membrane perforation or myringotomy tube in place. A diagnosis of CSF otorrhea should be considered particularly if there is a history of head trauma, surgery, cholesteatoma, temporal bone or brain tumor, or radiation therapy and in patients with a high BMI.

B High-resolution computed tomography of the temporal bone (axial and coronal) reveals absence of the tegmen, or bone separating the temporal lobe and ear, at the sites of CSF leaks. Magnetic resonance imaging (MRI) is useful for the detection of temporal encephaloceles that are often associated with defects in the lateral skull base. The presence of β_2-transferrin, a protein found only in CSF, confirms the diagnosis of CSF otorrhea. However, this test requires a large volume of fluid without red cells

and so may be difficult to collect. An audiogram should be performed, because hearing status significantly affects the approach to surgical repair.

C In general, patients with CSF leaks who are at risk for acute or chronic otitis media should receive the *Streptococcus pneumonia* vaccine. *Streptococcus pneumonia* is a commensal bacterial species of the nose and throat that can enter the CSF through interruptions in the temporal bone and dura, causing meningitis.

D Although uncommon, congenital labyrinthine abnormalities may result in CSF otorrhea. There are four main types: cochlear malformations, enlarged and patent cochlear aqueducts, tympanomeningeal (Hyrtl's) fissures, and enlarged petrosal Fallopian canals. The most common cochlear anomaly associated with CSF otorrhea is the Mondini malformation, which includes cochlear dysplasia with a normal basal turn and cystic apex, enlarged vestibular aqueduct, and vestibular anomalies; in these patients, CSF leaks occur through an abnormal stapes footplate. The cochlear aqueduct is a normal structure that connects the perilymph space with the CSF space, but which is not typically patent. With an enlarged cochlear aqueduct, conduction of CSF to the middle ear occurs through the oval window. A tympanomeningeal fissure is a perilabyrinthine channel extending from the posterior cranial fossa to the middle ear just inferior to the round window niche, which can transmit CSF directly into the middle ear space. The arachnoid may extend into the petrosal Fallopian canal laterally to the geniculate ganglion or tympanic segment of the facial nerve. The bone surrounding the facial canal becomes thinned due to CSF pressure and may form fistulas that lead into the middle ear cavity. These congenital fistulas can be repaired with soft-tissue grafts.

Perilymphatic fistulas (PLFs), which can occur after trauma to the stapes, oval window, and round window, are also sometimes associated with inner ear anomalies. The PLFs will not be associated with significant otorrhea or middle ear effusion since the total volume of perilymph is 75 µL.

E Arachnoid granulations, protrusions of the arachnoid through the dura mater that drain CSF into the venous circulation, can form over the temporal bone during development. With increased age and physical activity, arachnoid granulations can enlarge. Increases in pressure from pulsations of CSF through the granulations can weaken the dura and erode the surrounding bone, resulting in spontaneous CSF leaks. These leaks present in patients ≥ 50 years with unilateral CSF otorrhea and/or rhinorrhea and are more common in patients with a high BMI and those with OSA. Repair involves suturing the dural defects, if possible, placing a soft-tissue graft or flap or dural substitute over the dural defect, and repairing the tegmen defect.

F Iatrogenic CSF leaks are often due to incomplete closure of the dura during surgery. Lumbar drain placement is used initially to divert CSF flow and allow for healing of the dura. If CSF diversion fails, definitive treatment involves suture approximation of dura (if possible), coverage of the dural defect with a soft-tissue graft or dural substitute, and securing the tissue graft in place with absorbable packing.

G Temporal bone fractures may lead to CSF otorrhea. In these cases, otorrhea may not be clear due to the presence of blood. Other findings may include damage to the meninges, otic capsule, ossicles, and tympanic membrane. Most of these CSF leaks will resolve with several weeks of bed rest and avoidance of straining. Lumbar CSF drainage or surgical exploration and repair are reserved for recalcitrant CSF leaks due to a fracture that does not resolve after conservative treatment.

H The temporal bone and its surrounding structures can be eroded by malignant tumors. When the dura is damaged by the tumor, CSF leaks from the arachnoid space into the middle ear cavity. The draining CSF is often blood-tinged due to the necrosis caused by the tumor. Depending up on the location of the tumor, patients will present with additional symptoms, including unilateral peripheral facial paralysis, vertigo, and hearing loss. Squamous cell carcinoma, basal cell carcinoma, and primary cancers of the parotid that have extended to the temporal bone are the most common primary tumors found in these cases. However, metastatic cancer from the breast, lungs, kidneys, prostate, and stomach, as well as lymphoma and leukemia, can cause similar damage. Treatment typically entails surgical removal of the tumor, repair of the tegmen, and postoperative chemoradiation.

I Cholesteatomas are keratinized masses that can destroy bone of the middle ear and mastoid, including the bone of the tegmen. Cholesteatomas are often associated with chronic infections caused by Pseudomonas aeruginosa. Treatment entails surgical resection of the cholesteatoma, reconstruction of the tegmen and dura, and treatment for associated infection. Similarly, chronic otitis media in the absence of cholesteatoma can lead to erosion of the tegmen and CSF otorrhea and are treated similarly.

Granulomatous infections that can lead to CSF otorrhea include tuberculosis and nontuberculoid mycobacterial mastoiditis. Patients can present with fevers, unilateral facial paralysis, and vertigo.

SUGGESTED READING

Bauer CA, Jenkins HA. Otologic symptoms and syndromes. In: Flint PW, Haughey BH, Lund VJ, et al. (Eds). Cummings Otolaryngology Head and Neck Surgery, 5th edition. Philadelphia, PA: Elsevier Health Sciences; 2010.

Clark JL, DeSanto LW, Facer GW. Congenital deafness and spontaneous CSF otorrhea. Arch Otolaryngol. 1978;104(3):163-166.

Hoffman RA, Pappas D. Cerebrospinal fluid leak of temporal bone origin. In: Jackler RL, Brackmann DE (Eds). Neurotology, 2nd edition. Philadelphia, PA: Elsevier Health Sciences; 2005. pp. 926-933.

Hornibrook J. Perilymph fistula: fifty years of controversy. ISRN Otolaryngol. 2012;2012:248-281.

Jégoux F, Malard O, Gayet-Delacroix M, et al. Hyrtl's fissure: a case of spontaneous cerebrospinal fluid otorrhea. AJNR Am J Neuroradiol. 2005;26:963-966.

Petrus LV, Lo WW. Spontaneous CSF otorrhea caused by abnormal development of the facial nerve canal. AJNR Am J Neuroradiol. 1999;20:275-277.

Teufert KB, Slattery WH. Cerebrospinal fluid leak of the fallopian canal. Ear Nose Throat J. 2013;92(3):e20-23.

Otosclerosis

Douglas A Chen

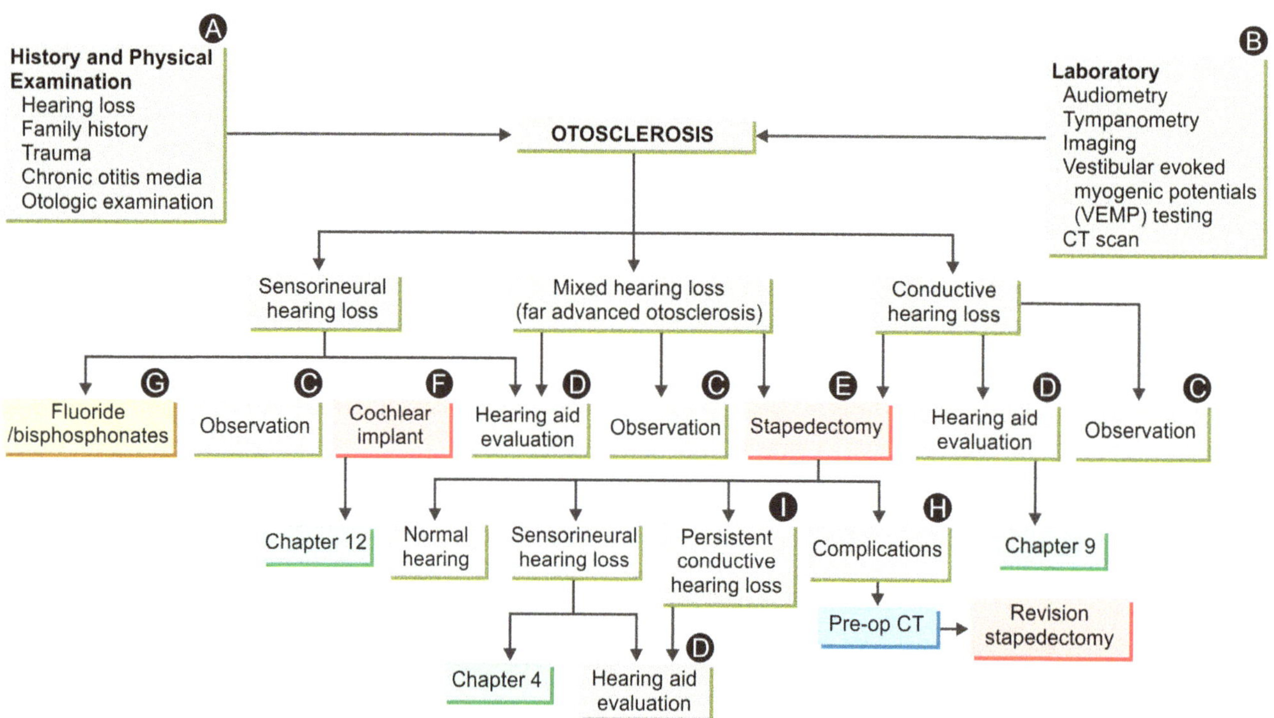

Otosclerosis is a common cause of hearing loss, usually conductive, but also sensorineural and mixed, depending upon whether the lesion involves the stapes or cochlea. Initially, a spongiotic phase occurs, followed by sclerosis. Otosclerosis is thought to be an inherited disease with variable penetrance, with environmental triggers such as measles.

Ⓐ Otosclerosis classically presents in a young adult woman with a history of bilateral hearing loss without trauma or ear infections and normal tympanic membranes. Frequently, there is a family history of hearing loss. There is evidence that the contemporary presenting signs and symptoms of otosclerosis are changing. For example, unilateral otosclerosis at presentation is more common now than what had classically been described. An examination of the ears using a microscope as well as tuning fork testing is absolutely essential.

Ⓑ Accurate audiometry is critical. Otosclerosis can produce conductive, sensorineural, or mixed hearing loss. Conductive hearing loss from stapedial otosclerosis is easily diagnosed. Absent stapedial reflexes are the rule; however, a negative on-off reflex may be present when minimal footplate fixation is present. Tympanometry is frequently normal. Radiographic imaging with fine-cut computed tomography (CT) scans of the temporal bone can be helpful, especially if a diagnosis of cochlear otosclerosis is being considered. Cochlear otosclerosis usually increases the density of the bone of the normal otic capsule, and otospongiosis decreases it. A CT scan is especially useful in children to identify coexisting inner ear abnormalities. If stapedial reflexes are present, superior canal dehiscence should be ruled out with vestibulo-evoked myogenic potential and a CT scan.

Ⓒ Patients with otosclerotic hearing loss have three options: Observation, hearing aid fitting and stapedectomy. Options are discussed with the patient, who, of course, must make the final decision. Some patients, either by their own decision or by medical considerations, are not candidates for a hearing aid or stapedectomy. Periodic audiologic evaluation is recommended for all patients regardless of treatment.

Ⓓ Hearing aids are offered as a treatment option to all patients. The advantage of a hearing aid is that it will improve hearing without the risk of surgery. The disadvantage includes occlusion effects, difficulty with background noise, feedback, external otitis, and cosmetic concerns. The ultimate decision to use a hearing aid is left to the discretion of the patient.

Ⓔ The expectations of stapes surgery should be explained to the patient. Some patients will have normal hearing restored. In others, hearing will be improved but a hearing aid may still be helpful. Some patients will be able to use a hearing aid more effectively after a stapedectomy. Patients with far-advanced otosclerosis have extensive sensorineural and conductive hearing loss. They classically have good voice quality and obtain unexpected benefits from hearing aids despite hearing losses at profound levels. After stapedectomy, these patients are very grateful because they can use a less powerful hearing aid with fewer feedback problems.

Patients are considered candidates for stapes surgery if they have the following characteristics:

1. Good general health; age not a critical factor.
2. The poorer hearing ear is the ear that is being contemplated for surgery.
3. Rinne sign is negative (air conduction < bone conduction) at 512 Hz on tuning fork examination or there is a minimum of 20-dB air-bone gap as averaged in the speech frequency on audiogram.
4. Stapedectomy should not be performed in patients with coexisting active Meniere's disease, tympanic membrane perforation, otitis externa or otitis media in the better hearing ear.

F For those patients who have severe-to-profound sensorineural hearing loss and whose hearing aids provide minimal-to-no benefit, cochlear implantation has proven beneficial. Patients who have evidence of an obliterated cochlea on radiographic imaging should be advised of difficulty in electrode placement and possible reduced benefits.

G Fluorides and bisphosphonates have been reported for medical treatment of sensorineural hearing loss from otosclerosis. Their use is controversial and not widespread.

H All patients should be counseled preoperatively about possible complications. Either partial or total hearing loss occurs in <1% of patients. Trauma, labyrinthitis, fistula, and reparative granulomas can cause postoperative sensorineural hearing loss. Tinnitus can occur in the absence of postoperative hearing loss. Dizziness is common postoperatively; however, typically it is neither prolonged nor severe. Disturbance of taste from manipulation of the chorda tympani is common, but severe symptoms are unusual. Facial paralysis is usually from local anesthesia and consequently temporary. Permanent facial paralysis is quite unusual. Tympanic membrane perforations heal spontaneously and, if not, can be closed using various grafts.

I Patients with conductive hearing loss after stapedectomy may undergo revision stapedectomy. The success rate for a primary stapedectomy in experienced hands is ~90%, but it is significantly lower for revision stapedectomy and the incidence of total hearing loss is higher. Patients with persistent conductive hearing loss following routine stapes surgery may be evaluated with CT for superior canal dehiscence. The usefulness of laser in stapedectomy, especially in revision, has been described.

SUGGESTED READING

Brookler K. Medical treatment of otosclerosis: rationale for the use of bisphosphonates. Int Tinnitus J. 2008;14(2):92-96.

Halmagui GM, Aw ST, McGarvie LA. Superior canal dehiscence simulating otosclerosis. J. Laryngol Otol. 2003;117:553-557.

Hannley MT. Audiologic characteristics of the patient with otosclerosis. Otolaryngol Clin North Am. 1993;26:373-387.

Hom KL, Gherini SG, Griffin GM. Argon laser stapedectomy using an endo-otoprobe system. Otolaryngol Head and Neck Surg. 1990;102:193-198.

House HP, Kwartler JA. Total stapedectomy. In: Brackmann DE (Ed). Otologic Surgery. Philadelphia: WB Saunders; 1994. p. 291.

Lesinski SG, Palmer A. Lasers for otosclerosis: CO_2 vs. argon and KTP-532. Laryngoscope. 1989;99(Suppl 46):1-8.

Lippy WH, Berenholz LP, Burley JM. Otosclerosis in the 1960s, 1970s, 1980s and 1990s. Laryngoscope. 1999;109:1307-1309.

Shambaugh GE Jr. Adult fluoride therapy for otosclerosis. Arch Otolaryngol. 1983;109:353.

Valvassori EG. Imaging of otosclerosis. Otolaryngol Clin North Am. 1993;26:359-371.

Meniere's Disease

Peter C Weber

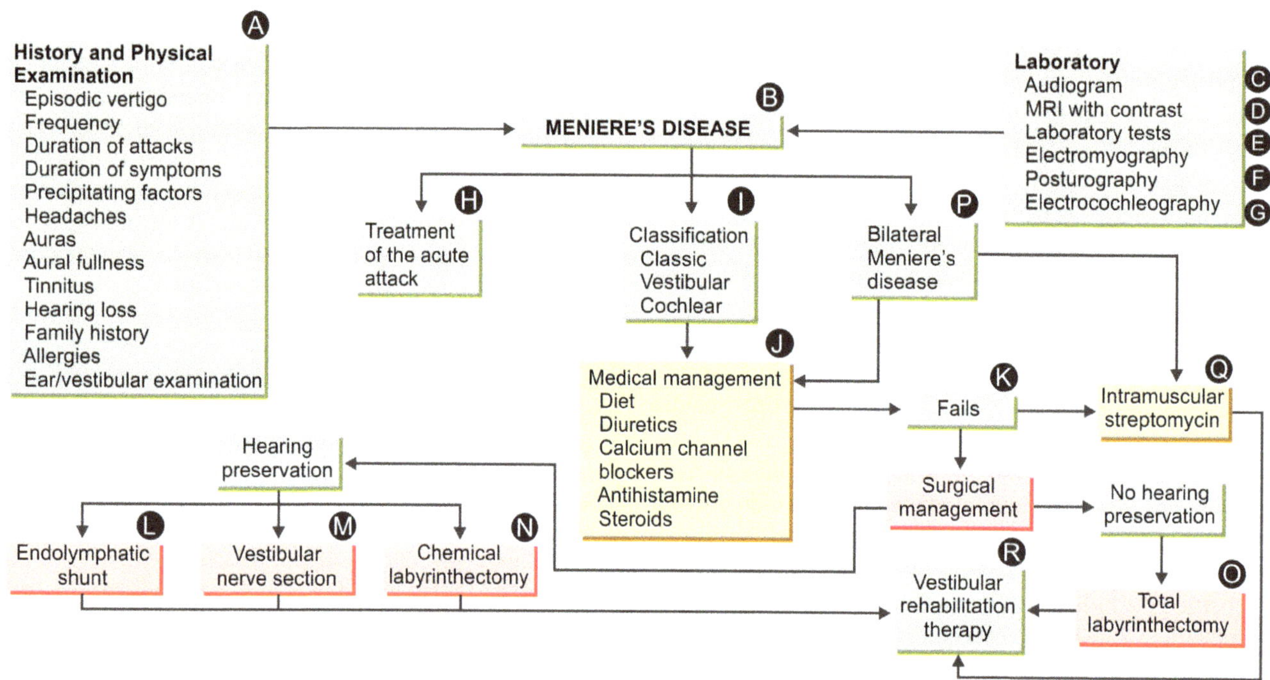

Meniere's syndrome is a chronic condition consisting of episodic vertigo associated with aural fullness, tinnitus, and hearing loss that last hours at a time. Affected patients have a highly variable clinical course, some are able to be managed easily with conservative measures, whereas for others, the symptoms are life-altering and require more aggressive management. Many etiologies (e.g. migraines, allergies, and autoimmune) may cause the symptoms associated with Meniere's syndrome. These should be treated appropriately (such as Topomax or Effexor for migraines), but when the etiology is idiopathic, it is then called Meniere's disease. Classically, Meniere's disease is thought of as a build-up of excess fluid in the inner ear system for unknown reasons. Accurately ascertaining triggers for the attacks often assists in selecting appropriate management.

A The history is key in making the diagnosis. Although classically the episodic attacks of vertigo are associated with aural fullness, tinnitus, and fluctuating hearing loss that last hours at a time, sometimes only a few of these symptoms are present. In addition, the fullness, tinnitus, and hearing loss normally resolve after the attack has subsided. However, with long-standing disease, the associated symptoms of hearing loss, tinnitus, and fullness may become permanent.

B When the patient is not having an attack of vertigo, the otologic examination and office vestibular examination are normal. However, during an attack, the patient will typically have nystagmus, with the fast component beating toward the affected ear.

C The patient will have a normal audiogram during the symptom-free time between attacks early in the disease. As the disease progresses a low-frequency sensorineural hearing loss will typically develop, which will become permanent and will eventually progress to include the other frequencies.

D A magnetic resonance imaging (MRI) scan with gadolinium is required, because Meniere's disease is a diagnosis of exclusion. Various disease entities such as tumors can mimic Meniere's disease. MRI with gadolinium is normal in Meniere's disease.

E Because Meniere's disease is a diagnosis of exclusion, evaluation for hypo- and hyperthyroidism, syphilis, autoimmune disorders, anemia, white blood cell dysplasias, and diabetes should be considered. Because of the possible treatment entities, a baseline potassium level may be helpful.

F When the patient is not having an attack, videoelectronystagmography (VNG) and posturography are invariably normal. Over time, unilateral vestibular weakness may be seen. There is a higher propensity for patients with Meniere's disease to experience benign positional vertigo. This may be noted either in office vestibular testing or on the VNG during Hallpike's maneuver. The benign paroxysmal positional vertigo is treated in the usual positional maneuvers.

Ⓖ Classically, an increased summation potential/action potential ratio is seen; however, electrocochleography is a nonspecific test and, like other tests (glycerol), is not used universally.

Ⓗ Treatment of an acute attack of Meniere's disease is supportive. Vestibular suppressants, such as benzodiazepines, may be used as well as antiemetics. These fall into the category of anticholinergics-antidopaminergics-antihistamines. The new antiemetic, ondansetron hydrochloride may also be used but this is not as useful for vertigo as it is for nausea from chemotherapy and anesthesia.

Ⓘ Meniere's disease may be categorized into three different subgroups. Classical Meniere's disease consists of episodic vertigo, aural fullness, tinnitus, and hearing loss. Vestibular Meniere's disease consists of episodic attacks of vertigo without the aural fullness, tinnitus, or hearing loss (or maybe just one or two associated symptoms). Cochlear Meniere's disease consists of fluctuating hearing loss without the episodic vertigo.

Ⓙ Medical management of Meniere's disease classically consists of diet modifications to reduce the intake of sodium in hopes of preventing the attacks of vertigo. A salt-restrictive diet (about 2000 mg of sodium per day) is recommended. Intake of caffeine, alcohol, nicotine, and chocolate is restricted. Because Meniere's disease is thought to be due to an accumulation of excess fluid in the inner ear system, diuretics are usually employed, the most common of which is a combination of hydrochlorothiazide and triamterene. Occasionally, a potassium supplement may be needed. Other medications that can be effective in the treatment of Meniere's disease include calcium channel blockers, antihistamines (because 10–20% of cases may be allergy-induced), vasodilators, angiotensin-converting enzyme inhibitors, lipoflavins, and vitamins. In many other countries (not in the United States) β-histamine (Serc) is used with good success. When vertiginous attacks occur frequently (i.e. every day or every other day), treatment with steroids may also be beneficial.

Ⓚ Medical management of Meniere's disease will fail in about 10–30% of cases in that in these patients the frequency of vertiginous attacks significantly interferes with the patient's lifestyle. Once this occurs, the patient should be considered for surgical management or chemoablation. Surgical management consists of either hearing preservation or nonhearing preservation approaches. Decisions regarding further therapy require considerable discussion with the patient to include all options. Prior to surgical options, the use of intratympanic injections (typically 1–3 injections) of dexamethasone is very useful to abate these breakthrough spells. The use of intratympanic injections has reduced the number of patients requiring surgical intervention to about 5–10% of cases.

Ⓛ Endolymphatic shunt will control vertigo spells in about 60% of cases. It is hypothesized to work by allowing excess fluid to drain out of the endolymphatic sac. In skilled hands, it has a very low risk for facial nerve paralysis or hearing loss. Long-term success rates vary, but if it works initially, then there is only about a 20% relapse rate.

Ⓜ Vestibular nerve section eliminates the episodic vertigo spells at least 95% of the time. The possibility of hearing loss is <5%, and the risk of facial nerve paralysis is also quite low. This is an intracranial procedure, however, and intracranial complications may occur.

Ⓝ Chemical labyrinthectomy is a procedure that ablates the vestibular end organs by injection of gentamicin into the middle ear, allowing absorption into the inner ear. This is an office procedure that is well tolerated. It will control dizzy spells up to 80% of the time, but is associated with a 20–30% chance of significant hearing loss.

Ⓞ Total labyrinthectomy is an excellent method for treating Meniere's disease, especially if the patient has no hearing or negligible, nonuseful hearing. It eliminates vertigo 95% of the time and has a very low incidence of facial nerve paralysis. These patients may be implanted with a cochlear implant at the same time to enhance their hearing.

Ⓟ Meniere's disease may affect both ears. Some report this incidence to be 30% or more.

Ⓠ The treatment for bilateral Meniere's disease that fails traditional medical management, including steroids and intratympanic injections, has included endolymphatic shunts, vestibular ablation on one side and nonablative treatments on the other (which usually happens because the ablative surgery is done prior to the second side becoming a problem), and intramuscular injection of streptomycin. The streptomycin is given until the vertiginous spells are controlled but there is a risk of significant hearing loss and oscillopsia.

Ⓡ Vestibular rehabilitation therapy is very useful in minimizing the long-term effects of vestibular ablation or weakness (unilateral or bilateral). Patients undergoing vestibular nerve section, chemical labyrinthectomy, labyrinthectomy, or intramuscular streptomycin should be offered vestibular rehabilitation therapy to enhance compensation for the loss of the unilateral vestibular system.

SUGGESTED READING

Arnold SA, Stewart AM, Moor HM, et al. The effectiveness of vestibular rehabilitation interventions in treating unilateral peripheral vestibular disorders: a systematic review. Physiother Res Int. 2015;Jun 25. doi: 10.1002/pri.1635. [Epub ahead of print].

Hirsch BE, Kamerer DB. Intratympanic gentamicin therapy for Meniere's disease. Am J Otol. 1997;18:44-51.

Silverstein H, Wannamaker H, Flaeager J. Vestibular neurectomy in the U.S.—1990. Am J Otol. 1992;13:23-30.

Sood AJ, Lambert PR, Nguyen SA, et al. Endolymphatic sac surgery for Meniere's disease: a systematic review and meta-analysis. Otol Neurotol. 2014;35:1033-1045.

Syed MI, Ilan O, Nassar J, et al. Intratympanic therapy in Meniere's syndrome or disease: up to date evidence for clinical practice. Clin Otolaryngol. 2015;40:682-690.

Weber PC. Meniere's disease. Otolaryngol Clin North Am. 1997; 30:977-986.

Vestibular Neuritis

Douglas M Hildrew, Andrew A McCall

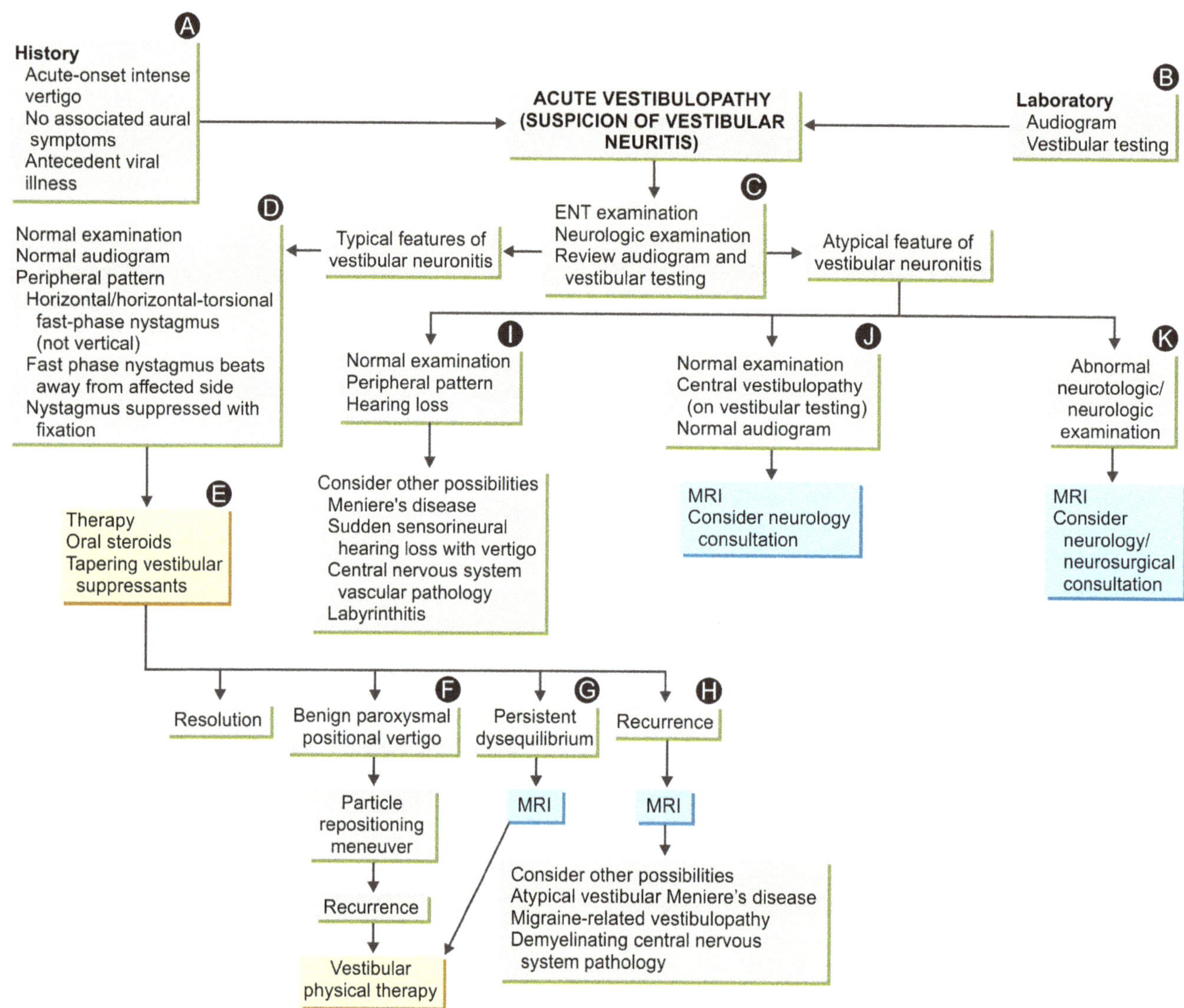

Vestibular neuritis (VN) is an acute unilateral vestibulopathy, associated with an acute onset of rotatory vertigo that can last from days to weeks. The key symptoms associated with VN include acute or subacute onset of sustained rotatory vertigo, gait, and postural unsteadiness with a tendency to fall toward the affected ear, nausea, and vomiting. While VN is thought to be associated with herpes simplex virus (HSV)-1 and some patients report antecedent upper respiratory tract infection (URI) symptoms, many patients have no antecedent triggers or prodromal symptoms. Because the superior division of the vestibular nerve is thought to be most vulnerable, one should expect to see horizontal-rotatory spontaneous nystagmus with a fast phase that beats toward the nonaffected ear.

A torsional component is often seen, beating with the pole at the 12-o'clock position directed toward the nonaffected ear. Clinical recovery is achieved through spontaneous recovery of peripheral vestibular function (which is often incomplete), sensory substitution, and central compensation. Even though corticosteroids are the mainstay of therapy, many studies indicate that while they may hasten the initial rate of recovery, they do not affect the ultimate clinical outcome.

A Vestibular neuritis is characterized by acute or subacute onset of intense rotatory vertigo associated with nausea and vomiting. The symptom of vertigo should be sustained, and will last from days to weeks. Associated aural symptoms (decreased hearing, aural pressure, and tinnitus) are typically absent. Patients are frequently younger (30s to 40s) without a significant medical history. Some patients may experience an antecedent viral upper respiratory infection several days to weeks before the onset of vertiginous symptoms.

B Standard initial laboratory evaluation includes audiometric testing and vestibular testing. The presence of new onset hearing loss is generally inconsistent with VN. Vestibular testing is helpful in distinguishing between peripheral and central vestibular dysfunction, and can reveal which side is involved. A full battery of vestibular testing may include electronystagmography (oculomotor testing, positional/positioning testing, and response to caloric irrigation of the labyrinth), rotational chair testing, vestibular-evoked myogenic potential (VEMP), and computerized dynamic posturography. Oculomotor examination classically reveals a horizontal-rotatory spontaneous nystagmus that beats toward the nonaffected ear with a torsional component, beating with the pole at the 12-o'clock position directed toward the nonaffected ear. This nystagmus will increase in intensity when gaze is directed toward the nonaffected ear. Caloric testing typically shows reduced function of the affected horizontal canal. Head-impulse testing will reveal an inability to maintain fixation during a head-thrust toward the affected side. Since the majority of patients presenting with VN will have an onset of disease that is thought to originate within the superior vestibular nerve, one should expect ocular vestibular-evoked myogenic potential (oVEMP) studies to have reduced or absent amplitudes. In the less common case that the cervical vestibular-evoked myogenic potential (cVEMP) is reduced or absent in amplitude involvement of the inferior vestibular nerve is suspected.

C While an in-depth history is often the most instructive component for suggesting the diagnosis, a thorough otolaryngologic and neurological examination should never be omitted. The use of a binocular microscope and pneumatic otoscopy may be useful in ruling out infectious disease. From a neurologic standpoint, one should assess the cranial nerves, evaluate the motor and sensory systems, perform coordination testing, Romberg's test, and gait assessment.

D Patients evaluated during the acute phase may demonstrate spontaneous nystagmus and a peripheral vestibulopathy pattern on vestibular testing. The nystagmus is expected to be horizontal or horizontal-torsional (with the fast-phase nystagmus beating away from the affected side) and suppressed with visual fixation. Nystagmus should not be vertical in VN, as this finding suggests a central origin of disease. Examination after the acute phase has subsided will usually demonstrate no spontaneous nystagmus, but findings consistent with peripheral vestibulopathy on vestibular testing will typically persist.

E Vestibular suppressants, such as meclizine, dimenhydrinate, scopolamine, and benzodiazepines can be helpful for the first several days after onset, but their use should be restricted there after, as they may ultimately delay central nervous system (CNS) compensation mechanisms

and prolong vestibular symptoms. Treatment with a high-dose oral steroid taper (such as prednisone, prednisolone, or methylprednisolone) may hasten the initial rate of recovery, but has not been proven to alter the ultimate clinical outcome. Clinical recovery may be achieved within a 6- to 8-week time frame through spontaneous recovery of peripheral vestibular function (which is often incomplete), sensory substitution, and central compensation. Because VN is often characterized by an incomplete vestibular recovery, peripheral weakness as seen on vestibular testing may persist indefinitely.

F It is not uncommon for patients to develop benign paroxysmal positional vertigo weeks to months after developing VN. Typically, they can be treated in the office with a particle repositioning maneuver; patients suffering from intermittent recurrences can be managed well with vestibular physical therapy.

G Infrequently, persistent dysequilibrium can occur after the acute vertigo has subsided due to impaired central compensation mechanisms. Vestibular physical therapy is the mainstay for therapy. Magnetic resonance imaging (MRI) testing should be considered to evaluate whether CNS disease is present.

H Although VN is classically described as a single episode of self-limiting symptoms, a small subset of patients can develop infrequent recurrences of intense vertigo. Such recurrent vestibular symptoms should prompt clinicians to consider atypical vestibular Meniere's disease, migraine-related vestibulopathy, demyelinating CNS disease, and CNS vascular disease. Retrocochlear and CNS pathology should be excluded by way of MRI.

I Hearing loss is not a symptom typically seen with VN. Patients with a peripheral vestibular weakness, hearing loss, and a normal physical examination are unlikely to be suffering from an isolated episode of VN. In this case, one should explore an alternate diagnosis, such as Meniere's disease, sudden sensorineural hearing loss with vertigo, serous labyrinthitis, and CNS vascular diseases.

J Central nervous system disease may present with vestibular abnormalities in spite of a normal physical examination and audiometric testing. In this setting, one should consider both MRI testing and consultation with a Neurologist who has knowledge of balance disorders.

K Any physical examination findings consistent with a retrocochlear or central etiology of disease should be diagnosed with MRI, and may warrant neurotologic and/ or neurosurgical consultation. Such findings include cranial nerve palsies, motor/sensory asymmetries, asymmetric sensorineural hearing loss, and poor speech discrimination scores.

SUGGESTED READING

Fishman JM, Burgess C, Waddell A. Corticosteroids for the treatment of idiopathic acute vestibular dysfunction (vestibular neuritis). Cochrane Database Syst Rev. 2011;(5):CD008607.

Goudakos JK, Markou KD, Franco-Vidal V, et al. Corticosteroids in the treatment of vestibular neuritis: a systematic review and meta-analysis. Otol Neurotol. 2010;31(2):183-189.

Strupp M, Magnusson M. Acute unilateral vestibulopathy. Neurol Clin. 2015;33(3):669-685.

Ototoxicity

CY Joseph Chang

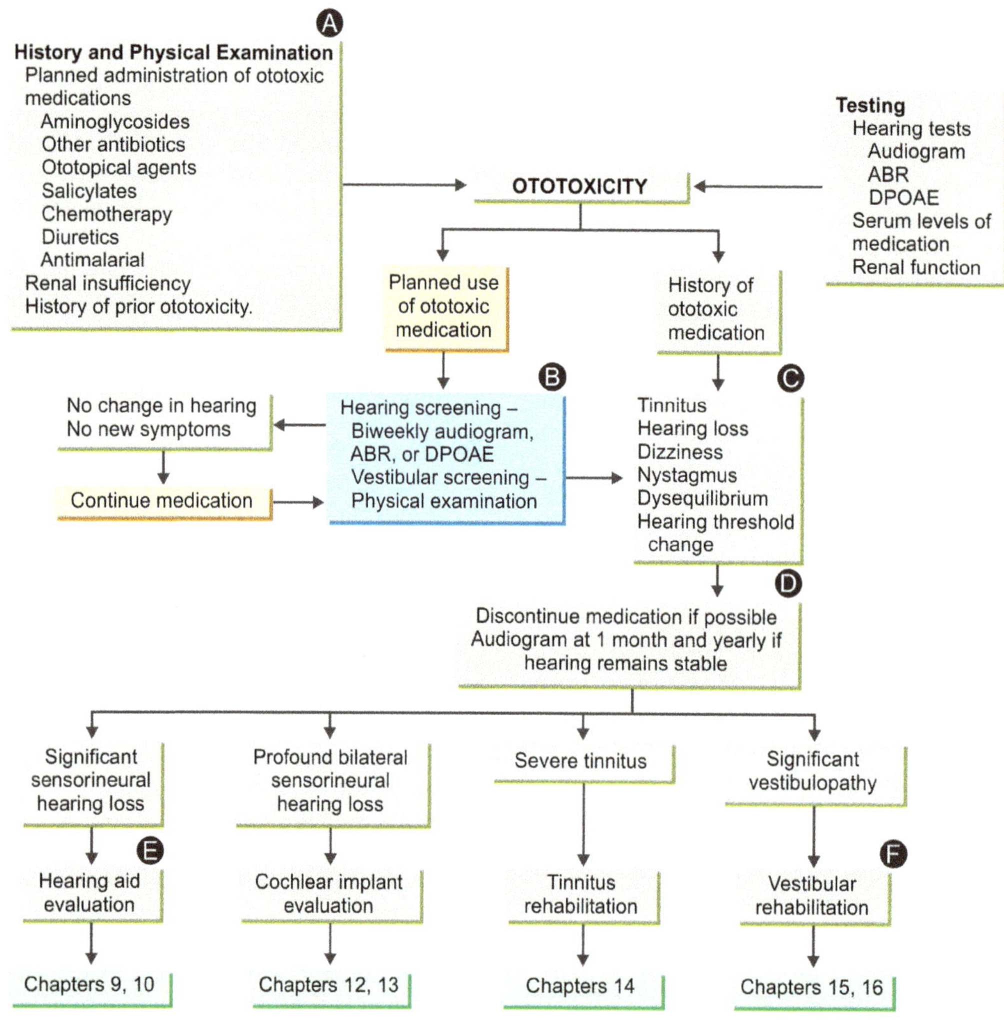

There are numerous agents that are known to have ototoxic properties; hence, the incidence of drug-induced ototoxicity is quite significant (*see* Table 41.1). The prevalence of ototoxicity with aminoglycosides is estimated to be 10%, and even higher with cisplatin administration. Because treatment options for ototoxicity are limited, it is important to institute policies and procedures to prevent irreversible damage during the administration of potentially ototoxic medications. Early detection of inner ear damage may be possible in some cases, however, many patients will incur significant ototoxic damage and require treatment for this condition.

A A history of prior ototoxicity and renal insufficiency is thought to increase the risk of additional ototoxic damage. No definitive set of risk factors has been identified that seems to be effective for screening. Factors that can potentiate the ototoxic effects of known ototoxic agents include coadministration of multiple ototoxic drugs and poor control of dosing and serum levels. Genetic factors have recently been implicated in individual susceptibility to aminoglycoside and cisplatin ototoxicity. Additional advances in personalized medicine with sophisticated genetic testing may eventually provide new strategies for predicting and preventing ototoxicity.

B There are various agents under investigation that may ameliorate the ototoxic effects of medications such as aminoglycosides and cisplatin. There are numerous candidate protective agents that have been evaluated in animal studies with variable success. There are a few protective agents against neurotoxicity, nephrotoxicity, and bone marrow toxicity that have shown promise in limited human studies, and these include steroids, d-methionine, l-N-acetylcysteine, and amifostine. These agents have not

Table 41.1: Medications with ototoxic potential.

Classes – ototoxic	Medications	Notes
Aminoglycosides	Gentamicin, neomycin, tobramycin, amikacin, kanamycin	Directly toxic to hair cells even with therapeutic dosages.
Other antibiotics	Erythromycin, vancomycin	Ototoxicity reported with high doses.
Topical otologic medications	Neomycin, polymixin B	Ototoxicity demonstrated in animal studies, suspected but not substantiated cause of ototoxicity in humans. New nono-totoxic topical agents such as ofloxacin should obviate the need to use ototoxic topical agents in most cases.
Salicylates	Aspirin	Ototoxic effects are reversible.
Chemotherapy	Cisplatin	Newer agents such as carboplatin are less ototoxic.
Diuretics	Furosemide (loop diuretics), hydrochlorothiazide	Main ototoxicity risk when coadministered with other agents, i.e. aminoglycosides.
Antimalarial	Quinine, chloroquine	Ototoxicity reported with high doses.

yet been studied adequately for widespread clinical use to reduce or prevent ototoxicity. There is also a concern that these protective agents could decrease the efficacy of treatment with aminoglycoside or cisplatin. Transtympanic administration of these protective agents may eliminate this concern, but more investigations are needed to show if this approach is feasible or effective.

Monitoring during treatment with a potentially ototoxic drug should include daily questioning for symptoms such as tinnitus, hearing loss, and dizziness, as well as physical examination aimed at detecting vestibular changes. Biweekly hearing screening with audiograms, auditory brainstem response (ABR), or distortion-product otoacoustic emissions (DPOAE) should also be considered. Pure tone audiograms offer the most definitive method of hearing loss detection, and high-frequency testing above 8 kHz may lead to detection of ototoxicity prior to development of hearing loss in the speech range, although this latter testing is not routinely available ABR and OAE (otoacoustic emission) offer a less labor-intensive screening method. These latter technologies may provide early indications of cochleotoxicity prior to the advent of hearing loss detectable on audiometry. This potential is under investigation at this time.

Screening for vestibulotoxicity is problematic since there are no established screening tests that are simple to perform, low-cost, and reliable. Bedside clinical evaluation for spontaneous nystagmus, post-headshake nystagmus, and balance function remain critical methods for detecting early onset of vestibulotoxicity.

(C) At the first sign of inner ear damage, the administration of the suspected ototoxic medication should be discontinued or replaced if it is clinically safe to do so. For example, carboplatin is associated with a much lower incidence of neurotoxicity compared to cisplatin. If the medication cannot be discontinued, dosing will need to be optimized to reduce its ototoxic effect by monitoring serum drug levels closely.

(D) Hearing evaluations should be carried out after discontinuation of the ototoxic medication as some patients recover cochlear function to varying degrees.

(E) Hearing loss present 1–2 months after ototoxic exposure is usually permanent, and the main treatment option is amplification. If the hearing loss is too severe for adequate amplification, cochlear implantation should be considered. The treatment of severe subjective tinnitus continues to be problematic. The treatment algorithm for tinnitus due to ototoxicity is the same as for tinnitus associated with sensorineural hearing loss.

(F) Vestibular dysfunction is often quite debilitating. Initial symptoms may include vertigo, which often subsides. Permanent vestibular dysfunction typically consists of dysequilibrium, gait dysfunction, and sometimes oscillopsia. Episodic vertigo, especially with certain head or body motion, may also occur. The vertigo symptoms can sometimes be managed medically with meclizine or diazepam, but prolonged use of vestibular suppressants can delay recovery of balance function. In most cases, balance evaluation followed by vestibular rehabilitation therapy represents the most helpful form of intervention. The prognosis for full recovery of balance function depends on the severity of deficits and symptoms, but most patients improve slowly over time.

SUGGESTED READING

Abi-Hachem RN, Zine A, Van De Water TR. The injured cochlea as a target for inflammatory processes, initiation of cell death pathways and application of related otoprotectives strategies. Recent Pat CNS Drug Discov. 2010;5:147-163.

De Lauretis A, De Capua B, Barbieri MT, et al. ABR evaluation of ototoxicity in cancer patients receiving cisplatin or carboplatin. Scand Audiol. 1999;28:139-143.

Fausti SA, Larson VD, Noffsinger D, et al. High-frequency audiometric monitoring strategies for early detection of ototoxicity. Ear Hear. 1994;15(3):232-239.

Halmagyi GM, Fattore CM, Curthoys IA, et al. Gentamicin vestibulotoxicity. Otolaryngol Head Neck Surg. 1994;111:571-574.

Hobbie SN, Akshay S, Kalapala SK, et al. Genetic analysis of interactions with eukaryotic rRNA identify the mitoribosome as target in aminoglycoside ototoxicity. Proc Natl Acad Sci USA. 2008;105:20888-20893.

Hotz MA, Harris FP, Probst R. Otoacoustic emissions: an approach for monitoring aminoglycoside-induced ototoxicity. Laryngoscope. 1994;104:1130-1134.

Mukherjea D, Rybak LP, Sheehan KE, et al. The design and screening of drugs to prevent acquired sensorineural hearing loss. Expert Opin Drug Discov. 2011;6:491-505.

Rybak LP, Brenner MJ. Vestibular and Auditory Ototoxicity. In Flint P (Ed.) Cummings Otolaryngology-Head and Neck Surgery, 6th ed. Philadelphia, PA: Elsevier, 2014. pp. 2369-2382.

Tumors of the Ear and Temporal Bone

Moisés A Arriaga

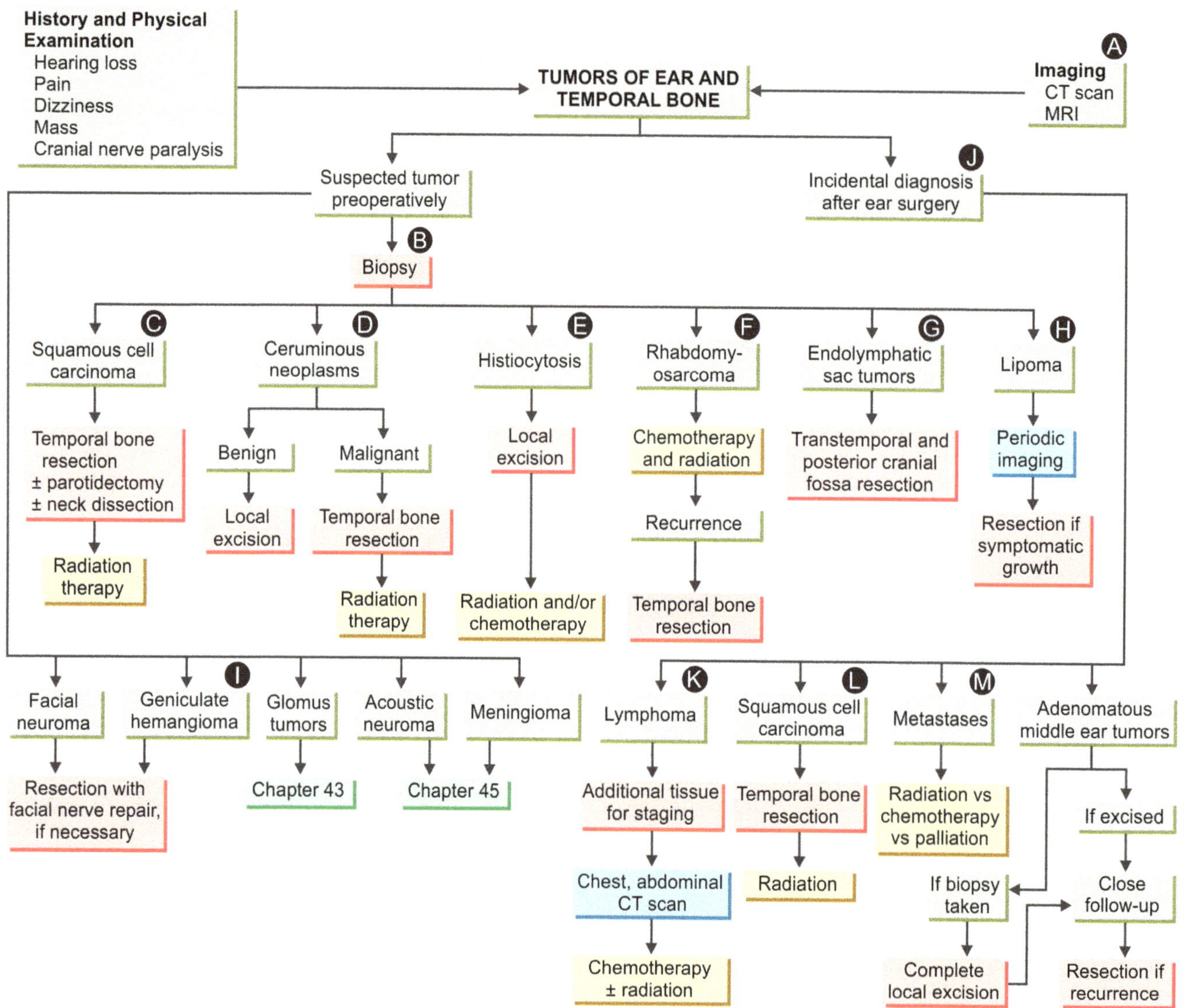

The temporal bone may be the site of primary tumors or neoplasms extending from the adjacent skull base. In this location, such tumors produce a broad range of symptoms related to the audiovestibular system, cranial nerves traversing the skull base and adjacent brain parenchyma. The clinical management of these tumors includes observation, surgery, radiation, and chemotherapy depending on the histology, size and clinical presentation of the lesion.

A Computed tomography (CT) and magnetic resonance imaging (MRI) are the imaging modalities of choice for tumors of the temporal bone. CT provides detail of bone erosion. MRI with contrast discloses soft tissue lesions, neural involvement, and subclinical tissue infiltration. Both studies are usually required.

B Biopsy of lesions of the ear canal or middle ear can be considered after CT confirms that important vascular or neural structures are not involved. Biopsy of middle ear lesions is specifically discouraged before imaging studies.

C Temporal bone carcinoma can be staged:

Stage I: Ear canal soft tissue only

Stage II: Limited ear canal bone erosion

Stage III: Middle ear/mastoid involvement or deep erosion of the ear canal

Stage IV: Extensive tumor with deep soft tissue, dura, or facial nerve involvement.

The most important prognostic factor is the status of surgical margins. The choice of partial (lateral), subtotal, and total temporal bone resection depends on the tumor stage. Postoperative radiation is usually recommended for advanced stage tumors.

D The histology of ceruminous neoplasms determines the aggressiveness of therapy. Local excision is adequate for benign lesions, whereas more aggressive surgery is necessary for malignant tumors.

E Histiocytosis X (Langerhans cell histiocytosis) represents a spectrum of neoplastic lesions (eosinophilic granuloma, Hand-Schüller-Christian disease, Letterer-Siwe disease) characterized by local bone destruction. These are usually managed by tumor debulking and chemotherapy and/or radiation.

F Rhabdomyosarcoma is managed primarily with chemotherapy and radiation. Surgery is used only for biopsy or treatment of recurrent tumor.

G Tumors of the endolymphatic sac often erode beyond the mastoid into the posterior cranial fossa. Histologically, these are usually low-grade adenocarcinomas. Team management with Neurosurgery is recommended as obtaining clear margins usually requires resection of dura.

H Temporal bone lipomas are very adherent to adjacent nerves. Because they are slow growing, lipomas are usually managed expectantly with periodic imaging and resection only in patients who are symptomatic.

I Hemangiomas often arise adjacent to the geniculate ganglion. Middle fossa exposure is usually needed for complete excision and facial nerve repair, if necessary.

J When the histopathologic diagnosis of malignancy is unexpected, the surgeon must obtain adequate imaging and confirm the histology before further treatment planning.

K Lymphoma is usually an unexpected diagnosis during surgery for presumptive chronic otitis media. The lesions are usually pale, infiltrative, and poorly vascularized. Chest and abdominal CT and bone marrow biopsy are necessary before treatment (chemotherapy or radiation or both).

L The diagnosis of squamous carcinoma of the temporal bone usually occurs in advanced stages with involvement of the middle ear and mastoid. Surgery requires an extensive temporal bone resection followed by radiation therapy. Alternatively, palliative radiation may be offered.

M Metastatic adenocarcinoma to the temporal bone is uncommon. Consultation with a medical oncologist for staging, identification of primary tumor, and treatment planning is necessary.

SUGGESTED READING

Arriaga M, Curtin H, Takahashi H, et al. Staging proposal for external auditory meatus carcinoma based on preoperative clinical examination and computed tomography findings. Ann Otol Rhinol Laryngol. 1990;99:714-721.

Arriaga M. Anatomy of Transtemporal Surgery. In: Janecka IP, Tiedemann K (Eds). Skull Base Surgery: Anatomy, Biology, and Technology. Philadelphia: Lippincott Williams and Wilkins; 1997.

Arriaga MA, Brackmann D. Posterior Fossa Neoplasms. In: Flint PW, Haughey BH, Lund VJ, et al. (Eds). Cummings Otolaryngology: Head & Neck Surgery, 6th edition. Philadelphia, PA: Elsevier Mosby Saunders; 2015.

Brackmann D, Shelton D, Arriaga M. Otologic Surgery, 4th edition. Philadelphia: Elsevier; 2015.

Jackler RK, Brackmann ED (Eds). Neurotology, 2nd edition. St. Louis: Mosby; 2004.

Moody SA, Hirsch BE, Myers EN. Squamous cell carcinoma of the external auditory canal: an evolution of a staging system. Am J Otol. 2000;21(4):582-588.

Glomus Tumors of the Temporal Bone and Skull Base

Craig A Buchman, Jacques Herzog

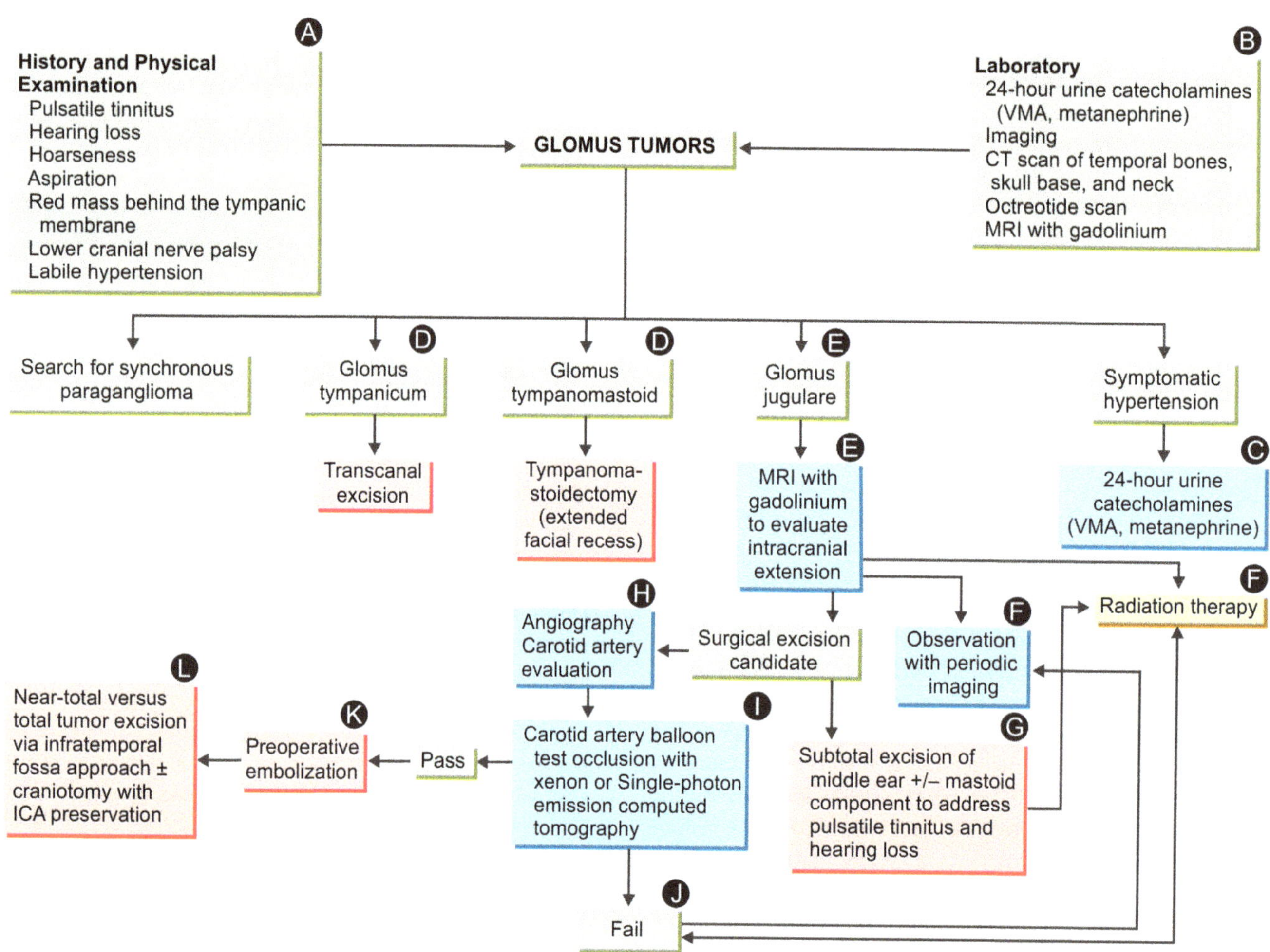

Glomus tumors of the temporal bone and skull base (also known as paragangliomas) are rare, slow-growing, hypervascular tumors, arising from glomus bodies that serve as baroreceptors in the middle ear or in the jugular vein. There are two types of glomus tumors related to the ear: glomus tympanicum and glomus jugulare. Although glomus tumors are rare, they are among the most common benign tumors of the ear. Glomus tumors occur predominantly in women in the fifth and sixth decades of life. Because of the slow onset of symptoms, these tumors often go unnoticed, and diagnosis is delayed. Because of the location and extent of involvement, glomus jugulare tumors present a significant challenge in diagnosis and management.

A A patient with a glomus tumor of the temporal bone most commonly presents with pulsatile tinnitus and a red mass behind or involving the tympanic membrane with or without associated lower cranial nerve dysfunction. A positive family history may be present in patients with these tumors and should arouse suspicion for multiple paragangliomas.

B High-resolution computed tomography (CT) with contrast can be used to differentiate these lesions from vascular malformations and to delineate extension of the tumor. Octreotide scanning is also useful for confirming the diagnosis as well as identifying synchronous tumors throughout the body. With these tests, diagnostic biopsy of these lesions is unnecessary and thus should be avoided, because profuse bleeding may occur.

C Although secreting glomus tumors or synchronous pheochromocytomas are rare (1–3%), all patients with glomus tumors involving the jugular foramen (jugulare) or those with signs and symptoms of catecholamine hypersecretion (episodic flushing and labile hypertension) should undergo 24-hour urine collection for catecholamine metabolites [5-hydroxyindoleacetic acid and vanillylmandelic acid (VMA)]. All patients with catecholamine-secreting tumors require medical intervention before definitive management of the glomus tumor to prevent intraoperative, hypertensive crisis.

D Glomus tumors confined to the middle ear (tympanicum) or mastoid (tympanomastoid or mastoid) require no further diagnostic studies (see the prior discussion) and can be resected via transcanal or tympanomastoid approaches, with recurrence rates of <5% and minimal complications.

E Patients with glomus jugulare tumors should undergo magnetic resonance imaging (MRI) with gadolinium infusion to determine the degree of intracranial extension. The tumors typically demonstrate a "salt and pepper" pattern after infusion of contrast. Intracranial extension with significant brainstem compression is important in that it may require surgical intervention.

F In general, older patients, those with substantial medical comorbidities or small tumors, and those without associated symptoms should be considered for nonsurgical management (i.e. observation or radiation therapy). The use of external beam radiation and stereotactic radiosurgery is becoming commonplace with excellent long-term control in these cases. Annual imaging to assess tumor growth in nonsurgical patients recommended.

G In patients who are significantly bothered by pulsatile tinnitus and conductive hearing loss, there remains a role for surgical debulking of the middle ear/mastoid tumor to reduce or alleviate symptoms. In such cases, surgery can be followed by radiation therapy with excellent rates of tumor control.

H In very young patients, those with secreting tumors, those with extensive intracranial involvement, and those in whom the risk of further morbidity related to additional cranial neuropathies appears unlikely, definitive surgical excision can still be considered an option. In such patients, angiography establishes the vascular supply of these tumors and allows for assessment of the internal carotid artery (ICA). Patients without ICA involvement should proceed to preoperative embolization, because this procedure substantially decreases intraoperative blood loss and may allow greater visualization during tumor removal.

I Patients with significant tumor involvement of the ICA (i.e. pseudoaneurysm, thrombosis, critical compression, or encasement) should be assessed for adequacy of collateral cerebral blood flow with ICA balloon test occlusion (BTO) followed by either xenon or single photon emission CT scanning. To pass this test, patients should tolerate at least 30 minutes of temporary ICA occlusion without neurologic symptoms and demonstrate no associated decrement in cerebral blood flow on xenon or single photon emission CT.

J Patients who fail the BTO procedure should be managed with a procedure that avoids ICA manipulation (i.e. observation, radiation therapy, and subtotal tumor removal with ICA preservation) or should undergo an ICA bypass procedure before tumor removal. The optimal choice between these management modalities remains controversial and treatment should be individualized.

K Those patients with significant tumor involvement of the ICA in whom the BTO procedure succeeds can be considered for a total tumor removal procedure with or without an ICA isolation procedure using detachable proximal and distal intra-arterial balloons. The choice between these particular interventions should also be individualized. Even in these circumstances, carotid artery sacrifice carries with it a risk of catastrophic stroke.

L For patients with glomus jugulare tumors without surgical contraindications, gross total removal with preservation of neurologic function provides recurrence rates of <10%. Mortality rates for glomus jugulare tumors at most institutions are <1%, and morbidity is usually related to the associated cranial nerve dysfunction. In general, complications are related to the degree of preoperative cranial nerve dysfunction and the extent of tumor involvement. Complications may include facial weakness, hearing loss, hoarseness, aspiration, dysarthria, or intracranial complication such as meningitis, hemorrhage, stroke, or death.

SUGGESTED READING

Carlson ML, Sweeney AD, Pelosi S, et al. Glomus tympanicum: a review of 115 cases over 4 decades. Otolaryngol Head Neck Surg. 2015;152(1):136-142.

Carlson ML, Sweeney AD, Wanna GB, et al. Natural history of glomus jugulare: a review of 16 tumors managed with primary observation. Otolaryngol Head Neck Surg. 2015;152(1):98-105.

Jacob JT, Pollock BE, Carlson ML, et al. Stereotactic radiosurgery in the management of vestibular schwannoma and glomus jugulare: indications, techniques, and results. Otolaryngol Clin North Am. 2015;48(3):515-526.

Miller JP, Semaan MT, Maciunas RJ, et al. Radiosurgery for glomus jugulare tumors. Otolaryngol Clin North Am. 2009;42(4):689-706.

Telischi FF, Bustillo A, Whiteman MLH, et al. Octreotide scintigraphy for the detection of paragangliomas. Otolaryngol Head Neck Surg. 2000;122(3):358-362.

Wanna GB, Sweeney AD, Haynes DS, et al. Contemporary management of jugular paragangliomas. Otolaryngol Clin North Am. 2015;48(2):331-341.

Petrous Apex Lesions

CY Joseph Chang

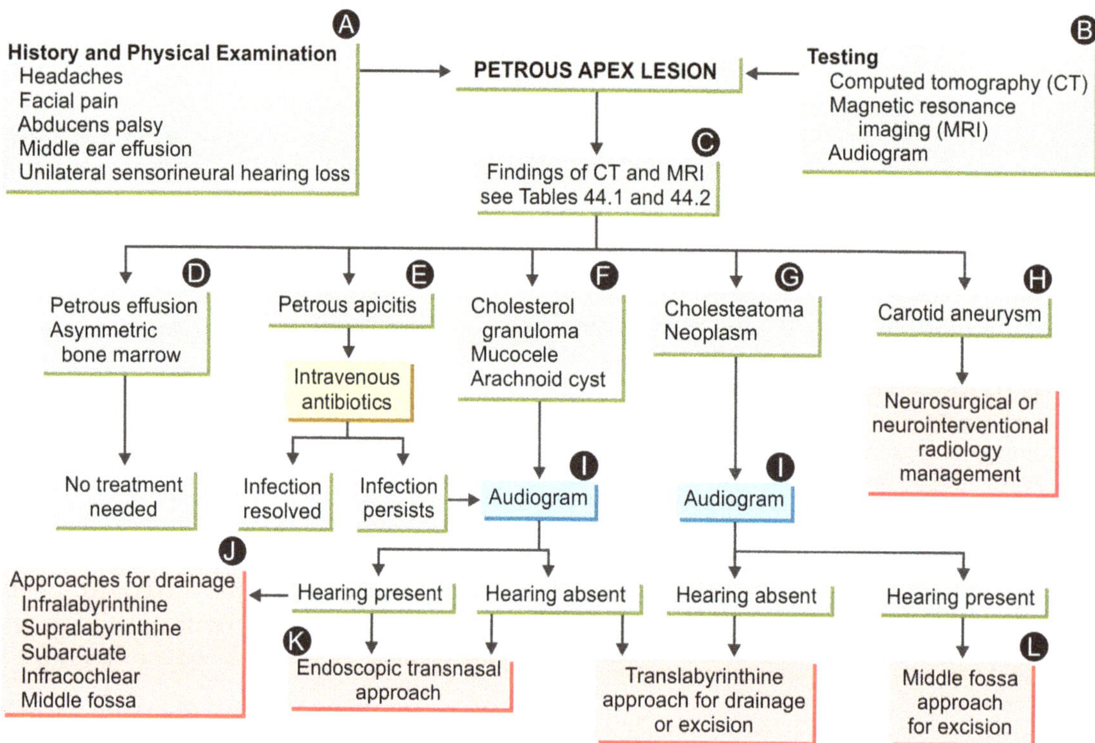

Petrous apex lesions are encountered infrequently and are in an anatomical location with limited accessibility. The major goal of the evaluation is to determine whether the petrous apex abnormality can be observed or whether a drainage procedure or excision is needed.

A The presenting symptoms are often nonspecific, especially if the lesion is a slow-growing noninflammatory lesion, such as a mucocele or benign neoplasm. Many of the lesions are discovered incidentally during scans performed for other reasons. Otherwise, the diagnosis of a petrous apex lesion is often not made until regional cranial nerve deficits such as abducens palsy or trigeminal nerve dysfunction, or serous effusion from Eustachian tube blockage occur.

B When a petrous apex lesion is suspected, the first radiographic study obtained is the computed tomography (CT) scan with contrast. This scan will detect the majority of petrous apex abnormalities that require further evaluation. Any changes in the surrounding bone will also be delineated.

C Magnetic resonance imaging (MRI) with gadolinium provides additional information regarding the characteristics of any soft-tissue abnormalities. Based on the CT and MRI, a tentative diagnosis can be made. The diagnosis in some cases will not be completely clear so the surgeon will need to be prepared to deviate from the proposed algorithm based on the individual patient.

D Asymmetric bone marrow and effusion do not require treatment. A repeat CT or MRI can be performed in 1 year to ensure that the effusion does not expand into a mucocele.

E Petrous apicitis is usually associated with an acute febrile illness and evidence of otitis media. Antibiotic therapy is essential, but the duration of medical treatment prior to considering surgical drainage is controversial. A reasonable course is an initial trial of intravenous antibiotics with surgical intervention reserved for those who do not respond adequately to medical therapy.

F Cholesterol granulomas and mucoceles can be observed or drained depending on size and symptoms. A more limited surgical exposure can be used for drainage. Arachnoid cysts are either observed, drained, or excised.

G Cholesteatomas and neoplasms in general require excision. A surgical approach with relatively wide exposure is required. Although most neoplasms are treated with complete excision, there will be cases such as lymphoma in which biopsy alone is warranted.

H Vascular lesions usually require involvement of neurosurgical and neurointerventional teams.

Table 44.1: Imaging characteristics and surgical management of petrous apex lesions.

| Lesion | Computed tomography (CT) | | Magnetic resonance imaging (MRI) | | | Surgical management |
	Bone erosion	Contrast enhancement	T1	T2	Gadolinium enhancement	
Effusion	None	None	Hypo	Hyper	Rim or none	None
Mucocele	Smooth	Rim or none	Hypo	Hyper	Rim or none	Drainage
Arachnoid cyst	Smooth	None	Hypo	Hyper	None	Drainage/ excision
Bone marrow	None	None	Hyper	Hypo	None	None
Cholesterol granuloma	Smooth	None	Hyper	Hyper	None	Drainage
Cholesteatoma	Smooth	None	Hypo	Hyper	None	Excision
Petrous apicitis	Irregular	Rim	Hypo	Hyper	Rim	Drainage
Neoplasm	Var	Yes	Iso or var	Hyper or var	Yes	Excision or biopsy
Carotid aneurysm	Smooth	Yes	Hypo	Inhomogenous	Rim	Embolization/ clipping

Rim, enhancement at the periphery of the lesion; Hypo, hypointense to brain; Hyper, hyperintense to brain; Iso, isointense to brain; Var, variable. The imaging characteristics of these lesions presented here are those typically found, but a definitive diagnosis cannot be made without supporting pathologic and clinical information.

Table 44.2: Types of neoplasms.

Neoplasms

Chordoma

Chondrosarcoma

Osteosarcoma

Meningioma

Schwannoma

Paraganglioma

Nasopharyngeal carcinoma

Metastases from other sites

I Regardless of whether drainage or excision is required, the presence or absence of useful hearing has a significant impact on the surgical approach. For those patients without useful hearing, the translabyrinthine exposure provides relatively wide access to the various areas of the petrous apex for either drainage or excision without the need to retract intracranial structures. There is some risk of postoperative dizziness and long-term imbalance if there is significant residual vestibular function so a labyrinth sparing procedure may still be considered. The definition of "useful" hearing is somewhat controversial and depends on the pure tone hearing level, discrimination score, contralateral hearing function, and the nature of the skull base lesion. In general, hearing preservation may be attempted if the patient's hearing is better than in cases in which a cochlear implant would be considered. Current criteria are a discrimination score of 50% on sentence testing. There are no specific pure tone threshold criteria, but patients who have a cochlear implant generally have a worse than 70 dB PTA loss. Of course, if the hearing preservation approach is contraindicated, cannot be performed, or would have little chance of preserving hearing, then the surgeon may elect to sacrifice the labyrinth regardless of hearing level.

J If the hearing is to be preserved for a drainage procedure, several transtemporal approaches are available. These procedures can usually be performed without significant retraction of any intracranial structures. The infralabyrinthine and infracochlear approaches can be used for access to the inferior portion, whereas the supralabyrinthine and subarcuate approaches can be used for access to the superior portion of the petrous apex.

K More recently, a transnasal endoscopic approach has been used in some cases, mostly for drainage but sometimes for excision. The feasibility and limitations of each approach depend mainly on the variable anatomy of the temporal bone and associated vascular and neural structures, the details of which are beyond the scope of this chapter.

L If these transtemporal or transnasal approaches are not feasible, the middle cranial fossa approach can be used. This approach requires a craniotomy with extradural temporal lobe retraction. If hearing is to be preserved in a case requiring excision, the middle cranial fossa approach will typically be needed, although the endoscopic transnasal approaches are evolving.

SUGGESTED READING

Arriaga MA, Brackmann DE. Differential diagnosis of primary petrous apex lesions. Am J Otol. 1991;12(6):470-474.

Chole RA. Petrous apicitis: surgical anatomy. Ann Otol Rhinol Laryngol. 1985;94:251-257.

Curtin HD, Som PM. The petrous apex. Otolaryngol Clin North Am. 1995;28:473-496.

Fong BP, Brackmann DE, Telischi FF. The long-term follow-up of drainage procedures for petrous apex cholesterol granulomas. Arch Otolaryngol Head Neck Surg. 1995;121:426-430.

Jackler RK, Parker DA. Radiographic differential diagnosis of petrous apex lesions. Am J Otol. 1992;13:561-574.

Muckle RP, De la Cruz A, Lo WM. Petrous apex lesions. Am J Otol. 1998;19:219-225.

Zanation AM, Snyderman CH, Carrau RL, et al. Endoscopic endonasal surgery for petrous apex lesions. Laryngoscope. 2009; 119(1):19-25.

Cerebellopontine Angle Tumors

Barry E Hisrch

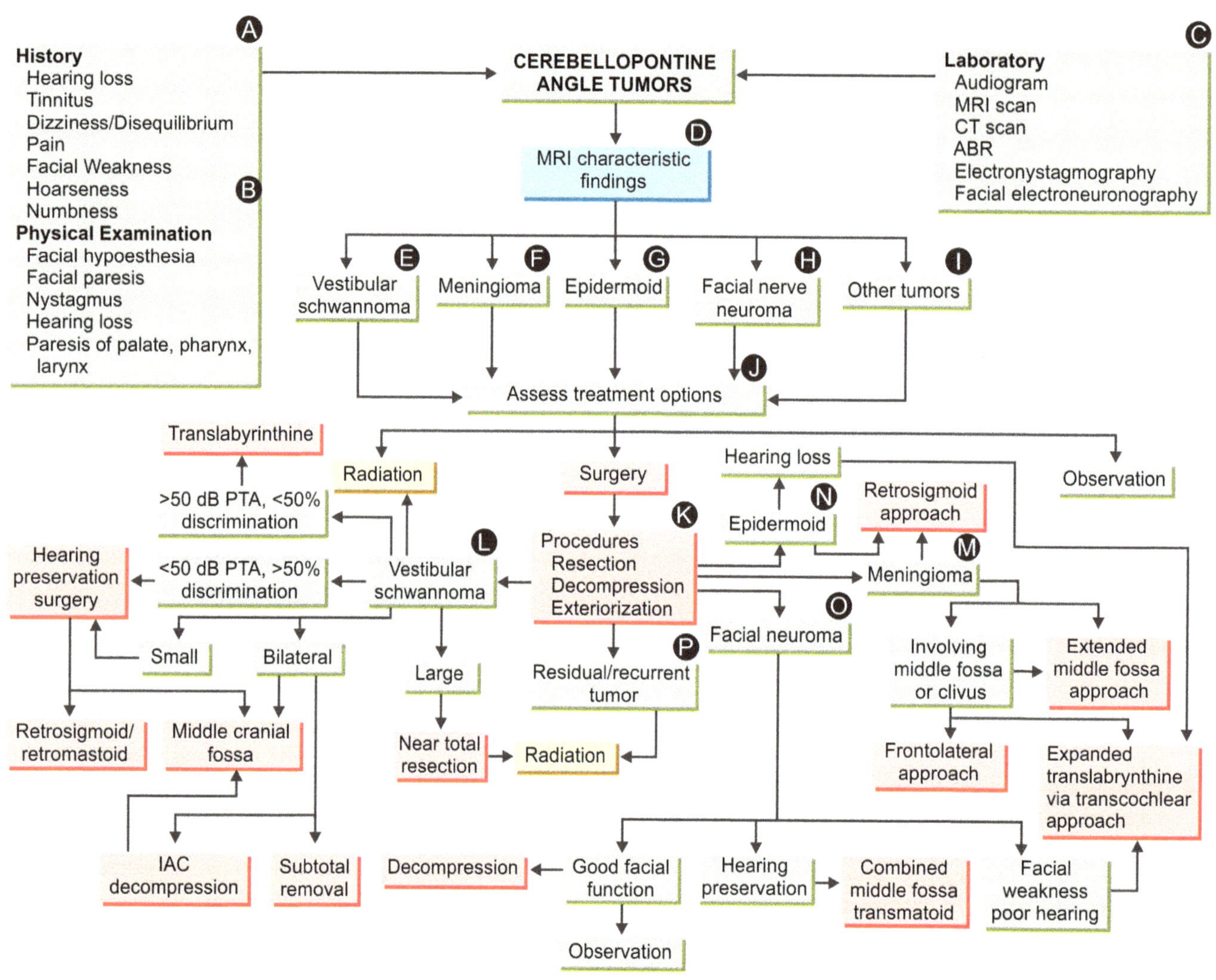

Patients with a tumor of the cerebellopontine angle (CPA) present with symptoms referable to cranial nerves V through XI. The most common tumor of the CPA is the vestibular schwannoma (acoustic neuroma) (90%), followed by meningioma and epidermoid tumors.

A Patients with vestibular schwannoma typically present with unilateral hearing loss and tinnitus. Facial numbness implies involvement of the trigeminal ganglion. A history of progressive facial weakness with synkinesis and twitching raises suspicion of a schwannoma of the facial nerve.

B Physical examination focuses on the cranial nerves. Careful assessment of cranial nerves V to XI can be helpful in judging the origin and extent of a tumor. However, large tumors can be present despite few symptoms and signs.

C An audiogram identifies the type and degree of hearing loss. Sensorineural hearing loss can be minimal to profound. Speech discrimination scores will influence management and the approach for tumor removal. Auditory brainstem response testing is often obtained if a hearing preservation procedure is anticipated. A baseline tracing provides a means for comparison during intraoperative monitoring.

Magnetic resonance imaging (MRI) is the gold standard for diagnostic testing of CPA tumors. Computed tomography (CT) imaging provides information regarding the pneumatization of the temporal bone, status of the Fallopian canal and geniculate ganglion region, identifying potential erosion of the otic capsule, and relationship of the sigmoid sinus and jugular bulb to the internal auditory canal (IAC). Facial electroneuronography and electromyography testing can also provide information about the integrity of the facial nerve. The results of caloric response vestibular testing can help to determine whether the inferior or superior vestibular nerve is more compromised.

D Magnetic resonance imaging is the study of choice for diagnosing CPA tumors. The important factors that determine the probable histopathology of the tumor are the signal characteristics, location, and shape of the tumor. Computed tomography imaging in certain situations can provide supplemental information such as depiction of bone expansion or destruction.

Vestibular schwannoma are typically centered on the meatus of IAC with variable extension toward the fundus. There may be expansion of the IAC. There can be limited medial extent or massive growth compressing the brainstem and cerebellum. The shape of the tumor is oval to spherical and makes an acute angle with the posterior wall of the temporal bone. The intensity of signal is hypodense relative to the brain but markedly enhances with intravenous contrast on T1-weighted imaging.

Meningiomas of the CPA take origin from the anterior or posterior wall of the temporal bone and are often eccentric to the IAC. There may be extension and enhancement within the IAC, although expansion is uncommon. The tumor appears plaque-like in origin and makes an obtuse angle with the temporal bone. The signal characteristics on T2-weighted imaging are variable. Similar to acoustic neuroma, meningiomas enhance on T1-weighted imaging with contrast. A dural tail, manifested by a thinning wedge of enhancing tumor trailing from the tumor mass along the dural surface, is characteristic of meningioma. There may be hyperostotic changes evident on CT scanning.

Epidermoid tumors, or cholesteatomas, of the CPA are not malignant but can achieve considerable size before they are detected. The diagnosis of a CPA epidermoid is usually evident on MRI. These lesions are typically hypointense to moderately intense on T1-weighted imaging and hyperintense on T2-weighted imaging and do not enhance with contrast. Some tumors may have a cystic component that brightens the T1 signal. Advances in MRI software permit easier differentiation of epidermoid tumor from arachnoid cyst. Computed tomography scanning defines the status of the temporal bone with regard to the integrity of the petrous apex and IAC, demonstrating evidence of bone erosion. Computed tomography and MRI are complementary when trying to determine whether the tumor originated with the CPA or temporal bone.

Schwannomas (neuroma) of the facial nerve, primarily located in the CPA, are rare. They typically involve the region of the geniculate ganglion with extension superiorly to the middle cranial fossa. These tumors can extend into the CPA via the IAC. Tumor involvement along the course of the facial nerve is manifested as a bright signal on enhanced T1-weighted MRI. It may be difficult to distinguish an acoustic neuroma from facial nerve neuroma when originating within the IAC. Computed tomography imaging is often helpful in diagnosing facial nerve neuroma when bone erosion, enhancement around the geniculate ganglion, and expansion of the Fallopian canal are identified.

E Vestibular schwannoma is the most common tumor arising in the CPA, accounting for 80–90% of all tumors. Sporadic tumors are unilateral (95%), and those associated with neurofibromatosis (NF) II are typically bilateral. The most common presenting symptoms are unilateral progressive hearing loss and tinnitus. Vestibular dysfunction is often present. Facial nerve signs and symptoms are infrequent.

F Meningioma accounts for approximately 10% of tumors in the CPA, with a female predominance for this location. They tend to be larger than acoustic neuroma at the time of diagnosis. Meningioma may be seen with other tumors in patients with NF II. Similar to vestibular schwannoma, hearing loss, vertigo or imbalance, tinnitus, and occasionally facial pain are the most common presenting symptoms.

G Epidermoid tumors account for 2–7% of the CPA tumors, which is the most common site for their intracranial occurrence. They are often identified in patients younger than 40 years of age and present with symptoms of the trigeminal, facial, and auditory nerves.

H Neuroma of the facial nerve typically involves the temporal bone around the geniculate ganglion but may extend into the CPA. Hearing loss is the most frequent presenting symptom followed by facial nerve dysfunction and tinnitus. Sudden-onset facial paralysis may be the presenting sign, but progressive paresis and twitching are more common.

I Other lesions that can occur in the CPA include lipoma, aneurysm, lower cranial nerve neuroma, metastatic lesion, plasmacytoma, arachnoid cyst, and primary neoplasms of the brain and arterial aneurysm.

J There is no requirement for urgent intervention, because these tumors are benign (unless mass effect has caused hydrocephalus or significant shift of the brainstem) and slow growing. Numerous factors must be considered in formulating a treatment plan: patient's age, health status, presumed histology based on imaging characteristics, size and location of the tumor, previous treatment, presence of multiple tumors, hearing status of both ears, balance and facial nerve function, and status of the lower cranial nerves.

Patients with small vestibular schwannoma or meningioma who are elderly or have significant health problems can often be monitored with serial imaging. These tumors often demonstrate slow rates of growth when identified in the elderly. Appropriate intervention can be determined by observing the rate of growth with biannual and then annual scans if the size of the tumor remains stable. Evidence of growth warrants intervention by surgery or radiation. The presence of a substantial tumor within the CPA (>1.5 cm) warrants either surgical removal or treatment with radiation. Stereotactic radiation appears to be effective in controlling tumor growth of vestibular schwannoma and less of meningioma. Long-term (>10 years) tumor control has been established using lower dosing protocols that were modified since this form of therapy was initially offered. Stereotactic radiation is also used to treat bilateral acoustic tumors, meningioma, and residual tumor after subtotal resection when tumor growth has occurred. Epidermoid tumors have not been treated with radiation therapy. There is limited data on radiation for therapy due to the rarity of facial neuroma. Patients with facial nerve neuroma and minimal facial weakness warrant observation of their tumor over time. Progressive facial paresis and synkinesis hasten the decision for surgical intervention.

(K) Surgical options include complete or subtotal resection (all tumors), decompression (vestibular schwannoma, facial nerve neuroma), and occasionally exteriorization of epidermoid tumors.

(L) Choosing the appropriate surgical approach is predicated on various factors. Patients who have a small vestibular schwannoma with good auditory function can be offered a hearing preservation procedure using either the middle cranial fossa or retrosigmoid (retromastoid) approach. (The definition of good auditory function is controversial. Some advocate that hearing pure-tone thresholds >30 dB and word discrimination <70% justify the more direct translabyrinthine approach. I use 50-dB pure-tone average [PTA] and <50% discrimination.) The most lateral aspect of the IAC (fundus) may not be completely exposed with either technique. The translabyrinthine approach provides complete exposure of the IAC but includes loss of hearing in that ear. Patients with bilateral tumors and reasonable hearing may be offered decompression of the IAC via a middle fossa approach or subtotal removal if they wish to delay further loss of hearing.

(M) Meningiomas of the posterior fossa can involve the IAC. Unlike vestibular schwannoma, preoperative hearing is often preserved. Their more common location along the posterior face of the petrous bone with extension toward the petrous apex is usually addressed via a retrosigmoid approach. Meningiomas involving the middle fossa or clivus require additional exposure through an extended middle fossa or frontolateral approach. The translabyrinthine approach can be expanded by transcochlear dissection to gain access to the lateral and anterior brainstem.

(N) Epidermoid tumors of the posterior fossa can be difficult to excise completely. The matrix is often adherent to the brainstem, cerebellum, and blood vessels and insinuates between the fibers of the cranial nerves. If sensorineural hearing loss is present as a result of erosion of the temporal bone, a translabyrinthine (transcochlear) approach may permit exteriorization.

(O) Patients who have a neuroma of the facial nerve with significant facial weakness and poor hearing are managed by a translabyrinthine approach and, if needed, a transcochlear approach. This combination provides the necessary exposure to the CPA and temporal bone portions of the tumor, permitting reconstruction by nerve rerouting and direct anastomosis or interposition nerve grafting. A combined middle fossa/transmastoid approach provides access for tumor resection, cable graft reconstruction, and hearing preservation. Patients with good facial function may be offered temporizing treatment by decompression of the surrounding bone (IAC).

(P) In cases of schwannoma, neuroma, and meningioma, there may be residual tumor left behind at the time of surgery. This is often when complete resection would injure the facial nerve or brainstem. Should growth or recurrence be demonstrated on subsequent imaging, strong consideration is given toward stereotactic radiosurgery.

SUGGESTED READINGS

Bartels IA, Arrington JR. Rare tumors of the cerebellopontine angle. In: Jackler RJ, Brachmann DE (Eds). Neurotology. St Louis, MO: CV Mosby; 1994. p. 835.

Boari N, Bailo M, Gagliardi F, et al. Gamma knife radiosurgery for vestibular schwannoma: clinical results at long-term follow-up in a series of 379 patients. J Neurosurg. 2014;121(Suppl): 123-142.

Calzada AP, Go JL, Tschirhart DL, et al. Cerebellopontine angle and intracanalicular masses mimicking vestibular schwannomas. Otol Neurotol. 2015;36(3):491-499.

Hasegawa M, Nouri M, Nagahisa S, et al. Cerebellopontine angle epidermoid cysts: clinical presentations and surgical outcome. Neurosurg Rev. 2016;39(2):259-266.

Mcrackan TR, Wilkinson EP, Brackmann DE, et al. Stereotactic radiosurgery for facial nerve schwannomas. Otol Neurotol. 2015;36(3):393-398.

Nager GT. Epidermoids involving the temporal bone: clinical, radiological and pathological aspects. Laryngoscope. 1975;2(Suppl): 1-21.

O'Donoghue GM, Brachmann DE, House JW, et al. Neuromas of the facial nerve. Am J Otol. 1989;10(1):49-54.

Pollock BE, Link MJ. Vestibular schwannoma radiosurgery after previous surgical resection or stereotactic radiosurgery. Prog Neurol Surg. 2008;21:163-168.

Walter GF. Pathobiology and neuropathology of meningiomas. In: Samii M, Ammirate M (Eds). Surgery of Skull Base Meningiomas. Berlin: Springer-Verlag; 1992. pp. 123-142.

Xiang D, Liu L, Li Y, et al. Near-total removal of facial nerve schwannomas: long-term outcomes. Am J Otolaryngol. 2015;36(3): 390-392.

Vestibular Disorders in Older People

Jameson K Mattingly, Stephen P Cass

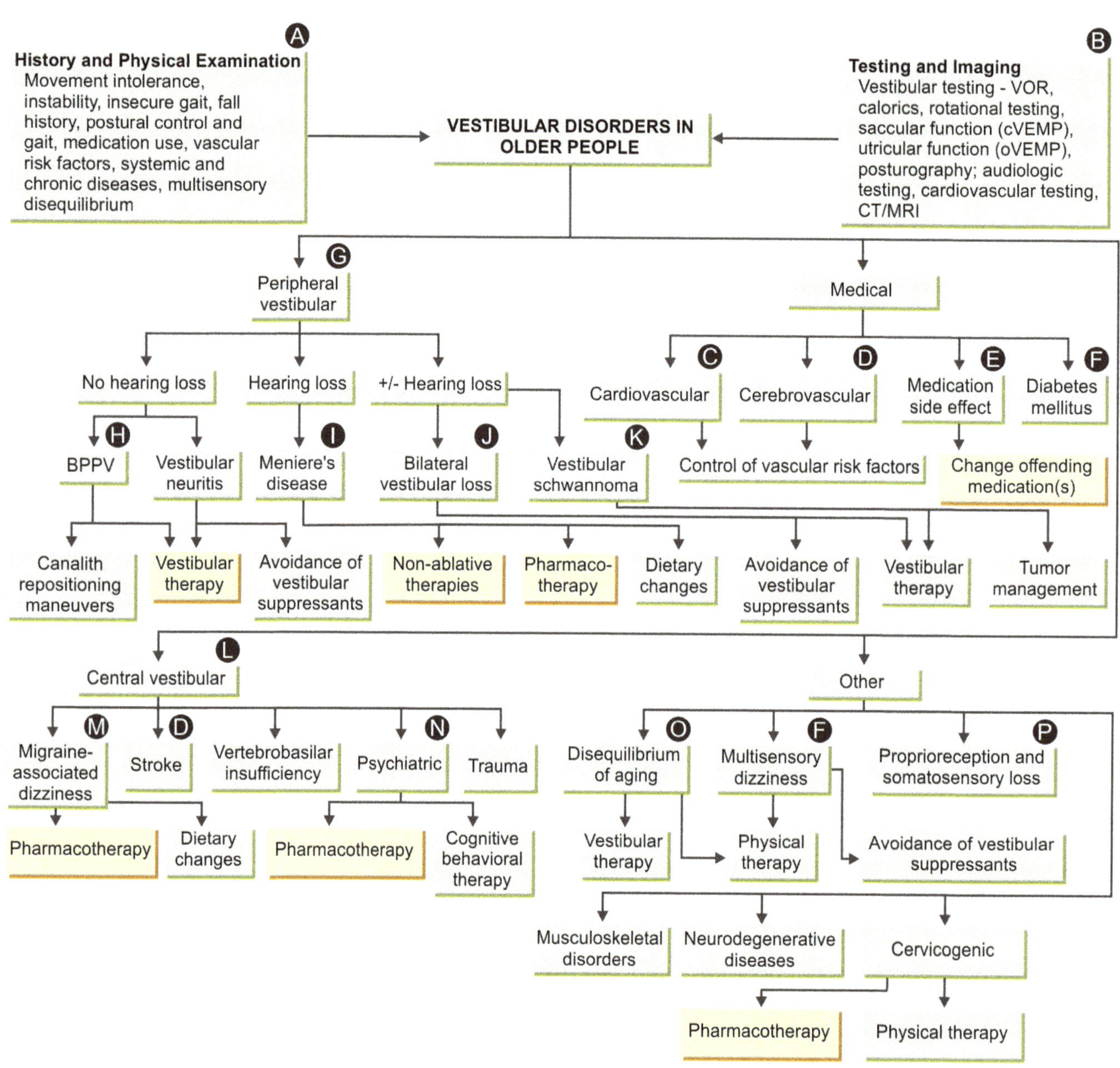

Dizziness and imbalance are common in the aging population. Decline of sensory and motor pathway and peripheral vestibular functions are considered to be a part of the normal aging process. This issue is concerning because patients with these symptoms are at an increased risk of falls and subsequent injury (i.e. fractures).

Although the same etiologies can affect both younger and older patients, vestibular symptoms in the aging population tend to be multisensory deficits, multifactorial etiologies, and disequilibrium of aging secondary to microvascular disease.

A History and physical examination should include neurologic, neurotologic, and general medical examinations. Elderly patients may have less reports of rotary vertigo, and instead more commonly report movement intolerance, instability, and insecure gait. Thus, the physical examination should emphasize postural control and gait. An accurate history should focus on comorbidities, use of medications, vascular risk factors, and a thorough description of symptoms.

B Testing may include vestibular, audiologic, imaging, and cardiovascular testing. Computed tomography and magnetic resonance imaging are indicated for focal signs and symptoms that suggest a retrocochlear lesion or acute vascular insult. Laboratory evaluation should be ordered selectively, dictated by medical history and test results.

C Cardiovascular causes include heart failure, arrhythmias, medications treating these conditions, and orthostatic hypotension. Examination should always include vital and orthostatic signs.

D Cerebrovascular disease is common in the elderly patients. Stroke presents a potentially life-threatening form of dizziness, and therefore must be thoroughly investigated in the older patient presenting with acute onset of dizziness or vestibular complaints. Vertebrobasilar insufficiency is characterized by vertigo, vision changes, drop attacks or weakness, visceral sensations, diplopia, and other transient neurologic deficits.

E Medications can be a major sole or a contributing factor to dizziness and falls in the elderly population. These medications include anticonvulsants, antidepressants, antihypertensives, anxiolytics, sedatives, muscle relaxants, and antiarrhythmics. Vestibular suppressant medications (i.e. meclizine, promethazine, and benzodiazepines) are frequently inappropriately used to treat dizziness and vertigo. These must be used cautiously in older patients in whom sedation and drug-induced central vestibular dysfunction must be avoided. Thus, an effort should be made to reduce the number of medications used (including over-the-counter medications).

F Multisensory dizziness/disequilibrium is common in the elderly population. This is typically a diagnosis of exclusion, and is often multifactorial in nature involving both peripheral and central functions. This can be commonly seen in patients with diabetes mellitus as the result of vestibulopathy, retinopathy, and peripheral neuropathy. Treatment includes optimizing sensory input available, reducing the use of vestibular suppressant medications, and training patients how to use their remaining sensory inputs for balance.

G Peripheral vestibular disorders are common in the elderly population and are suggested by the presence of vertigo, vestibular nystagmus, decreased vestibulo-ocular reflex function, normal neurologic examination, reduced caloric responses, and normal brain imaging.

H Benign paroxysmal positional vertigo is the most common peripheral vestibular disorder at any age in adults, with a significant increase in prevalence with aging. The Dix-Hallpike maneuver may need to be modified in those with musculoskeletal issues. Particle repositioning maneuvers are highly effective in treating this condition, but as coexisting vestibular hypofunction can be present, vestibular physical therapy can be helpful.

I Meniere's disease is characterized by episodic vertigo, fluctuating hearing loss, tinnitus, and aural fullness. Recent studies have reported that 15% of patients with Meniere's disease are older than 65 years; 40% of these cases are the result of decompensation of previously compensated disease and 60% de novo. Due to impaired compensation in this population, non-ablative treatments are preferred, such as steroid injections, symptomatic relief, and dietary controls.

J Bilateral vestibular loss can be severely debilitating. Investigating for a history of ototoxicity and autoimmune disease should be performed. Age >65 is a major risk factor for occurrence of bilateral vestibulopathy when using ototoxic medications. This manifests as Dandy's syndrome (oscillopsia and gait ataxia). Treatment includes cessation of vestibular suppressant medications and referral for vestibular physical therapy.

K Vestibular schwannomas can present at any age but are more commonly found in older people. Important diagnostic clues include asymmetric high-frequency sensorineural hearing loss with poor speech perception and tinnitus. Treatment options include surgery, stereotactic radiosurgery, and observation.

L Central vestibular disorders are suggested by symptoms referable to the central nervous system and abnormalities on neurologic examination, eye movement testing, and brain imaging. Additionally, these changes may affect the ability to compensate for vestibular losses.

M Migraine-associated dizziness as the primary cause of dizziness is uncommon in the older population. Dizziness may or may not be temporally associated with migraine headache, and may present as a migraine equivalent or acephalgic migraine.

N Psychiatric conditions can be a contributing factor in the elderly population, with anxiety a common finding.

O Disequilibrium of aging, presbystasis, or disequilibrium of the elderly population is thought to be due to abnormal sensory processing by the central nervous system, a decline in peripheral vestibular function, abnormal sensory signals, abnormal control of balance mechanisms, and an aged musculoskeletal system. Vestibular physical therapy, and education on prevention of falls are useful in this disorder.

P Proprioception and somatosensory functions demonstrate age-related decline, such as decreased vibration and touch thresholds, ability to detect position and direction of joint movements, and postural stability. Medical conditions such as neuropathies can contribute to decline in these functions.

SUGGESTED READING

Furman J, Cass S, Whitney S. Vestibular Disorders: A Case Study Approach to Diagnosis and Treatment, 3rd edition. New York: Oxford University Press; 2010.

Furman J, Raz Y, Whitney S. Geriatric vestibulopathy assessment and management. Curr Opin Otolaryngol Head Neck Surg. 2010;18:386-391.

Iwasaki S, Yamasoba T. Dizziness and imbalance in the elderly: age-related decline in the vestibular system. Aging Dis. 2015;6(1):38-47.

Katsarkas A. Dizziness in aging: a retrospective study of 1194 cases. Otolaryngol Head Neck Surg. 1994;110(3):296-301.

Maarsingh O, Dros J, Schellevis F, et al. Causes of persistent dizziness in elderly patients in primary care. Ann Fam Med. 2010;8(3):196-205.

Nose, Paranasal Sinuses and Nasopharynx

Nasal Obstruction

Stella E Lee, David E Eibling

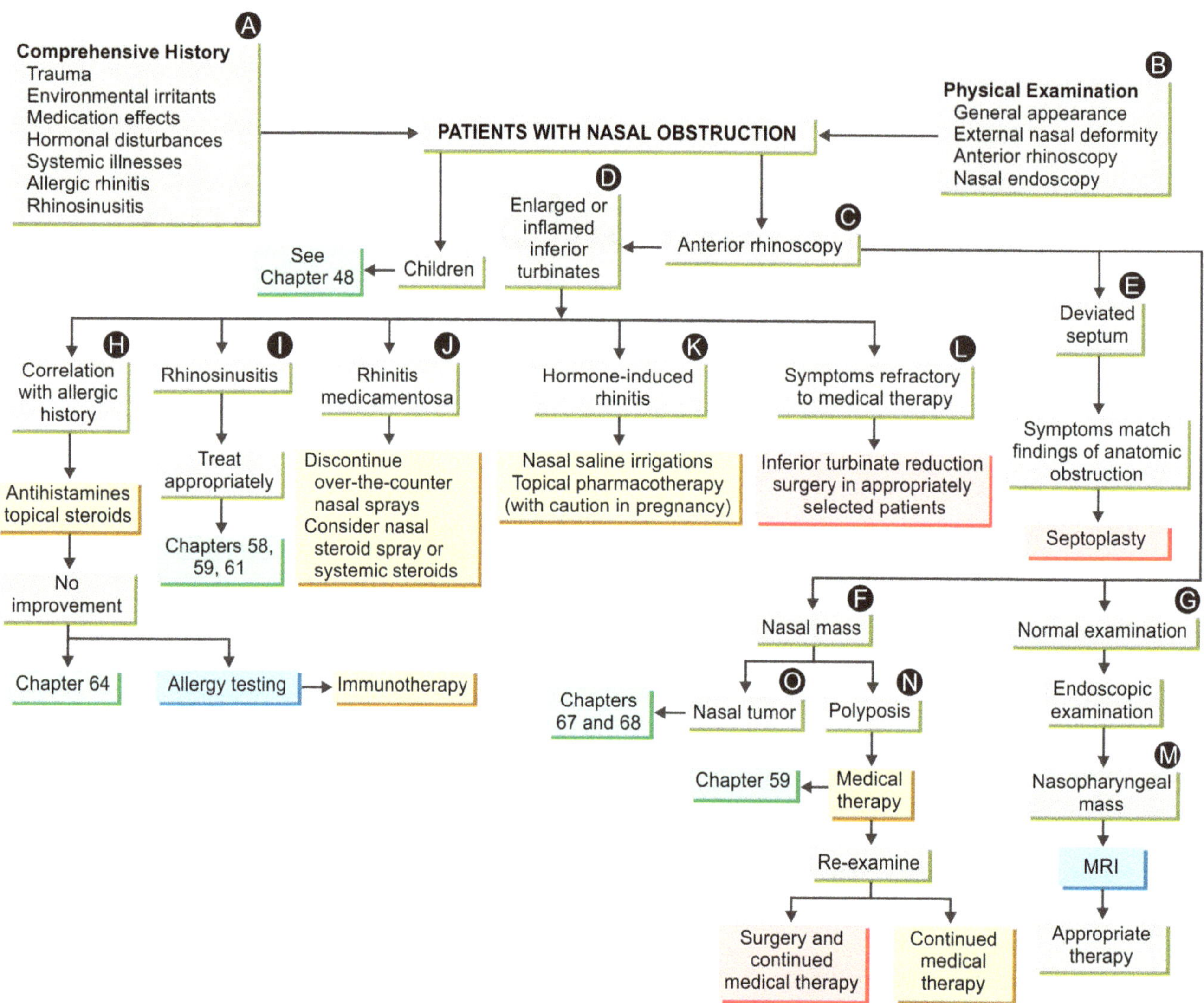

Nasal obstruction is a common symptom that can result from diverse and overlapping etiologies. An understanding of the wide differential diagnosis of nasal obstruction is important to arrive at a correct diagnosis and direct appropriate management. Anterior rhinoscopy in conjunction with comprehensive nasal endoscopy may be necessary to obtain an accurate evaluation of the patient with nasal obstruction.

A This chapter addresses nasal obstruction in adults. Refer to Chapter 48 for an in-depth discussion of nasal obstruction in infants and children. The history should include onset, duration, incidence, laterality, and precipitating events or environmental triggers. A history of surgery or nasal trauma, known allergies, systemic illnesses, and medications, either those used currently or in the past should be noted.

B Initial examination should include the overall status of the patient, particularly with note to dyspnea that may be due to pulmonary and not nasal cause. The nose should be examined for external deformity. Further evaluation will be directed by the results of anterior rhinoscopy. In most instances, nasal endoscopy and nasopharyngoscopy will be required.

C Findings on anterior rhinoscopy may quickly identify the etiologic factor responsible for the obstruction.

D Finding of inferior turbinate enlargement should prompt further investigation of allergic rhinitis or rhinosinusitis. The use of over-the-counter sympathomimetic nasal sprays should also be explored.

E A deviated nasal septum may be readily apparent on anterior rhinoscopy or may require nasal endoscopy.

If symptoms correlate with endoscopic findings, septoplasty can be helpful to correct the anatomic obstruction.

F A nasal mass may be visible and may represent either polyp or tumor, either benign or malignant. In most instances, polyposis can be readily identified on anterior rhinoscopy. It must be noted that unilateral polyposis suggests another cause, such as an underlying tumor such as inverted papilloma. A dedicated CT scan of the paranasal sinuses should be performed. Children with a history of nasal polyposis should be tested for cystic fibrosis.

G When anterior rhinoscopy is normal, nasal endoscopy is required for a complete examination. Nasal endoscopy should include visualization of the middle meatus, the sphenoethmoid recess, olfactory cleft, nasopharynx, as well as the characteristics of the nasal valve including the septum and inferior turbinates that may contribute to nasal obstruction. Endoscopy may reveal an unexpected deviated nasal septum, nasal mass, or a mass in the nasopharynx.

H Patients with a history of allergy should be treated appropriately. Suspected allergic rhinitis can be evaluated by different modalities of testing (epicutaneous, intradermal, or in vitro). Refer to Chapter 64 for further discussion of allergic rhinitis.

I Patients may have acute, subacute, or chronic rhinosinusitis. The differentiation is based on the duration of symptoms and/or objective findings. Refer to Chapters 58, 59, and 61.

J Rhinitis medicamentosa can be particularly difficult to manage. Many patients are unable to discontinue the use of nasal spray and often benefit from a short course of systemic steroids and the use of nasal steroid sprays.

K Hormone-induced rhinitis is typically accompanied by the hormone surge of puberty and pregnancy, and can oftentimes be managed with nasal saline irrigations. Evidence is scarce regarding topical pharmacotherapy in pregnancy and should be approached with caution.

L Inferior turbinate reduction can be helpful in alleviating symptoms in patients with persistent nasal blockage refractory to medical therapy.

M The finding of a nasopharyngeal mass on endoscopy will usually require imaging. Symptomatic relief can often be obtained by removal of the nasopharyngeal mass, be it a Thornwaldt cyst, nasopharyngeal cyst, or adenoid tissue. Nasopharyngeal malignancy rarely presents as nasal obstruction until late in the course. Juvenile nasopharyngeal angiofibroma typically presents in adolescent males and should not undergo biopsy because of the risk of significant bleeding. Refer to Chapter 66.

N Bilateral nasal polyposis is usually a manifestation of chronic rhinosinusitis but cystic fibrosis is also a possibility. Polyposis in a child should prompt evaluation for cystic fibrosis. A polypoid middle turbinate can be seen in patients with severe allergic rhinitis. Refer to Chapter 59.

O Nasal tumors are addressed in Chapters 67 and 68.

SUGGESTED READING

Chhabra N, Houser SM. Surgery for allergic rhinitis. Int Forum Allergy Rhinol. 2014;4(Suppl 2):S79-83.

Fokkens WJ, Lund VJ, Mullol J, et al. EPOS 2012: European position paper on rhinosinusitis and nasal polyps 2012. A summary for otorhinolaryngologists. Rhinology. 2012;50(1):1-12.

Osborn JL, Sacks R. Nasal obstruction. Am J Rhinol Allergy. 2013;27 (Suppl 1):S7-8.

Rosenfeld RM, Piccirillo JF, Chandrasekhar SS, et al. Clinical practice guideline (update): adult sinusitis. Otolaryngol Head Neck Surg. 2015;152(2 Suppl):S1-39.

Seidman MD, Gurgel RK, Lin SY, et al. Clinical practice guideline: allergic rhinitis. Otolaryngol Head Neck Surg. 2015;152 (1 Suppl):S1-43.

Nasal Obstruction in the Child

Joshua B Silverman, Richard M Rosenfeld

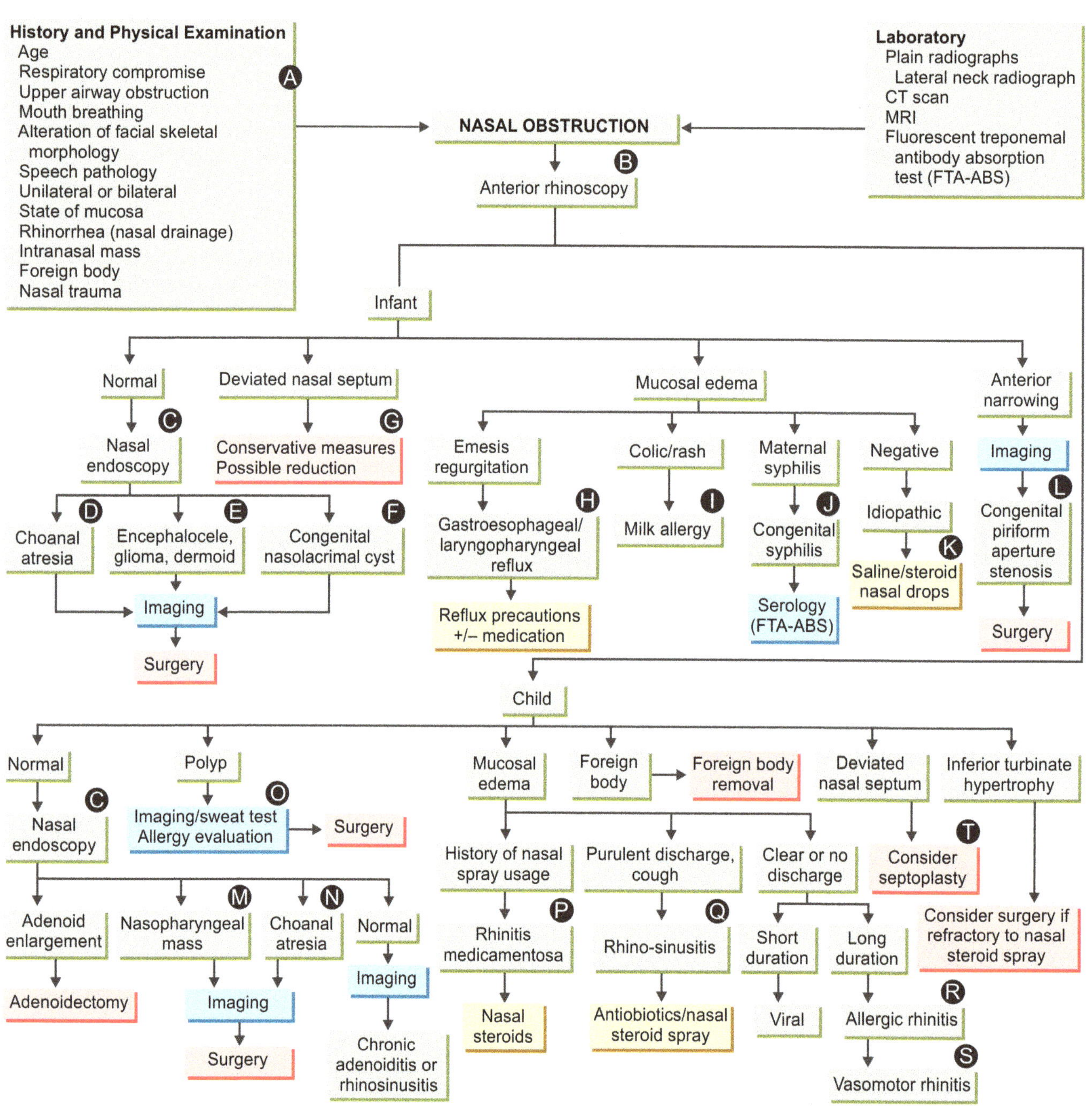

Nasal obstruction in infants can cause significant respiratory compromise due to obligate nasal breathing. Older children will not have severe respiratory compromise from nasal obstruction alone, although obstructive sleep apnea may result. Chronic mouth breathing may alter facial skeletal morphology and may impair speech intelligibility due to decreased nasal airflow.

A The evaluation of any infant with nasal obstruction must include assessment for respiratory compromise.

B Anterior rhinoscopy is best performed with a standard otoscope and ear speculum to evaluate nasal mucosa, presence and quality of secretions, and alignment of the septum.

C Evaluation of the posterior nasal cavity, nasopharynx, and adenoid requires nasal endoscopy, typically with a flexible pediatric nasopharyngoscope. A lateral neck radiograph is not recommended to evaluate adenoid size because the two-dimensional view correlates poorly with endoscopic findings and will vary depending on head position and respiratory phase.

D Choanal atresia in infants is typically bony and bilateral, and is associated with severe respiratory difficulty relieved by crying. Failure to pass an 8-French catheter through the nose of a newborn suggests atresia; CT scan and nasal endoscopy can confirm. Treatment involves enlarging the choanae by transnasal or transpalatal approach. The child must be evaluated for CHARGE association or other syndromes.

E Congenital midline nasal mass includes encephalocele, glioma, or dermoid. Biopsy of these masses should be avoided. CT and MRI are required to diagnose and plan treatment.

F Congenital obstruction of the nasolacrimal duct can result in cystic dilatation presenting as an intranasal bluish mass, treated with marsupialization. Nasoalveolar cysts can present with similar obstruction.

G Septal injury may result from intrauterine positioning or from birth trauma. Symptomatic septal deviation of the newborn can be treated conservatively with sprays and suctioning and will usually self-correct by 4–6 months. Severe deflection or subluxation can usually be gently "popped" back into position.

H Repeated emesis from reflux may contribute to nasal obstruction and rhinitis. Reflux precautions may be instituted, though antireflux medication should be reserved for refractory cases, as evidence to support medication for nasal symptoms alone is empiric.

I Milk allergy is an adverse immunological reaction induced by cow's milk protein and is relatively common during infancy. The diagnosis is suggested with a history of colic or rashes, excessive secretions, and positive allergy or elimination diet tests. Treatment involves avoidance of cow's milk.

J Concern for syphilis may warrant fluorescent treponemal antibody testing. Physical findings include flattening of the nasal dorsum. Treatment is with penicillin and nasal steroid drops.

K Before making an idiopathic diagnosis, a nasal culture must be obtained to rule out bacterial rhinitis and other causes, such as congenital chlamydial infection. Treatment involves saline and steroid sprays, and suctioning. Consider nasal stenting for refractory cases.

L Congenital stenosis of the piriform aperture produces a shelf-like projection at the anterior aspect of the nasal cavity, making nasal endoscopy difficult. CT scan confirms the diagnosis by measuring the aperture width; surgery (sublabial approach) corrects the problem. A geneticist should rule out holoprosencephaly.

M Juvenile nasopharyngeal angiofibromas are benign yet aggressive vascular tumors that occur in older male children and present with obstruction and epistaxis. Other nasopharyngeal masses include rhabdomyosarcoma, lymphoma, and nasopharyngeal carcinoma.

N Unilateral choanal atresia will typically not be diagnosed in the newborn and will present in older children with unilateral nasal obstruction and rhinorrhea.

O Cystic fibrosis testing is mandatory for any child with bilateral nasal polyps; other causes include severe allergic rhinitis and Samter's triad (asthma, aspirin sensitivity) and nasal polyps. Unilateral nasal polyps are most likely antrochoanal or allergic fungal sinusitis. Management typically consists of CT scan followed by endoscopic sinus surgery.

P Rhinitis medicamentosa (rebound) is caused by overuse of topical sympathomimetic sprays. Treatment includes adding a topical intranasal steroid, then discontinuing the sympathomimetic spray with possible systemic steroids.

Q Acute bacterial rhinosinusitis in children manifests as an acute upper respiratory infection that is prolonged (>10 days), worsens after initial improvement, or severe (concurrent fever and purulent discharge for >3 days). Chronic rhinosinusitis causes symptoms including cough, nasal obstruction, facial pain, and purulent discharge for >3 months.

R Allergic rhinitis is IgE-mediated and is characterized by nasal congestion, rhinorrhea, sneezing, and/or nasal itching. Initial treatment is avoidance of the offending allergen and use of nasal steroid spray, with possible oral antihistamine. Severe cases may require skin testing and immunotherapy.

S Vasomotor rhinitis is caused by abnormal autonomic nasal stimulation, possibly from mechanical irritation (pollution), temperature changes, hormonal effects (puberty), or anxiety. It is a diagnosis of exclusion and is treated with topical nasal steroid sprays.

T Septoplasty with cartilage resection should be avoided until middle teenage years; cartilage-sparing or repositioning surgeries may be performed when nasal obstruction effects exercise—tolerance or quality of life.

SUGGESTED READING

Brietzke SE, Shin JJ, Choi S, et al. Clinical consensus statement: pediatric chronic rhinosinusitis. Otolaryngol Head and Neck Surg. 2014;151:542-553.

Chohan A, Lal A, Chohan K, et al. Systematic review and meta-analysis of randomized controlled trials on the role of mometasone in adenoid hypertrophy in children. Int J Pediatr Otorhinolaryngol. 2015;79(10):1599-1608.

Gnagi SH, Schra SA. Nasal obstruction in newborns. Pediatr Clin North Am. 2013;60(4):903-922.

Ramsden JD, Campisi P, Forte V, et al. Choanal atresia and choanal stenosis. Otolaryngol Clin North Am. 2009;42(2):339-352.

Wald ER, Applegate KE, Bordley C, et al. Clinical practice guideline for the diagnosis and management of acute bacterial sinusitis in children aged 1 to 18 years. Pediatrics. 2013;132(1):262-280.

Congenital Nasal Masses

Amanda L Stapleton

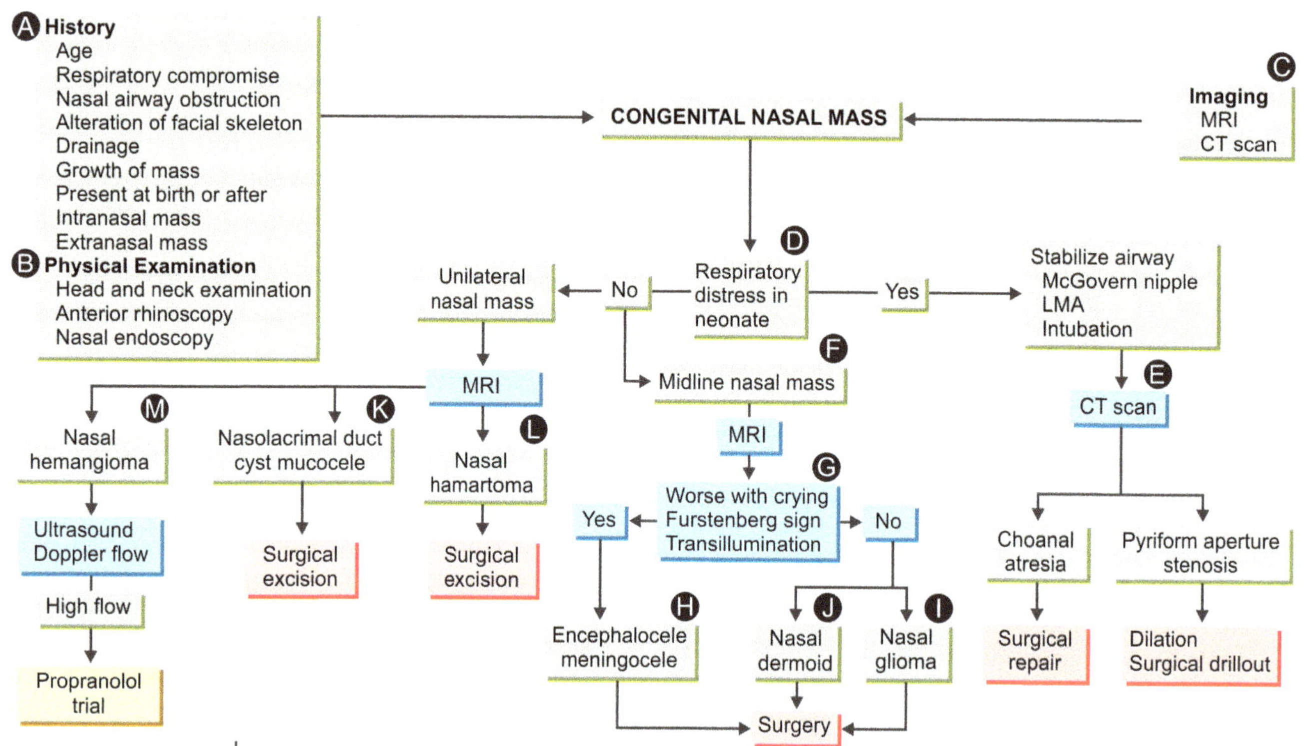

Congenital nasal masses are uncommon but can present with significant clinical consequences in the newborn, infant, and young child. The patient may present with nasal obstruction, cosmetic deformity, presence of a lesion, or respiratory compromise. Thorough and careful evaluation of the lesion prior to intervention can improve the outcome.

A A thorough history and physical examination can quickly narrow down the differential diagnosis of nasal masses. Presence at birth, growth of the lesion, respiratory compromise, nasal obstruction, and extranasal deformity are all key parts of the history and physical examination. A complete examination of the head and neck with nasal endoscopy is required.

B Anterior rhinoscopy is used in the initial evaluation. Nasal endoscopy is recommended to evaluate the entire nasal cavity, choana, and nasopharynx.

C Imaging: Computed tomography (CT) scan is ideal for the evaluation of bony lesions and the relationship between a mass and the surrounding bone. Generally, CT is the imaging modality of choice for lesions that are associated with airway obstruction (choanal atresia, pyriform aperture stenosis). Magnetic resonance imaging (MRI) is ideal for imaging nasofrontal masses where intracranial communication is suspected. They are complementary procedures and are frequently both required for eventual surgical management if indicated.

D Respiratory compromise in a neonate is a medical emergency. Inability to pass a nasogastric tube through the nasal cavity and nasopharynx is suggestive of choanal atresia. Nasal obstruction due to a mass obstructing the nasal airway should be managed conservatively with an oral airway until appropriate imaging and evaluation are complete. Use of a McGovern nipple, Laryngeal Mask Airway (LMA), or orotracheal intubation may be required to stabilize the patient until further evaluation is complete. A CT scan is recommended to evaluate for choanal atresia or pyriform aperture stenosis, whereas MRI is required to evaluate nasofrontal congenital masses.

E Bilateral choanal atresia or pyriform aperture stenosis is associated with severe respiratory difficulty in the neonate that is relieved by crying and placement of a McGovern nipple (bottle nipple with the tip cut off). The diagnosis is suggested by the inability to pass an 8-French catheter through the nose and confirmed by nasal endoscopy and CT scan. See Chapter 50 for further discussion and management.

F A midline nasal mass with or without an external nasal deformity/mass requires an MRI with contrast to evaluate size, depth, and possible intracranial component. A CT scan should also be performed to evaluate the bony integrity of the skull base, widening of the crista galli, and location in relation to the septum.

G Physical examination is also essential in narrowing the differential diagnosis. If the mass enlarges with crying or straining, transilluminates, or enlarges with jugular vein compression (+Furstenberg Sign) then it is likely an encephalocele or meningocele. Nasal dermoids and gliomas do not enlarge with straining, have negative Furstenberg's sign, and do not transilluminate.

H Nasal encephalocele/meningocele is a protrusion of cranial contents through a defect in the skull base. Nasoethmoidal encephaloceles are due to a herniation of dural diverticulum through the foramen cecum into the prenasal space. Frontonasal encephaloceles present with a glabellar mass and are a result of herniation of main tissue and dura through both the foramen cecum and the fonticulus frontalis. These lesions transilluminate and have a positive Furstenberg's sign. They are also associated with meningitis. The CT scan can demonstrate the bony defect, but MRI will reveal the connection with the intracranial compartment. The treatment of choice is surgical excision with a Neurosurgeon to help manage the intracranial component. Endoscopic or open resections are both appropriate approaches for resection depending on the skill set of the skull base team.

I Nasal gliomas are nonhereditary, benign, congenital midline nasal masses composed of heterotopic neuroglial tissue. They are isolated brain tissue that was displaced by closure of the anterior neuropore during development. On examination they are firm, noncompressible, gray, or purple lesions. They can obstruct the nasal cavity or cause extranasal deformity. They do not transilluminate and are not affected by crying. Negative Furstenberg sign (distend with jugular venous compression). Sixty percent are extranasal, 30% intranasal, 10% both. Fifteen to twenty-five percent have an intracranial extension via a fibrous stalk to the intracranial space. They are treated with surgery alone. Extranasal gliomas can be excised via a bicoronal approach, midline nasal excision, or external rhinoplasty. Intranasal gliomas with no intracranial extension can be resected endoscopically.

J Nasal dermoids are teratomatous lesions composed of ectoderm and mesoderm. They present with a cutaneous midline dimple/sinus that typically contain hair or have sebaceous discharge. They can expand the nasal septum or form a bifid septum. Twenty to thirty percent of dermoids can have intracranial extension via the foramen cecum or cribriform plate. The CT scan can reveal a widened foramen cecum, bifid crista galli, or bony destruction of the glabella. The MRI can define intracranial extension. Surgical excision is the treatment of choice. There are multiple surgical approaches in the literature: open rhinoplasty approach, midline vertical (elliptical) direct excision, transverse excision, bicoronal with excision of the tract, endoscopic with elliptical external excision of the sinus tract have all been reported.

K Nasolacrimal duct cyst/mucoceles: Result from distal obstruction of the nasolacrimal duct at the level of Hasner's valve. They present with a dacrocystocele, dilation of the nasolacrimal duct and a mass in the inferior meatus consistent with a mucocele. Treatment is excision (see Chapter 51).

L Nasal hamartomas: Benign masses of excess tissue that is indigenous to the site of origin. Nasal hamartomas are composed of mesenchymal tissue and typically arise in the midline. They are associated with Pai syndrome. Excision is the treatment of choice.

M Nasal hemangiomas can be confused with nasal gliomas or dermoids. An ultrasound examination with Doppler flow can help differentiate these lesions. If ultrasound shows arterial flow through the lesion it is likely a hemangioma. The natural history of hemangiomas is rapid growth in the first year of life and then gradual involution until age 5. A trial of propranolol is the recommended first-line treatment. If the lesion does not respond to propranolol, steroid injection or surgical excision is additional treatment option if the mass is obstructing or causing other functional deficits.

SUGGESTED READING

Ajose-Popoola O, Lin HW, Silvera VM, et al. Nasal glioma: prenatal diagnosis and multidisciplinary approach. Skull Base Rep. 2011;1:83-88.

Dasgupta NR, Bentz ML. Nasal gliomas: identification and differentiation from hemangiomas. J Craniofacial Surg. 2003;14(5):736-738.

Ginat DT, Robson CD. Diagnostic imaging features of congenital nose and nasal cavity lesions. Clin Neuroradiol. 2015;25:3-11.

Rahbar R, Shah P, Mulliken JB, et al. The presentation and management of nasal dermoid. Arch Otolaryngol Head Neck Surg. 2003;129:464-471.

Wang IJ, Lin SL, Tsou KI, et al. Congenital midline nasal mass: case series and review of the literature. Turkish J Pediatrics. 2010;52:520-524.

CHAPTER 50

Choanal Atresia and Congenital Nasal Pyriform Aperture Stenosis

Todd M Wine

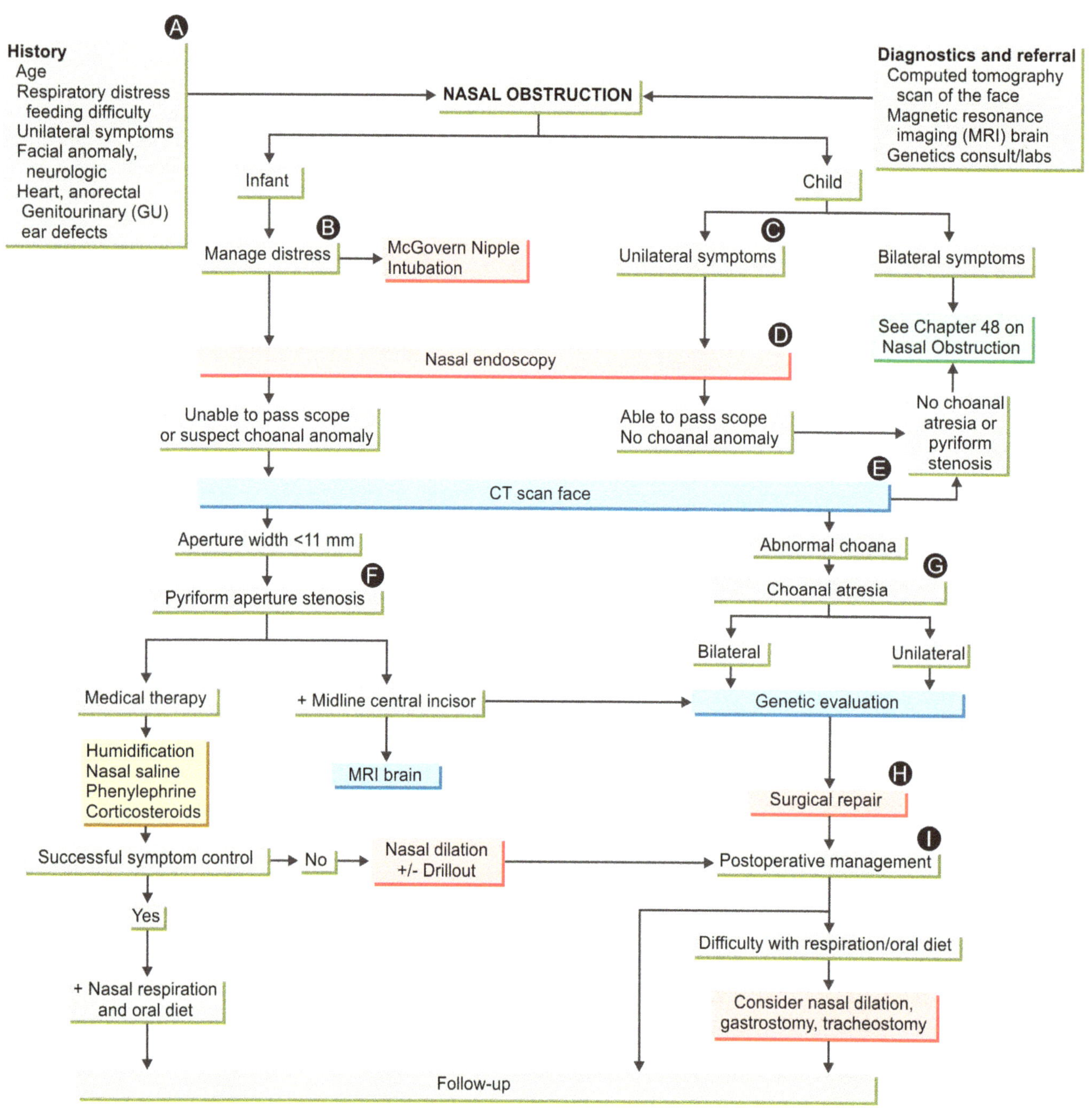

Nasal obstruction secondary to choanal atresia (CA) and pyriform aperture stenosis (PAS) can present with varying degrees of severity in a child. Bilateral CA and congenital nasal PAS can cause severe respiratory distress in infants due to inhibition of obligate nasal respiration. Inability to pass a 5-French suction catheter and difficulty in feeding are often reported. Unilateral CA is more commonly present in an older child presenting with unilateral nasal symptoms.

A The history of nasal obstruction should include the age of onset. The differential diagnoses of infant and later childhood nasal obstruction are not similar.

B Assessment and management of neonatal respiratory distress is the first priority. If severe distress is noted, endotracheal intubation will likely be required. Mild-to-moderate distress can be improved with the use of an oral airway or a Mc-Govern nipple (modified pacifier/nipple with the open-end).

C Older children with unilateral symptoms require anterior rhinoscopy and nasal endoscopy to rule out unilateral CA or other unilateral problems.

D In older children, nasal endoscopy can accurately detect the presence of a choanal anomaly. In neonates, it will be very difficult or impossible to pass the scope through the nose in PAS or CA. Otherwise, nasal endoscopy can rule out CA and PAS.

E If CA or PAS are suspected based on nasal endoscopy, computed tomography (CT) of the face will either confirm or rule out the diagnosis.

F Pyriform aperture stenosis is diagnosed when the pyriform aperture is less than 11 mm. Other CT features commonly seen in PAS are triangular-shaped palate, midline palatal ridge, and sometimes a maxillary median central incisor. Once the diagnosis is made, medical therapy is initiated. This consists of humidification, nasal saline spray or drops, topical decongestion with phenylephrine, and topical nasal corticosteroids. If a midline central incisor is present, brain magnetic resonance imaging (MRI) and genetics evaluation are recommended to rule out median maxillary central incisor syndrome or holoprosencephaly. If medical therapy fails, surgical therapy is recommended. Classically, a sublabial approach is performed to drill out the pyriform aperture. Alternatively, nasal dilation with Hegar dilators or balloon dilation can be performed to improve the nasal airway in a less invasive manner.

G Unilateral or bilateral CA is confirmed by the CT scan. CA will often be bony in 30% and mixed membranous or bony in 70%. Associated findings on CT scan include medialization of the pterygoid plates, widened vomer, and other defects of the skull base. CA can be associated with Coloboma, Heart defect, Atresia choanae, Retarded Growth and development, genital abnormality, and Ear abnormality (CHARGE) or other syndromes, thus genetic evaluation is warranted.

H Choanal atresia repair is most often performed via transnasal or transoral endoscopic approach to remove the atretic plate and partially resect the posterior septum or vomer. Postoperatively, many, but not all surgeons use nasal stents. Unilateral CA is treated similarly with the exception that it is performed electively and stenting is less likely to be required.

I Postoperative management of CA and PAS in neonates requires close follow-up. Revision procedures are sometimes necessary. When surgical therapy fails to allow proper respiration and feeding, tracheostomy and gastrostomy need to be considered. In an older child with unilateral atresia repair, in office endoscopy can assess the functional status of the repair.

SUGGESTED READING

Arlis H, Ward RF. Congenital nasal pyriform aperture stenosis. Isolated abnormality vs. developmental field 17 defect. Arch Otolaryngol Head Neck Surg. 1992;118(9):989-991.

Belden CJ, Mancuso AA, Schmalfuss IM. CT features of 13 congenital nasal piriform aperture stenosis: initial 14 experience. Radiology. 1999;213(2):495-501.

Brown OE, Myer CM III, Manning SC. Congenital nasal 10 pyriform aperture stenosis. Laryngoscope. 1989;99(1):86-91.

Hengerer AS, Brickman TM, Jeyakumar A. Choanal atresia: embryologic analysis and evolution of treatment, a 30-year experience. Laryngoscope. 2008;118(5):862-866.

Newman JR, Harmon P, Shirley WP, et al. Operative management of choanal atresia: A 15-year experience. JAMA Otolaryngol Head Neck Surg. 2013;139(1):71-75.

Ramsden JD, Campisi P, Forte V. Choanal atresia and choanal stenosis. Otolaryngol Clin North Am. 2009;42(2):339-352.

Reeves TD, Discolo CM, White DR. Nasal cavity dimensions in congenital pyriform aperture stenosis. Int J Pediatr Otorhinolaryngol. 2013;77(11):1830-1832.

Saafan ME. Endoscopic management of congenital bilateral posterior choanal atresia: value of using stents. Eur Arch Otorhinolaryngol. 2013;270(1):129-134.

Wine TM, Dedhia K, Chi DH. Congenital nasal pyriform aperture stenosis: is there a role for nasal dilation? JAMA Otolaryngol Head Neck Surg. 2014;140(4):352-356.

Disorders of the Nasolacrimal Apparatus

Susan Tonya Stefko

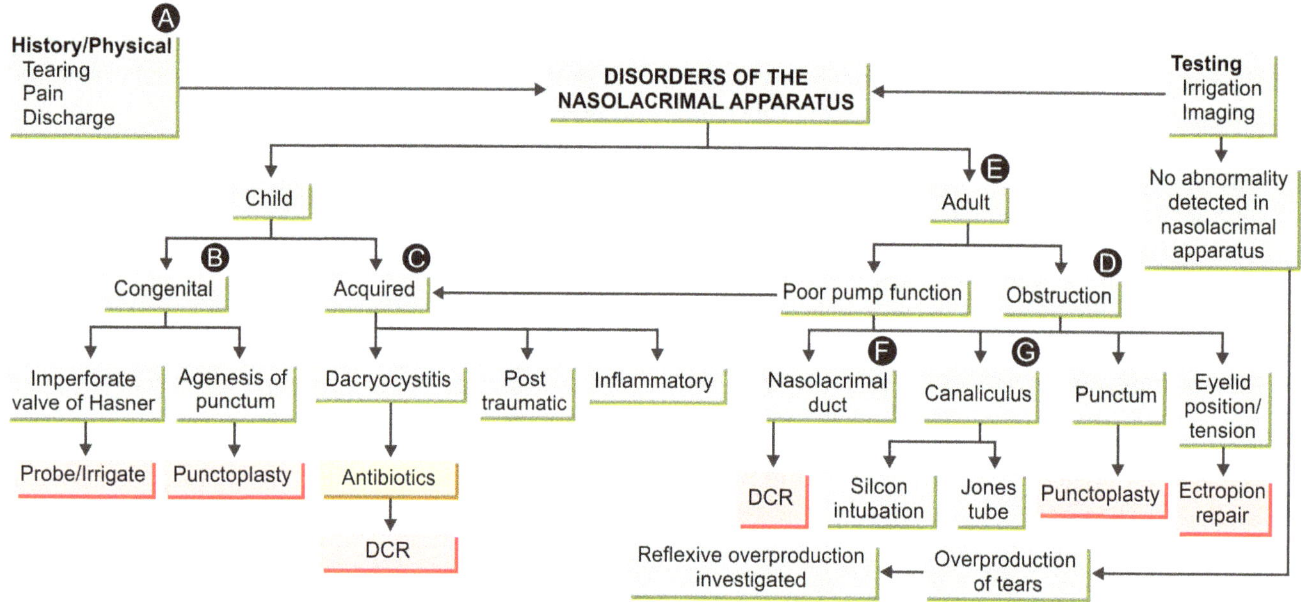

Epiphora, or tearing, is a common complaint among patients presenting to either an Ophthalmologist or an Otolaryngologist. This overflow may be due to overproduction of tears (usually reflexive), underdrainage of tears (a disorder of the nasolacrimal apparatus), or both.

A Most nasolacrimal disorders present with tearing. It is advantageous to have an examination by an Ophthalmologist to identify any ocular surface causes for overproduction of tears. If reflex tearing is not the cause, failure/obstruction at some level of the drainage system is suspected. These have much different causes in children and adults.

B By far the most common cause of congenital tearing is an imperforate valve of Hasner (distally under the inferior turbinate). This is present in approximately 6% of infants, though this incidence is higher in Down syndrome and in craniofacial anomalies. Approximately 90% of these will resolve with conservative treatment by the age of 1 year, so the recommendation is to observe, in the absence of infection, until that time. In those patients where this fails to resolve spontaneously or with massage of the lacrimal sac by the parents, the sec may be probed under general anesthetic. The probing is easily performed via the upper or lower punctum, is generally reported to be about 80–90% successful at resolution of symptoms on the first attempt, and use of balloon dilation of the duct or silicon intubation increases the success rate modestly. At this time, absence of puncta would be apparent and could be addressed with a 25-gauge needle punctoplasty and

irrigation, with or without placement of silicon stents. In general, however, patients lacking puncta tear but do not have discharge and crusting of the lashes.

C A congenital dacryocele, or lacrimal sac cyst, is present in approximately 1/4,000 infants, and, in the absence of infection, may be prescribed Crigler massage and observation. Infection requires immediate probing. Bilateral nasolacrimal duct cysts (found in about 25% of those with dacryocystoceles) have been reported to present at birth with bilateral nasal obstruction, rendering this a surgical emergency. The portion of the cyst extending into the nose must be excised, in addition to decompression of the sac by probing.

D In an older child who develops tearing, a low threshold for imaging must be kept. If there is no clear history of trauma, infection, or congenital problems, a computed tomography (CT) of the orbits should be assessed. Trauma to the lids, such as by a dog bite, can transect the canaliculus and present a problem for reconstruction. Any inflammation, such as nasal congestion caused by allergic rhinitis, should be treated appropriately.

E The lower eyelid must have appropriate tension and position to effectively pump tears into the nasolacrimal duct. Poor snap-back of the lid, malposition, or excessive distraction (>1 cm from the globe) requires surgical repair. This may include a horizontal tightening procedure, with or without a skin graft if there is a cicatricial or mechanical component present.

F Irrigation with saline via one punctum will delineate the level of outflow obstruction; if all reflux occurs from the same punctum, that canaliculus is obstructed. If reflux occurs from the opposite lid, the patient is obstructed distal to the common canaliculus and a dacryocystorhinostomy (DCR) may be appropriate. If the patient tastes the saline, but there is some reflux from the upper system, there may be functional obstruction (with pressure, the system works, but at the normal physiologic pressure of about –4 mm Hg, minimal flow occurs), and a DCR may, again, be necessary.

G Canalicular obstruction may be caused by inflammation (such as post-viral), trauma, and some medications (5-fluorouracil, taxotere, and I131 among them). Treatment of complete obstruction requires a conjunctivodacryocystorhinostomy with placement of a Lester Jones tube. Incomplete or early obstruction can sometimes be treated with prompt bicanalicular silicon tube placement.

Mass of the lacrimal sac or nasolacrimal duct mandates an external approach to biopsy/DCR.

SUGGESTED READING

Esmaeli B, Amin S, Valero V, et al. Prospective study of incidence and severity of epiphora and canalicular stenosis in patients with metastatic breast cancer receiving docetaxel. J Clin Oncol. 2006;24(22):3619-3622.

Kapadia MK, Freitag SK, Woog JJ. Evaluation and management of congenital nasolacrimal duct obstruction. Otolaryngol Clin North Am. 2006;39(5):959-977.

Olitsy S. Update on congenital nasolacrimal duct obstruction. Int Ophthalmol Clin. 2014;54(3):1-7.

Schnall BM. Pediatric nasolacrimal duct obstruction. Curr Opin Ophthalmol. 2013;24(5):421-445.

Stefko ST, Snyderman CH. Dacryocystorhinostomy. In: Myers E (Ed). Operative Otolaryngology: Head and Neck Surgery, 2nd edition. Elsevier, 2008, pp: 967-972.

Rhinorrhea

Sean D Houston

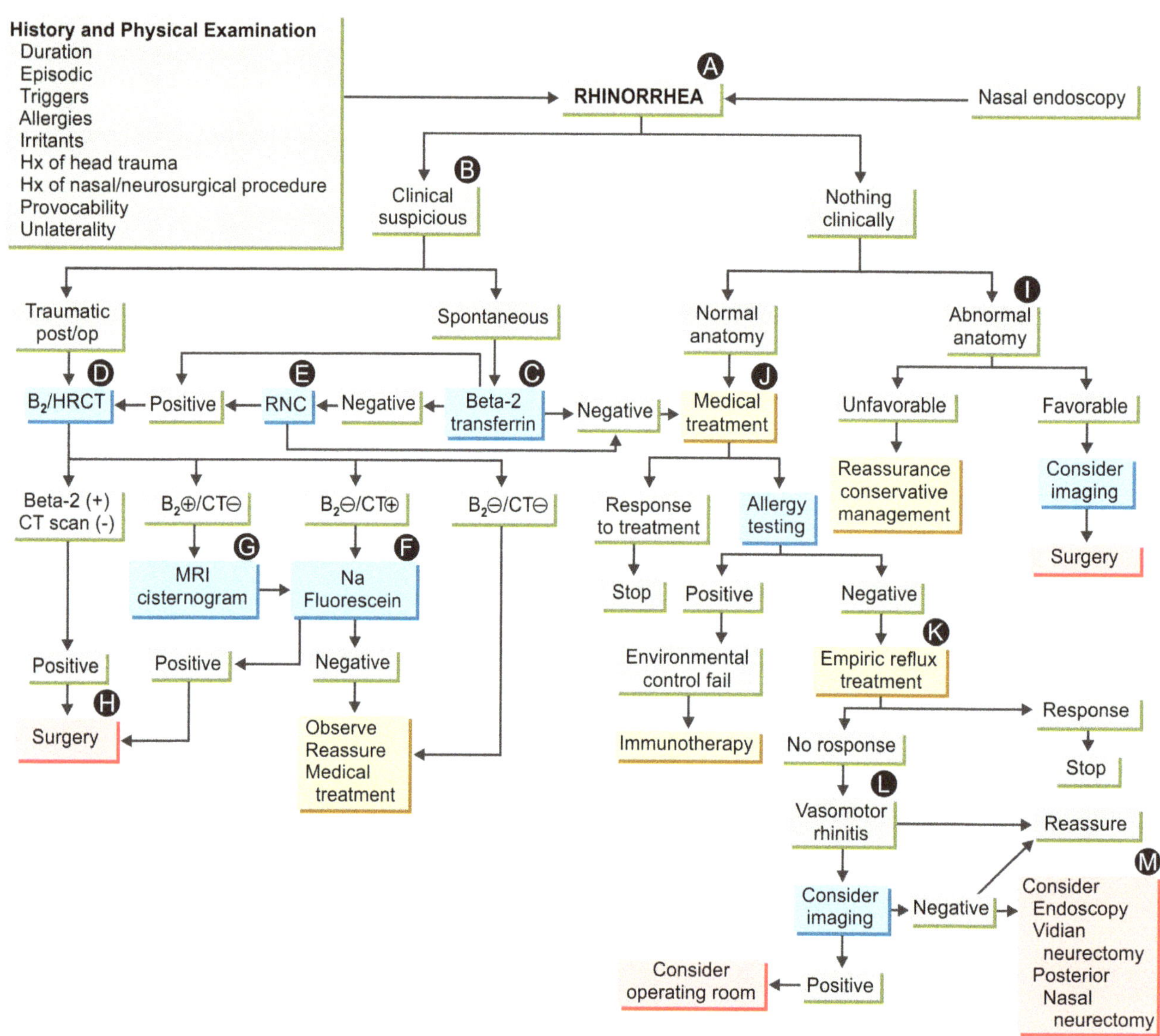

Rhinorrhea is defined as a clear nasal discharge that is not suppurative or acute in nature. The former suggests infection and will be discussed under the chronic sinusitis algorithm. Concerning the latter patients rarely come to the Otolaryngologist for upper respiratory tract infection (URI) or allergic symptoms that have been present for less than one week. Another practical approach used in our office is to get the patient who complains of chronic postnasal drip to pinpoint where they first localize the sensation of the drip. If the patient points to the midline of their cricoid cartilage, silent reflux is suspected and the algorithm for hoarseness/dysphagia/reflux is considered.

A The two arms of the algorithm diverge primarily on an appropriate history. Cues that should alert the physician to the cerebrospinal fluid (CSF) arm of the algorithm are unilateral rhinorrhea that is more producible on exertion, Valsalva or bending over. A history of trauma, skull fracture, or recent nasal surgery that preceded the rhinorrhea is also a concern. The patient with a history of benign intracranial hypertension or history suggestive of it and chronic rhinorrhea is clinically suspicious.

B Rhinorrhea suspicious for CSF can be categorized into traumatic, nontraumatic, and spontaneous/idiopathic. A history of significant head trauma, specifically skull base fracture, raises concerns for the clinician. Traumatic (including surgical) CSF fistulas are the most common of the subgroups. Postoperative CSF fistulas may present late when surgical swelling decreases. Nontraumatic sources include infection, neoplasm, meningoencephalocele, and hydrocephalus. Spontaneous CSF fistulas are least common and are associated with papilledema, CSF pressures >200 m H_2O, benign intracranial pressure and empty sella syndrome. Spontaneous CSF rhinorrhea are subtle and intermittent in nature.

C β2-transferrin is currently the laboratory study of choice and is a highly sensitive diagnostic tool to confirm CSF leaks.

D High-resolution computed tomography (HRCT) findings include pneumocephalus and fracture dislocation >3 mm and unilateral opacification along the skull base. Anterior skull fractures, specifically the cribriform plate, is the most common site of spontaneous CSF fistulas.

E Radionuclide cisternography (RNC): Extravasation of radionuclide onto cotton pledgets placed within the nasal cavity is a positive result.

F Na fluorescein: Direct intraoperative visualization of extravasated fluorescein into the sinonasal cavity after intrathecal administration is a positive result.

G In cases where HRCT and magnetic resonance imaging cisternography are used, multiple studies have shown the combined sensitivity, specificity, and accuracy of CSF defect site detection is 95%, 100%, and 96%, respectively.

H Untreated CSF leaks related to head trauma have a 10–25% risk of meningitis with a subsequent 10% mortality. When localization/identification of the CSF leak's anatomical origin occurs preoperatively/intraoperatively the surgical success rates of closure are >90% regardless of the method of repair chosen.

I Abnormal anatomy that potentially contributes to the patients symptoms of rhinorrhea includes polyps, tumor, septal perforation with crusting, ulcerative mucositis, deviated nasal septum, synechiae, turbinate resection, foreign body, unilateral atresia, and adenoid hypertrophy. Not all have favorable surgical options. For instance, a septoplasty done primarily for rhinorrhea should be considered carefully. Septal perforations can cause crusting and mucosal irritation but good local care is easier than repair which is more difficult with defects >2 cm. There are no good surgical options for resected turbinates.

J Medical treatment includes saline, hypertonic saline, antibiotic rinses, nasal steroid sprays, antihistamine nasal sprays, and ipratropium bromide (Atrovent). These therapies can be issued individually or in combination as tolerated by the patient.

K Even with a history and physical finding that does not suggest reflux, at this point the algorithm should be considered.

L Vasomotor rhinitis may include drug induced, pregnancy, change in menstrual-related hormones, hypothyroidism, temperature mediated, or may be due to hyperactive parasympathetic system, a hypoactive parasympathetic system or imbalance between the two. Reassurance and avoidance of potential triggers needs to be considered.

M It is reasonable that the majority of patients with rhinorrhea are not symptomatic enough to require surgical intervention.

However, surgical options do exist. Endoscopic Vidian neurectomy has demonstrated effectiveness in alleviating symptoms of vasomotor rhinitis in most patients and that the benefit is maintained over a period of 2–5 years.

SUGGESTED READING

Bachmann-Harildstad G. Diagnostic values of beta-2 transferrin and beta-trace protein as markers for cerebrospinal fluid fistula. Rhinology. 2008;46:82-86.

Halderman A, Sindwani R. Surgical management of vasomotor rhinitis: a systematic review. Am J Rhinol Allergy. 2015;29:128-134.

Kim SW, Rhee CS. Nasal septal perforation repair: predictive factors and systematic review of the literature. Curr Opin Otolaryngol Head Neck Surg. 2012;20:58-65.

Meco C, Oberascher G. Comprehensive algorithm for skull base dural lesion and cerebrospinal fluid fistula diagnosis. Laryngoscope. 2004;114:991-999.

Oakley GM, Alt JA, Schlosser RJ, et al. Diagnosis of cerebrospinal fluid rhinorrhea: an evidence—based review with recommendation. Int Forum Allergy Rhinol. 2016;6:8-16.

Shetty PG, Shroff MM, Sahani DV, et al. Evaluation of high resolution CT and MR cisternography in the diagnosis of cerebrospinal fluid fistula. AJNR Am J Neuroradiol. 1998;19:633-639.

Zapalac JS, Marple BF, Schwade ND. Skull base cerebrospinal fluid fistulas: a comprehensive diagnostic algorithm. Otolaryngol Head and Neck Surg. 2002;126:669-676.

CHAPTER 53

Epistaxis

Andrea M Hebert, Carl H Snyderman

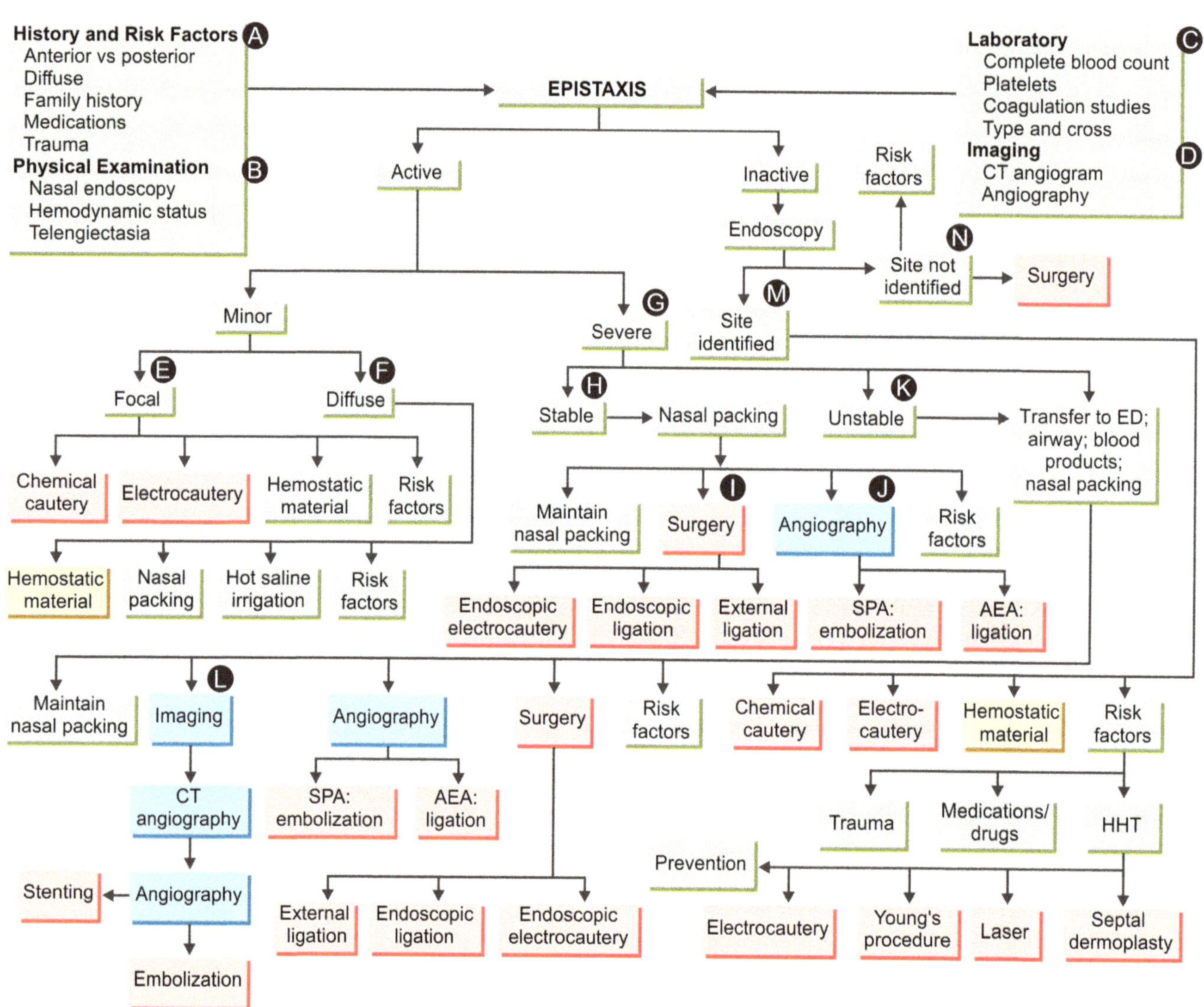

Epistaxis is a common otolaryngologic problem that affects all age groups. Although most episodes are benign and self-limited, epistaxis can be an indicator of sinonasal malignancy or a vascular emergency. The treatment strategy depends on the etiology and severity of hemorrhage.

A The history should establish the characteristics of the bleeding and elicit risk factors. Anterior bleeding is more likely to be from the nasal septum or anterior ethmoid artery (AEA). Posterior bleeding is more likely to be from the sphenopalatine artery (SPA). Diffuse bleeding suggests a coagulopathy. Associated symptoms may indicate a neoplasm. Comorbidities and family history may suggest an underlying cause. A careful drug history is especially important since patients are often unaware of the anticoagulant effects of medications and other products (blood thinners, antiplatelet drugs, nonsteroidal anti-inflammatory drugs, alcohol, vitamin D, fish oil, and herbal products). Recent head trauma or sinus surgery is a risk factor for injury of the internal carotid artery (ICA).

B In addition to identifying the site of the bleeding by nasal endoscopy, an assessment should be made of the patient's hemodynamic status (hypertension, acute hypovolemia). Examination for the characteristics of hereditary hemorrhagic telangiectasia (HHT), also known as Osler-Weber-Rendu disease, should include examination of the lips and oral cavity for telangiectasia.

C Laboratory studies are required only for patients with severe hemorrhage or a history of recurrent bleeding.

These should include a complete blood count, platelets, and coagulation studies. Matched blood should be available if bleeding is severe.

D Routine imaging is not recommended unless there are associated symptoms or endoscopic findings suggestive of a neoplasm. In such cases, computed tomography with angiographic (CTA) visualization should be performed for diagnosis and to assess vascular involvement. If there is a recent history of sinus surgery or head trauma, angiography should be considered to rule out a pseudo-aneurysm of the ICA.

E Focal sites may include a small arteriole, mucosal abrasion, or angioma. A temporizing measure can be the application of external pressure and topical vasoconstrictive agents. Chemical cautery with $AgNO_3$ is adequate for most focal sites. Topical hemostatic materials such as oxidized cellulose may be applied to the site. Electrocautery is an option but may not be available in an office setting. Common risk factors include self-induced trauma (nose-picking) and medications.

F Diffuse bleeding is usually due to a coagulopathy (congenital or acquired) and treatment of the underlying condition is the primary goal. Placement of hemostatic material or an anterior pack may be necessary but additional mucosal trauma should be avoided.

G The first priority is to assess the overall condition of the patient. If the airway is compromised, vital signs are unstable, or the patient has significant comorbidities, management in the emergency department is preferred. Temporary control of bleeding is best accomplished with a balloon inflated with water that compresses the anterior and posterior nasal cavity. If active bleeding persists, surgical intervention or embolization is indicated once the patient is stabilized.

H If the patient is stable, treatment options include nasal packing for 3–5 days, surgery, or angiography with embolization (A&E). Of these, surgery is the most cost-effective treatment, has minimal morbidity, and is well tolerated by patients. Nasal packing is uncomfortable, compromises pulmonary function, and has the highest failure rate. A&E is not universally available, is more costly, has more severe complications, and does not address bleeding from the ethmoidal arteries. Risk factors should also be addressed but anticoagulation is not a contraindication to surgery.

I The SPA is the most likely source for idiopathic severe epistaxis. If the bleeding site is indeterminate at the time of surgery, endoscopic cauterization and/or ligation of the SPA and AEA are recommended. In patients with facial trauma, the AEA is a more common source. External ligation of the AEA is an option based on surgeon preference.

Recurrent epistaxis after surgery may be due to incomplete ligation of multiple vascular branches exiting through separate foramina or failure to recognize the source. Treatment options include repeat surgery with ligation of additional vessels or embolization.

J The source of bleeding cannot be identified unless there is active bleeding at the time of surgery. Embolization of the SPA is usually performed along with more proximal branches of the internal maxillary artery; branches of the facial artery may also be embolized. Bleeding from the AEA requires surgical ligation, as embolization could cause blindness.

K If the patient is unstable, priorities include securing a safe airway with oral intubation, controlling the hemorrhage with a nasal balloon, volume replacement with blood transfusion, and treatment of medical comorbidities. Treatment options include nasal packing for 3–5 days, surgery, or A&E. Surgery should be delayed until the patient is stable. A&E is preferred in patients with significant medical comorbidities.

L In unstable patients, additional imaging can help guide management. If CTA demonstrates neoplastic involvement of the ICA, angiography is performed for embolization of tumor vessels or stenting of the ICA.

M If the site of bleeding is identified but not active (mucosal trauma, prominent vessel, angioma), the site may be cauterized (chemical or electrical) or covered with a hemostatic material. Risk factors should be addressed to prevent recurrence (mucosal trauma, medications, and humidification). If HHT is diagnosed, treatment is problematic. In most instances, laser cautery (Nd:YAG or KTP) may control bleeding. Other options include sclerotherapy, bipolar electrocautery and coblation. If bleeding is persistent, a septal dermoplasty should be considered. In life-threatening epistaxis, where septal dermoplasty has been unsuccessful, closure of the nasal vestibule, or Young's procedure, can be performed. Bevacizumab, a monoclonal antibody inhibitor of the vascular endothelial growth factor A receptor (VEGF-A), and estrogen therapy have been used for prevention of epistaxis with promising results. These patients require further evaluation to rule out intestinal telangiectasia and pulmonary arteriovenous malformations.

N If a site is not identified, risk factors are addressed to prevent recurrence. If the episodes of epistaxis are significant and frequent, elective ligation of the SPA may be offered.

SUGGESTED READING

Gede LL, Aanaes K, Collatz H, et al. National long-lasting effect of endonasal endoscopic sphenopalatine artery clipping for epistaxis. Acta Otolaryngol. 2013;133(7):744-748.

Lin G, Bleier B. Surgical management of severe epistaxis. Otolaryngol Clin North Am. 2017;49(3):627-637.

McDermott AM, O'Cathain E, Carey BW, et al. Sphenopalatine artery ligation for epistaxis: factors influencing outcome and impact of timing of surgery. Otolaryngol Head Neck Surg. 2016;154(3):547-552.

Pant H. Hemostasis in sinus surgery. Otolaryngol Clin North Am. 2017;49(3):655-676.

Sautter NB, Smith TL. Treatment of hereditary hemorrhagic telangiectasia-related epistaxis. Otolaryngol Clin North Am. 2017;49(3):639-654.

Soyka MB, Nikolaou G, Rufibach K, et al. On the effectiveness of treatment options in epistaxis: an analysis of 678 interventions. Rhinology. 2011;49(1):474-478.

Tassler A, Kaye R. Preoperative assessment of risk factors. Otolaryngol Clin North Am. 2017;49(3):517-529.

CHAPTER 54

Nasal Foreign Bodies

Julia E Noel, Jayakar V Nayak

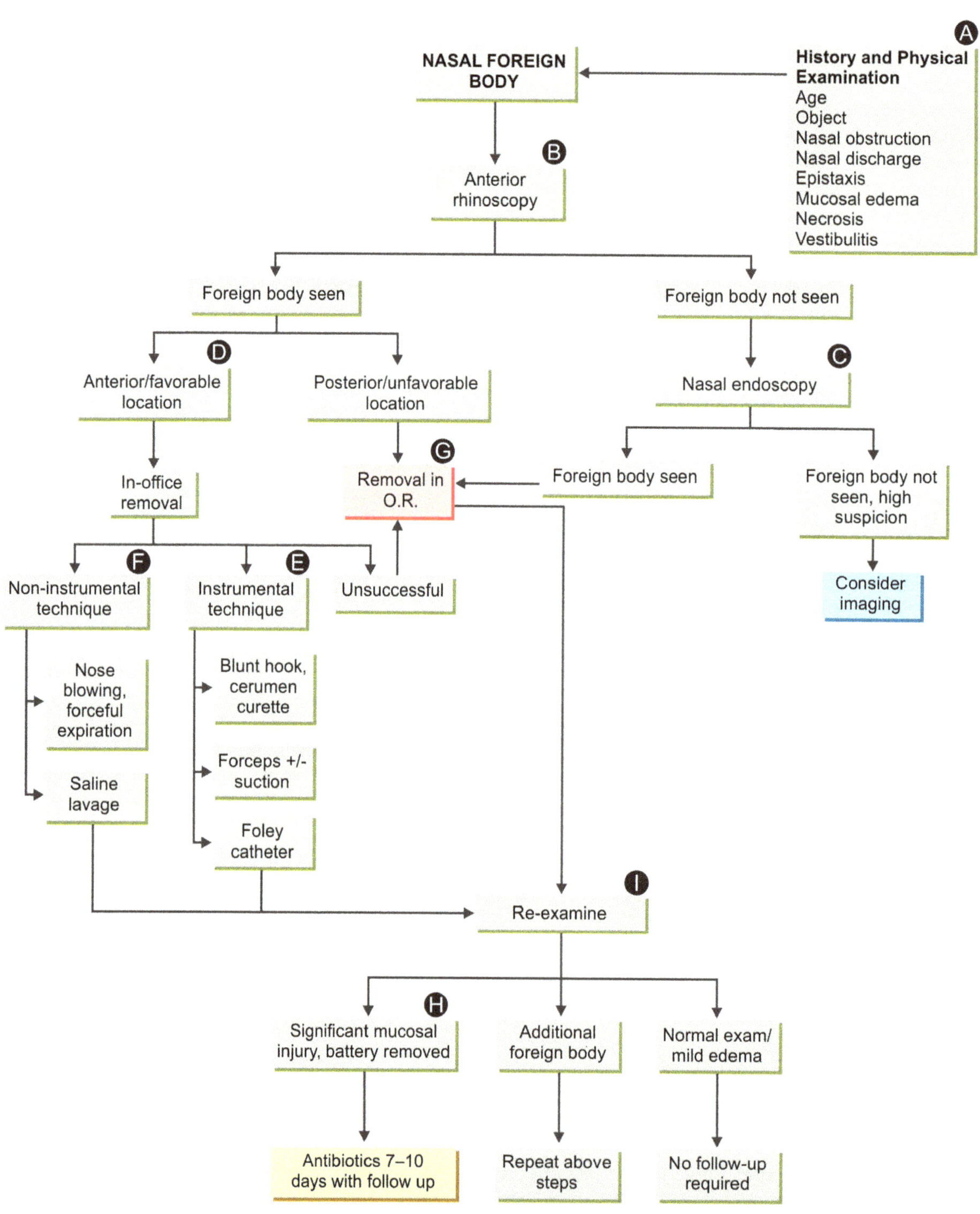

Nasal foreign bodies (FB) are common, especially in young children (3–5 years). Although not typically life threatening, an early diagnosis is important to avoid potential complications due to the nature of the FB itself, chronicity of irritation, bronchoaspiration, or superinfection.

A Most patients will present with a family member or caretaker who witnessed the insertion of the FB. It is important to elicit the nature of the object, as some (i.e. button batteries) require prompt removal. Those with unwitnessed placements will often come to attention only when a foul odor and unilateral discharge has persisted despite antibiotic treatment, or with new epistaxis or nasal obstruction.

B Anterior rhinoscopy is best performed with an otoscope and ear speculum. Alternatively, the nasal tip may be gently lifted with the thumb to expose the nasal vestibule. The majority of nasal FBs will be evident on this examination because of narrowing of the nasal airways at the pyriform aperture.

C When history suggests a posterior location or there is concern for FB not revealed by anterior rhinoscopy, flexible nasal endoscopy is indicated. Rigid endoscopes may be used for older children or adults. Imaging is typically unnecessary unless there is high suspicion for a nonvisualized FB.

D Foreign objects in the nose are typically found on the nasal floor in front of, or just behind, the head of the inferior turbinate, or anterior to the middle turbinate head. When previous extraction has been attempted, they may be located more superiorly or posteriorly.

E When the FB is anterior and previous attempts have not compromised visualization, it may be removed in the clinic. Topical vasoconstriction and anesthesia are recommended. Firm round or cylindrical objects may be removed by passing a blunt hook or cerumen curette past the object, rotating, and slowly pulling forward. A 6 or 8-French Foley catheter, with the deflated balloon inserted past the object and then inflated with 1–2cc of water before retrieval, is also suitable in these cases. The FBs with a flat edge or soft consistency (foam, paper, or organic matter) are best removed with forceps. If this proves difficult, a Frazier suction can be used instead or in conjunction.

F In older children, instrument-independent measures may be used. Nose blowing or forced expiration with the mouth closed may dislodge the FB. A forceful saline lavage to the unaffected side can also be effective and is often the best choice when dealing with fragmented organic matter.

G When the child is uncooperative, office extraction has failed, or the position of the FB is unfavorable, general anesthesia may be required. After intubation, posterior displacement into the pharynx or fragmentation are additional options for removal of difficult objects.

H Button batteries, though rare, are special cases. They require immediate extraction due to the risk of mucosal ulceration and septal perforation. Antibiotics are recommended for 7–10 days following extraction.

I Following removal of any FB in the nose, careful re-examination of the affected and contralateral side of the nasal cavity is important to identify any previously unrecognized objects or signs of significant mucosal trauma.

SUGGESTED READING

Abou-Elfadl M, Horra A, Abada R-L, et al. Nasal foreign bodies: results of a study of 260 cases. Eur Ann Otorhinolaryngol Head Neck Dis. 2015;132(6):343-346.

Cetinkaya EA, Arslan İB, Cukurova İ. Nasal foreign bodies in children: types, locations, complications and removal. Int J Pediatr Otorhinolaryngol. 2015;79(11):1881-1885.

Figueiredo RR, Azevedo AA, Kós AO de A, et al. Nasal foreign bodies: description of types and complications in 420 cases. Braz J Otorhinolaryngol. 2006;72(1):18-23.

François M, Hamrioui R, Narcy P. Nasal foreign bodies in children. Eur Arch Otorhinolaryngol. 1998;255(3):132-134.

Gregori D, Salerni L, Scarinzi C, et al. Foreign bodies in the nose causing complications and requiring hospitalization in children 0-14 age: results from the European survey of foreign bodies injuries study. Rhinology. 2008;46(1):28-33.

Kiger JR, Brenkert TE, Losek JD. Nasal foreign body removal in children. Pediatr Emerg Care. 2008;24(11):785-792.

CHAPTER 55

Olfactory Disorders

Carl H Snyderman, Aron Z Pollack

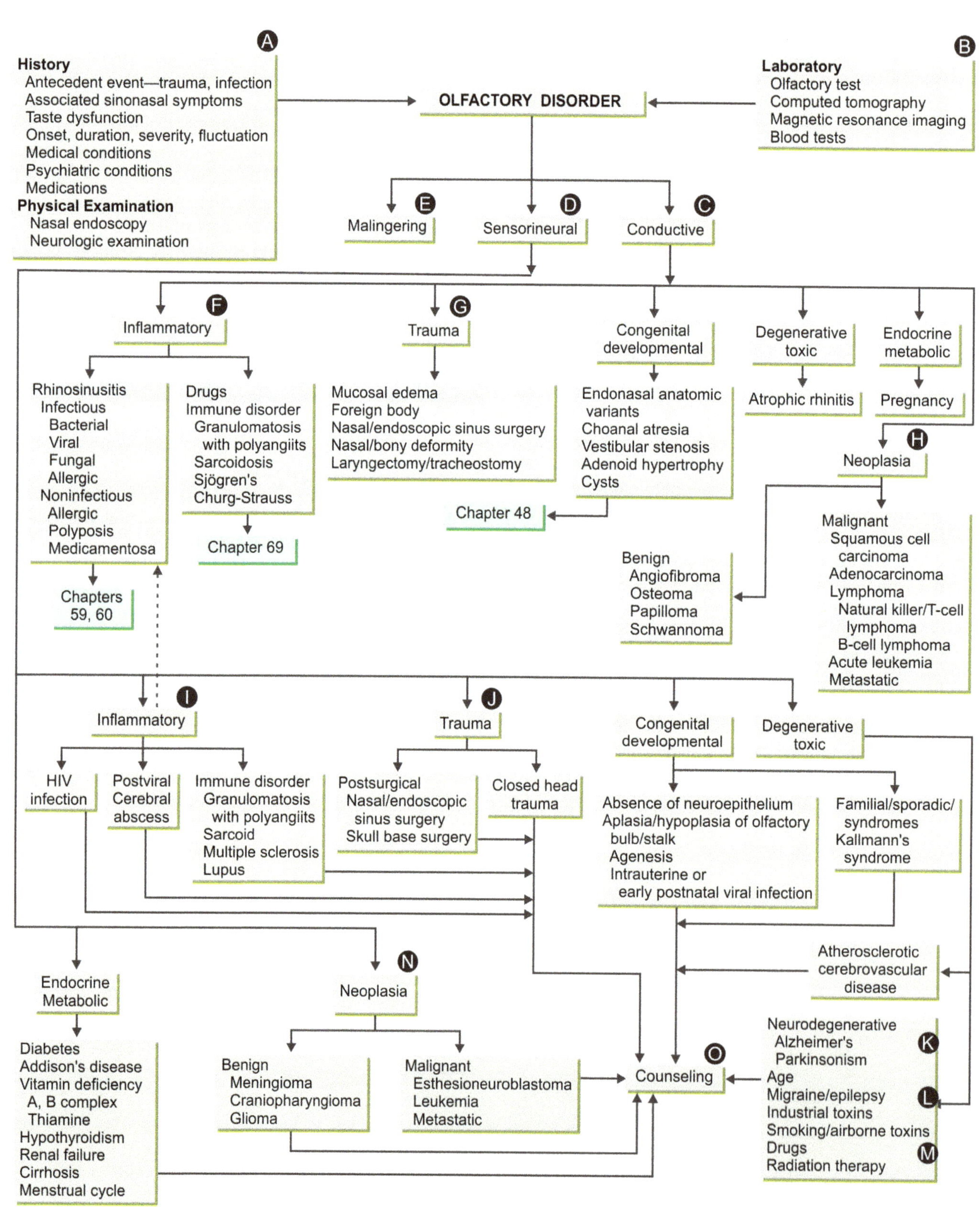

Olfactory function may be described as a complete loss (anosmia), diminished (hyposmia), enhanced sensitivity (hyperosmia), or distorted (dysosmia). Phantosmia is dysosmia with no stimulus present. Cacosmia is dysosmia described as a bad odor. Disorders of detection (anosmia, hyposmia) and identification often occur simultaneously.

A The most common antecedent events include trauma and upper respiratory tract infection. The onset is typically acute with these conditions. A slowly progressive onset may indicate a systemic illness or neoplastic process. Associated sinonasal symptoms, especially if olfactory function fluctuates, may indicate an inflammatory cause (chronic rhinosinusitis, allergic rhinitis, nasal polyposis, granulomatous disease). Patients often present with a complaint of decreased taste rather than olfactory loss. Olfactory loss has been associated with renal failure, liver disease, diabetes, and hypothyroidism, in addition to neuropsychiatric disorders (schizophrenia).

Olfactory dysfunction can be divided into conditions that prevent the access of odorants to the olfactory neuroepithelium (conductive) and those that affect the neuronal elements (sensorineural). Nasal endoscopy is required as a first step to look for a potential cause for a conductive loss.

B When a conductive etiology is not apparent, chemosensory testing should be performed. The detection threshold is the most dilute concentration of a specific odorant that an individual can detect. Identification tests are suprathreshold tests that allow the subject to differentiate a variety of odorants. [University of Pennsylvania Smell Identification Test (UPSIT; Sensonics, Haddon Heights, New Jersey)].

Imaging is not ordered routinely. Noncontrast computed tomography (CT) is helpful in diagnosing inflammatory sinonasal disease that is not apparent with endoscopy and CT with contrast or magnetic resonance imaging (MRI) can detect intracranial disease when the cause of olfactory dysfunction is not evident. In the absence of an identifiable cause, blood tests (thyroid-stimulating hormone, complete blood count, fasting glucose, renal function tests, autoimmune studies, allergy evaluation, nutrition panel) are obtained as indicated.

C Conductive loss can be due to inflammatory disease, anatomic deformities, or obstructive neoplasms. Conductive causes may respond to medical or surgical management of the obstruction.

D Sensorineural olfactory loss may be further divided into sensory loss—injury to the olfactory receptor region—and neural loss—damage of central olfactory pathways. Sensorineural loss of olfaction after a viral upper respiratory infection is the most frequently identified cause of permanent hyposmia or anosmia. The prognosis for recovery is generally poor.

E Malingering may be seen after head trauma (automobile accident) or toxic exposure. Malingerers may be detected by scoring worse than predicted by chance on multiple-choice tests such as the UPSIT and failure to detect noxious stimuli of the trigeminal (the most important), glossopharyngeal and/or vagal nerves.

F Conductive olfactory loss with rhinosinusitis may result from mucosal edema and/or polyps with obstruction of airflow to the olfactory region.

G Nasal and sinus trauma and surgery may result in conductive loss due to mucosal edema and/or synechiae. Diversion of airflow following tracheostomy or laryngectomy results in anosmia. Use of maneuvers to move air through the nasal cavity can successfully rehabilitate olfactory ability in patients following laryngectomy.

H Neoplasms, both benign and malignant, that obstruct airflow may cause a conductive loss of olfaction.

I Mild impairment in olfactory function might be an early indicator of immune suppression or of neurological disease (human immunodeficiency virus).

J Closed head trauma may cause either a traction injury of the fila olfactoria with retrograde neuronal degeneration or a contusion of the olfactory bulbs or other central processing region. Less than 10% of patients with post-traumatic anosmia will recover some olfactory function; dysosmia is frequent. Loss of olfactory neuroepithelium may occur with resection of the middle and superior turbinates. Shearing injury of the olfactory nerves may occur with manipulation of the septum and osteotomies. Transcranial surgery may cause direct trauma to the olfactory bulbs or tracts.

K Olfactory ability normally declines with age. Central loss of olfactory function may be one of the first detectable abnormalities of Alzheimer's and Parkinson's diseases. Suprathreshold deficits are common in epilepsy, with right-sided foci being more disruptive.

L Workplace exposure to organic compounds, nonmetallic inorganic compounds, metallurgical processing (cadmium, chromium, nickel, manganese), and dusts can cause olfactory dysfunction, particularly when such exposures have been chronic. Even common substances such as cigarette smoke and hairdressing chemicals can be associated with olfactory loss.

M Hundreds of medications have been associated with chemosensory disturbances. Major classes of drugs that may induce olfactory disturbances (either conductive and/or sensorineural) include antihypertensives (angiotensin-converting enzyme inhibitors, calcium channel blockers), antiarrhythmics (groups I and III), adrenergic stimulants, antiproliferatives, immunosuppressants, corticosteroids and statins. Chronic ethanol use has been associated with both reversible and nonreversible olfactory dysfunction.

N Neoplasia can cause direct destruction of the olfactory neuroepithelium or nerve tracts. Intracranial tumors (e.g. olfactory meningioma) are rarely a cause of anosmia in the absence of other symptoms or signs but must be ruled out with radiologic studies.

O With the exception of some drug-induced impairments, most sensorineural causes of olfactory loss cannot be effectively treated, and patients should be counseled regarding the implications of olfactory loss (decreased appetite and weight loss). Other risks include detection of smoke, natural gas, and spoiled food; appropriate safety measures are imperative.

SUGGESTED READING

Doty RL, Bromley SM. Effects of drugs on olfaction and taste. Otolaryngol Clin N Am. 2004;37:1229-1254.

Doty RL. The olfactory system and its disorders. Semin Neur. 2009;29:74-81.

Holbrook EH, Leopold DA. An updated review of clinical olfaction. Curr Opin Otolaryngol Head Neck Surg. 2006;6:23-28.

Kivity S, Ortega-Hernandez OD, Shoenfeld Y. Olfaction—a window to the mind. IMAJ. 2009;11:238-243.

Leopold DA, Holbrook EH. Physiology of olfaction. In: Flint PW, Haughey BH, Lund VJ, et al. (Eds). Cummings Otolaryngology: Head & Neck Surgery, 6th Edition. Philadelphia, PA: Elsevier/Saunders; 2015.

Treatment of Nasal Septal Perforation

Jonathan B Overdevest, Andrew N Goldberg

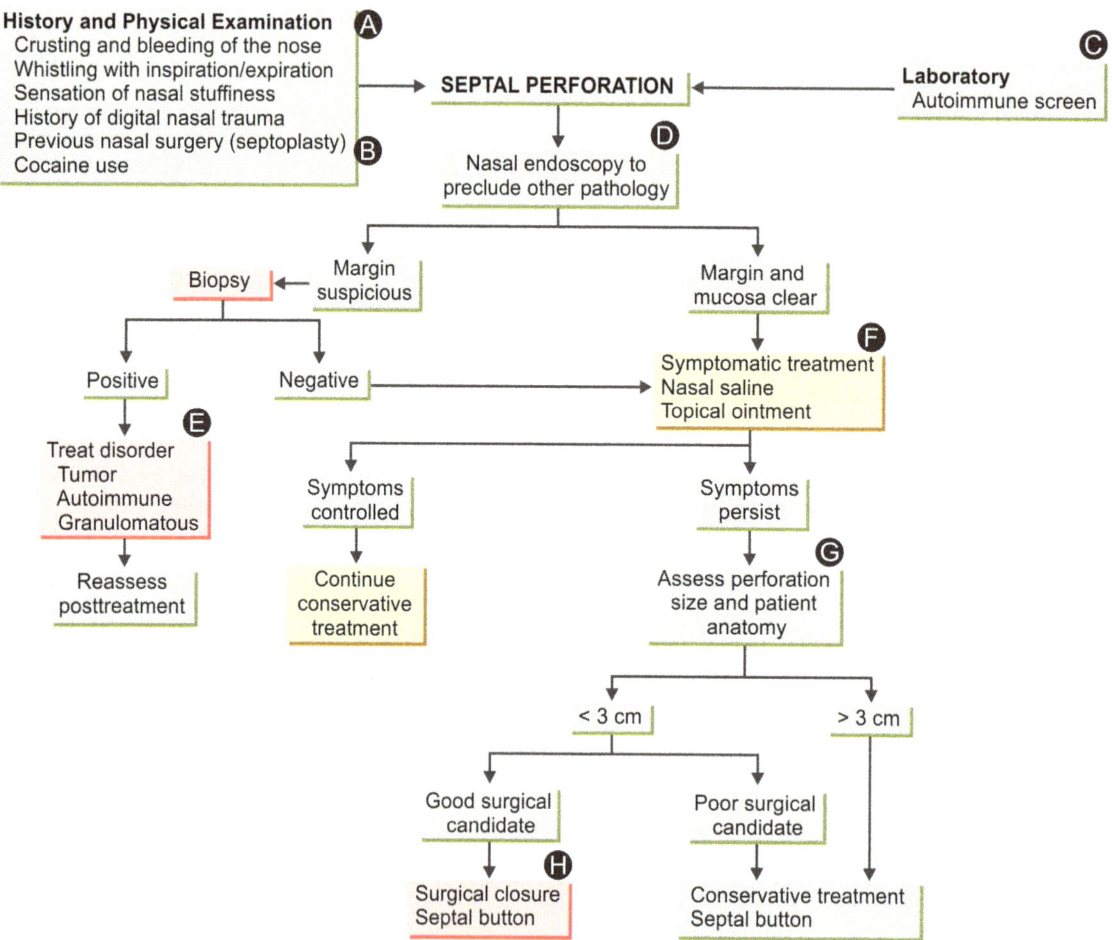

Nasal septal perforations are rare, with a prevalence of <1% in the general population. The majority of septal perforations are asymptomatic; however, patients with symptoms often experience significant deficits in their quality of life.

A Symptoms of septal perforations may depend on location and size. Posterior perforations are often asymptomatic; inspired air is already humidified by the time it reaches the perforation. Anterior perforations, however, commonly result in dryness, crusting, epistaxis, subjective obstruction and a high-pitched whistling sound. Larger, anterior perforations may compromise septal integrity, resulting in a saddle nose deformity (both cosmetically and functionally debilitating). A single institution review demonstrated that 12% of perforations were <1 cm, 57% were 1–2 cm and 31% were >2 cm.

B Gathering a detailed history will identify common causes of nasal septal perforations: trauma, infection, inflammatory, neoplastic and pharmacologic. A history of trauma or iatrogenic complications from cautery or prior nasal septal surgery precedes the majority of perforations. Because of the risk of perforation with septal cautery during the management of epistaxis, bilateral cautery should be avoided. Cocaine abuse is a common cause of perforation, and cessation of cocaine use should be verified before surgical repair to mitigate risks of failure. Reports suggest that nasal septal perforations are a rare side effect of intranasal corticosteroid sprays, where perforations are most commonly found during the first 12 months of treatment and in young women. Patients receiving bevacizumab as an adjuvant treatment for breast cancer and or for treatment of hereditary hemorrhagic telangiectasia should be advised of the risk of nasal septal perforation. Other pertinent topics to discuss with patients include nose picking, previous nasal instrumentation with nasotracheal or nasogastric tubes and tobacco smoking, which may potentiate the effects of other nasal insults and worsen symptoms. All potential etiologies for septal perforation are the result of mucoperichondrial devascularization and subsequent regression of underlying cartilaginous support.

C Laboratory testing is indicated only in a small subset of patients with septal perforations. Patients with a clear cause of perforation and well-healed, normal-appearing mucosa do not need further laboratory evaluation. Patients with unclear causes or abnormal-appearing mucosa/granulation tissue should undergo broad autoimmune testing, including cytoplasmic antineutrophil cytoplasmic antibody, erythrocyte sedimentation rate, C-reactive protein and specific autoantibodies depending on presenting symptoms to rule out sarcoidosis, granulomatosis with polyangiitis and other forms of vasculitis. Selected patients with systemic inflammatory disease should be referred for appropriate renal and pulmonary evaluations. Serum testing for syphilis may be indicated. Intranasal swab cultures are rarely useful, although culture of biopsy material may be indicated if there is a suspicion of an infectious cause (e.g. tuberculosis, leprosy and fungal invasion). Patients who are suspected of continuing cocaine use may warrant testing to confirm abstinence.

D Nasal endoscopy is recommended to rule out concomitant sinonasal pathology. If biopsies are necessary, they should be taken from the posterior portion of the perforation to prevent complicating eventual closure. A paper ruler placed on one side of the perforation and visualized through the contralateral nasal cavity is a simple method for documenting the initial size of the defect and changes over time. For complex and large perforations, sinus computed tomography (CT) imaging with fine slices may assist reconstructive planning.

E Positive biopsies should prompt appropriate treatment. Granulomatous diseases are particularly problematic because they can recur after long periods of quiescence. Patients with these disorders should understand that recurrence often results from reactivation of their disease, despite adequate primary surgical closure. Malignancies involving the septum are rare, but adequate treatment of the most common neoplasms—squamous cell carcinoma and T-cell lymphoma—often results in extremely large septal defects. Conservative therapy may be the best treatment for these patients to facilitate adequate surveillance for recurrence, with deferred surgical intervention until after the disease is definitively controlled.

F Asymptomatic septal perforations require no intervention. For symptomatic perforations, humidification is the primary goal. Copious nasal irrigation with saline is often helpful, and adding emollients such as mupirocin (Bactroban) or glycerin often potentiates the moisturizing effect. Commercially available moisturizing nasal gels are also helpful, used in this manner. Petrolatum ointment can be applied to the anterior nasal cavity with a cotton-tipped applicator to maintain humidification.

G Septal button prostheses may be used in patients who fail conservative therapy, are critically ill, continue to abuse nasal inhalants, or those patients who have failed prior surgical intervention due to septal perforations of >2 cm. Septal buttons made of Silastic materials and may be inserted in the office or operating room depending on patient's tolerance. The predominant issues with septal buttons are a propensity to become displaced over time

and a lack of intrinsic moisturizing properties. A recent systematic review suggests that septal buttons were tolerated and improved symptoms in 65% of patients with negligible complications. Newer technologies, including custom molded prosthetic buttons, based on CT results and septal buttons with embedded magnets have increased efficacy while improving patient satisfaction. Indeed, the growing omnipresence of 3D printing technology may accelerate accessibility and reduce the cost of customized prostheses.

H Surgical closure is highly successful in healthy patients with perforations <3 cm. Many different procedures have been described, with successful closure dependent on the size and location of the perforation. Studies though report high rates of early success; recurrence may be encountered 2 years following surgery. Perforation size is most predictive of surgical success, with most failures occurring in perforations of >2 cm resulting in a surgical success rate of 78%. Some authors have noted prior nasal trauma, specifically nasal surgery, as a risk factor for surgical failure. Principles of surgical repair include rotation of well-vascularized nasal mucosa from the floor of the nose, turbinates, or septum into the defect on both sides, closure without tension and placement of an interposition graft to stabilize the repair. Exposure can be obtained endonasally with endoscopes, through an open rhinoplasty approach or, rarely, a midface degloving approach. Many different uni- and bipedicled flaps have been described; tailoring of the surgical approach to the specific defect is very important. Temporalis fascia is the most popular autologous graft, although cartilage, bone and other fascial grafts have been described. Acellular human dermis and porcine small intestinal mucosa have been described as useful allo- and xenograft matrices. Use of an interposition graft will often aid mucosalization of areas that were not covered by the initial rotation flaps. Even in cases of failed surgical closure, recurrent perforations are often smaller than the original perforation, and patients may report significant symptomatic relief even from incomplete closure.

SUGGESTED READING

Cervin A, Andersson M. Intranasal steroids and septum perforation—an overlooked complication? A description of the course of events and a discussion of the causes. Rhinology. 1998;36:128-132.

Dosen LK, Haaye R. Surgical closure of nasal septal perforation. Early and long term observation. Rhinology. 2011;49:486-491.

Kim SW, Rhee CS. Nasal septal perforation repair. Curr Opin Otolaryngol Head Neck Surg. 2012;20:58-65.

Moon IJ, Kim SW, Han DH, et al. Predictive factors for the outcome of nasal septal perforation repair. Auris Nasus Larynx. 2011;38:52-57.

Oberg D, Akerlund A, Johansson L, et al. Prevalence of nasal septal perforation: the Skövde population-based study. Rhinology. 2003;41:72-75.

Pedroza F, Patrocinio LG, Arevalo O. A review of 25-year experience of nasal septal perforation repair. Arch Facial Plast Surg. 2007;9:12-18.

Taylor RJ, Sherris D. Prosthetics for nasoseptal perforations: a systematic review and meta-analysis. Otolaryngol Head Neck Surg. 2015;152:803-810.

Headache and Facial Pain

Robert G Kaniecki

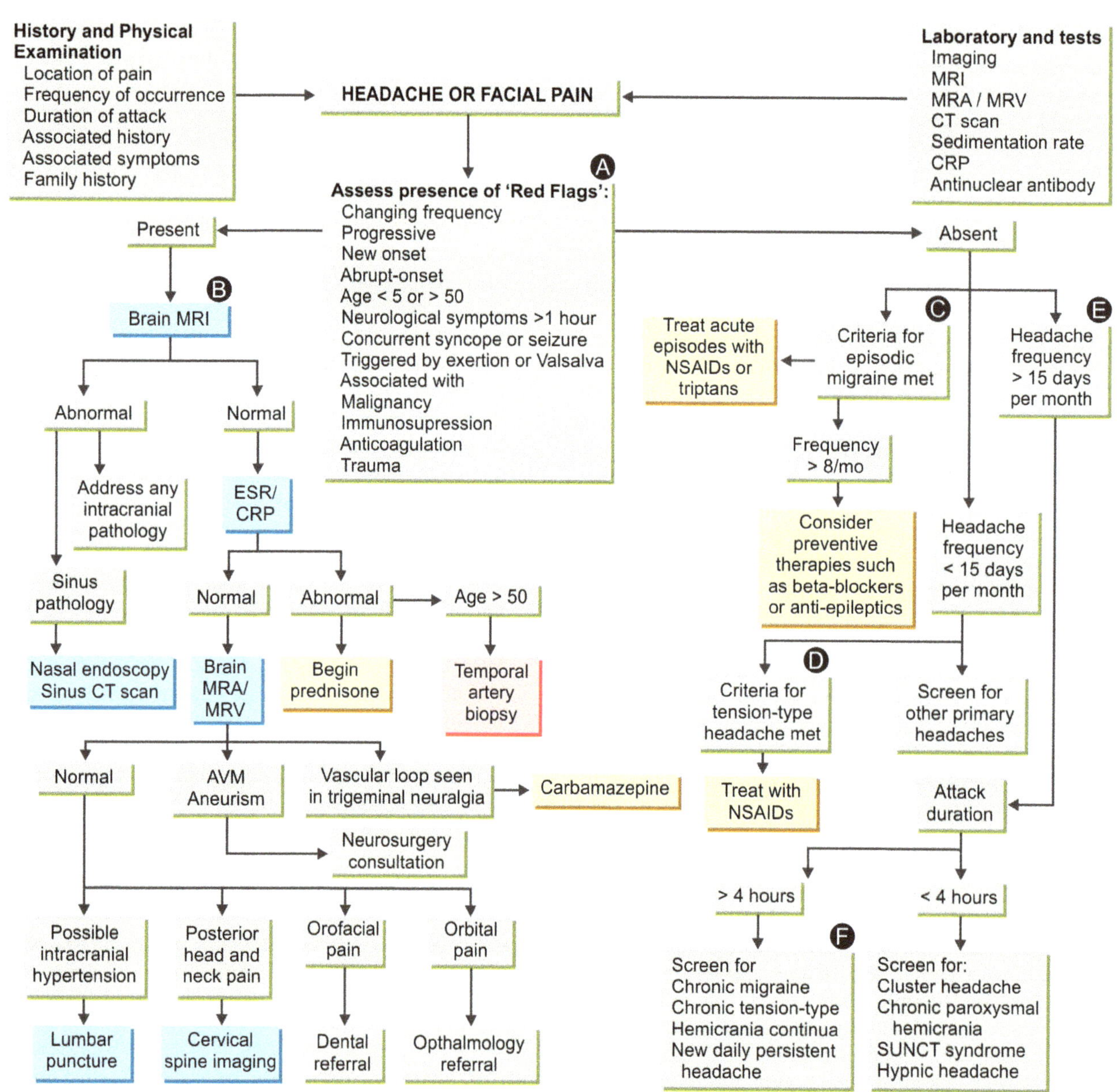

Although occasionally seen after an isolated incident, most patients with head or facial pain will present with patterns of recurrent or chronic discomfort. The vast majority will present with a primary headache disorder arising from a biological disorder of the brain. Although less prevalent, those with secondary headache conditions must be recognized early to limit potential morbidity or mortality from the responsible pathology.

A Indicators for secondary headaches include the following: changing or progressive headache frequency; first/ worst or abrupt-onset headache; headaches in patients under age 5 or over age 50; neurological symptoms with headache of duration >1 hour or associated syncope or seizure; abnormal physical examination findings; headache triggered by exertion or Valsalva; and headache in significant medical settings such as malignancy, immunosuppression, anticoagulation, or trauma.

B Brain magnetic resonance imaging is considered the imaging modality of choice for evaluation of suspected secondary headache disorders. Intracranial and extracranial structural causes of headache may be identified. Those patients over age 50 should also undergo screening for giant cell arteritis with erythrocyte sedimentation rate, C-reactive protein, and potential temporal artery biopsy. Magnetic resonance arteriography and venography may reveal vascular lesions responsible for the headaches. Compression of the trigeminal nerve from a vascular loop of the superior cerebellar artery may be seen in trigeminal neuralgia. Those with intracranial pressure abnormalities may be diagnosed following lumbar puncture.

C Migraine headache annually affects 18% of women and 6% of men in the United States but represents >90% of those presenting for medical attention for recurrent headaches. Episodes may last 4–72 hours. The pain is typically unilateral, throbbing, moderate to severe, and worsened by physical activity. Criteria require the presence of two of these four pain features as well as either nausea or a combination of light and noise sensitivity. Up to 50% display facial pressure, nasal congestion, or tearing with some attacks, frequently leading to the misdiagnosis of "sinus" headache. Guidelines recommend the use of nonsteroidal anti-inflammatory drugs (NSAIDs) or triptans as acute therapy. Evidence is best for β-blockers and the antiepileptics topiramate and valproate for migraine prevention.

D Episodic tension-type headache annually affects 40% of adults but represents only 3% of those consulting for headache. Like migraine each headache may last hours to days, but unlike migraine tension-type headache is rarely disabling. The criteria mandate the prior exclusion of migraine, (two of four required) with pain that is bilateral, nonthrobbing, mild to moderate, and not worsened by activity. Neither nausea nor both photophobia and phonophobia can be present. Acetaminophen, aspirin, and NSAIDs all have proven benefit in treatment.

E Nearly 5% of the population suffers from headache >15 days per month, and most will report individual headaches of >4 hours in duration. Those with untreated attack duration of <4 hours typically fall into the category of "trigeminal autonomic cephalalgias." These are characterized by episodes of severe unilateral frontal or temporal pain associated with ipsilateral ocular or nasal autonomic features. Cluster attacks occur 1–8 times daily and last 15–180 minutes. Chronic paroxysmal hemicrania (CPH) attacks generally last 2–30 minutes and episodes of short-lasting unilateral neuralgiform headache with conjunctival injection and tearing (SUNCT) syndrome 1–600 seconds. Cluster cycles may respond to prednisone and verapamil, whereas attacks are treated with oxygen and subcutaneous sumatriptan. CPH invariably responds to indomethacin, while SUNCT may respond on occasion to lamotrigine. Hypnic headache is a rare nocturnal headache condition seen among the elderly which often possess migraine features and responds to lithium.

F Those patients with daily headache disorders and individual attacks of duration >4 hours most commonly suffer from chronic migraine (2% of adult population) or chronic tension-type headache (2.5% of adults). Those with chronic migraine often describe some headaches suggestive of tension-type or sinus pathology, but have a background of headaches meeting migraine criteria. Hemicrania continua should be considered in any patient with a side-locked continuous headache. It often displays ipsilateral autonomic features and responds to indomethacin. New daily persistent headache (NDPH) involves spontaneous abrupt-onset daily headache pain persistent without significant variation for >3 months. It may last months to years and has no known medical management.

SUGGESTED READING

Evans R. Diagnostic testing for migraine and other primary headaches. Neurol Clin. 2009;27:393-415.

Fumal A, Schoenen J. Tension-type headache: current research and clinical management. Lancet Neurol. 2008;7:70-83.

Headache Classification Committee of the International Headache Society. The International Classification of Headache Disorders, 3rd edition (beta version). Cephalalgia. 2013;33(9):629-808.

Kaniecki R. Headache assessment and management. JAMA. 2003;289:1430-1433.

Loder E, Weizenbaum E, Frishberg B, et al. American Choosing Wisely Task Force. Choosing wisely in headache medicine: the American Headache Society's list of five things physicians and patients should question. American Headache Society Choosing Wisely Task Force. Headache. 2013;53:1651-1659.

Maarbjerg S, Gozalov A, Olesen J, et al. Trigeminal neuralgia—a prospective systematic study of clinical characteristics in 158 patients. Headache. 2014;54:1574-1582.

May A. Diagnosis and clinical features of trigemino-autonomic headaches. Headache. 2013;53:1470-1478.

Smith J, Swanson J. Giant cell arteritis. Headache. 2014;54:1217-1289.

Acute and Subacute Bacterial Rhinosinusitis

Jonathan B Overdevest, Andrew N Goldberg

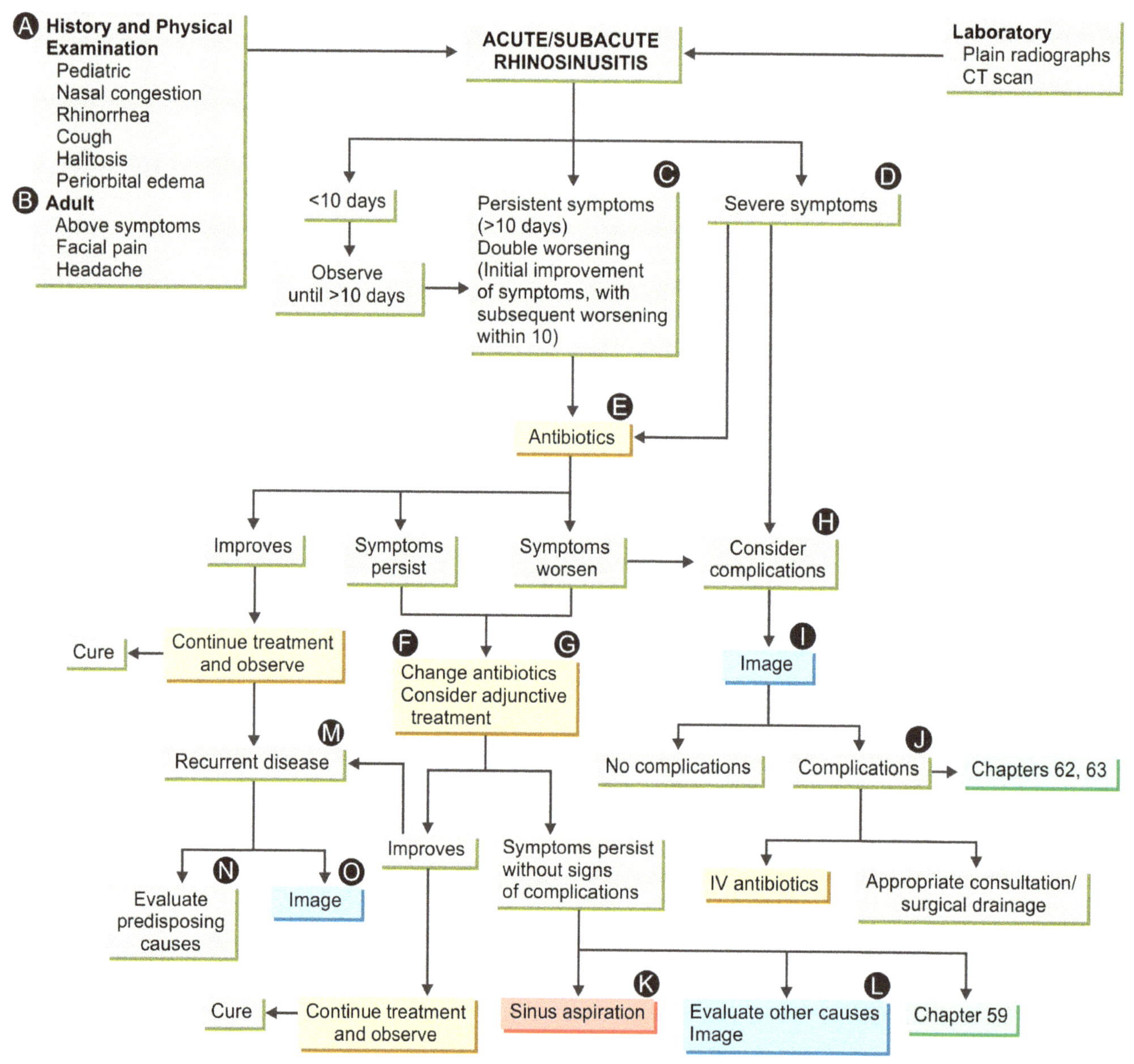

Recent clinical practice guidelines have placed an increased onus on clinicians to differentiate acute bacterial rhinosinusitis (ABRS) from acute rhinosinusitis (ARS) of viral and noninfectious etiologies in an effort to reduce unnecessary antibiotic treatment. This differentiation rests on identification of key symptom characteristics and duration.

A Children with ABRS present with nasal congestion or rhinorrhea, or both, as well as cough. The rhinorrhea may be thick, thin, clear, or purulent. The cough is typically of greater severity at night but is present throughout the day. Halitosis and mild periorbital edema also are encountered frequently in this population. The physical examination in children is helpful in identifying either allergic disorders or physical stigmata that predispose to ABRS.

B Adults experience similar symptoms as children, but also frequently complain of headache, facial pain, and dental pain. Facial tenderness on palpation of regions overlying the sinuses or the maxillary teeth suggests ABRS, but is a relatively nonspecific finding. Purulent exudate from the middle meatus may be more easily visualized in adults than children and, if present, is a more specific finding for ABRS.

C To prevent over prescription of unnecessary antibiotics, ABRS must be differentiated from common acute viral rhinosinusitis (VRS), which results from common viral infection. Clinical practice guidelines suggest ABRS may be diagnosed in patients with acute upper respiratory tract infection symptoms that have: (1) persisted for 10 days without improvement, or (2) initially improved, then worsened within 10 days (double worsening), where key symptoms include purulent nasal drainage (anterior, posterior, or both) and nasal obstruction, facial pain-pressure-fullness, or both. Thus, failure of symptom improvement within 10 days or a double worsening phenomenon is important in differentiating ABRS from VRS. Typically, presentations with symptoms that last <4 weeks are categorized as ABRS, and those presentations with symptoms that persist for >4 weeks, but <12 weeks are termed subacute bacterial rhinosinusitis.

D Acute bacterial rhinosinusitis may also present with severe symptoms, a presentation more commonly observed in the pediatric population. Severity is defined by concurrent fever (temperature ≥39°C/102.2°F) and purulent nasal discharge for at least 3 consecutive days. These patients are more likely to have headache, facial pain, and periorbital swelling. In contrast, a simple "cold" may or may not be accompanied by fever; if fever is present, it is usually only present for the first day of symptoms. The importance of distinguishing ABRS from nonbacterial causes lies in a potential for developing serious sequelae, including orbital cellulitis, intracranial complications such as meningitis, cavernous sinus thrombosis, or intraparenchymal abscesses.

E Antibiotic recommendations are structured upon the prevalence of three bacterial species that account for the vast majority of cases of acute and subacute bacterial rhinosinusitis: *Streptococcus pneumoniae*, *Haemophilus influenzae*, and *Moraxella catarrhalis*. Although clinical outcomes demonstrate no significant variation based on antibiotic regimen, regional variations in resistance patterns prevent full generalization of these results. Nevertheless, current practice guidelines suggest amoxicillin as first-line therapy for uncomplicated ABRS due to safety, efficacy, and low cost availability. Initial dosing should begin at 45 mg/kg per day, in twice daily dosing for 10 days or for 7 days following resolution of symptoms. In communities with high levels of resistance, high-dose amoxicillin treatment may be initiated at 90 mg/kg per day, in twice daily dosing, not to exceed 2 g per dose. Alternatively, amoxicillin–clavulanate (90 mg/kg per day, in twice daily dosing, not to exceed 2 g per dose) is a reasonable first-line antibiotic choice in clinical practice community with demonstrated high resistance, in patients with antibiotic use in the past month, those presentations consistent with more severe infection, or the presence of immune-compromising comorbidities and advanced age. For penicillin-allergic patients, doxycycline (100 mg twice daily) or respiratory fluoroquinolones such as levofloxacin (500 mg daily) or moxifloxacin (400 mg daily) are reasonable first-line antibiotic regimen selections. More nuanced recommendations for antibiotic selection may be found in a recent practice guideline from the Infectious Disease Society of America.

F Increasing bacterial resistance is a consideration in patients who fail to respond to traditional treatments. Patients categorized as nonresponders based on lack of clinical improvement within 7 days following diagnosis and initiation of treatment in adults (72 hours in children) should transition to an alternate antibiotic. Indeed, β-lactamase producing, penicillin-resistant *H. influenzae* has an estimated prevalence of >30%, and regional variations in *S. pneumoniae* resistance are similarly high. Second-line antimicrobial agents should either have activity against β-lactamase, such as amoxicillin with clavulanate, or utilize alternate mechanisms of action as is the case with using a fluoroquinolone or the combination of clindamycin and cefpodoxime or cefuroxime.

G The role of adjunctive therapies in the treatment of ABRS remains limited due to a deficit of generalizable data in our literature. The best evidence for adjuvant therapies involves the use of intranasal corticosteroid sprays. Although these effects are notably modest, the preponderance of evidence supporting likely efficacy in reducing symptomatology paired with a limited adverse event profile should provide clinicians the confidence to offer this class of therapeutics to select patients. Systemic corticosteroids, however, are typically avoided in primary treatment of acute disease. Decongestants, including topical oxymetazoline and phenylephrine and oral pseudoephedrine may diminish mucosal swelling and provide some relief of symptoms but should not be used for >3–5 days due to the potential for rebound congestion.

H Complications of ABRS are rare and involve propagation of infection to the orbit, bone, and central nervous system (CNS), typically via the venous drainage system. Involvement of the orbit is most common, resulting in a range of symptoms from mild periorbital edema, erythema of the eyelids and low-grade fever, to subperiosteal and orbital abscesses. In rare cases, osteomyelitis may develop in the frontal bone with swelling (Pott's puffy tumor), erythema, and tenderness over the involved area. Complications involving the CNS such as epidural abscess, subdural empyema, brain abscess, and meningitis are typically associated with deep-seated headaches, mental status changes, nuchal rigidity, high fever, and a toxic appearance.

I Patients should not undergo routine imaging as part of the diagnostic workup of uncomplicated ABRS, as the diagnosis remains rooted in clinical presentation. However, all patients with suspected complications of ABRS should obtain contrast-enhanced computed tomography (CT) imaging of the head and paranasal sinuses including axial, coronal, and sagittal imaging, in bone and soft tissue windows, to determine the extent of orbital, CNS, or bony involvement. After intracranial mass lesion is ruled out, a lumbar puncture should be considered in patients with symptoms suggestive of meningitis.

J Patients with complications of ABRS should be treated with parenteral antibiotics, subspecialty consultation, and surgical drainage when appropriate. The pediatric population, particularly adolescent males, is most predisposed to the development of orbital complications including orbital or subperiosteal abscess, where surgical intervention may be indicated. The specific management of these issues is outside the scope of this guideline; these helpful references may serve as a starting point. For the inpatient setting, ideal antibiotic regimens include broad coverage of aerobes and anaerobes with either amoxicillin-sulbactam or a third-generation cephalosporin (such as ceftriaxone), and either clindamycin or vancomycin to provide methicillin-resistant *Staphylococcus aureus* coverage. Anecdotal evidence from our institutional experience suggests increased rates of clindamycin resistance among isolates of *S. aureus*. Aspiration of fluid from the sinus or endoscopically directed middle meatus culture may facilitate identification of the infecting organism in order to provide targeted antimicrobial therapy.

K Patients who fail to improve with second-line antibiotic therapy should be considered for sinus aspiration or endoscopically guided culture to identify the infecting organism. Bacterial isolates should be tested for their sensitivity to antibiotics to ensure the use of appropriate antibiotic therapy. The recovery of bacteria in a density of at least 10^4 colony-forming units/mL is considered to represent true infection.

L Alternative diagnoses for respiratory symptoms should be sought in patients who fail to improve on appropriate antibiotic therapy. Tumors, invasive fungal disease, allergic fungal sinusitis, allergic rhinitis, or granulomatous disease can present with symptoms similar to ABRS. The evaluation of alternative diagnoses may require further evaluation including CT or magnetic resonance imaging and biopsy of the sinus mucosa. Importantly, persistent unilateral disease is associated with neoplasm or dental origin in some patients and warrants further investigation.

M Patients who have complete recovery of symptoms between episodes of ABRS are said to have recurrent ABRS defined as four or more episodes per year without signs or symptoms of rhinosinusitis between episodes. Clinicians should consider a diagnosis of chronic rhinosinusitis in patients whose symptoms persist for >12 weeks and meet the following criteria: (1) two or more of the following symptoms: (i) mucopurulent drainage (anterior, posterior, or both), (ii) nasal obstruction (congestion), (iii) facial pain–pressure–fullness, or (iv) decreased sense of smell, and (2) documentation of inflammation via (i) purulence visible from middle meatus, (ii) presence of nasal cavity polyps, or (iii) radiographic evidence of inflammation.

N Patients with recurrent ABRS should be evaluated for predisposing factors such as (1) significant anatomic or structural abnormalities, (2) cystic fibrosis, (3) immunodeficiency, or (4) chronic inflammation resulting from allergens or irritants.

O Imaging studies of the paranasal sinuses have the greatest utility in patients with recurrent ABRS or patients with suspected complication. The role of plain radiographs in this group is increasingly obsolete and CT imaging of the paranasal sinuses using high-resolution thin-cut reconstruction is typically the study of choice. This is best performed after completion of antibiotic therapy during an asymptomatic period to determine whether persistent obstruction of the osteomeatal complex, polypoid changes, or bony abnormalities is present to predispose to recurrent rhinosinusitis. Rarely, CT scanning may be indicated in uncomplicated suspected ARS to resolve a diagnostic dilemma and confirm sinus inflammation.

SUGGESTED READING

Ahovuo-Saloranta A, Rautakorpi UM, Borisenko OV, et al. Antibiotics for acute maxillary sinusitis in adults. Cochrane Database Syst Rev. 2015;10:CD000243.

Bedwell JR, Choi SS. Medical versus surgical management of pediatric orbital subperiosteal abscesses. Laryngoscope. 2013;123: 2337-2338.

Chow AW, Benninger MS, Brook I, et al. IDSA clinical practice guideline for acute bacterial rhinosinusitis in children and adults. Clin Infect Dis. 2012;54:1041-1045.

Fairbanks DNF. Pocket Guide to Antimicrobial Therapy in Otolaryngology – Head and Neck Surgery, 13th edition. Alexandria, VA: American Academy of Otolaryngology – Head and Neck Surgery Foundation, Inc., 2007.

Gordts F, Halewyck S, Pierard D, et al. Microbiology of the middle meatus: a comparison between normal adults and children. J Laryngol Otol. 2000;114:184-188.

Hoban DJ, Doern GV, Fluit AC, et al. Worldwide prevalence of antimicrobial resistance in *Streptococcus pneumoniae*, *Haemophilus influenzae*, and *Moraxella catarrhalis* in the SENTRY Antimicrobial Surveillance Program, 1997–1999. Clin Infect Dis. 2001;32(Suppl 2):S81-93.

Liao JC, Harris GJ. Subperiosteal abscess of the orbit: evolving pathogens and the therapeutic protocol. Ophthalmology. 2015; 122:639-647.

Rosenfeld RM, Andes D, Bhattacharyya N, et al. Adult sinusitis (Update). Otolaryngol Head Neck Surg. 2015;137:S1-31.

Wald ER, Applegate KE, Bordley C, et al. Clinical practice guideline for the diagnosis and management of acute bacterial sinusitis in children aged 1 to 18 years. Pediatrics. 2013;32:e262-280.

Zalmanovici Trestioreanu A, Yaphe J. Intranasal steroids for acute sinusitis. Cochrane Database Syst Rev. 2013;(12).

Chronic Rhinosinusitis

David E Eibling

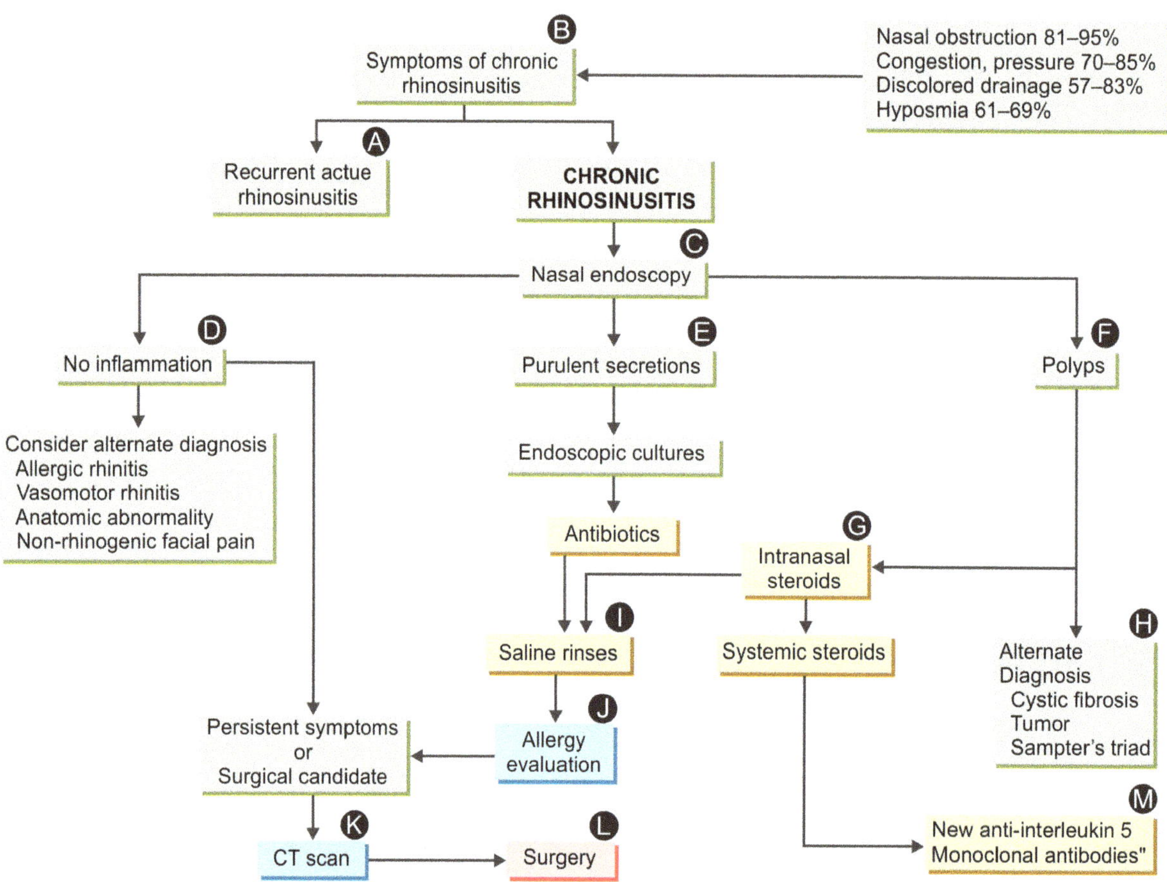

In 2015, the American Academy of Otolaryngology—Head and Neck Surgery updated the pre-existing (2007) Clinical Practice Guideline (CPG) addressing rhinosinusitis in the adult. Rhinosinusitis is classified as acute, recurrent acute, subacute, or chronic (CRS—chronic rhinosinusitis) based on duration of symptoms. Patients are considered to have chronic rhinosinusitis if symptoms persist for ≥12 weeks. One in eight Americans will have had at least one episode of rhinosinusitis in the past 12 months, and CRS alone accounts for over 7% of all primary care visits at which an antibiotic is prescribed.

A "Recurrent acute rhinosinusitis" is defined as four or more episodes per year with each episode lasting > 7 days with absence of intervening signs and symptoms of chronic sinusitis between episodes. Patients with recurrent acute rhinosinusitis frequently respond promptly to antibiotics; however, the entity is less well studied than that of patients with chronic rhinosinusitis.

B Diagnosis is made on the basis of the history of persistent symptoms, including two or more "major factors," (one of which must be either nasal drainage or obstruction), and at least one objective indicator of inflammation such as visualization of purulent secretions on endoscopy or findings of mucosal disease on computerized tomography (CT). A widely used validated quality-of-life tool that assesses the impact of chronic rhinosinusitis is the 22 item Sino-Nasal Outcome Test SNOT-22.

C Nasal endoscopy should be performed on all patients with symptoms of chronic rhinosinusitis. The presence and the source of purulent drainage, mucosal edema, and the presence of polyps should be noted. Nasal endoscopy raises the odds ratio (OR) of the presence of CRS from 1.1 to 4.6 (over symptoms alone).

D The absence of inflammation, purulence, or polyposis on nasal endoscopy suggests an alternative diagnosis such as allergic rhinosinusitis, vasomotor rhinitis, or an anatomic abnormality such as a deviated septum.

E Purulent exudate, if seen, should be cultured using endoscopic control to assure accurate sampling. Broad-spectrum antibiotics can be initiated immediately and changed to culture directed when cultures are available.

There is no evidence supporting prolonged use of anti-biotics in CRS; however, most opinion leaders suggest a 28-day course of a broad-spectrum or culture-directed antibiotic in the presence of purulence.

F Polyps can be staged as stage 1, not extending to the end of the middle turbinate; stage 2, extending beyond the middle turbinate; stage 3, extending to the level of the inferior turbinate; or stage 4, extending to the floor of the nose.

G First-line therapy for CRS with (or without) polyps is topical nasal steroids. For persistent and recurrent polyps, oral steroids may be effective in the managent of symptoms.

H Polyps in a child should prompt an evaluation for cystic fibrosis or primary ciliary dyskinesia syndromes. Polyps in adults are commonly associated with asthma, particularly aspirin-sensitive asthma (also known as aspirin triad syndrome or Samter's triad).

I High-level evidence supports saline irrigations as effective in removing inspissated mucus, enhancing ciliary function, and reducing symptoms.

J The 2015 CPG lists allergy evaluation as an option (Statement 9); however, most authorities recommend allergy evaluation in patients with CRS, since 40–84% will be found to have allergy on testing.

K The diagnosis of CRS is based on objective evidence of inflammation in the setting of appropriate symptoms.

Hence, CT may be avoided if endoscopic evidence of CRS exists. The CT scan may be indicated if endoscopic examination is unrevealing in the face of convincing symptoms, or if disease persists despite treatment, or if surgery is being considered.

L Endoscopic sinus surgery should be directed to the disease present on CT or by examination. Nasal polyps frequently recur postoperatively. Preoperative preparation and postoperative care, including long-term intranasal topical steroids, enhance the effectiveness of surgery.

M New anti-interleukin 5 monoclonal antibodies such as omalizumab and dupilumab have shown dramatic effect on CRS with polyps in early clinical trials, and may soon be available for clinical use. The primary contraindication may be price.

SUGGESTED READING

Harvey R, Hannan SA, Badia L, et al. Nasal saline irrigations for the symptoms of chronic rhinosinusitis. Cochrane Database Syst Rev. 2007;3:CD006394.

Kennedy JL, Hubbard MA, Huyett P, et al. Sino-nasal outcome test (SNOT-22) a predictor of post-surgical improvement in patients with chronic rhinosinusitis. Ann Allergy Asthma Immunol. 2013;111:246-251.

Rosenfeld RM, Piccirillo JF, Chandrasekhar SS, et al. Clinical practice guideline (update) adult sinusitis. Otolaryngol Head Neck Surg. 2015;152:S1-39.

Fungal Rhinosinusitis

Berrylin J Ferguson, Stella E Lee

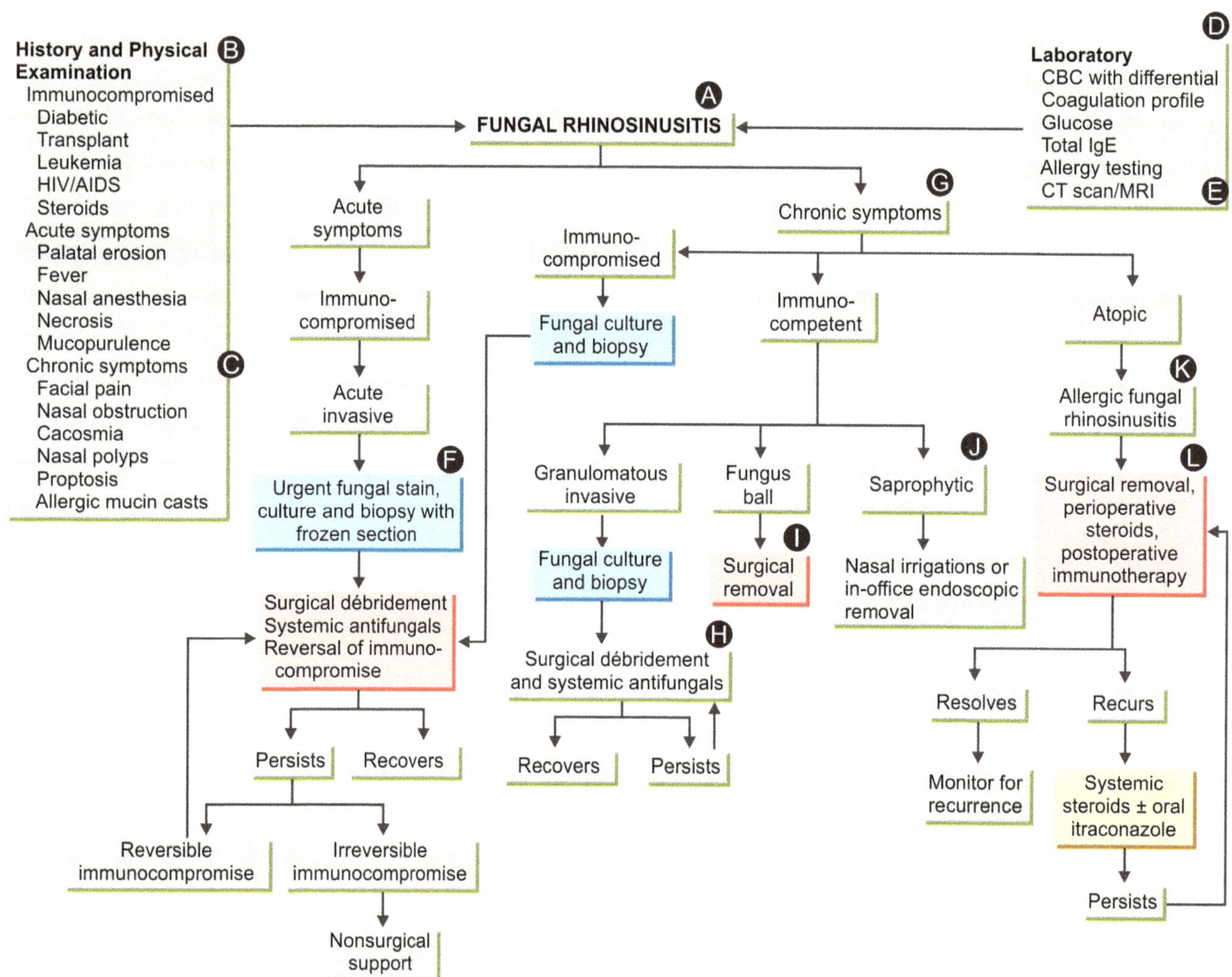

Fungal rhinosinusitis expresses itself in distinct forms that are related to the immunocompetency of the host. The most important distinction is whether the fungus is invasive or noninvasive. The immunocompromised patient is at most risk for invasive fungal rhinosinusitis and must be aggressively and expediently evaluated for this possibility. In contrast, patients with fungus balls of the sinus (a noninvasive manifestation) may be asymptomatic for months to years. Allergic fungal rhinosinusitis (AFRS) is a noninvasive hypersensitivity response by the host to the fungus and paradoxically responds to systemic steroids; however, in the invasive form of the disease, steroids may be one of the precipitating factors.

A This algorithm discusses the management of the patient with regard to whether the fungal infection is (1) invasive, (2) a fungus ball, (3) saprophytic colonization, or (4) AFRS. The immunologic status of the host is an important consideration. Noninvasive fungal rhinosinusitis (i.e., a fungus ball) may become invasive if the patient becomes immunocompromised.

B Any patient who is immunosuppressed is at risk for invasive fungal sinusitis. Symptoms of invasive fungal rhinosinusitis may be subtle. Mucopurulence is variable depending on host neutropenia. A wide variety of fungi can cause invasive sinusitis, most commonly Aspergillus species and Mucorales (causing mucormycosis). One must assess for palatal erosion, impairment of vision, reduced extraocular movement, nasal necrosis, or facial anesthesia. The diabetic patient is at increased risk for invasive mucormycosis. Anesthesia of the face or intranasal area frequently precedes necrosis in mucormycosis.

C In the patient with chronic symptoms of sinusitis and no source of immunocompromise, fungus balls and AFRS are suspected. Fungus balls are frequently asymptomatic but may cause facial pain or cacosmia, whereas AFRS occurs in patients with allergic hypersensitivity to fungus, nasal polyposis, and eosinophilic mucin.

D The complete blood count (CBC) with differential is important for a complete evaluation. In the immunosuppressed patient, it may reveal neutropenia or evidence of a left shift. In the patient with AFRS, it may reveal eosinophilia. Laboratory evaluation in acutely ill patients includes assessment of a coagulation profile: platelets, bleeding time, prothrombin time, and partial thromboplastin time. Significant abnormalities must be corrected before biopsy. One should check glucose because an elevation makes the diagnosis of invasive mucormycosis more likely. Total immunoglobulin (Ig)E is usually elevated in AFRS, along with fungus-specific IgE. Unfortunately, there are many fungi that cause AFRS, and one may not be able to obtain a laboratory value for each fungus commercially. Total IgE may be normal in AFRS when the disease is quiescent.

E A dedicated maxillofacial sinus computed tomography (CT) scan is required before surgery on any patient with suspected fungal rhinosinusitis. The initial scan does not require contrast unless invasive fungal rhinosinusitis shows bony erosion or intracranial or orbital extension. In invasive disease, a sinus CT may show only minimal abnormality with no evidence of bone invasion. Magnetic resonance imaging (MRI) may serve as a more sensitive imaging modality but it is possible that in early stage disease, both CT and MRI may not reveal any abnormalities. Fungus balls usually show total or subtotal sinus opacification and rarely bony erosion. AFRS shows heterogeneity of tissue densities within the sinuses. Half of cases will be unilateral. Bone erosion and intracranial or intraorbital extension are common.

F If invasive fungal rhinosinusitis is suspected, one should perform an endoscopic culture with immediate stains for fungus and biopsy of the abnormal region with frozen section. If the patient is an operative candidate, then surgical debridement is performed.

G Chronic indolent invasive fungal sinusitis is of two forms: granulomatous and nongranulomatous. Both progress over weeks to months and occasionally years. The former is most common in Sudan and infects the immunocompetent, whereas in the latter patients usually have some source of immunocompromise, which is mild and allows continued slow invasive fungal growth. The diagnosis is made by biopsy with special fungal stain. These patients often require repeated courses of antifungal therapy and surgical debridement, because the disease will be quiescent during treatment and will often recur when the antifungal agent is stopped. Every attempt to control any underlying cause of immunocompromise must be made.

H The treatment for invasive fungal sinusitis is reversal of immunocompromise, conservative debridement, and systemic and topical antifungals appropriate for the cultured fungus. Systemic amphotericin B is begun while awaiting fungal growth. If the culture grows Pseudallescheria boydii, then amphotericin should be stopped and ketoconazole or itraconazole instituted. If the patient's source of immunocompromise cannot be reversed, as in a bone marrow transplant patient in whom ingraft fails, heroic surgical measures should not be undertaken, because they will be futile. The patient whose immunocompromised state can be reversed may need repeated surgical debridement to conservatively remove necrotic tissue. If the orbit is involved but the patient is not blind, then orbital exenteration is not usually required. There are several case reports of patients surviving blindness secondary to mucormycosis invasion without undergoing orbital exenteration.

I A fungus ball is diagnosed at surgical removal and can be suspected by imaging. Cultures will often be negative. If the diagnosis is suspected and cultures and routine pathology are negative, then special stains for fungus should be obtained. Recurrence after complete surgical removal is rare.

J Saprophytic fungal growth refers to fungus growing on mucocrusts that often are present in patients who have undergone endoscopic sinus surgery. Treatment consists of removing the crusts. If the growths recur, the patient can be instructed to irrigate the nose weekly with sterile saline as well as to implement appropriate environmental controls.

K Allergic fungal rhinosinusitis is diagnosed by characteristic histopathology, which includes hyphae present in eosinophil-rich mucin. There is no evidence of fungal tissue invasion. If the pathologist assesses only the polyps and not the mucin, then the diagnosis will be missed. Type I hypersensitivity to fungus should also be present as well as characteristic CT findings as described in step "E."

L After removing all allergic mucin and polyps, immunotherapy directed toward the patient's fungal hypersensitivity can be helpful if instituted within 4–8 weeks to prevent recurrence. Recurrence or persistent disease is common. If the disease recurs while the patient is on immunotherapy, then repeated surgical removal of the mucin combined with perioperative steroids is recommended. The role of oral itraconazole (ranging from 200 to 400 mg daily while monitoring liver functions monthly) shows promise, but there are no controlled studies regarding its use.

SUGGESTED READING

Ferguson BJ. Fungus balls of the paranasal sinuses. Otolaryngol Clin North Am. 2000;33(2):389-398.

Gan EC, Thamboo A, Rudmik L, et al. Medical management of allergic fungal rhinosinusitis following endoscopic sinus surgery: an evidence-based review and recommendations. Int Forum Allergy Rhinol. 2014;4(9):702-715.

Halderman A, Shrestha R, Sindwani R. Chronic granulomatous invasive fungal sinusitis: an evolving approach to management. Int Forum Allergy Rhinol. 2014;4(4):280-283.

Rupa V, Maheswaran S, Ebenezer J, et al. Current therapeutic protocols for chronic granulomatous fungal sinusitis. Rhinology. 2015;53(2):181-186.

Turner JH, Soudry E, Nayak JV, et al. Survival outcomes in acute invasive fungal sinusitis: a systematic review and quantitative synthesis of published evidence. Laryngoscope. 2013;123(5):1112-1118.

Rhinosinusitis in the Pediatric Age Group

Scott C Manning

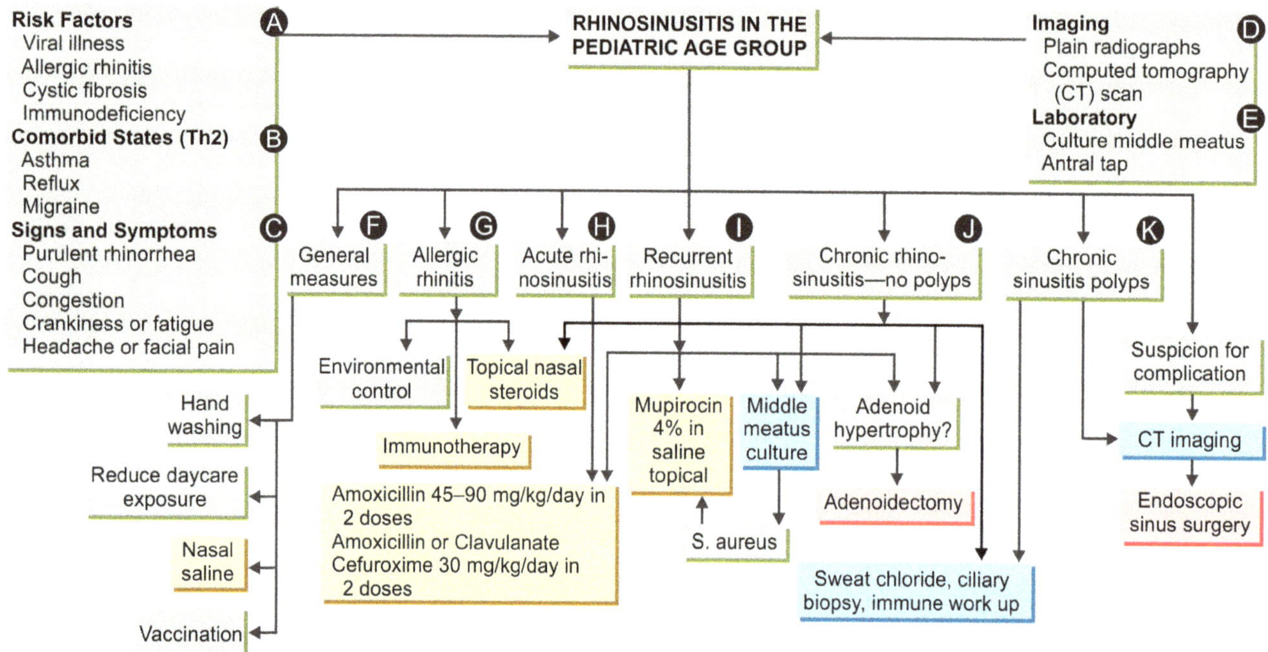

Imaging studies have shown that the sinuses and nasal cavity usually function as one entity in terms of inflammation and thus rhinosinusitis has become a more standard term than sinusitis. Rhinosinusitis in the pediatric age group is a common problem and often a source of frustration to parents and primary care providers. Modern living may be shifting more people to a Th2-dominated immune balance with an increase in asthma, reflux, eczema, migraine, type I diabetes and Hashimoto's thyroiditis, in addition to allergic rhinitis and rhinosinusitis. In terms of treatments for pediatric rhinosinusitis, the pendulum is shifting away from antibiotics towards therapeutic regimens that include immune modulation (allergy management).

A The most common risk factors for pediatric rhinosinusitis are viral illness and allergic rhinitis. Day-care attendance can triple the number of viral respiratory infections for children under age of 3 years. Allergic rhinitis by skin prick testing and asthma are both associated with rhinosinusitis in older children. Allergy testing is relatively insensitive in younger children but "local allergy", mucosal eosinophilia with negative skin test or serology, is associated with both rhinosinusitis and adenoid hypertrophy. Rhinosinusitis is a common presentation of primary immunodeficiency such as common variable immunodeficiency. Heterozygous cystic fibrosis may present initially as severe rhinosinusitis.

B The hygiene hypothesis may explain the Th1-to-Th2 immune dysregulation seen increasingly with asthma, eczema, gastritis, reflux, migraine headache, and rhinosinusitis. Vaccines, early exposure to food antigens such as cow's milk, early antibiotic exposure, air pollution, and small family size have all been shown to promote a Th1-to-Th2 shift with increased predisposition to eosinophil-mediated disease. The background is the Th2 shift and the associated diseases are not necessarily causally-related. For example, evidence does not support gastroesophageal reflux as a cause of rhinosinusitis nor sinusitis as a cause of migraine.

C The most common signs and symptoms of pediatric rhinosinusitis are congestion, postnasal drip, fatigue, and nighttime cough with all symptoms, especially congestion and fatigue, potentially-associated with allergic rhinitis. Rhinosinusitis flares and resolves. Congestion that is chronic and unremitting implies an anatomic cause such as adenoid hypertrophy or turbinate hypertrophy. Persistent headache implies migraine or other primary headache diagnosis. Assessment by examination, endoscopy and/or imaging of secretions, turbinates, septum, and adenoids is necessary for determining a diagnosis. Defining sinusitis by the symptoms that are of greatest importance to the parents and patients is the key to successful treatment that improves quality of life.

Sinusitis is a vague concept and in many languages at least colloquially, the word does not exist. Families and patients are thinking about specific symptoms when they present to their doctors with "sinusitis" and the clinician must determine what specific diagnosis corresponds to those symptoms in order to make an effective treatment plan. With quality of life studies, the domain of nasal obstruction is the most sensitive to treatment (most likely to see improvements with treatment) while the domain of headache is the least sensitive (not usually related to sinusitis). For patients with chronic lung disease such as severe asthma or cystic fibrosis, successful treatment of rhinosinusitis can go beyond improving quality of life and actually improve the patients health.

D Imaging is indicated for suspected suppurative complications, as a roadmap for planned surgery, as part of the evaluation for polyps or as a way to rule out sinusitis during evaluation of headaches. Usually computed tomography (CT) with its high-sensitivity and ability to define bony anatomy is the modality of choice. However plain radiographs still have a role as a low-cost screen (especially as a rule-out test) and a way to evaluate for adenoid hypertrophy.

E Culture is indicated for severe or recurrent cases of rhinosinusitis, especially in this age of resistant *Staphylococcus aureus* and other organisms. Endoscopic (or otoscopic)-guided culture of obvious purulent discharge will allow for the appropriate selection of antibiotics. Even occasional culturing can give a good indication of antibiotic-resistance patterns in your community. Maxillary sinus taps have been largely supplanted by endoscopically-guided culture of the middle meatus. For suspected cystic fibrosis (polyps), a sweat chloride test should be performed. Ciliary biopsy of the inferior meatus or other non-inflamed airway mucosa should be performed for suspected ciliary dyskinesia (persistent middle ear effusions, bronchitis).

F Reducing day-care exposure with smaller class size if possible is a reasonable goal for young children. Promoting hand hygiene at home and reducing dust mite exposure (no pets on the bed) may also have benefit. Nasal saline lavage has been shown to reduce symptoms of rhinosinusitis in pediatric patients. Antihistamines and acid blockers have not been shown to improve the resolution of documented rhinosinusitis.

G The biggest change over the last 15 years in the philosophy of management of rhinosinusitis has been a shift away from repetitive courses of antibiotics and towards attempts to blunt Th2 inflammation that is often a predisposing condition. Topical steroid nasal sprays have Food and Drug Administration (FDA) approval to age of 3 years in some cases and combined with nasal saline, are usually part of any management for recurring symptoms of rhinosinusitis. Antihistamines combined with leukotriene inhibitors such as montelukast may have nearly the same benefit as topical steroids for chronic congestion and rhinorrhea. Allergy testing is relatively insensitive at young ages but has value especially when keeping in mind that negative results at a young age do not rule out allergy. Immunotherapy injections are generally considered for older children, especially those with asthma. Sublingual immunotherapy drops may prove to be a practical alternative to injections but that treatment is not yet FDA-approved in the United States.

H This is more of an issue for primary care providers than Otolaryngologists but studies have shown definite benefit from antibiotic treatment in symptom resolution for image-proven acute rhinosinusitis. The organisms are similar to those causing acute otitis media with nontypeable *Haemophilus influenzae* and *Moraxella catarrhalis,* most commonly isolated. Amoxicillin 45–90 mg/kg/day divided in 2 doses, or amoxicillin or clavulanate or cefuroxime 30 mg/kg/day in 2 doses are commonly recommended as first-line antibiotics. Culture of *Streptococcus pneumoniae* species should trigger inquiries about vaccination status or possibly further testing for immunodeficiency.

I Recurrent symptom flare ups with temporary improvement with medical therapy constitutes the most common reason for presentation to the Otolaryngologist. Imaging at some point is needed to confirm the diagnosis. In addition to general measures and allergy management, topical antibiotic treatment can be considered. For the Th2 spectrum patients (asthma, eczema, reflux), staphylococcal organisms can serve as superantigens. Topical anti-staphylococcal therapy such as 4% mupirocin in saline irrigations can have benefit both as an initial treatment and as a way of preventing the next infection, allowing for recovery of local mucosal immune defense and thus breaking a cycle of recurrence.

J This entity is the most difficult to define but is usually described as persistent symptoms for at least 6 weeks. Studies do show that chronic rhinosinusitis is not defined by imaging or culture abnormalities. Persistent congestion as a primary symptom in a pediatric patient usually means adenoid or inferior turbinate hypertrophy with first-line treatment with topical nasal steroids and second-line treatment with adenoidectomy or conservative turbinate reduction. Persistent headache requires imaging to rule out sinusitis as a cause.

K Polyps are relatively unusual in children and their presence should trigger an evaluation for cystic fibrosis, ciliary dyskinesia or severe allergy. Imaging with CT is indicated with a low threshold for endoscopic sinus surgery, both for diagnosis and treatment. Unilateral polyposis in children should suggested the possibility of rhabdomyosarcoma.

SUGGEST READING

Chang GU, Jang TY, Kin KS, et al. Nonspecific hyper-reactivity and localized allergy: cause of discrepancy between skin prick and nasal provocation test. Otolaryngol Head Neck Surg. 2014;150:194-200.

Fokkens WJ, Lund VJ, Mullol J, et al. EPOS 2012: European Position Paper on Rhinosinusitis and nasal polyps 2012. A summary for otorhinolaryngologists. Rhinology 2012;50:1-12.

Kennedy JL, Borish L. Chronic rhinosinusitis and antibiotics: the good, the bad and the ugly. Am J Rhinol Allergy. 2013;27:467-472.

Lin SY, Baugher KM, Brown DJ, et al. Effects of nasal saline lavage on pediatric sinusitis symptoms and disease-specific quality of life: a case series of 10 patients. Ear Nose Throat J. 2015;94:E13-18.

Sedaghat AR, Phipatanakul W, Cunningham MJ. Prevalence of and associations with allergic rhinitis in children with chronic rhinosinusitis. Int J Pediatr Otorhinolaryngol. 2014;78:343-347.

Complications of Bacterial Sinusitis

Nicholas R Rowan, Barry M Schaitkin

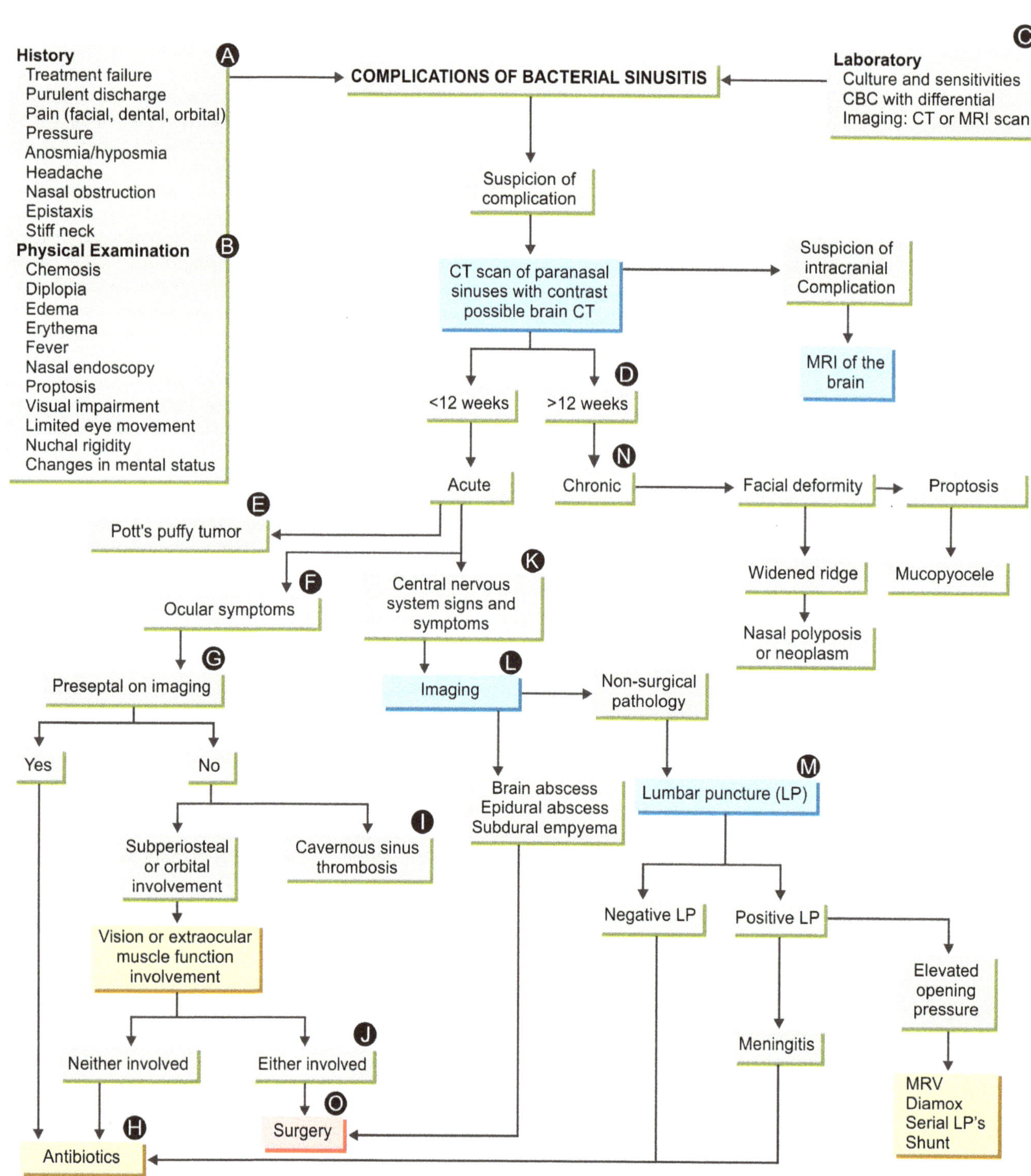

Complications of bacterial sinusitis are largely infectious in nature. Given the critical structures adjacent to the paranasal sinuses, persistent sinus symptoms should be evaluated promptly as intravenous antibiotics or surgical intervention may be warranted.

Ⓐ A high index of suspicion allows the practitioner to intervene early in patients with symptoms of impending complications.

Ⓑ Nasal examination must include nasal endoscopy. Cultures from the middle meatus should be obtained endoscopically with a protected swab or aspirator.

Ⓒ Imaging is dictated by circumstances. Contrast-enhanced fine cut computed tomography (CT) scans are the primary modality to evaluate paranasal sinus disease and orbital involvement, while gadolinium-enhanced magnetic resonance imaging (MRI) better delineates involvement of the central nervous system. A complete blood count with differential is useful to assess and follow clinical severity. Blood cultures should be considered in the presence of fever and leukocytosis.

Ⓓ Most complications of sinusitis are the result of an isolated acute infection or an acute infection in the setting of chronic sinusitis.

Ⓔ Acute suppurative frontal sinusitis may present with swelling of the forehead resulting from a subperiosteal abscess (Pott's puffy tumor).

Ⓕ In the setting of ocular symptoms, a complete ophthalmologic examination must be performed, including evaluation of visual acuity, measurements of exophthalmos, examination of the optic disk, and assessment of extraocular muscle function.

Ⓖ Preseptal cellulitis can be treated nonoperatively and usually resolves with oral antibiotics.

Ⓗ Initial antibiotics should be intravenous, high dose, broad spectrum, and started immediately. We prefer ampicillin-sulbactam as a drug of choice and then narrow to fit the results of the endoscopic culture. Infectious disease consultants should be included early in the setting of orbital or intracranial complications.

Ⓘ Cavernous sinus thrombosis will manifest with orbital pain, proptosis, photophobia, and deficits of cranial nerves II, III, IV, and VI.

Ⓙ Involvement of vision or extraocular muscle function usually requires surgery.

Ⓚ Severe frontal headache, focal neurologic or systemic signs should prompt concern for meningitis, the most common intracranial complication of bacterial sinusitis.

Ⓛ Central nervous system symptoms warrant radiographic evaluation with either CT or MRI to determine whether there is a need for operative intervention.

Ⓜ Bacterial meningitis is typically identified on lumbar puncture with increased opening pressures (>25 cm H_2O), cloudy or purulent cerebrospinal fluid, a white blood cell >100 cells/μL ($>90\%$ neutrophils), low glucose levels, and elevated protein levels.

Ⓝ Chronic sinusitis presents primarily with insidious complications related to mass effect. Although patients with chronic sinusitis are less likely to experience acute complications, if they present with facial deformity, nasal polyposis, a mucopyocele, a neoplasm must be in the differential diagnoses.

Ⓞ Surgical drainage is dictated by many factors, including the aggressiveness of the disease, the health of the patient, the particular sinus involved, and the surgeon's skill and training. Most cases of orbital abscess can be treated endoscopically. Acute frontal sinusitis may require trephination with or without endoscopic drainage once the acute infection is resolved.

SUGGESTED READING

Chadha NK. An evidence-based staging system for orbital infections from acute rhinosinusitis. Laryngoscope. 2012;122:s95-96.

Collet S, Grulois V, Eloy P, et al. Pott's puffy tumor as a late complication of a frontal sinus reconstruction: a case report and review of the literature. Rhinology. 2009;47(4):470-475.

Demuri GP, Wald ER. Complications of acute bacterial sinusitis in children. Pediatr Infect Dis J. 2011;30(8):701-702.

Kastner J. Orbital and intracranial complications after acute rhinosinusitis. Rhinology. 2010;48:457-461.

Osborn MK, Steinberg JP. Subdural empyema and other suppurative complications of paranasal sinusitis. Lancet Infect Dis. 2007;7(1):62-67.

Rosenfeld RM, Piccirillo JF, Chandrasekhar SS, et al. Clinical practice guideline (update): adult sinusitis. Otolaryngol Head Neck Surg. 2015;152:s1-39.

Vairaktaris E, Moschos MM, Vassiliou S, et al. Orbital cellulitis, orbital subperiosteal and intraorbital abscess. Report of three cases and review of the literature. J Craniomaxillofac Surg. 2009;37(3):132-136.

Pediatric Orbital Subperiosteal Abscess

Amanda L Stapleton, Sukgi S Choi

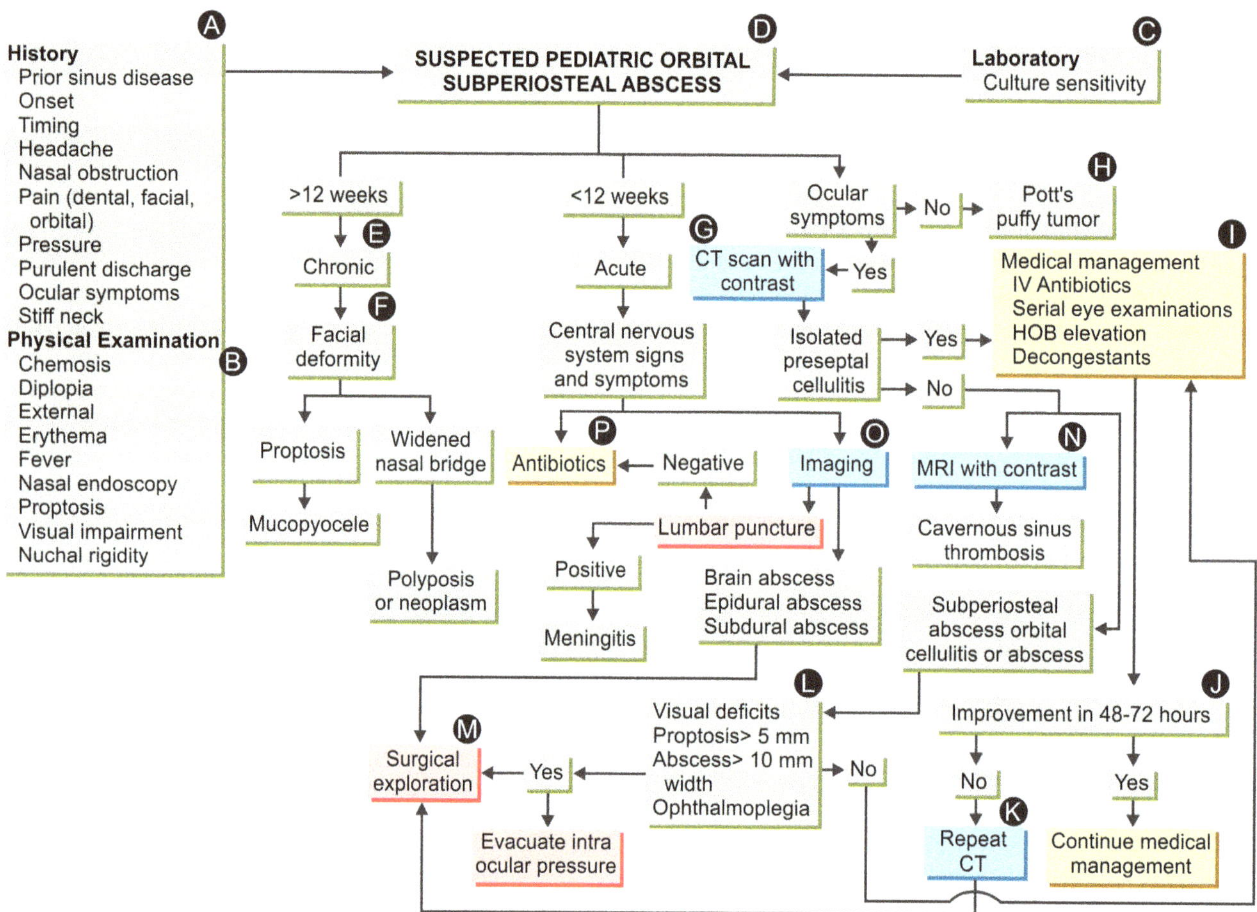

Subperiosteal orbital abscess is a known complication that arises from acute bacterial sinusitis in children. A subperiosteal abscess is a collection of purulent fluid beneath the periosteum of the ethmoid, frontal, and maxillary bone. The Chandler classification of orbital complications of sinusitis identifies this as a group 3 complication along the progression from preseptal cellulitis to cavernous sinus thrombosis.

A The onset and severity of symptoms, as well as the physical examination findings, are keys to making the correct diagnosis. Early intervention can help limit progressive complications.

B Physical examination should include nasal endoscopy.

C If possible cultures should be taken prior to initiation of antibiotic therapy.

D An orbital subperiosteal abscess is typically seen in the setting of acute sinusitis or an acute exacerbation of chronic sinusitis.

E Chronic sinusitis presents primarily with complications related to mass effect. Patients with chronic sinusitis are less likely to experience acute complications except after surgical intervention with alteration of mucociliary flow or introduction of scar tissue.

F The patient must have a complete ophthalmologic examination, including visual acuity, measurement of exophthalmos, extraocular movements, and examination of the optic disc. Evaluation for an afferent pupillary defect is also required.

G Computed tomography (CT) scan with contrast +/− image navigation protocol is the initial imaging modality of choice in the pediatric patient. The CT has 91% sensitivity for diagnosing orbital complications from sinusitis. Magnetic resonance imaging (MRI) should be performed if the CT scan is negative if there is a concern for intracranial complications due to its higher sensitivity for detecting intracranial processes. The CT had a 93% accuracy rate for diagnosing intracranial processes, whereas MRI had 100% accuracy rate in a recent study evaluating the role of CT versus MRI in sinusitis in patients with complications.

H Acute suppurative frontal sinusitis can lead to a subperiosteal abscess of the frontal bone leading to swelling of the forehead. This requires surgical drainage.

I Medical management can be used for 48–72 hours and include IV antibiotics, serial eye examinations, elevation of the head of the bed and nasal decongestants. Most common pathogens are those that are seen in acute and chronic sinusitis. Broad-spectrum, high-dose, IV antibiotic coverage against *Streptococcus pneumoniae*, *Haemophilus influenzae*, *Staphylococcus aureus*, and anaerobes should be given until culture results return.

J Isolated preseptal cellulitis should be managed initially with antibiotic therapy. If symptoms progress after 48 hours of intravenous (IV) antibiotic treatment then repeat imaging and evaluation for possible subperiosteal abscess should be performed. Recommended therapy is IV clindamycin with third-generation cephalosporin with central nervous system penetration.

K Worsening of symptoms within 24 hours or lack of improvement after 48 hours of medical therapy is an indication for repeat CT scan imaging and possible surgical exploration/drainage.

L Visual deficits, elevated intraocular pressure, extraocular muscle involvement, optic nerve deficits, proptosis >5 mm, or an abscess measuring >10 mm in size require surgical exploration and drainage.

M Ethmoidectomy, maxillary antrostomy, and opening of the lamina papyracea to drain the abscess can be performed endoscopically in most cases. Open drainage, using a Lynch incision, with external ethmoidectomy and drainage is reserved for cases with challenging endoscopic anatomy. Combined endoscopic and open surgical drainage with our oculoplastics colleagues can help address superior and lateral orbital disease.

N Symptoms include orbital pain, proptosis, photophobia, and cranial nerves III, IV, V1, V2 and VI deficits. Suspicion on CT should be further evaluated with an MRI with contrast or MR angiography/MR venography.

O The CT scan with contrast to evaluate for mass effect or signs of increased intracranial pressure should be done prior to lumbar puncture.

P Treat the case as if it is an acute uncomplicated sinusitis.

SUGGESTED READING

Bedwell JR, Bauman NM. Management of pediatric orbital cellulitis and abscess. Curr Opin Otolaryngol Head Neck Surg. 2011;19:467-473.

Bedwell JR, Choi SS. Medical versus surgical management of pediatric orbital subperiosteal abscesses. Laryngoscope. 2013;123:2337-2338.

Brook I. Microbiology and antimicrobial treatment of orbital and intracranial complications of sinusitis in children and their management. Int J Pediatr Otorhinolaryngol. 2009;73:1183-1186.

Hurley PE, Harris GJ. Subperiosteal abscess of the orbit: duration of intravenous antibiotic therapy in nonsurgical cases. Ophthal Plast Reconstr Surg. 2012;28(1):22-26.

Ryan JT, Preciado DA, Bauman N, et al. Management of pediatric orbital cellulitis in patients with radiographic findings of subperiosteal abscess. Otolaryngol Head Neck Surg. 2009;140:907-911.

Tabarino F, Elmaleh-Berges M, Quesnel S, et al. Subperiosteal orbital abscess: volumetric criteria for surgical drainage. Int J Pediatr Otorhinolaryngol. 2015;79:131-135.

Younis RT, Anand VK, Davidson B. The role of computed tomography and magnetic resonance imaging in patients with sinusitis with complications. Laryngoscope. 2002;12:224-229.

Nasal Allergy

Amanda L Stapleton

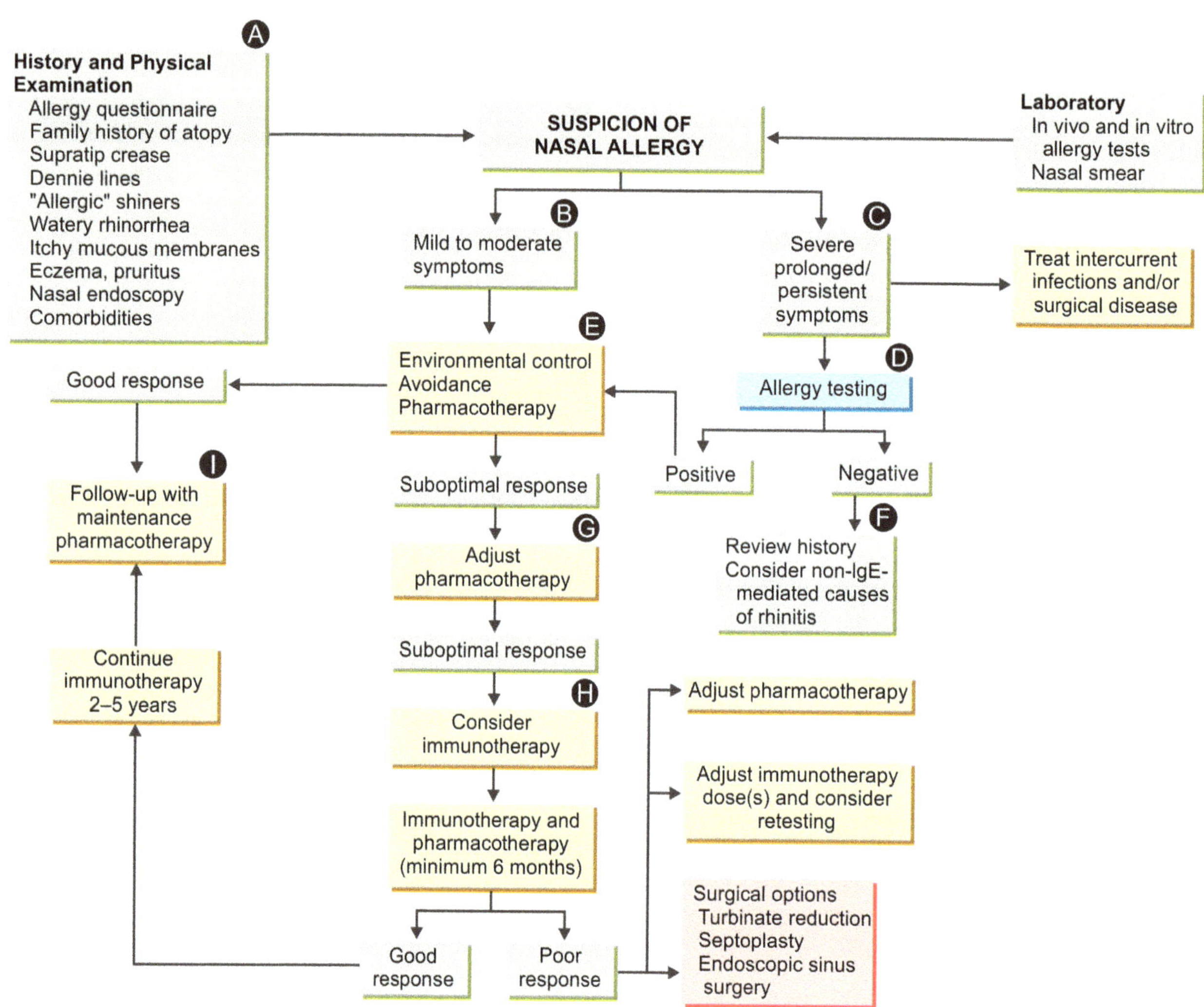

Nasal allergy (rhinitis) is one of the most common diseases affecting adults and children in the United States. It can diminish quality of life by affecting work and school productivity. Allergic rhinitis is an IgE mediated-inflammatory response of the nasal mucosal membranes after exposure to inhaled allergens. Correct diagnosis and treatment can lead to significant improvement in symptoms and quality of life.

A A detailed history is the key element in the diagnosis of nasal allergy. The temporal relationship between environmental factors and the occurrence of symptoms is important. A standard allergy questionnaire provides information about the environment at home and at work. Severity of symptoms and their impact on the patients quality of life should be assessed. Physical examination may show signs of allergy and chronic nasal congestion. Swollen, bluish turbinates, polypoid mucosa, and nasal polyps are common in allergic rhinitis. If there is concern for adenoid hypertrophy or chronic sinusitis, nasal endoscopy should be performed. The presence of other signs of allergy (dermatographism, eczema, skin dryness, conjunctival injection) should be noted. Screening for asthma, atopic dermatitis, sleep-disordered breathing, conjunctivitis, sinusitis, and otitis media is recommended. Assessment of growth percentiles for children may be used to document a baseline value, because therapy with some intranasal steroids may affect growth velocity in the short-term.

B Seasonal symptoms (3–6 months) with limited impact on quality of life are considered mild to moderate and are usually associated with seasonal allergic rhinitis.

C Perennial allergic rhinitis or symptoms persisting over a period of 6 months or more (multiple seasonal allergic rhinitis) with severe impact on quality of life are considered severe forms of nasal allergy, which require a combination of treatment modalities. Acute or chronic sinus infections must be treated with antibiotics. In cases of extensive nasal polyposis or anatomic abnormalities predisposing to nasal congestion or sinusitis, surgical management should be considered.

D Allergy testing is recommended for patients with a clinical diagnosis of allergic rhinitis who do not respond to medical therapy, when the diagnosis is uncertain, or when knowledge of the specific causative allergen is needed to target therapy. Allergen selection is guided by history. Routine allergy screening consists of two of the trees, weeds, grasses, molds, and dust mites common to the area as well as any pertinent animal dander. This usually results in a panel of 9–10 antigens that can detect the majority of atopic subjects. In vitro tests (radioallergosorbent test and enzyme-linked immunosorbent assay) to measure allergen-specific immunoglobulin (Ig) E and total IgE in serum providing quantitative results can be used to calculate immunotherapy (IT) doses. A total IgE level in and of itself is not an effective screening test. Total IgE may be normal and the patient may still have significant allergy. Interpretation of test results has to be done in light of clinical findings and history.

E Topical intranasal steroids and oral antihistamines are the recommended first-line therapy to treat allergic rhinitis. Use of oral second generation/less sedating (loratadine, fexofenadine) antihistamines for patients with primary complaints of sneezing and itching is recommended. Clinicians have the option of offering topical intranasal antihistamines as combination therapy to help with symptom control. It has a more rapid onset of action. Patients should be instructed to direct the intranasal spray nozzle laterally to avoid epistaxis and the very rare complication of septal perforation. Nasal saline irrigations can also be an important component of allergy therapy—typically used before topical medications are applied. Oral leukotriene receptor antagonists are not recommended as primary therapy for allergic rhinitis. A positive allergy test can be used as a dramatic educational tool to reinforce the importance of avoidance and environmental control as well as to increase the compliance with medications.

Cromolyn is very safe and is the preferred drug during pregnancy and for small children. The anticholinergic spray ipratropium can be used to relieve excessive rhinorrhea but is not effective for other symptoms. All nasal sprays may be used with other nasal sprays, but the general guideline is to titrate the patient to the most cost-effective medication or medications that control symptoms.

F If the screen panel is negative, further testing rarely provides useful information. After a careful review of the history, non-IgE-mediated causes of rhinitis, including infectious (viral, bacterial) rhinosinusitis, vasomotor rhinitis, nonallergic rhinitis with eosinophilia syndrome, drug-induced rhinitis (antihypertensives, aspirin, nonsteroidal anti-inflammatory drug, oral contraceptives, nasal decongestants, cocaine), occupational rhinitis (may be allergic or nonallergic), hormonal rhinitis (pregnancy, menstrual cycle, hypothyroidism), reflex-induced rhinitis (gustatory rhinitis, nasal cycle, posture reflexes, emotional, chemical, or irritant induced), should be considered.

G Combination therapy or variable medication formulations may elicit different responses in each individual. Individual response to various antihistamines is variable; therefore, control of symptoms with modified doses and different agents should be tried. Patient compliance must be assessed and addressed. Compliance is enhanced when fewer daily doses are required and written instructions are given to the patient.

H Immunotherapy (sublingual or subcutaneous) should be offered to patients who have inadequate response to symptoms with pharmacologic therapy with or without environmental controls. Patients should be considered candidates for immunotherapy based on the severity and duration of symptoms, presence of comorbid conditions, and response to previous treatment options. Immunotherapy should be initiated only in individuals with rhinitis of allergic cause, resulting from allergens for which potent extracts or sublingual tablets are available.

I Maintenance pharmacotherapy consists of the minimum amount of medications that control symptoms.

SUGGESTED READING

Dykewicz MS, Fineman S. Executive summary of joint task force practice parameters on diagnosis and management of rhinitis. Ann Allergy Asthma Immunol. 1998;81:63-68.

Dykiewicz MS, Fineman S, Skoner DP. Diagnosis and management of rhinitis: complete guidelines of the joint task Force on practice parameters in allergy, asthma and immunology. Ann Allergy Asthma Immunol. 1998;81:478-518.

Jutel M, Agache I, Bonini S, et al. International consensus on allergy immunotherapy. J Allergy Clin Immunol. 2015;136:556-568.

Mener DJ, Shargorodsky J, Varadhan R, et al. Topical intranasal corticosteroids and growth velocity in children: a meta-analysis. Int Forum Allergy Rhinol. 2015;5:95-103.

Scadding GK. Optimal management of allergic rhinitis. Arch Dis Child. 2015;100:576-582.

Seidman MD, Gurgel RK, Lin SY, et al. Clinical practice guideline: allergic rhinitis executive summary. Otolaryngol Head Neck Surg. 2015;152(2):197-206.

Nonallergic Rhinitis

Nicholas R Rowan, Stella E Lee

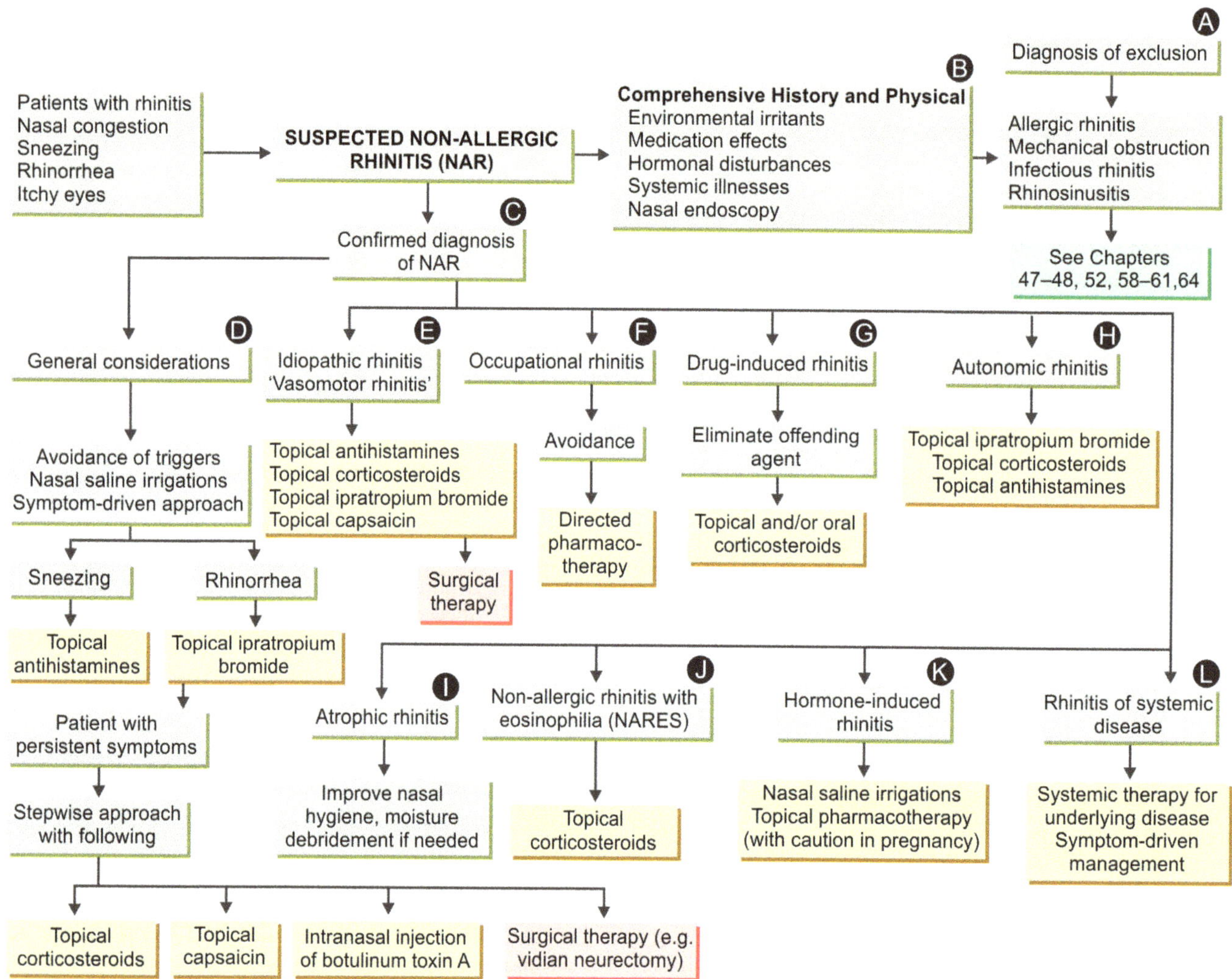

Nonallergic rhinitis (NAR) is an umbrella category that includes a wide range of disease processes with different underlying pathophysiologies but similar clinical manifestations.

A Nonallergic rhinitis is a diagnosis of exclusion and must be differentiated from patients with an underlying allergic, anatomical, or infectious etiology. Allergic rhinitis should be ruled out by negative history and confirmed by skin or in vitro testing. Nonallergic rhinitis is more common in women and typically presents with symptoms of nasal congestion and rhinorrhea.

B A comprehensive history and physical examination are the key to diagnosis of NAR. Specific inquiries regarding the multiple etiologies of NAR including environmental irritants, hormonal disturbances, medication effects, systemic illnesses, autonomic, or age-related dysfunction must be obtained. Nasal endoscopy is helpful in diagnosis.

C Once a diagnosis of NAR is made an attempt to identify an underlying cause should be undertaken, though the etiology may be mixed.

D In general, avoidance should be pursued if there is an obvious inciting factor, otherwise topical therapies (e.g. nasal saline irrigations and topical corticosteroids) are the mainstay of treatment. A symptom-driven approach can also be helpful to manage the patient.

E Idiopathic rhinitis or "vasomotor rhinitis" is the most common cause of NAR and may represent an array of pathologies. Topical antihistamines, corticosteroids, and ipratropium bromide are the mainstay of treatment, while surgical therapies such as inferior turbinate reduction and vidian neurectomy may be appropriate for recalcitrant disease. Recent review suggests that topical capsaicin may also be helpful.

F Occupational rhinitis is characterized by symptoms limited exclusively to the workplace and is best treated with avoidance. Directed symptom-driven pharmacotherapy is indicated when complete avoidance is not possible.

G Drug-induced rhinitis may stem from a range of medications such as topical decongestants (rhinitis medicamentosa) to systemic medications (e.g. antihypertensives and erectile dysfunction medications). Avoidance, if possible, and elimination of the causative agent is the optimal treatment strategy.

H Autonomic rhinitis may occur in response to diverse stimuli and is typically characterized by profuse watery rhinorrhea. Ipratropium bromide is the first-line treatment.

I Atrophic rhinitis, which may also be known as ozena or empty nose syndrome is characterized by the symptom of severe nasal obstruction in the setting of a widely patent nasal cavity. Treatment is challenging and involves improved nasal hygiene and debridement of nasal crusting.

J Nonallergic rhinitis with eosinophilia must be considered in patients with allergic-type symptoms, but in the absence of systemic atopy. Diagnosis is made by a nasal smear (>20% eosinophils). Topical corticosteroid therapies are typically effective.

K Hormone-induced rhinitis is typically accompanied by the hormone surge associated with puberty and pregnancy, and can oftentimes be managed with nasal saline irrigations. Evidence is scarce regarding topical pharmacotherapy in pregnancy and should be approached with caution.

L Rhinitis of systemic disease (e.g. granulomatosis with polyangiitis or sarcoid) should be managed by treatment of the underlying systemic illness with referral to rheumatology and symptom-driven management of nasal and upper airway symptoms by the Otolaryngologist.

SUGGESTED READING

Fokkens WJ. Thoughts on the pathophysiology of nonallergic rhinitis. Curr Allergy Asthma Rep. 2002;2(3):203-209.

Gevorgyan A, Segboer C, Gorissen R, et al. Capsaicin for non-allergic rhinitis. Cochrane Database Sys Rev. 2015;7:CD010591.

Heilings PW, Scadding G, Alobid I, et al. Executive summary of European Task Force document on diagnostic tools in rhinology. Rhinology. 2012;50(4):339-352.

Molgaard E, Thomsen SF, Lund T, et al. Differences between allergic and nonallergic rhinitis in a large sample of adolescents and adults. Allergy. 2007;62:1033-1037.

Moscato G, Rolla G, Siracusa A. Occupational rhinitis: consensus on diagnosis and medicolegal implications. Curr Opin Otolaryngol Head Neck Surg. 2011;19(1):36-42.

Nyenhuis S, Matheur SK. Rhinitis in older adults. Curr Allergy Asthma Rep. 2013;13(2):171-179.

Orban N, Maughan E, Bleach N. Pregnancy-induced rhinitis. Rhinology. 2013;51(2):111-119.

Ricardo L Carrau

CHAPTER 66
Juvenile Nasopharyngeal Angiofibroma

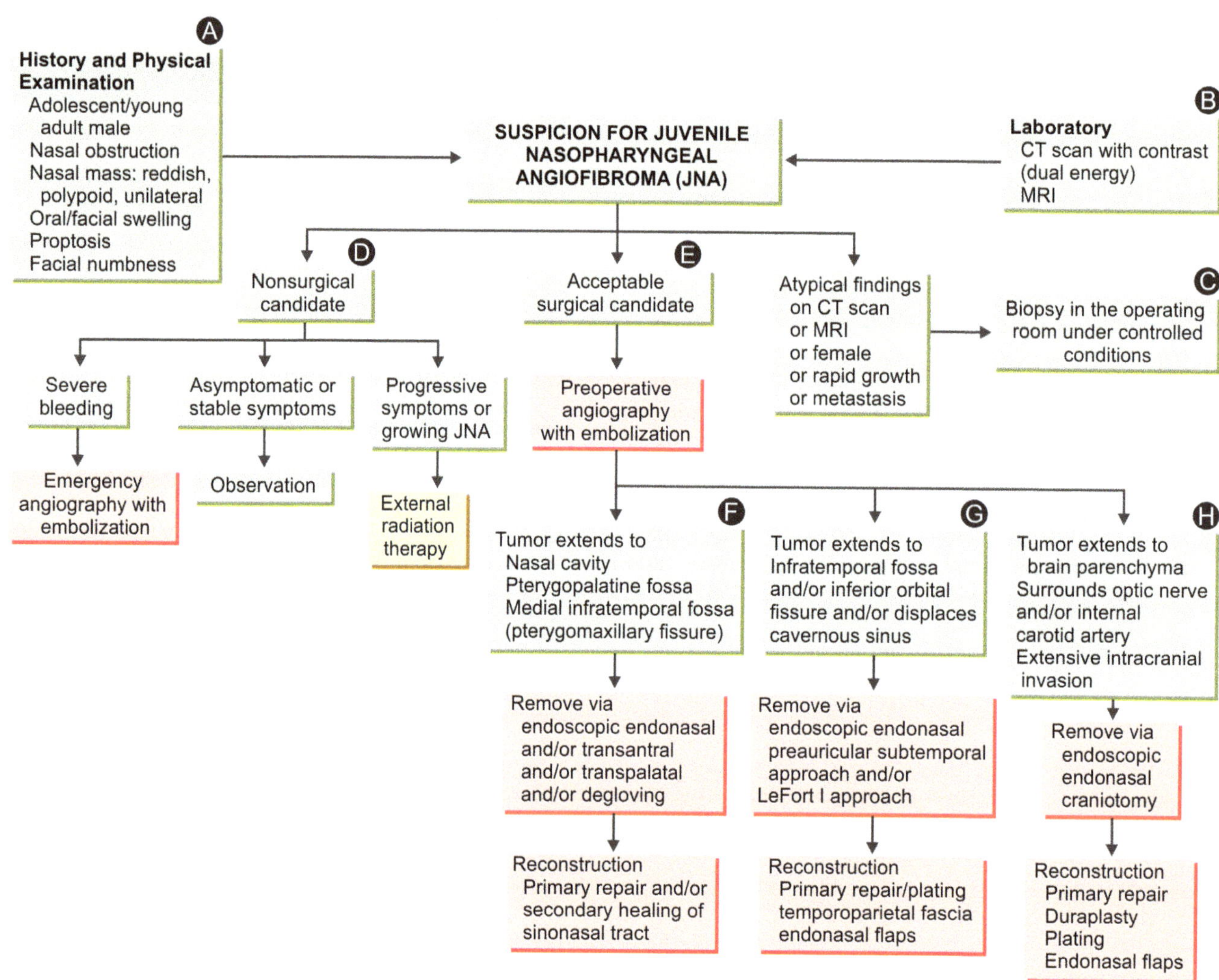

Juvenile nasopharyngeal angiofibroma (JNA) is a rare benign tumor that arises exclusively in adolescent males. Its incidence varies around the world, with a higher frequency in South America, the Middle East, and Asia. Its origin is controversial but Schick suggested that it represents a vascular atavism due to the incomplete regression of the artery of the first branchial arch, around the area of the sphenopalatine foramen.

Juvenile nasopharyngeal angiofibromas grow by displacement of surrounding structures, forming a pseudocapsule that facilitates its surgical dissection. Its high vascularity, comprising vessels that lack contractility, accounts for its hallmark characteristic of profuse bleeding. Most patients with a JNA present with unilateral epistaxis or mass effect (i.e. nasal obstruction, facial deformity, and proptosis).

A A unilateral polypoid reddish mass associated with epistaxis in a preadolescent or adolescent male should be considered a JNA until proven otherwise.

B A clinical diagnosis of JNA is confirmed with imaging such as a computed tomography (CT) scan or magnetic resonance imaging (MRI). CT is superior in defining the bony architecture and provides a clear "surgical map." Magnetic resonance imaging is advantageous in those patients with JNA that invade the orbit or middle cranial fossa, or involve neurovascular structures. A contrasted dual energy CT provides an definition of both the tumor and the bony architecture; therefore, it has become our first choice for preoperative imaging. MRI is preferred for postoperative surveillance as it avoids further radiation exposure.

C Biopsy is usually unnecessary and potentially dangerous; however, it should be considered in patients with JNA presenting rapid growth, infiltrative pattern on imaging studies, or lymphadenopathy, and in female patients.

It is best performed in the operating room under general anesthesia with blood replacement available.

D Patients who are poor surgical candidates as a result of significant comorbidities, or those who refuse surgery, can be offered a variety of nonsurgical options according to their age and presenting symptoms. Patients presenting severe bleeding can undergo angiography and embolization.

Patients who are asymptomatic can be monitored with sequential imaging. If the tumor grows or extends to vital areas or if the symptoms progress, external radiation therapy may be considered. Testosterone receptor blockers may reduce the tumor and bleeding in postpubertal patients; thus, temporizing or ameliorating problems; or as a preoperative adjunct. Its use is more practical and seems more effective in late adolescent patients. Reports of stabilization of symptoms and growth with antiangiogenic agents such as bevacizumab, are anecdotal.

E Surgery is considered the mainstay therapy for JNA and is advocated for all patients who are acceptable surgical candidates. Critical surgical aspects include control of bleeding (early control of feeding vessels and centripetal resection) and avoidance of sequelae (JNA is a benign tumor in patients with an expected long-term survival). Hemostasis and blood replacement are important considerations in the surgical planning. Ideally, patients undergo angiography and embolization 24 hours before surgery (avoids revascularization). Its role has been questioned mostly in developing countries where the technology and expertise are not widely available. Patients are usually typed and cross-matched for 2–4 units of packed red blood cells. Autotransfusion is possible but is not commonly applied.

F JNA limited to the nasal cavity, nasopharynx, paranasal sinuses, pterygopalatine fossa, and medial infratemporal fossa can be removed through a variety of limited approaches. The choice of approach greatly depends on the experience and preference of the surgeon; however, the transnasal endoscopic approach has gained remarkable popularity. In may experience most of these tumors can be removed using a transnasal-endoscopic approach. Transpalatal and transantral approaches may provide adequate exposure with limited morbidity.

Mucosal defects arising from the removal of a JNA can be left to heal by secondary intention. If an open approach is used, all incisions are closed primarily.

G A JNA that extends to the lateral or anterior infratemporal fossa, or the inferior orbital fissure, or displaces the cavernous sinus may require a wider surgical approach, or a combination of approaches. One should take into consideration cosmetic, functional, and oncologic factors, as well as the ability to control bleeding. Removal of a JNA only requires its enucleation as it grows by displacement rather than invasion thus, wide exposure of all the areas of extension is unnecessary. In experienced hands, tumors with significant extensions can be removed via an endoscopic endonasal approach.

Tumors with broad nasopharyngeal and sphenoid bone attachments, but with limited extension to the infratemporal fossa, can be managed via a LeFort I osteotomy approach, a transpalatal approach or a combination of endoscopic endonasal and anterior maxillotomy approaches. In patients with significant extension of the JNA, e.g. bilateral intracranial extension, the resection can be divided in two or more stages. The need to stage the surgery is usually dictated by intraoperative blood loss. If this possibility is anticipated, I follow a pattern that allows me to abort the resection and complete hemostasis, leaving the removal of the remnants for a second intervention. The most common paradigm is to remove the nasal, nasopharyngeal and paranasal sinuses components (i.e. the resulting corridor can be packed and the surgery aborted), followed by the infratemporal fossa (i.e. somewhat amenable to packing and its blood supply is relatively accessible) and lastly the intracranial and intraorbital components (i.e. this area cannot be packed, therefore the tumor has to be completely removed or hemostasis completed).

Closure of the surgical defect requires primary repair of incisions, reapproximation of the soft tissue in the deeper planes, plating of those maxillofacial buttresses disrupted by osteotomies, and the use of vascularized tissue to obliterate the dead space or to achieve separation of the cranial cavity and the upper aerodigestive tract.

H JNA that extends to the brain parenchyma, surrounds the optic nerve or the internal carotid artery, or has extensive intracranial invasion may require a craniotomy to fully expose and control the neurovascular structures.

SUGGESTED READING

El Sharkawy AA. Endonasal endoscopic management of juvenile nasopharyngeal angiofibroma without angiographic embolization. Eur Arch Otorhinolaryngol. 2013;270(7):2051-2055.

Fagan JJ, Snyderman CH, Carrau RL, et al. Nasopharyngeal angiofibromas: selecting a surgical approach. Head Neck. 1997;19: 391-399.

Hackman T, Snyderman CH, Carrau R, et al. Juvenile nasopharyngeal angiofibroma: the expanded endonasal approach. Am J Rhinol Allergy. 2009;23(1):95-99.

López F, Suárez V, Costales M, et al. Treatment of juvenile angiofibromas: 18-year experience of a single tertiary centre in Spain. Rhinology. 2012;50(1):95-103.

Nicolai P, Villaret AB, Farina D, et al. Endoscopic surgery for juvenile angiofibroma: a critical review of indications after 46 cases. Am J Rhinol Allergy. 2010;24(2):e67-72.

Schick B, Tahan ERA, Brors D, et al. Experiences with endonasal surgery in angiofibroma. Rhinology. 1999;37:80-85.

Snyderman CH, Pant H, Carrau RL, et al. A new endoscopic staging system for angiofibromas. Arch Otolaryngol Head Neck Surg. 2010;136(6):588-594.

Thakar A, Gupta G, Bhalla AS, et al. Adjuvant therapy with flutamide for presurgical volume reduction in juvenile nasopharyngeal angiofibroma. Head Neck. 2011;33(12):1747-1753.

Malignant Sinonasal Neoplasms

John V Segas, Efthymios E Kyrodimos

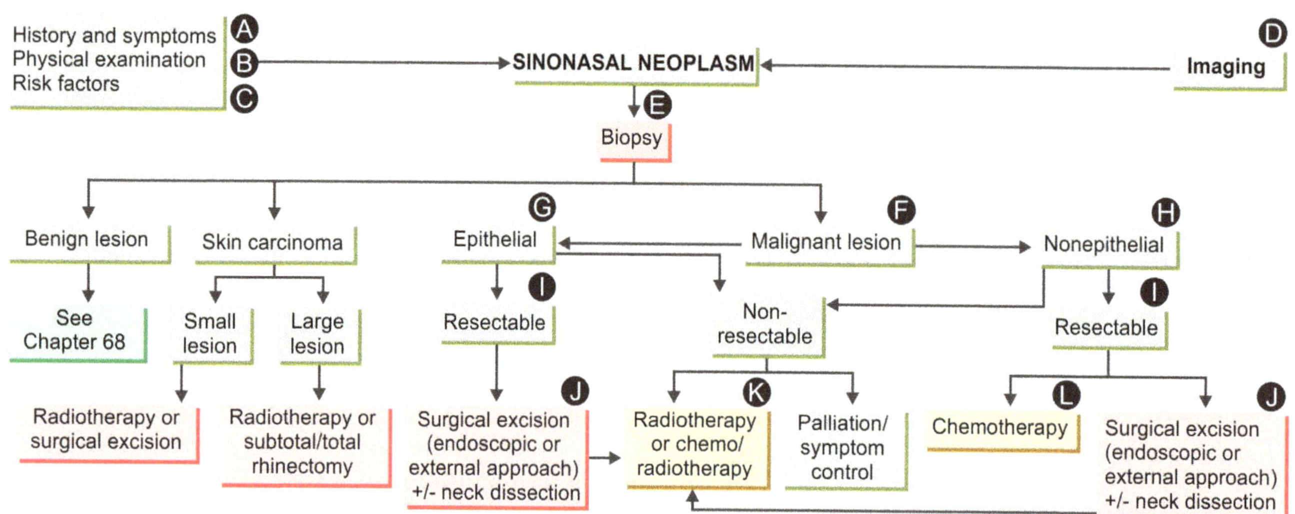

Over the past two decades, significant technologic advances such as the introduction of office endoscopy and high-resolution imaging techniques has revolutionized the diagnosis of malignant sinonasal neoplasms.

Ⓐ A number of signs and symptoms may suggest sinonasal malignancy even in the presence of a normal physical examination. Local symptoms are the most common presenting symptoms (nasal obstruction, nasal bleeding, discharge, and hyposmia or anosmia). Regional and locoregional symptoms (mass in the cheek, mass in the neck, proptosis, diplopia, epiphora, loose maxillary teeth, hypesthesia of the infraorbital nerve, anesthesia of the palate, and cranial nerve dysfunction) highlight the importance of clinical suspicion especially in patients with no previous history of inflammatory sinonasal disease. Unilateral Eustachian tube dysfunction and middle ear effusion may also be present. Distant metastases are relatively uncommon for these tumors.

Ⓑ Rhinoscopy and/or endoscopy reveal a neoplasm within the nasal cavity.

Ⓒ Exposure to wood dust and industrial chemicals are considered prominent risk factors in the development of sinonasal malignancy. Hardwood particle dusts (ebony, oak, beech) are associated with an increased incidence of adenocarcinoma. Tobacco abuse, nickel and chromate particles from the metal industry, leather products, chrome pigments from the textile industry, thorium dioxide, and imaging agents are all considered high-risk factors for the development of squamous cell carcinoma. The role of human papillomavirus as a primary carcinogen in the sinonasal tract still remains unclear yet additional studies are required to obtain conclusive evidence.

Ⓓ Computed tomography (CT) and magnetic resonance imaging (MRI) are used for accurate diagnosis. Both modalities are required since T1 MRI with contrast demonstrates tumor expansion and T2 MRI can distinguish secretions and mucous retention from tumor and CT can reveal bone erosion. Expansion to the orbit, dura, and brain can be defined by both CT and MRI. Proof of perineural invasion and involvement of brain parenchyma may require the use of detailed MRI or high-resolution CT images. Involvement of the internal carotid artery can be defined by MR angiography or CT angiography. Regional and distant metastatic cancer can be defined by the use of 18 fluorodeoxyglucose–positron emission tomography CT scan.

Ⓔ The different variations in pathology of intranasal lesions require specific caution when a biopsy is indicated. Biopsy can be transnasal, transantral (creation of an antrostomy), through an endoscopic or by an open approach. Extra care must be taken in an office setting especially when the lesion is located behind the middle turbinate where a vascular lesion or a meningocele can be expected. Biopsy technique should be focused on obtaining formalin fixed tissue samples and fresh tissue samples when a lymphoma is suspected.

Ⓕ Malignancy of the sinonasal tract is uncommon and accounts for only 1% of all malignancies and 5% of head and neck malignancies. Malignant neoplasms in the sinonasal tract can be defined as epithelial or nonepithelial in origin. Nasopharyngeal carcinoma is not considered part of this group.

Ⓖ Based on WHO classification of sinonasal neoplasms as described in 2005, the epithelial neoplasms are the most common, and squamous cell carcinoma, adenocystic carcinoma, and adenocarcinoma are the prominent subtypes.

H In nonepithelial neoplasms there is a wide range of tumors which originate from different types of epithelium as hematolymphoid (lymphoma), neuroectodermal (olfactory neuroblastoma, mucosal melanoma), malignant tumors from bone and cartilage (chondrosarcoma), neuroendocrine tumors (carcinoid), malignant soft-tissue tumors (sarcomas), germ cell tumors, and secondary tumors arising from lung, breast, and renal area.

I Surgery is advocated for resectable cancer with clear margins. Anatomic landmarks are crucial and determine the degree of surgical resection. Proximity of the tumor to the orbit, internal carotid artery, dura, brain, palate, and cranial nerves are of vital importance and influence surgical planning.

J Endoscopic resection is, in general, advocated for lesions involving the nasoethmoidal box and more recently for lesions expanded to the dura or the anterior skull base. Tumors largely involving the frontal sinus, extension beyond the posterior inferior maxillary sinus wall, penetrating the floor of the nose and hard palate, involving orbital content and lacrimal complex, and finally large tumors extending from the ethmoids to the skull base require an external approach. External approaches include medial maxillectomy, inferior maxillectomy, total maxillectomy, osteoplastic frontal sinus approach, and craniofacial resections. Aggressive treatment is mandatory to achieve maximum local control of the primary site. The risk of nodal metastases correlates with extension of the primary tumor to the nasopharynx, palate, or the oral cavity, and elective treatment of the neck is crucial to detect nodal metastases. Nodal metastases are a very poor prognostic factor and should be addressed at the time of the primary resection.

K Radiotherapy is used for local or locoregional disease through prevention of tumor spread to the complex and extensive lymphatic drainage of the paranasal sinuses and skull base. Radiotherapy can be administrated prior to surgery (neoadjuvant) or following surgery (adjuvant). Chemotherapy can be added synchronous to radiotherapy targeting in encashment of radiotherapy results, controlling of micrometastases and reducing tumor growth. A combination of radiotherapy and chemotherapy is generally the modality of choice in nonresectable tumors or nonclear margins targeting in minimizing the risk of tumor expansion. In large nonresectable tumors, the therapeutic effort must be focused on control of the patient's symptoms. In all cases, initial staging must be followed meticulously.

L Chemotherapy prior to surgery, especially in sensitive tumors such as olfactory neuroblastoma, can minimize the tumor volume making resection less technically demanding and electively control bleeding.

SUGGESTED READING

Lund VJ, Stammberger H, Nicolai P, et al. European position paper on endoscopic management of tumors of the nose, paranasal sinuses and skull base. Rhino Suppl. 2010;22:1-143.

Myers E, Kennedy D. Rhinology, Part III: Techniques for Removal of Neoplasms. Philadelphia, PA: Wolters Kluwer; 2016. pp. 209-262.

Myers E, Kennedy D. Rhinology, Part V: Open Sinus Surgery Techniques. Philadelphia, PA: Wolters Kluwer; 2016. pp. 307-360.

Myers E, Suen J, Myers J, et al. Cancer of the Head and Neck, Cancer of the Nasal Cavity, Paranasal Sinus and Orbit, 4th edition. Philadelphia, PA: Saunders; 2003. pp. 162-178.

Nylander LA, Dement JM. Carcinogenic effects of wood dust: review and discussion. Am J Ind Med. 1993;24(5):619-647.

Rushton L, Hutchings S, Brown T. The burden of cancer at work: estimation as the first step to prevention. Occup Environ Med. 2008;65(12):789-800.

Wenig BM. Recently described sinonasal tract lesions/neoplasms: considerations for the new world health organization book. Head Neck Pathol. 2014; 8(1):33-41.

Benign Sinonasal Neoplasms

John I Song

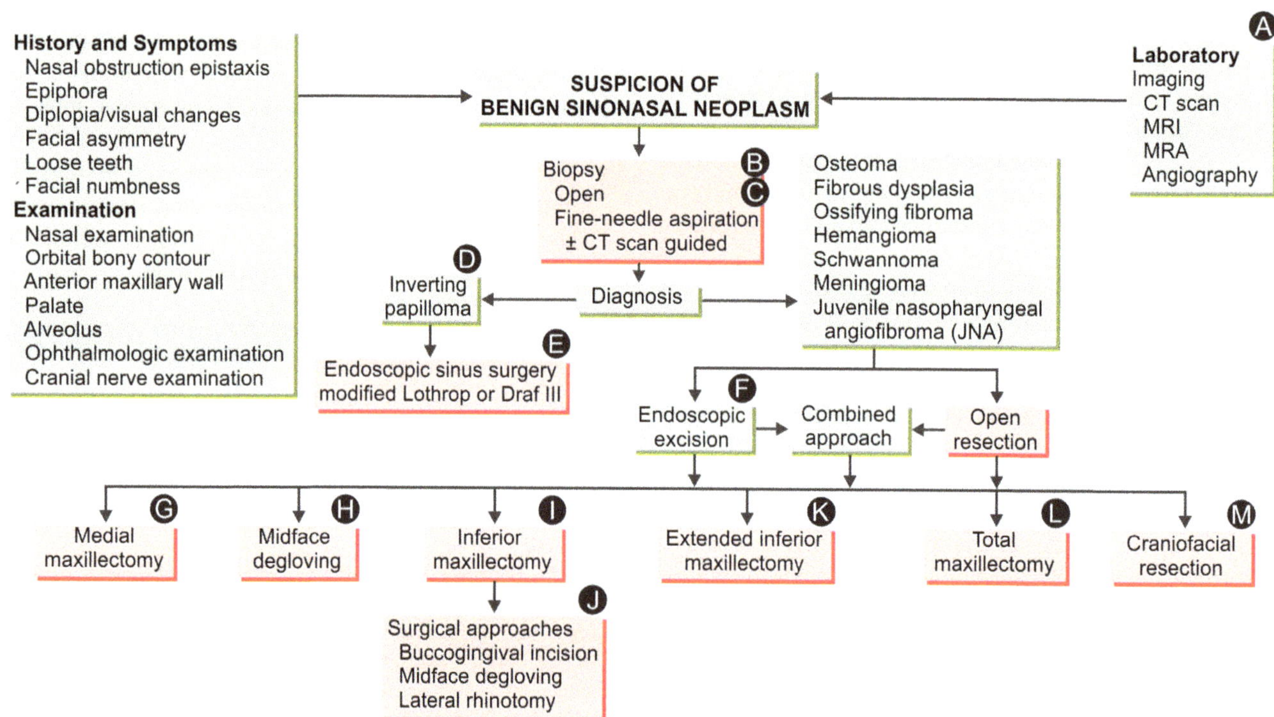

Benign tumors of the sinonasal tract are rare, but they represent a diverse group of neoplasms. These tumors can arise from the fibro-osseous, vascular, neural, odontogenic, and epithelial tissues surrounding the paranasal sinuses. Evaluation and treatment of these tumors should be individualized in order to maximize clinical outcomes and minimize morbidity to the facial skeleton, orbits, and central nervous system (CNS).

A Computed tomography (CT) scan (with or without contrast) is used to visualize the extent of disease within the bony anatomy of the paranasal sinuses and orbital apex. For example, bone erosion and osteitis can pinpoint the attachment site for an inverting papilloma. Magnetic resonance imaging (MRI) is superior to CT for soft-tissue tumors and vascular tumors [Juvenile nasopharyngeal angiofibroma (JNA)], in differentiating tumor from retained sinus secretions, cysts from cerebrospinal fluid (CSF), and assessing dural and CNS involvement. Magnetic resonance angiography (MRA) or angiography is indicated, if the lesion enhances on CT or abuts the carotid artery.

B Unilateral nasal masses should not be assumed to be inflammatory or allergic in origin and a biopsy should be considered. Careful review of the imaging studies can narrow the category of tumor with many fibro-osseous tumors diagnosed by imaging alone. Encephaloceles and vascular tumors should be ruled out before biopsy is made. Biopsies should be done in the operating room if one is concerned about a possible hemorrhage.

C Most nasal masses are accessible using endoscopic instruments alone and only rarely is an open-procedure (i.e. external ethmoidectomy, Caldwell-Luc, frontal trephination) indicated for biopsy and diagnosis. Any open-procedure should be planned in order not to compromise a definitive en-bloc resection.

D Inverting papillomas (IPs) are associated with high rates of recurrence, are locally aggressive, and have malignant potential. Malignancy rates from 3.6% to 7.1% have been reported. Most IPs can be managed via an endoscopic approach with complete removal of the involved mucosa and the underlying mucoperiosteum to reduce recurrence. Polypectomy or local excision alone can result in recurrence rates which may be as high as 50%.

E Extended frontal recess approaches (modified-Lothrop or Draf III) may be needed for IP's extending into the frontal sinus. Relative contraindications to endoscopic approaches include: (1) extensive involvement of the frontal sinus, (2) new bone formation or scarring of the frontal recess, and (3) malignancy.

F *Osteomas*: Treatment is based on the size and location of the tumor and may require an endoscopic, open- or combined-surgical approach. An open-approach is preferred if the tumor is attached to the anterior table of the frontal sinus or completely fills the frontal sinus. *Meningiomas*: Intranasal meningiomas are rare and arise from ectopic arachnoid tissue while the anterior skull base accounts for 40% of all intracranial meningiomas. Increasingly, endoscopic endonasal skull base approaches have been used successfully in these cases. *Juvenile nasopharyngeal angiofibroma*: MRA or angiography (if embolization is considered) may be needed for diagnosis. Preoperative embolization reduces intraoperative bleeding by 60–70% and can reduce the need for transfusions. JNAs have traditionally been treated via an open-approach. Endoscopic approaches to the pterygopalatine fossa and the infratemporal fossa have allowed for better control of vessels while advances in cautery and coblation have allowed for successful piecemeal resection of these tumors.

G Medial maxillectomy via an external approach (lateral rhinotomy vs midface degloving) is indicated when extensive bone involvement or lateral extension of tumor is present. Medial maxillectomy allows en-bloc removal of the lateral nasal wall, medial maxilla, ethmoid sinuses, and lacrimal sac. A lateral rhinotomy incision is favored because it provides both good exposure and good cosmetic and functional results.

H Midface degloving is used only if the tumor is isolated to the inferior turbinate or inferior aspect of the nasal cavity and nasal septum. This exposure is limited superiorly, especially for tumors involving the anterior ethmoid air cells and the frontoethmoidal recess.

I Indications for an inferior maxillectomy includes tumors limited to the infrastructure of the maxillary sinus without extension to the floor of the orbit or infraorbital rim. All patients are evaluated preoperatively by a maxillofacial prosthodontist, and a surgical obturator is fabricated. The inferior turbinate is removed to prevent hypertrophy and interference with the obturator. Maxillary sinus mucosa is judiciously removed to prevent mucoperiosteal thickening and chronic infection.

J Tumors on the inferior aspect of the maxilla can be approached through a buccogingival sulcus incision, tumors in the midportion of the nose using a midface degloving, and tumors in the superior aspect of the nasal cavity approached through a lateral rhinotomy incision.

K Extension through the posterior maxillary wall into the infratemporal fossa or pterygomaxillary fossa is an indication for an extended inferior maxillectomy.

L Tumor extension to the orbital floor or orbital rim (anterior orbit) requires near-total or total maxillectomy. A lateral rhinotomy incision is preferred for better cosmesis and function. A Weber-Fergusson incision is not required unless orbital exenteration is performed.

M Endoscopic approachs have largely supplanted craniofacial resection except to treat a small fraction of sinonasal neoplasms. A craniofacial approach is indicated if there is extension superiorly into the frontal lobe or posteriorly into the orbital apex or pterygopalatine fossa. A combination of bicoronal, anterior, and lateral facial incisions can be used for this exposure.

SUGGESTED READING

Bielamowicz S, Calcaterra TC, Watson D. Inverting papilloma of the head and neck: the UCLA update. Otolaryngol Head Neck Surg. 1993;109(1):71-76.

Douglas R, Wormald PJ. Endoscopic surgery for juvenile nasopharyngeal angiofibroma: where are the limits? Curr Opin Otolaryngol Head Neck Surg. 2006;14(1):1-5.

Han JK, Smith TL, Loehrl T, et al. An evolution in the management of sinonasal inverting papilloma. Laryngoscope. 2001;111(8): 1395-1400.

Johnson JT. Inferior maxillectomy. In: Myers EN (Ed). Operative Otolaryngology: Head and Neck Surgery. Philadelphia, PA, USA: WB Saunders; 1997. p. 110.

Kassam AB, Gardner P, Snyderman C, et al. Expanded endonasal approach: fully endoscopic, completely transnasal approach to the middle third of the clivus, petrous bone, middle cranial fossa, and infratemporal fossa. Neurosurg Focus. 2005;19(1):E6.

Kingdom TT, Delgaudio JM. Endoscopic approach to lesions of the sphenoid sinus, orbital apex, and clivus. Am J Otolaryngol. 2003;24(5):317-322.

Myers EN. Medial maxillectomy. In: Myers EN, Carrau RL, Cass SP (Eds). Operative Otolaryngology: Head and Neck Surgery. Philadelphia, PA, USA: WB Saunders; 1997. p. 101.

Inflammatory Lesions of the Nose

Nivedita Sahu, Eric W Wang

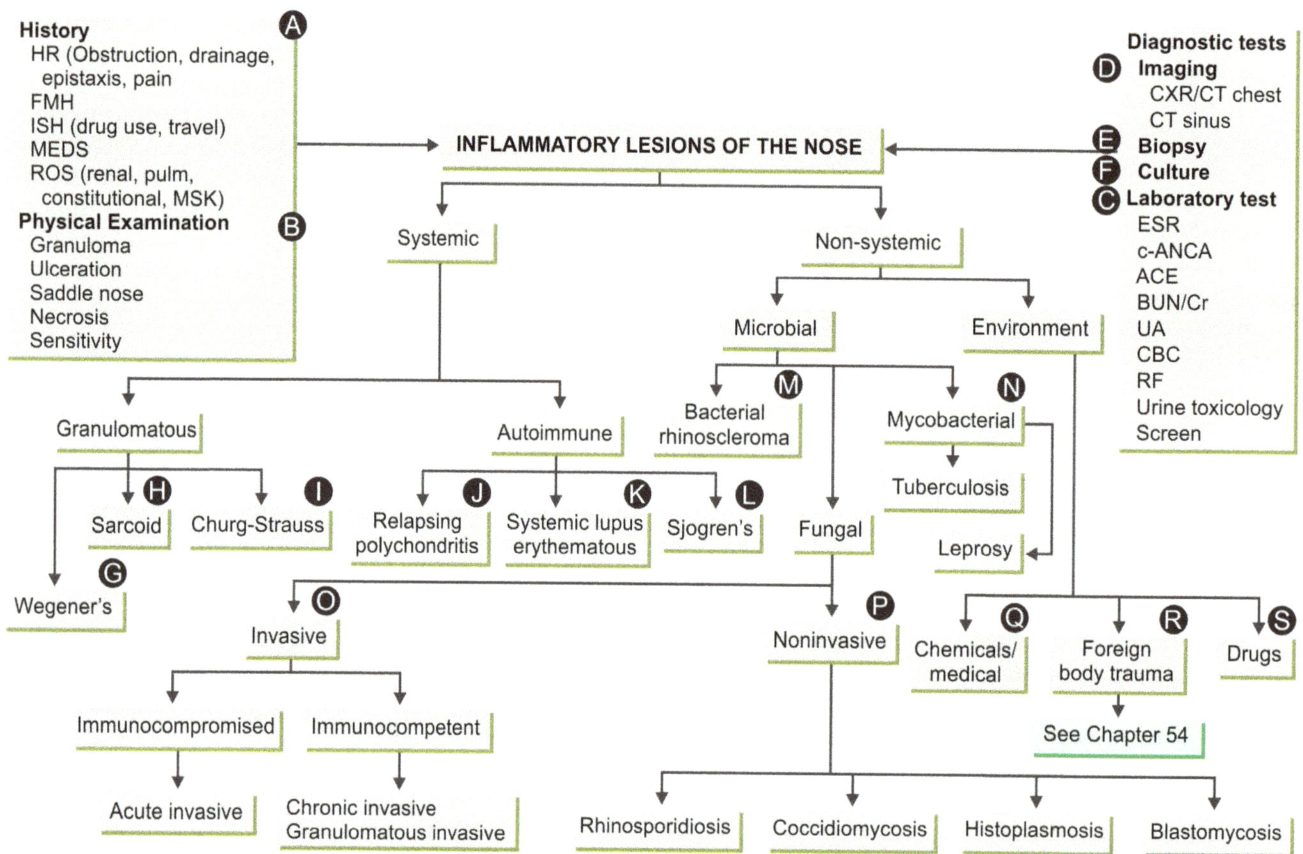

Nasal lesions arise from multiple etiologies including inflammatory processes, and specific historical elements, laboratory, and imaging studies can be used to establish the diagnosis. The underlying condition can range from systemic and autoimmune cases to infectious and foreign body related.

A The patients history is invaluable in the diagnosis of inflammatory lesions of the nose. While many lesions present with findings such as nasal obstruction, foul drainage, epistaxis, and pain, elements of the social history and review of systems can aid in developing an accurate differential diagnosis. Occupation, travel, and illicit drug use should be elicited. Review of systems should question renal, pulmonary, constitutional, and musculoskeletal issues.

B The physical examination should include examination of the external nose, anterior rhinoscopy, and nasal endoscopy. Findings may include granuloma, ulceration, bleeding, septal perforation, necrotic tissue, and saddle nose deformity (dorsum). Insensate mucosa is concerning for acute invasive fungal disease.

C Laboratory testing is targeted toward establishing a rheumatologic or autoimmune diagnosis. These include erythrocyte sedimentation rate and C-reactive protein (markers of inflammation), c-ANCA (positive in the setting of Wegener's Granulomatosis), angiotensin converting enzyme levels (elevated in sarcoidosis), BUN/Cr and urine analysis (markers of kidney function), RF (rheumatoid factor), SS-a and SS-b (Sjogren's antibodies), complete blood count, and urine toxicology.

D Imaging should include computed tomography of the paranasal sinuses to determine the effect of the lesion on the surrounding bone (erosion, expansile, confined) and may reveal associated sinusitis. Imaging of the chest (CT chest or chest radiography) is used to diagnose perihilar adenopathy in sarcoidosis or other abnormalities associated with Wegener's, tuberculosis (TB), coccidioidomycosis, and histoplasmosis.

E Biopsy is warranted when laboratory testing is inconclusive.

F If purulent exudate is noted, a nasal culture should be obtained to direct antimicrobial therapy. Tissue and swabs should be sent for acid-fast stains, fungal cultures, as well as aerobic and anaerobic bacterial cultures.

G Wegener's granulomatosis is a systemic vasculitis with a triad of necrotizing granulomas of the upper respiratory tract and lungs, glomerulonephritis, and disseminated vasculitis. c-ANCA is typically positive. Saddle nose deformity secondary to septal perforation is not uncommon in this disease.

H Sarcoidosis is a systemic granulomatous disease with associated perihilar lymphadenopathy. Subcutaneous nodules are common. Biopsy is characterized by noncaseating granulomas with histiocytes and multinucleated giant cells.

I Churg–Strauss syndrome is a triad of asthma, systemic vasculitis, and tissue and peripheral eosinophilia. Nasal polyps show necrosis and eosinophilic exudate.

J Relapsing polychondritis is an autoimmune disorder and is suspected when the patient has a history of cartilaginous involvement in the ribs, ears, joints, or trachea. Saddle nose deformity may be present.

K Systemic lupus erythematous is a chronic inflammatory disease with positive antinuclear antibodies (ANA). Nasal manifestations include intranasal ulcerations and is often associated with a malar rash involving the bridge of the nose.

L Sjogren's syndrome is an autoimmune disorder in which exocrine glands are destroyed leading to sicca syndrome (xerophthalmia, xerostomia) with associated joint pain and fatigue. SS-a and SS-b are associated with this disease, with SS-b being the more specific of the two. Sjogren's antibody tests are often falsely negative. Nasal dryness, crusting, and ulcerations can be present.

M Rhinoscleroma is caused by *Klebsiella rhinoscleromatis*, which progresses from a foul smelling catarrhal phase to an atrophic then granulomatous phase, and finally a sclerotic phase. The entire upper respiratory tract may be involved. It is endemic in Central and South America, Eastern Europe, and India.

N Tuberculosis and leprosy are mycobacterial infections leading to granulomatous lesions. TB is caused by *Mycobacterium tuberculosis* and presents with chronic cough, blood-tinged sputum, fever, night sweats, and weight loss. Leprosy is caused by *Mycobacterium leprae*. Infection may remain dormant for years and eventually present as granulomas of the skin, nerves, and respiratory tract. Both are associated with HIV.

O Invasive fungal sinusitis can be divided into two groups based on immunocompetence. Immunocompromised individuals (organ transplant, HIV, poorly controlled diabetes mellitus) can develop acute invasive fungal sinusitis, characterized by rapid onset, invasiveness, and tissue destruction. Typically, patients are severely ill and require hospitalization. Mucosa is often necrotic appearing and insensate. *Rhizopus*, *Rhizomucor*, and *Mucor* species are causative organisms. Immunocompetent patients can develop chronic or granulomatous fungal sinusitis and is associated with *Aspergillus fumigatus* and *Aspergillus flavus*.

P Noninvasive fungal disease can be divided into geographic regions, thus a travel history is warranted. Rhinosporidiosis (South India, Sri Lanka, South America, and Africa). Coccidioidomycosis (Southwest United States).

Histoplasmosis (Ohio River valley United States, caves in southern and East Africa). Blastomycosis (eastern North America).

Q Myospherulosis is asscociated with petroleum-based ointment in the sinonasal tract, resulting in inflammatory tissue. Alcohol, antithyroid drugs, aspirin, estrogen, phenothiazines, and ephedrine may cause nasal obstruction and inflammation. Rhinitis medicamentosa is a result of prolonged use of nasal decongestant sprays, in which rebound nasal inflammation and obstruction develop after discontinuation.

R Nasal foreign bodies lead to a localized inflammation response. Any history of nasal trauma should raise suspicion for giant cell reparative granuloma, which is typically a midline, septal lesion. It is the result of a reactive process thought to occur due to intraosseous hemorrhage following trauma.

S Drug abuse with cocaine or other nasal inhalants and chemical exposure (cigarette smoke, pollution) are other potential sources of nasal inflammation. Inhalation of prescription opioid-acetaminophen medications has been reported recently. Recognition of this entity is important. Typical findings include nasal pain, tissue necrosis, potential septal perforation, and noninvasive fungal colonization. Treatment includes abstinence and debridement of associated fibrinous necrotic tissue.

SUGGESTED READING

Adelson BF, Marple MW, Ryan. Fungal rhinosinusitis. In: Johnson JT, Rosen CA (Eds). Bailey's Head and Neck Surgery—Otolaryngology, 5th edition. Philadelphia, PA: Wolters Kluwer Health/Lippincott Williams & Wilkins; 2014. pp. 557-572.

Gubbels SP, Barkhuizen A, Hwang PH. Head and neck manifestations of Wegener's granulomatosis. Otolaryngol Clin North Am. 2003;36(4):685-705.

Jackson RS, McCaffrey TV. Nasal manifestations of systemic disease. In: Flint PW, Haughey BH, Lund VJ, et al. (Eds). Cummings Otolaryngology Head & Neck Surgery, 6th edition. Philadelphia, PA: Saunders/Elsevier; 2015. pp. 201-207.

Schreiber BE, Twigg S, Marais J, et al. Saddle-nose deformities in the rheumatology clinic. Ear Nose Throat J. 2014;93(4-5):E45-47.

Sindwani R, Cohen JT, Pilch BZ, et al. Myospherulosis following sinus surgery: pathological curiosity or important clinical entity? Laryngoscope. 2003;113(7):1123-1127.

Spellberg B, Edwards J Jr, Ibrahim A. Novel perspectives on mucormycosis: pathophysiology, presentation, and management. Clin Microbiol Rev. 2005;18(3):556-569.

Vosler PS, Ferguson BJ, Contreras JI, et al. Clinical and pathologic characteristics of intranasal abuse of combined opioid-acetaminophen medications. Int Forum Allergy Rhinol. 2014;4(10):839-844.

Zimmer LA, Carrau RL. Neoplasms of the nose and paranasal sinuses. In: Johnson, JT, Rosen CA (Eds). Bailey's Head and Neck Surgery—Otolaryngology, 5th edition. Philadelphia, PA: Wolters Kluwer Health/Lippincott Williams & Wilkins; 2014. pp. 2044-2062.

Zopf DA, Zacharek MA. Systemic diseases that affect the nose and sinuses. In: Johnson JT, Rosen CA (Eds). Bailey's Head and Neck Surgery—Otolaryngology, 5th edition. Philadelphia, PA: Wolters Kluwer Health/Lippincott Williams & Wilkins; 2014. pp. 489-500.

Carcinoma of the Nasopharynx

Sheng-Po Hao

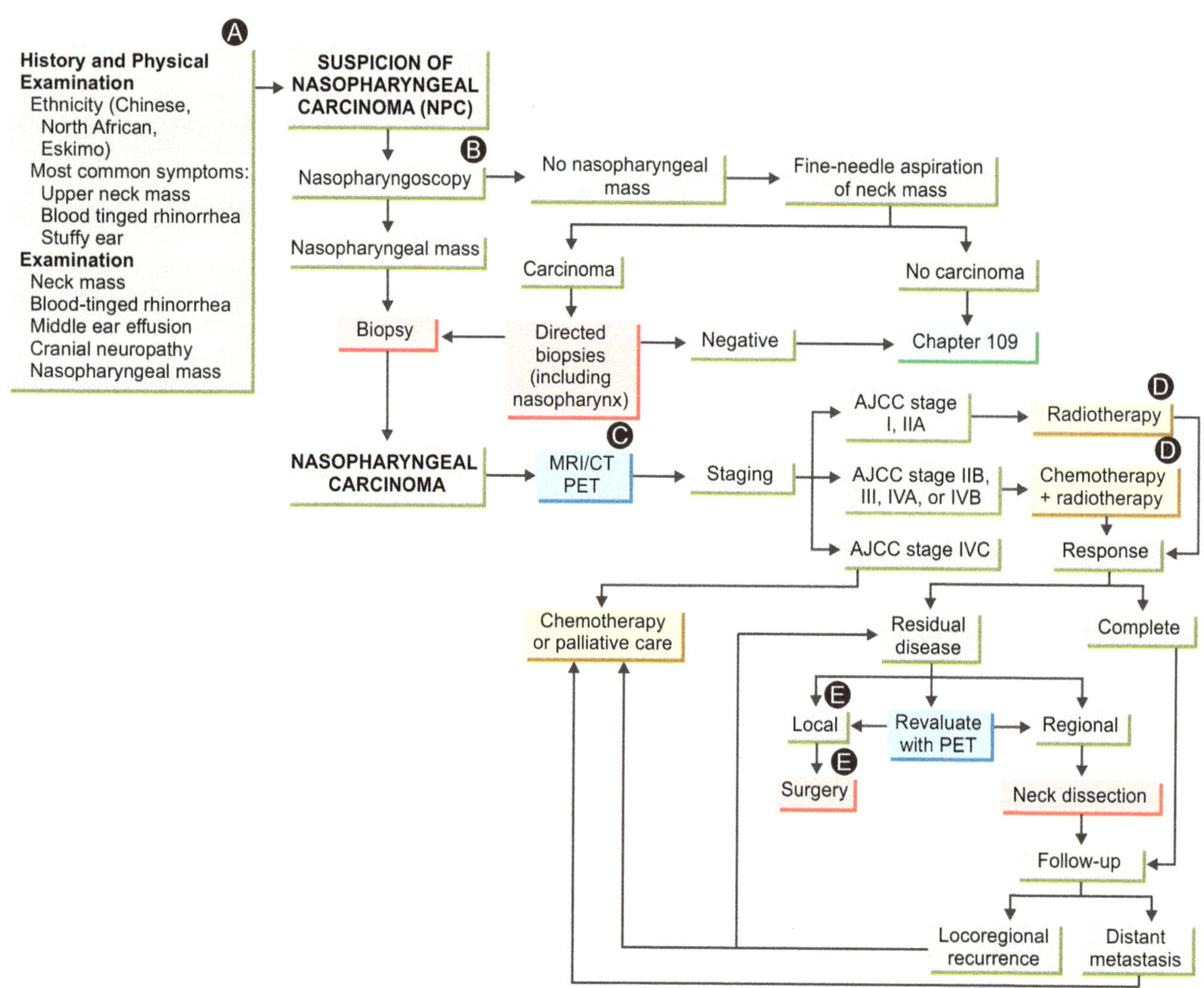

Nasopharyngeal carcinoma (NPC) is a squamous cell carcinoma arising from the nasopharynx. This neoplasm is frequently seen in the fossa of Rosenmüller posteromedial to the medial crura of the Eustachian tube opening in the nasopharynx.

NPC is a unique malignancy with an endemic distribution among certain ethnic geographic groups. The NPC is one of the most common head and neck cancers among Chinese. The NPC affects relatively younger patients, with a median age of 46 years old. The NPC is a male predominant cancer with a 3:1 male-to-female ratio.

NPC is a rare cancer among Caucasians. However, a high incidence of NPC is noted in American born Chinese, although the incidence is lower than that of China. These findings impose an interaction among geographic, ethnic, and environmental etiologic factors for NPC.

A Epstein–Barr virus (EBV), a double-stranded DNA virus, is closely related to NPC. Almost every NPC tumor cell carries clonal EBV genomes and expresses EBV proteins. The NPC becomes a model for EBV viral carcinogenesis. The EBV can be used as a biomarker in the screening, diagnosis, and monitoring of NPC. Serological markers such as EBC VCA IgA and DNase are used for general population screening. The EBV DNA copy numbers in plasma measured by real-time polymerase chain reaction methods could be used as a prognosticator to monitor treatment response and to follow up for recurrence. The main clinical symptomatology of NPC patients can be categorized into:

1. *Nasal symptoms*: Unilateral nasal obstruction with blood-tinged nasal discharge, epistaxis, and more

frequently blood-stained posterior nasal discharge in the early morning.

2. *Aural symptoms*: Stuffy ear, Eustachian tube dysfunction, or middle ear effusion is not rare. In endemic areas, adults presenting with middle ear effusion without obvious upper respiratory tract symptoms should raise the suspicion of NPC.

3. *Neck masses*: The most common mode of presentation of NPC is a painless unilateral or sometimes bilateral upper cervical masses, accounting for 60% of the NPC. The first echelon node of NPC is actually the retropharyngeal node, which is not palpable. The subdigastric or jugulodigastric nodes are commonly the first palpable nodes. The lymphatic metastasis can also happen along the spinal accessory chain to the posterior cervical triangle.

4. *Skull base and cranial nerves symptoms*: The patients may present with intractable headache when the skull base or dura are involved. Abducens palsy from VI cranial nerve involvement is not rare. Patients may also present with unilateral facial NPC, which poses a high distant metastatic rate (16%), mainly to bone, liver and lung.

B Appropriate diagnostic office-based procedures.
Inspection of the nasopharynx requires the use of a mirror or a fiberoptic nasopharyngoscope. Nasopharyngoscopy, both flexible and rigid, are important tools in examination of the nasopharynx. Rigid nasopharyngoscopy is usually used to guide a biopsy.

C Recommended imaging studies.
Computed tomography (CT) and/or magnetic resonance imaging (MRI) are for diagnosis, tumor extent, clinical staging, and treatment planning. The MRI appears to be better than CT for soft-tissue invasion, perineural invasion, retropharyngeal nodes, and skull base involvement. The MRI should be the imaging modality of choice for NPC. As distant metastases are not uncommon, a positron emission tomography is recommended for all patients with lymph node metastasis.

D Treatment
Currently available therapies for NPC are radiotherapy (RT), chemotherapy, or combination of both. NPC is highly radiosensitive. Early-staged patients have a high cure rate after RT. Concurrent chemoradiotherapy is the standard treatment for patients with advanced locoregional disease. Three-dimensional conformal RT and intensity-modulated radiation therapy (IMRT) technique spares normal tissues from a heavy radiation dose, thereby decreasing complications, but also offers excellent tumor control. The treatment of NPC with current techniques of RT can achieve >80% local control.

However, local failure (persistence and recurrence in the nasopharynx) occurs in 16% of the patients with NPC after initial RT.

E Salvage treatment after radiation failure.
Salvage nasopharyngectomy is the mainstay of treatment after radiation failure. Various surgical approaches to the nasopharynx have been developed, such as transpalatal, transmaxillary, mandibulotomy, facial translocation, and infratemporal fossa approaches. Recently, endoscopic nasopharyngectomy has gained popularity, especially for the small mucosal recurrence. Different approaches should be adopted on the basis of the tumor extent. In general, endoscopic approach is indicated in small or mucosal recurrence within the nasopharynx. Transfacial approaches, such as maxillary swing or (modified) facial translocation, are indicated in tumors with lateral extension. Involvement of the skull base or transcranial extension requires craniofacial resection. The surgical results of local control and overall survival rate for rNPC falls on 40–55%/5 years. Negative surgical margin is a most significant prognosticator for local control and survival. The recent introduction of a flexible robot seems promising in this setting.

SUGGESTED READING

Chang KP, Hsu CL, Chang YL, et al. Complementary serum test of antibodies to Epstein-Barr virus nuclear antigen-1 and early antigen: a possible alternative for primary screening of nasopharyngeal carcinoma. Oral Oncol. 2008;44:784-792.

Cheng SH, Liu TW, Jian JJ, et al. Concomitant chemotherapy and radiotherapy for locally advanced nasopharyngeal carcinoma. Cancer J Sci Am. 1997;3:100-106.

Hao SP, Myers E, Ferris R. Endoscopic nasopharyngectomy. Master techniques in otolaryngology—head and neck surgery. Head Neck Surg. 2013;2:271-277.

Hao SP, Tsang NM. Surgical management of recurrent nasopharyngeal carcinoma. Chang Gung Med J. 2010;33:361-369.

Hao SP, Tsang NM, Chang KP, et al. Nasopharyngectomy for recurrent nasopharyngeal carcinoma: a review of 53 patients and prognostic factors. Acta Otolaryngol. 2008;128:473-481.

Lin JC, Wang WY, Chen KY, et al. Quantification of plasma Epstein-Barr virus DNA in patients with advanced nasopharyngeal carcinoma. N Engl J Med. 2004;350:2461-2470.

Ng SH, Liu HM, Ko SF, et al. Posttreatment imaging of the nasopharynx. Eur J Radiol. 2002;44:82-95.

Ong YK. Endoscopic nasopharyngectomy and its role in managing locally recurrent NPC. Otolaryngol Clin N Am. 2011;44:1141-1154.

Wei WI. Surgical salvage of persistent or rNPC with maxillary swing approach—critical appraisal after 2 decades. Head Neck. 2011;33:969-975.

Intracranial Extension of Cancer of the Sinonasal Tract

Henry P Barham, Daniel W Nuss

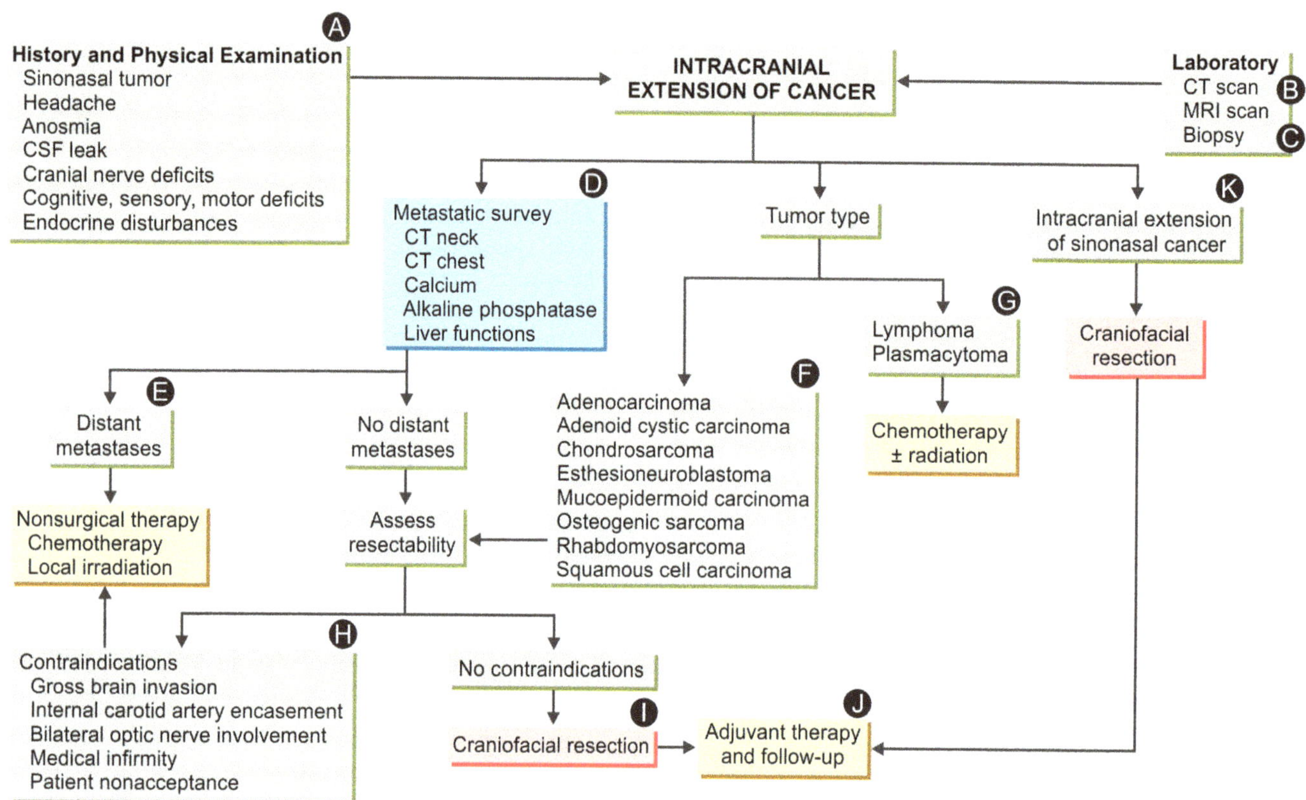

Cancer or tumors of the sinonasal tract (nasal cavity, paranasal sinuses, nasopharynx) can extend intracranially by several mechanisms: (1) direct erosion of bone; (2) through preexisting pathways (e.g. olfactory foramina); and (3) by involvement of adjacent compartments that have intracranial connections (e.g. orbit and orbital fissures; infratemporal fossa and foramen ovale).

A Symptoms are initially nonspecific, often beginning with headache, but may also include anosmia, cerebrospinal fluid (CSF) leak if dura has been invaded, and visual or oculomotor disturbance when the orbit is also involved. Cavernous sinus syndrome (ophthalmoplegia and facial numbness) may occur when the process extends to the orbital apex. Cognitive, sensory, and motor deficits may develop when intracranial mass effect is significant. Endocrinopathies may result from invasion of the sella or hypothalamus or from interference with their blood supply.

B Anatomic confirmation of intracranial extension of cancer relies on computed tomography (CT), magnetic resonance imaging (MRI), or both. CT demonstrates details of bony erosion of the cranial base and expansion of foramina or fissures. MRI affords better detail in imaging the brain and cranial nerves, especially the sometimes subtle appearance of early dural invasion. The two studies are complimentary, and often both are necessary.

C Histopathologic verification of cancer must be established by appropriate biopsy of a representative portion of the tumor, which may be accomplished by a direct transnasal route or via the affected sinus(es). When histopathology is indeterminate, immunohistochemical techniques may be necessary to accurately identify the tumor. This is especially important with small cell neoplasms, which can represent such diverse tumors as undifferentiated carcinoma, esthesioneuroblastoma, lymphoma, plasmacytoma, and embryonal rhabdomyosarcoma.

D Once intracranial extension of cancer has been diagnosed, a metastatic survey must be done to determine whether systemic disease is present (PET-CT scan). CT scans of the neck and chest (common sites of metastasis from sinonasal cancers), serum calcium and alkaline phosphatase levels (to detect bone metastasis), and liver function studies are suggested.

E Surgical resection is generally contraindicated if distant metastases are present. Depending on the histology, however, systemic chemotherapy can provide excellent responses with occasional cures (e.g. rhabdomyosarcoma, esthesioneuroblastoma). Local irradiation may also be used to achieve improved local disease control. If widespread metastasis has occurred with high-grade malignancies such as squamous cell carcinoma, consideration may be given to palliative treatment only, including pain control and nutritional support. Note that the presence of cervical (regional) metastases in the absence of distant metastases does not contraindicate surgical treatment of the primary lesion, but the metastasis to the neck will also need to be treated.

F Treatment of cancer involving the cranium varies significantly with tumor type. Lesions generally regarded as "surgical" (i.e. best survivals are observed in patients whose treatment includes surgical resection) include squamous cell carcinoma (SCCa), adenocarcinoma, adenoid cystic carcinoma, mucoepidermoid carcinoma, osteogenic sarcoma, and chondrosarcoma. Lesions for which complete resection improves survival but that respond well to chemotherapy/radiation, include esthesioneuroblastoma and rhabdomyosarcoma, the latter of which is nearly always treated with multimodality therapy.

G Lymphoma and plasmacytoma are treated with chemotherapy with or without radiation depending on the stage.

H Generally accepted contraindications to craniofacial resection include extensive invasion of brain parenchyma, encasement of the internal carotid artery by tumor, and bilateral involvement of the optic nerves, because surgery in these situations tends to produce limited oncologic benefit, high morbidity and poor functional outcomes. Extreme medical infirmity is a relative contraindication because of the risks of extensive surgery and anesthesia. Another relative contraindication is a patient's inability or unwillingness to accept the potential for substantial dysfunction.

I If no contraindications to surgery exist, surgical resection is recommended for tumor types mentioned in step F and other lesions that exhibit similar biological behavior. A variety of approaches to the anterior cranial base ("craniofacial resections") have been described that combine the neurosurgical and rhinological techniques. Collaboration with Neurosurgical colleagues preoperatively, intraoperatively, and postoperatively is imperative in the safe and successful management of sinonasal cancer that extends intracranially. Orbital exenteration may also be considered when cancer penetrates the periorbita, causing involvement of extraocular muscles and vision changes.

J When surgical resection is performed, it is imperative to follow a stepwise approach to reconstruction. If dura is resected, multilayered grafting techniques are employed to create an air and water tight closure to prevent CSF rhinorrhea or pneumocephalus. Various commercially available grafts (Alloderm, DuraGen, DuraMatrix) may be used to replace the section of resected dura. The pedicled rotational nasoseptal flap based on the posterior septal branch of the sphenopalatine artery has become the most widely used rhinological technique to reconstruct skull base defects.

K Sinonasal cancer invading the cranium represents advanced disease with high risk of recurrence. For this reason, adjuvant therapy is nearly always used postoperatively (and in some cases, preoperatively) even when surgical resection has been successfully accomplished. Adjuvant treatments may consist of radiation, chemotherapy, or both. Selection and timing of adjuvant treatments depend of tumor histopathology, initial tumor extent, and degree of expected radiosensitivity and chemoresponsiveness. Tumors in pediatric patients are often regarded as biologically different from the same tumors in adults; thus, pediatric patients are more commonly treated with adjuvant chemotherapy both pre- and postoperatively. After treatment, all patients should receive close follow-up at regular intervals for the long-term.

SUGGESTED READING

Bilsky MH, Kraus DH, Strong EW, et al. Extended anterior craniofacial resection for intracranial extension of malignant tumors. Am J Surg. 1997;174(5):565-568.

Carrau RL, Segas J, Nuss DW, et al. Squamous cell carcinoma of the sinonasal tract invading the orbit. Laryngoscope. 1999;109(2 Pt 1):230-235.

Harvey RJ, Malek J, Winder M, et al. Sinonasal morbidity following tumour resection with and without nasoseptal flap reconstruction. Rhinology. 2015;53(2):122-128.

Harvey RJ, Winder M, Davidson A, et al. The olfactory strip and its preservation in endoscopic pituitary surgery maintains smell and sinonasal function. J Neurol Surg B Skull Base. 2015;76(6):464-470.

Levine PA, Debo RF, Meredith SD, et al. Craniofacial resection at the University of Virginia (1976-1992): survival analysis. Head Neck. 1994;16(6):574-577.

Nuss DW, Rigby PL. Head and neck neoplasms with skull base involvement. In: Arriaga M, Day J. (Eds.) Neurosurgical Issues in Otolaryngology: Principles and Practice of Collaboration. Philadelphia: Lippincott Williams & Wilkins; 1999. pp. 309-340.

Shah JP, Kraus DH, Bilsky MH, et al. Craniofacial resection for malignant tumors involving the anterior skull base. Arch Otolaryngol Head Neck Surg. 1997;123(12):1312-1317.

CHAPTER 72

Approaches to Tumors of the Skull Base

Nicholas R Rowan, Eric W Wang

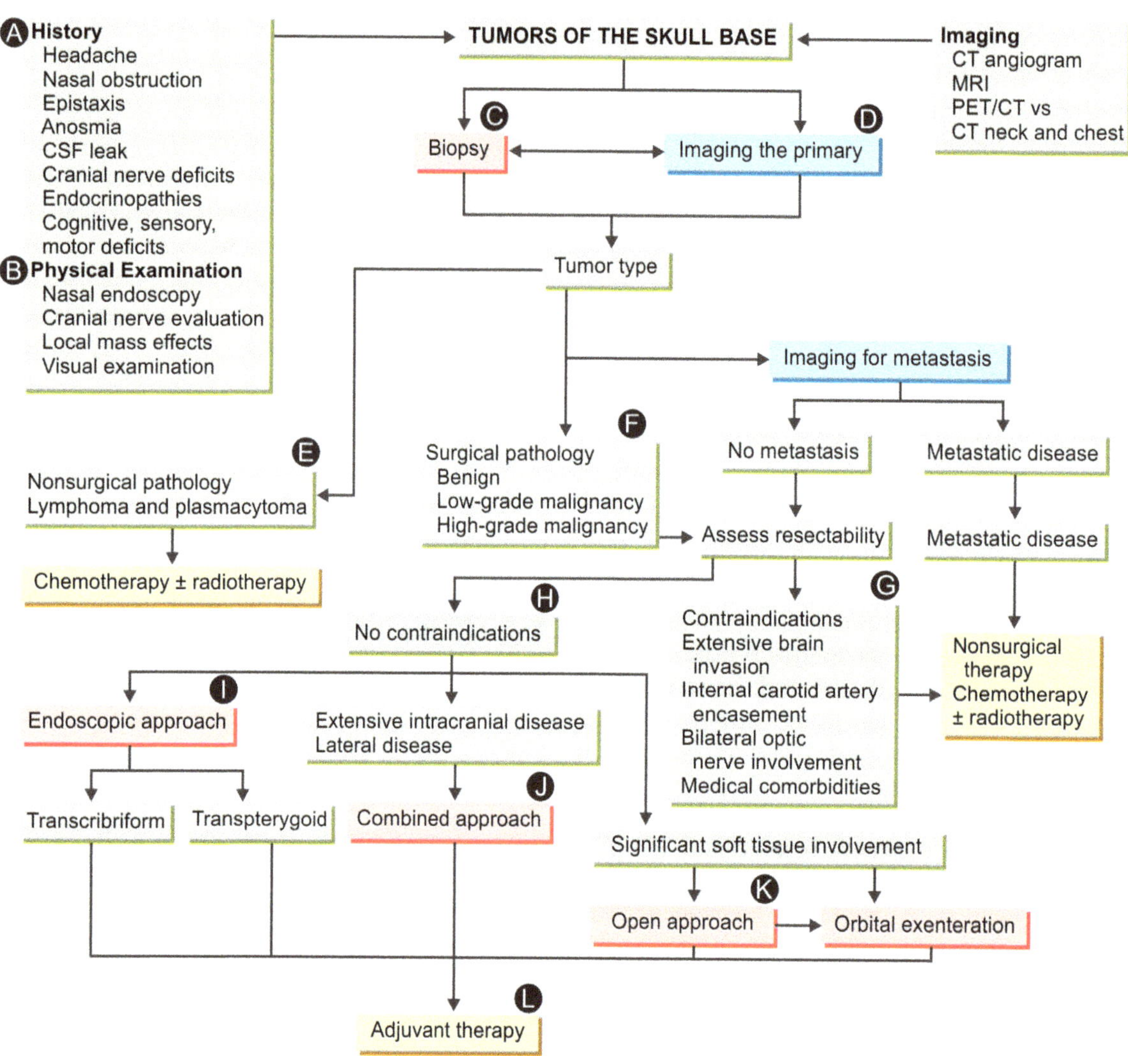

Tumors of the skull base encompass a diverse range of benign and malignant pathologies. Increasingly, the endoscopic endonasal corridor is used in the surgical management of these tumors. Due to the complex anatomy, patients should undergo multidisciplinary evaluation and management.

A Tumors of the nasal cavity and skull base may have an insidious onset and present most commonly with nasal obstruction. Nonspecific sinus-related complaints, epistaxis, or a nasal mass are also common at presentation. Symptoms vary depending on the involved anatomic subsite and may include but are not limited to, anosmia, facial pressure or pain, cerebrospinal fluid leaks, proptosis, visual disturbances, endocrinopathies, or rarely overt cognitive, sensory and motor deficits.

B Physical examination of the head and neck includes otoscopic evaluation for middle ear effusions, nasal endoscopy, complete cranial nerve evaluation, and palpation of the neck. Although findings may initially be largely unremarkable, cranial nerve deficits or local mass effects from tumor (e.g. proptosis) may be present with advanced disease.

C Tissue diagnosis can be obtained in an outpatient office setting or in an operating room setting in the case of vascular-appearing tumors (e.g. juvenile angiofibromas) with which caution should be used due to the potential bleeding. Biopsy should be deferred until after imaging is completed so that the characteristics of the lesion are better described.

D Extent of disease is best determined by evaluation with both computed tomography (CT) and magnetic resonance imaging (MRI), which are complementary. A CT angiogram with image guidance best demonstrates both bone involvement and vasculature involving the tumor; it is critical for preoperative planning and image-guided surgery. Meanwhile, MRI is more capable of depicting extent of soft-tissue disease and involvement of the orbit and dura. If tissue biopsy reveals malignancy, a metastatic evaluation including either positron emission tomography/CT or CT of the neck and chest is warranted.

E Primary chemotherapy, radiotherapy, or a combination thereof must be considered for nonsurgical disease processes such as lymphoma and plasmacytoma.

F Tumors of the skull base may be categorized as benign, low-grade malignancy, or high-grade malignancy as a guide for the type of primary and adjuvant therapy that will be required.

G There is no clear consensus regarding absolute contraindications to surgical resection; however, generally accepted contraindications include extensive invasion of the brain parenchyma, encasement of the internal carotid artery bilateral involvement of the optic nerves, and limited oncologic or functional benefit of surgery. Medical comorbidities may also be considered a relative contraindication given the serious risks associated with skull base surgery, the required anesthesia, and there are potential perioperative complications.

H If there are no contraindications to surgery, the surgical approach is dictated by the tumor pathology and the extent of the disease. Endoscopic approaches are preferred whenever possible given improved perioperative morbidities, excellent visualization, and equivalent survival rates as compared to traditional open techniques.

I Purely endoscopic approaches can be used to address a wide range of skull base pathologies of the anterior and middle cranial fossa. In general, unilateral or bilateral transcribriform approaches are used to address anterior cranial base pathologies while transpterygoid approaches are used to gain access to the pterygopalatine fossa, infratemporal fossa, and middle cranial fossa.

J Combined endoscopic and open approaches may be undertaken when the tumor cannot be accessed exclusively with an endonasal approach, such as cases with significant lateral extent of disease (past the midplane of the of the roof of the orbit), need for orbital exenteration, or an extensive intracranial component.

K Conventional open approaches are employed less commonly but may be required when there is significant soft-tissue involvement or the requirement for orbital exenteration. This can be combined with endoscopic approaches for the nasal component of the tumor.

L In cases where adjuvant therapy is required, selection and timing of therapy is dictated by tumor histopathology, initial tumor extent, surgical margins, and degree of expected radiosensitivity and chemoresponsiveness.

SUGGESTED READING

Carrau RL, Snyderman CH, Vescan AD, et al. Surgery of the anterior cranial base. Oper Otolaryngol Head Neck Surg. 2008;100: 979-996.

Farag A, Rosen M, Evans J. Surgical techniques for sinonasal malignancies. Neurosurg Clin of North Am. 2015;26(3):403-412.

Hanna E, DeMonte F, Ibrahim S, et al. Endoscopic resection of sinonasal cancers with and without craniotomy: oncologic results. Arch Otolaryngol Head Neck Surg. 2009;135(12):1219-1224.

Kassam A, Snyderman C2H, Mintz A, et al. Expanded endonasal approach: the rostrocaudal axis. Part I. Crista galli to the sella turcica. Neurosurg Focus. 2005;19:E3.

Kassam A, Snyderman CH, Mintz A, et al. Expanded endonasal approach: the rostrocaudal axis. Part II. Posterior clinoids to foramen magnum. Neurosurg Focus. 2005;19:E4.

Peng KA, Kita AE, Suh JD, et al. Sinonasal lymphoma: case series and review of the literature. Int Forum Allergy Rhinol. 2014;4: 670-674.

Complications of Endoscopic Sinus Surgery

Adam M Zanation, Dipan D Desai

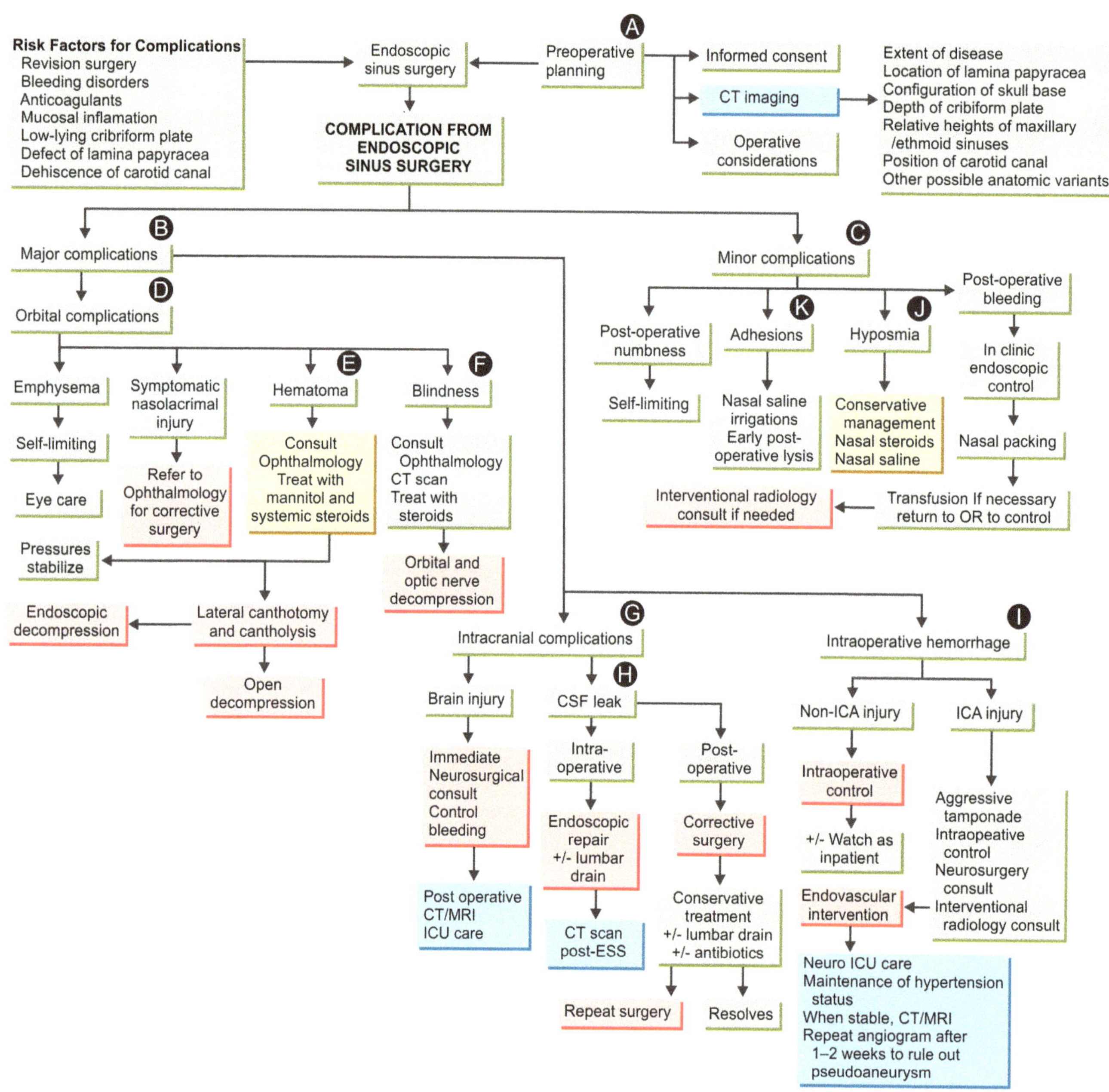

Prevention of complications is the optimal solution to the problem of adverse outcomes following endoscopic sinus surgery (ESS). Prevention begins with preoperative planning and extends throughout the surgical procedure. This algorithm begins when attempts at prevention have failed.

A A thorough understanding and preoperative review of the patient's anatomy is critical in preventing complications. Computerized tomography (CT) scan is the most commonly ordered preoperative imaging test and should be examined carefully in all three axis. Special attention should be given to evaluating the extent of disease, location and bony integrity of the lamina papyracea, configuration and height of the skull base, depth of the cribriform plate, relative heights of the maxillary/ethmoid sinuses, position and possible dehiscence of the carotid canal, and other possible anatomic variants. A discussion of potential complications, risks and benefits of the procedure with the patient is mandatory. Within the OR, interventions including the use of total intravenous anesthesia, reverse Trendelenburg positioning, local injections of lidocaine with 1:100,000 epinephrine, and nasal pledgets soaked in cocaine or epinephrine can improve surgical visualization. Finally, the use of image-guided navigation systems has become more routine and is appropriate for technically difficult and revision cases.

B There are three categories of major complications from ESS: orbital complications, hemorrhage, and intracranial injury. Major complications occur in <1.00% of ESS cases with hemorrhage being the most common.

C This group includes a variety of surgical complications that can typically be treated effectively and do not threaten the overall health of the patient. The combined incidence of minor complications following ESS has been shown to be 6.6% with postoperative bleeding comprising an estimated 75% of these.

D The close proximity of the orbit to the paranasal sinuses, as well as relative fragility of the lamina papyracea, predisposes this area to injury during ESS. These complications have been found to occur in 0.12% of ESS procedures and can be devastating. This group includes several potential complications that range in severity, including orbital hematoma, diplopia, emphysema, nasolacrimal injury, and blindness. Management of any of these complications begins with prompt Ophthalmologic consultation and measurement of intraocular pressures.

E Orbital hematoma is an Ophthalmologic emergency and requires prompt evaluation and treatment. This complication occurs when either a venous or arterial vessel, commonly the anterior ethmoidal artery which is located inferior to the skull base and is dehiscent in ~80% of patients, begins to bleed into the enclosed orbital space and increases orbital pressures. Elevated intraorbital pressures from arterial-fed hematomas can result in blindness within 1 hour if untreated, and physical signs such as proptosis, anisocoria, or opthalmoplegia indicate a need for urgent intervention. Administration of mannitol and steroids, elevation of the head, and removal of nasal packing are typically attempted initially. If these measures are not effective, a lateral canthotomy and cantholysis is typically performed to quickly lower intraocular pressure. Endoscopic or open orbital decompression with a simultaneous Ophthalmology consult is then performed.

F Blindness following ESS can be caused by increased orbital pressure, inflammatory neuropathy, or optic nerve injury at a location in the orbit, sphenoid sinus, or an Onodi cell. After obtaining Ophthalmologic consultation, orbital decompression and systemic steroid treatment may be helpful and can lead to improvement in visual acuity in some cases. A post-ESS fine-cut CT is mandatory to evaluate the bony confines of the optic canal.

G Intracranial complications are relatively rare and occur in ~0.13–0.17% of ESS cases. Violation of the anterior skull base most commonly occurs medially at the junction of the cribriform plate and roof of the ethmoid. Detailed preoperative assessment of imaging is required to prevent these complications during surgery. Specifically, surgeons should evaluate for disease involvement and dehiscence of the skull base, as well as type 3 Keros classification of the olfactory fossa.

H Cerebrospinal fluid leak is the most common intracranial complication and can potentially lead to serious sequelae, such as meningitis. Leaks discovered intraoperatively can be patched immediately using one of several options, including nasal vascularized flaps, adipose tissue, temporalis fascia, and acellular dermal grafts, and then sealed with fibrin glue. However, leaks discovered postoperatively are typically more difficult to locate and treat. A leak can be confirmed by detection of β-2 transferrin in secretions, and endoscopic examination or computed tomography cisternogram can be helpful with localizing the site of the leak. Persistent leaks that do not resolve with 1–2 weeks of conservative therapy consisting of strict bed rest and subarachnoid drainage via a lumbar drain should undergo surgical repair. In general, we recommend early surgical repair for persistent leaks instead of prolonged conservative management.

I Hemorrhage is a rare but serious complication of ESS. The most common sites of injury include the ethmoidal arteries and the posterior septal branches of the sphenopalatine artery; these injuries can typically be controlled effectively in the operating room. Internal carotid artery (ICA) injury most commonly occurs during sphenoid sinusotomy and can result in stroke or death. Suggested treatment of ICA injury begins with immediate, aggressive packing followed by transfer to interventional radiology for endovascular intervention. Postoperative imaging and ICU (intensive care unit) care are mandatory.

J The majority of ESS patients report preoperative hyposmia. Residual conditions such as infection or allergy can impair the sense of smell postoperatively; hence, patients should be counseled that symptoms of hyposmia might not improve after ESS.

K Postoperative adhesions can be prevented by regular saline nasal irrigations by the patient after surgery. Any loose crusting or adhesions in the nasal cavity or sinuses should be debrided during postoperative outpatient visits to prevent future dysfunction and scarring. However, debridement of fixed crusts can lead to mucosal damage and should be avoided.

SUGGESTED READING

Krings JG, Kallogjeri D, Wineland A, et al. Complications of primary and revision functional endoscopic sinus surgery for chronic rhinosinusitis. Laryngoscope. 2013;124(4):838-845.

Ramakrishnan VR, Kingdom TT, Nayak JV, et al. Nationwide incidence of major complications in endoscopic sinus surgery. Int Forum Allergy Rhinol. 2011;2(1):34-39.

Stankiewicz JA, Lal D, Connor M, et al. Complications in endoscopic sinus surgery for chronic rhinosinusitis. Laryngoscope. 2011;121(12):2684-2701.

Svider PF, Baredes S, Eloy JA. Pitfalls in sinus surgery. Otolaryngol Clin North Am. 2015;48(5):725-737.

Timperley D, Sacks R, Parkinson RJ, et al. Perioperative and Intraoperative maneuvers to optimize surgical outcomes in skull base surgery. Otolaryngol Clin North Am. 2010;43(4):699-730.

Dysphagia

Benjamin J Rubinstein, Craig S Derkay

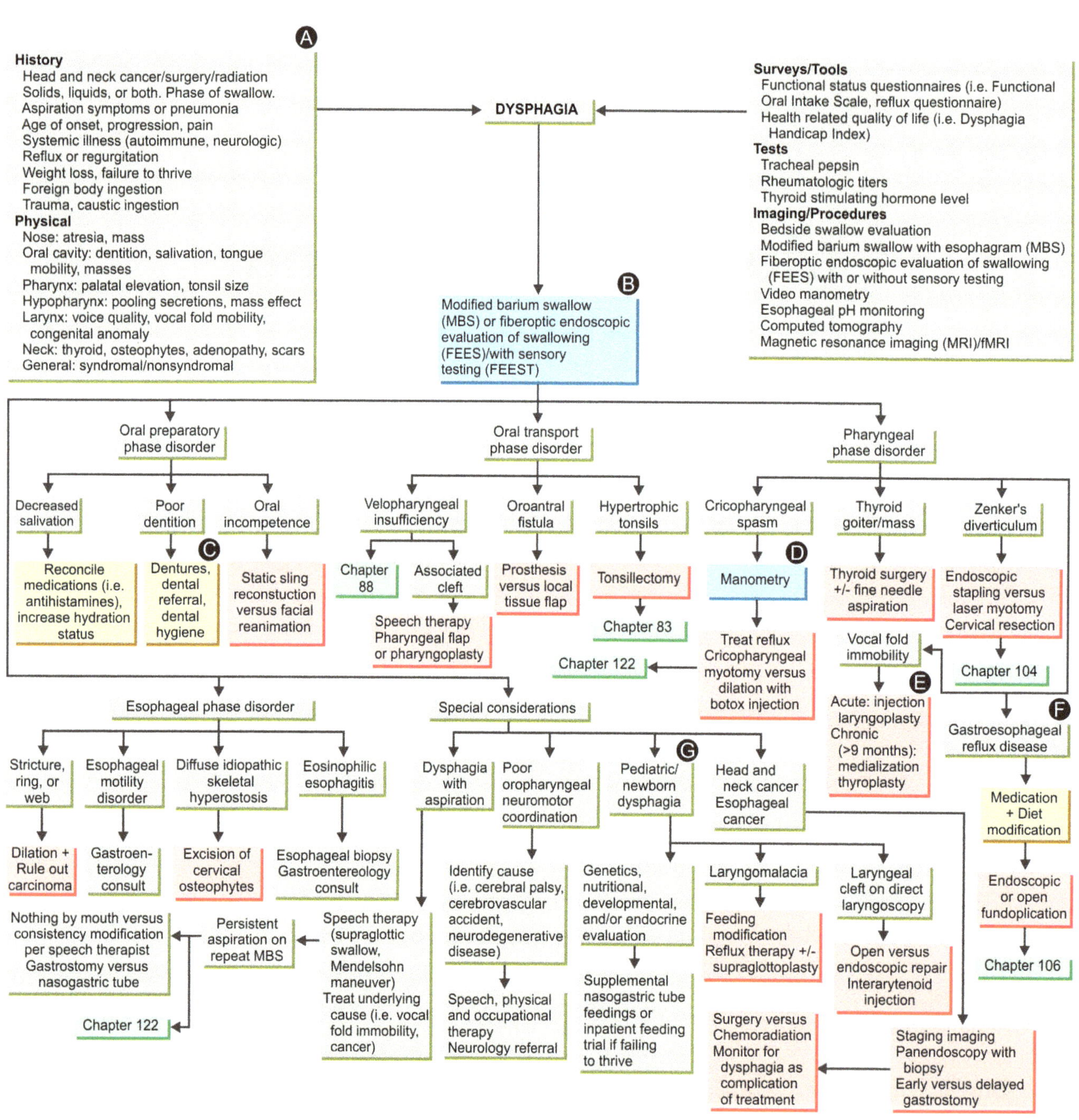

Dysphagia is a common complaint that can suggest dysfunction at any of the four phases of swallowing. A critical component in the evaluation is to rule out the presence of aspiration that can be confirmed by diagnostic testing. Due to the association of dysphagia with head and neck cancer, flexible fiberoptic laryngoscopy is always indicated, particularly when the patient presents with insidious onset, significant weight loss, and referred pain.

Ⓐ Onset of symptoms in the newborn period may suggest an underlying congenital abnormality of the nasal or oral cavity, larynx, trachea, esophagus, or great vessels. Rapid progression of dysphagia may indicate an associated infectious cause or the presence of a foreign body. Symptoms of odynophagia and referred otalgia should prompt a thorough investigation for neoplasm.

B Fiberoptic endoscopic evaluation of swallowing (FEES) with or without sensory testing provides a direct view of anatomic features of swallowing and can be performed at the bedside of a hospitalized patient by a sole practitioner. The FEES is limited by a whiteout period during the pharyngeal phase of swallowing when aspiration or penetration typically occurs. Modified barium swallow (MBS) visualizes all phases of swallowing and can also identify cervical spine pathology. The MBS is limited by radiation exposure and the need for a radiology suite staffed by a speech pathologist and radiologist.

C It is important to clarify a patient's use of dentures during feeding. Dentures are important for mastication in the edentulous patient, but many patients remove their dentures during eating as they interfere with sensation of the food bolus on the palate. Identifying such tendencies allows for counseling regarding dietary modification.

D Manometric studies can help to confirm the diagnosis of cricopharyngeal spasm and achalasia but may not be necessary if the history and the MBS findings are suggestive.

E Medialization laryngoplasty can be of benefit in patients with aspiration and hoarseness due to vocal fold immobility. Patients with decreased laryngeal sensation or pooling of secretions on fiberoptic examination are less likely to benefit. Postprocedure swallow evaluation is critical.

F Dysphagia predominantly associated with a globus sensation most often is due to gastroesophageal reflux disorder.

G Dysphagia associated with respiratory insufficiency in young children should alert the clinician to the possibility of an associated lesion. In newborns, this may include nasal masses or choanal atresia, because they are obligate nasal breathers. Outside the newborn period, vallecular cysts, respiratory papillomatosis disease, lymphangiomas, and hemangiomas need to be included in the differential diagnosis. Dysphagia associated with aspiration in children raises the suspicion for a laryngotracheal cleft or congenital vocal fold paralysis. Arnold–Chiari malformation should be considered if there is bilateral vocal fold paralysis and associated mediastinal abnormality or a history of cardiac surgery in unilateral vocal fold paralysis.

ACKNOWLEDGMENT

Authors acknowledge the contributions of John T Sinacori, MD, in revising this chapter.

SUGGESTED READING

Altman KW, Richards A, Goldberg L, et al. Dysphagia in stroke, neurodegenerative disease, and advanced dementia. Otolaryngol Clin North Am. 2013;46(6):1137-1149.

Arrese LC, Lazarus CL. Special groups: head and neck cancer. Otolaryngol Clin North Am. 2013;46(6):1123-1136.

Brady S, Donzelli J. The modified barium swallow and the functional endoscopic evaluation of swallowing. Otolaryngol Clin North Am. 2013;46(6):1009-1022.

Chokhavatia S, Alli-Akintade L, Harpaz N, et al. Esophageal pathology: a brief guide and atlas. Otolaryngol Clin North Am. 2013;46(6):1043-1057.

Giraldez-Rodriguez LA, Johns M 3rd. Glottal insufficiency with aspiration risk in dysphagia. Otolaryngol Clin North Am. 2013;46(6):1113-1121.

Kuhn MA, Belafsky PC. Management of cricopharyngeus muscle dysfunction. Otolaryngol Clin North Am. 2013;46(6):1087-1099.

Patel D, Vaezi MF. Normal esophageal physiology and laryngopharyngeal reflux. Otolaryngol Clin North Am. 2013;46(6):1023-1041.

Prisman E, Genden EM. Zenker diverticulum. Otolaryngol Clin North Am. 2013;46(6):1101-1111.

Roden DF, Altman KW. Causes of dysphagia among different age groups: a systematic review of the literature. Otolaryngol Clin North Am. 2013;46(6):965-987.

Speyer R. Oropharyngeal dysphagia: screening and assessment. Otolaryngol Clin North Am. 2013;46(6):989-1008.

Drooling

Sam J Daniel

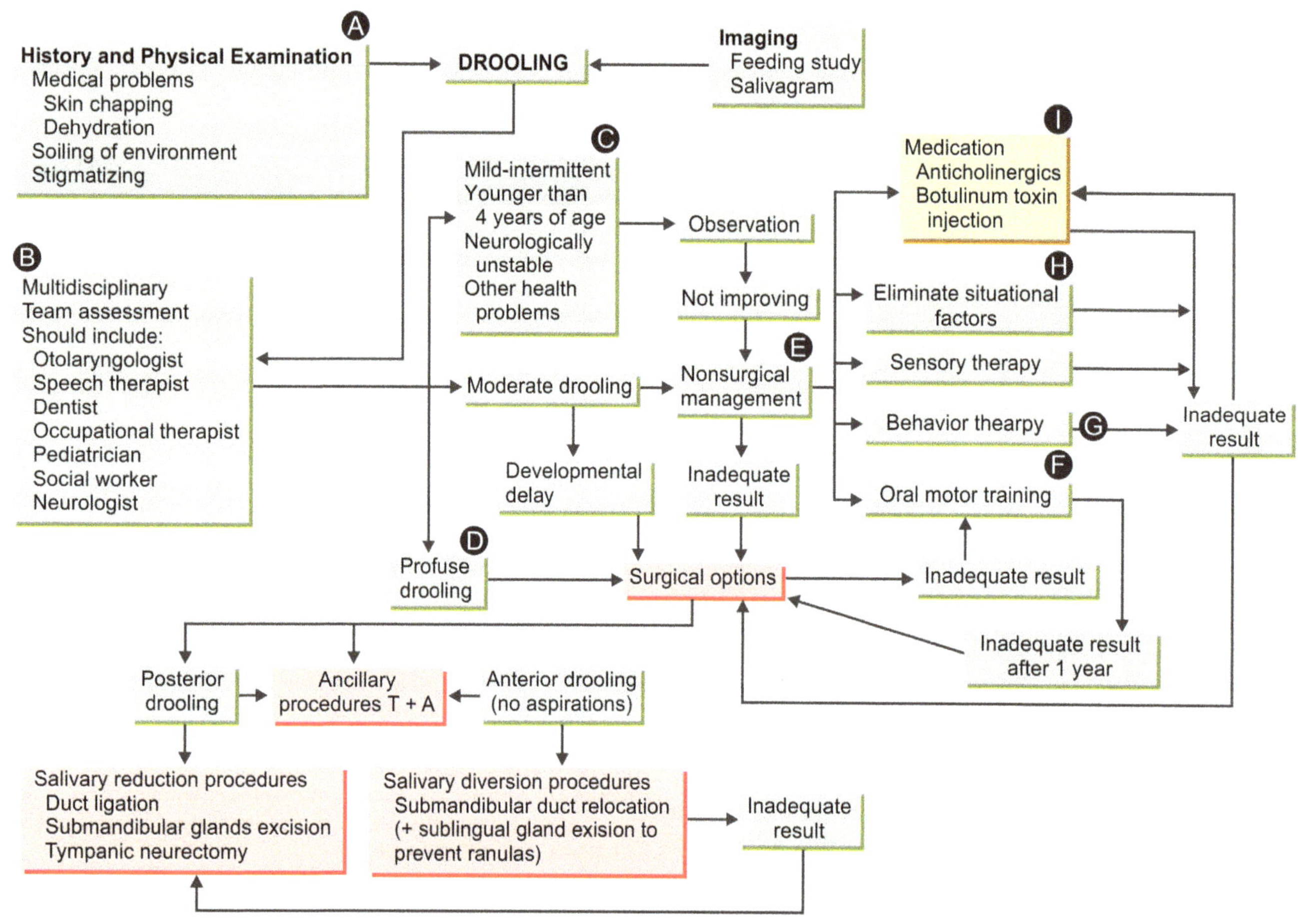

Drooling or sialorrhea is very common in young children and usually improves significantly by 2 years of age as oral motor skills and sensory function mature. It is seen more commonly in patients with associated neurological conditions, such as cerebral palsy or neuromuscular disorders, as it is typically caused by an inability to swallow saliva efficiently, rather than an overproduction of saliva. Drooling is considered pathological if it persists after the age of 4 years in healthy children with normal development.

A When evaluating a drooling patient, it is essential to classify them as having anterior or posterior drooling (could be both). In anterior drooling, saliva spills out of the oral cavity onto the lip and perioral areas. Patients with profuse anterior drooling may have chapping of the skin and dehydration. A disruptive component of soiling the environment can also be the stigmatizing impact on the patient and the burden on the caregivers. In posterior drooling, there is salivary spillage over the posterior tongue into the laryngeal area, which may manifest as a wet voice, congested breathing, gurgling, coughing, and at times, penetration into the airway, leading to aspiration pneumonia and pulmonary disease. The radionuclide salivagram is a sensitive imaging method for detecting pulmonary aspiration of saliva.

B In view of the complexity and multifactorial nature of drooling, patients should ideally be assessed by a multidisciplinary team that can present rehabilitative, medical, and surgical options to the patient and family.

C No treatment is recommended for patients who, on initial assessment, are having mild or intermittent drooling, are < 4 years, are not neurologically stable, and/or have other health problems of greater priority.

D Surgery is the treatment of choice in children with profuse anterior drooling, certain children with moderate drooling as some children improve over time with the maturation of their swallowing functions, and those who have failed adequate nonsurgical management. It is usually deferred until 6 years of age. Surgery is also the treatment of choice in patients with posterior drooling, and those requiring chronic and frequent care to manage secretions. Surgical options for drooling can be classified into procedures that reduce the quantity of saliva or those that divert saliva into the oropharynx. Salivary reduction procedures include excision of the submandibular gland, ligation of the duct and tympanic neurectomy. Salivary diversion procedures include submandibular duct rerouting and parotid duct rerouting. Ancillary surgical treatments that can help with drooling include tonsillectomy, adenoidectomy, turbinate reduction, tongue reduction, and craniofacial or orthodontic surgery.

E Nonsurgical treatment options consist of rehabilitation treatment options and pharmacotherapy. Rehabilitation treatment options include oral-motor therapy, sensory therapy to improve oral sensitivity, elimination of situational factors, and behavior therapy.

F Oral motor training designed to improve oral motor function (i.e. sucking, lip closure, lip and tongue mobility, jaw stability, oromotor coordination) is crucial. Ideally, all patients should receive a minimum of 6 months of such therapy.

G The goal of behavior therapy for drooling is to increase targeted behaviors, such as increasing the frequency of swallowing, closing the mouth, wiping the chin, and self-monitoring. It is best suited for patients with only a modest drooling problem and a high degree of cognitive function. Types of therapies include instruction, prompting, and positive reinforcement; cueing techniques; self-management procedures; and cognitive orientation to daily occupational performance.

H The elimination of situational factors may occasionally reduce drooling adequately. Such factors as poor seating (resulting in a head forward posture), dental or gingival disease (resulting in increased saliva production), correctable nasal airway obstruction (resulting in a mouth-open posture), or use of medications that result in increased saliva production should be addressed if possible.

I Medication options consist mainly of agents that block the cholinergic muscarinic parasympathetic receptors in the salivary glands such as glycopyrrolate, scopolamine and benzhexol. Using these drugs with significant side effects seems a poor long-term management choice in pediatric patients. I have extensive experience with botulinum toxin injections in the salivary glands as a safe and effective treatment option for sialorrhea. Injections can be done under local anesthesia, can avoid the systemic effects of oral agents, and the effect can last 3–9 months depending on the dosage, the injection technique, and the patient's response.

SUGGESTED READING

Cardona I, Saint-Martin C, Daniel SJ. Effect of recurrent onabotulinum toxin A injection into the salivary glands: an ultrasound measurement. Laryngoscope. 2015;125(10):E328-E332.

Cardona I, Saint-Martin C, Daniel SJ. Salivary glands of healthy children versus sialorrhea children, is there an anatomical difference? An ultrasonographic biometry. Int J Pediatr Otorhinolaryngol. 2015;79(5):644-647.

Crysdale WS, McCann C, Roske L, et al. Saliva control issues in the neurologically challenged. A 30-year experience in team management. Int J Pediatr Otorhinolaryngol. 2006;70(3):519-527.

Daniel SJ. Multidisciplinary management of sialorrhea in children. Laryngoscope. 2012;122:S67-68.

Daniel SJ. Controversies in the management of pediatric sialorrhea. Curr Otorhinolaryngol Rep. 2015;3(1):1-8.

Daniel SJ. Pediatric sialorrhea: medical and surgical options. Sataloff's Comprehensive Textbook of Otolaryngology: Head and Neck Surgery: Six Volume Set Hardcover – November 30, 2015.

Daniel SJ, Kanaan AA. Salivary gland disease in children. Cumm Pediatr Otolaryngol. 2014;22:293-308.

Rashnoo P, Daniel SJ. Drooling quantification: correlation of different techniques. Int J Pediatr Otorhinolaryngol. 2015;79(8):1201-1205.

Trismus

Peter N Demas

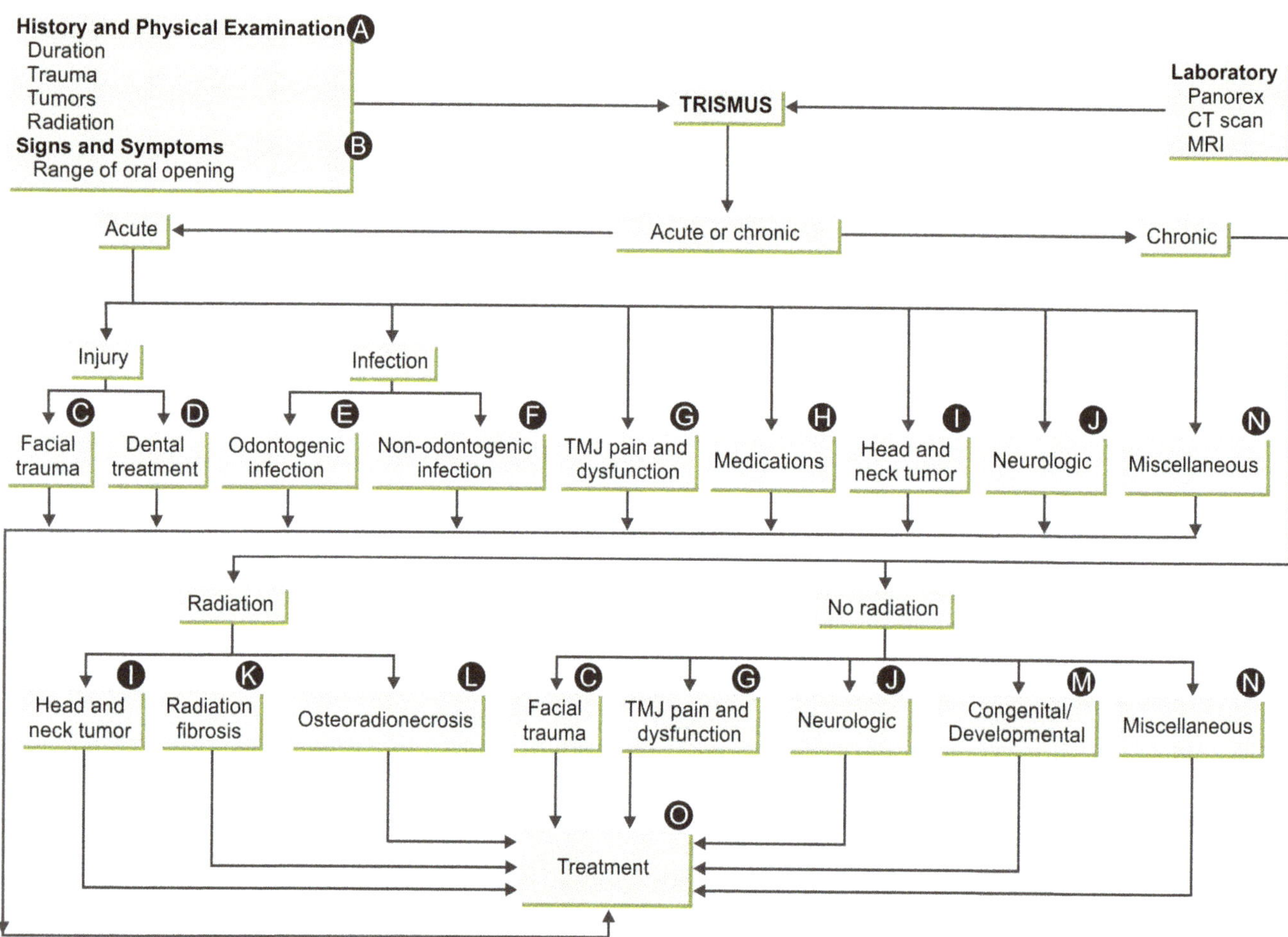

Trismus is defined as limited, painful opening of the oral cavity secondary to a spasm of the muscles of mastication. Trismus is less commonly used as a general term to describe restriction of mandibular opening movement, although alternatives such as mandibular hypomobility or temporomandibular joint (TMJ) ankylosis may be more accurate terms, if muscle spasm is absent.

The spasm or myotonic contraction causing pain originates in the involved muscles of mastication, which include the temporalis, masseter, and medial/internal and lateral/external pterygoid muscles.

Ⓐ The degree of associated muscle spasm and limitation of oral opening can vary with the etiology and present as an acute or chronic form. The acute form is of limited duration and resolves in 7–14 days after treatment, but resolving symptoms may linger for 1–2 months. Chronic trismus is associated with permanent altered tissue changes of the facial region effecting mandibular range of motion.

Ⓑ The normal range of oral opening between maxillary and mandibular incisors is > 40 mm. Limited oral opening can be classified as mild (30–40 mm), moderate (15–30 mm), and severe (< 15 mm). Generally males can open wider than females, based on increased dimension of the mandibular ramus and may open to 50–60 mm.

Ⓒ Trismus secondary to direct injury to the muscles of mastication may be associated with facial trauma of the adjacent mandible, maxilla, orbital bones, or the zygomatic arch. An isolated fracture of the zygomatic arch can cause trismus due to impingement of the arch on the medially positioned temporalis tendon inserting to the mandibular coronoid process.

Trismus can also occur in post-traumatic conditions with mandibular or condylar malunion, residual deformity of the zygomatic arch, infection of fixation plates, intraoral soft-tissue scar banding, masticatory muscle scarring, and disuse atrophy. Disuse atrophy in masticatory muscles occurs with prolonged intermaxillary fixation and results in chronic shortening of the muscle's myofibrils, causing pain and limited opening.

D Trismus subsequent to dental treatment may include local injection of an anesthetic, postsurgical edema after wisdom tooth extraction, dentoalveolar surgery, and prolonged dental therapy appointments (endodontics or complex restorative care).

Local anesthetic injection is one of the most common causes of trismus. It occurs acutely postdental treatment and is usually unilateral with minimal swelling, but significant muscle spasm, pain, and limitation of opening. The most common muscle involved is the medial pterygoid secondary to inferior alveolar nerve block, causing intramuscular bleeding and hematoma.

E Odontogenic infection is a frequent cause of trismus due to cellulitis from infection progressing from wisdom tooth pericoronitis or any dental infection advancing to the fascial spaces (buccal, submasseteric, medial pterygoid, infratemporal, lateral pharyngeal, retropharyngeal, superficial and deep temporal, sublingual, and submandibular). Treatment of Ludwig's Angina is often complicated by trismus.

F Nonodontogenic infections can involve the muscles of mastication, secondary to tonsillar or pharyngeal infection, parotitis, otitis, meningitis, osteomyelitis, TMJ (synovitis, infected prosthetic TM joint prosthesis), and the classic "lock jaw" of tetanus.

G Temporomandibular Joint dysfunction can cause acute or chronic trismus due to myofascial pain, TMJ dislocation, TMJ subluxation, bruxism, clenching, internal derangement of a displaced meniscus and intracapsular ankyloses, either fibrous or osseous. Rheumatoid arthritis or osteoarthritis degeneration can also have associated trismus.

H Medications can cause central nervous system extrapyramidal effects, inducing muscle spasm. The medications most often involved are antipsychotics (phenothiazines-haloperidol, fluphenazine), antiemetics (prochlorperazine, metoclopramide), and antidepressants (sertraline, fluoxetine).

I Tumors of the head and neck can infiltrate the muscles of mastication from the adjacent parotid gland, retromolar tissues, tonsils, infratemporal fossa, floor of mouth, submandibular or pharyngeal regions. The trismus may occur with primary or recurrent tumors. In addition, trismus may be associated with primary tumor of the condyle such as osteosarcoma or osteochondroma, betal nut-induced oral submucous fibrosis or Trotter's syndrome.

J Trismus from neurologic diseases associated with muscle spasticity can occur in seizures, cerebrovascular accident (CVA), Parkinson's disease, multiple sclerosis, amyotrophic lateral sclerosis, and dementia.

K Radiation treatment can cause trismus with muscle fiber stiffness and scarring within the temporalis, masseter, and internal and external pterygoid muscles. Radiation fibrosis is slowly progressive after the acute radiation tissue effects.

L Osteoradionecrosis can cause progressive infection of the mandible, maxilla, or cranial bones resulting in adjacent muscular trismus.

M Congenital and developmental conditions can have associated muscular trismus. These include a hyperplastic or hypertrophic coronoid process, TMJ ankylosis (fibrous or osseous), oral microstomia, hemifacial microsomia, epidermolysis bullosa, and Hecht's syndrome.

N Miscellaneous causes of trismus may include malignant hyperthermia, psychiatric hysteria, poisoning (Strychnine neurotoxin), facial burn contracture, giant cell arteritis, myositis ossificans, scleroderma (autoimmune), and chemotherapy-associated oral mucositis.

O Treatment depends on the inciting cause and can involve: analgesics, nonsteroidal anti-inflammatory drugs, antibiotics, warm or cold compresses, muscle massage, diet modification, muscle relaxants, physical therapy with active and passive range of motion activity using digital manipulation, tongue depressor guides, or commercial devices such as the Therabite by Atos Medical, bruxism splints, TENS with biofeedback therapy, botulinum toxin denervation and surgical intervention of drainage of infection, management of facial bone fractures, and treatment of cancers of the head and neck.

SUGGESTED READING

DeGowin EL, DeGowin RL. Bedside Diagnostic Examination. New York: Macmillan Publishing Company Inc; 1981.

Dolwick MF. Clinical diagnosis of temporomandibular joint internal derangement and myofascial pain and dysfunction. Oral Maxillofac Surg Clin North Am. 1989;1:1-11.

Hupp JR, Ellis E, Tucker MR. Contemporary Oral and Maxillofacial Surgery, 5th edition. St Louis, MO: Mosby Elsevier; 2008.

Online Dictionary.com. Dictionary.com, LLC. 2015.

Scully C, Bagan J, Carrozzo M, et al. Pocketbook of Oral Disease. New York: Churchill Livingstone-Elsevier; 2013.

Smith RA. Complications of local anesthesia in the oral and maxillofacial office. Oral Maxillofac Surg Clin North Am. 1990; 2:631-640.

Evaluation of Sleep-Disordered Breathing

David T Kent, Ryan J Soose

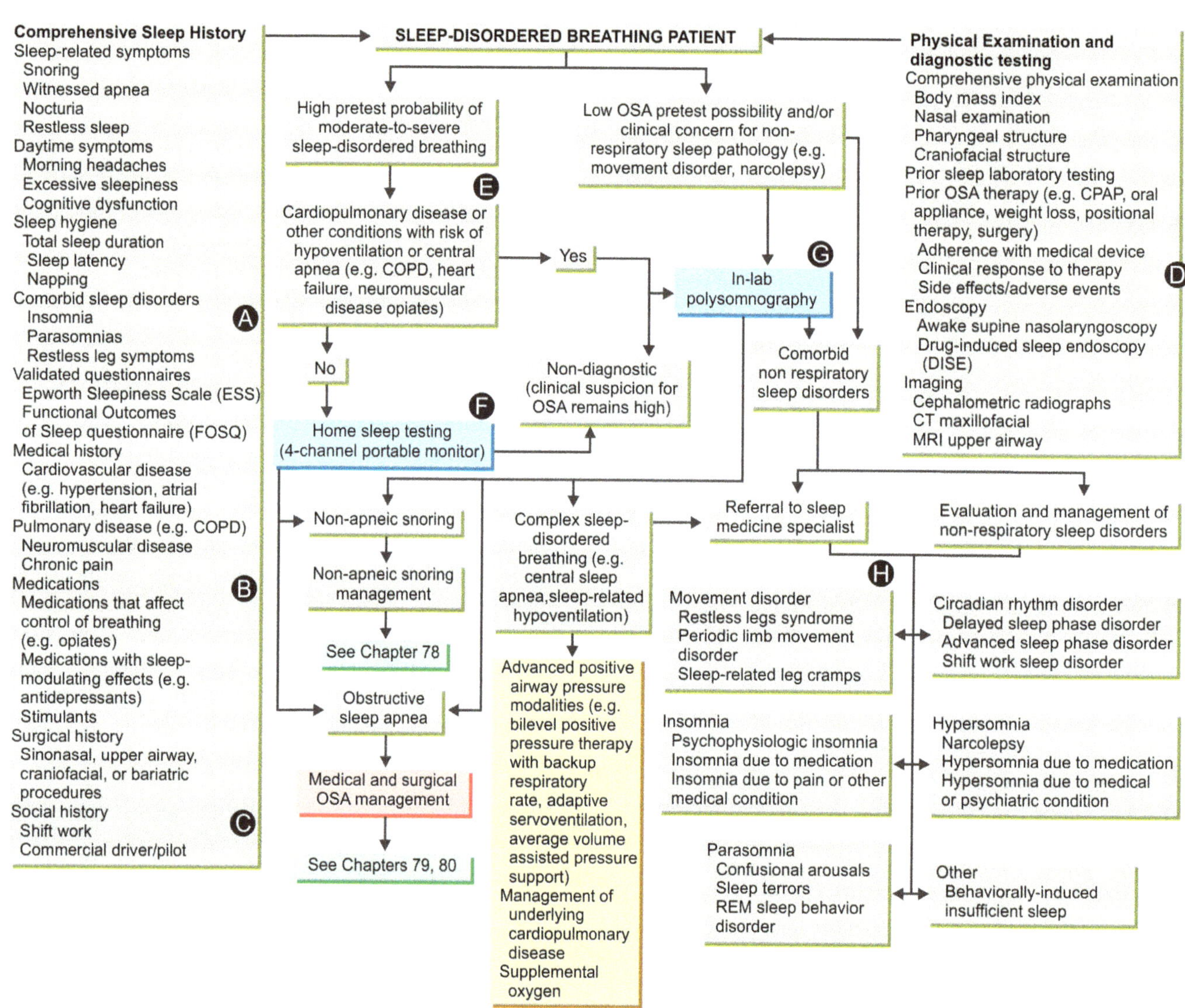

Sleep-disordered breathing (SDB) is one of the most common presenting conditions to the Otolaryngologist office. Although the pathophysiology of SDB may be complex and often varies greatly across the population, the goals of treatment remain consistent for the majority of SDB patients: to alleviate symptoms, to improve quality of life, and to reduce cardiovascular and general health risks. Sleep-disordered breathing is most often a chronic long-term condition that requires longitudinal care and constant re-evaluation and management throughout the lifespan. Obstructive sleep apnea (OSA) is only one of ~80 sleep disorders, including a dozen or so other sleep-related breathing disorders. A comprehensive sleep history and the appropriate use of diagnostic information are essential to customizing an effective treatment plan.

A A thorough sleep medicine history remains the cornerstone of the assessment of patients with sleep-related symptoms. The most common cause of excessive daytime sleepiness is inadequate total sleep duration. Validated sleep questionnaires serve as useful adjuncts to document the quality of life impact of the sleep disorder and to provide patient-reported outcome measures after treatment initiation.

B Many neuropsychiatric and medical conditions can contribute to both sleep disturbance and loss of control of breathing. Heart failure, stroke, pulmonary disease, morbid obesity, and neuromuscular disease each raise clinical concern for more complex SDB such as central sleep apnea, unstable ventilatory control (abnormal loop gain), or loss of lung volume. Furthermore, many vascular diseases (e.g. hypertension and cerebrovascular disease) may be consequences of the untreated OSA. Medications also have tremendous potential to negatively affect sleep and daytime function directly and/or can impact central and peripheral control of breathing.

C The management of OSA in truck drivers, pilots, and other specific occupations may have additional challenges and even medicolegal ramifications to protect public safety from the negative effects of hypersomnia. Shift workers also present a unique challenge in both the evaluation and management of OSA as the outcomes of OSA are often confounded by the shift work and associated disturbance of circadian rhythm.

D Otolaryngologists frequently see OSA patients struggling with continuous positive airway pressure (CPAP) who are interested in alternative treatments. In these patients, CPAP data download software should be accessed when available to provide objective data on adherence and effectiveness. A detailed assessment of the specific mask- or pressure-related side effects or psychosocial barriers may allow effective troubleshooting strategies to improve CPAP results.

E The sleep and medical history are synthesized to generate a pretest probability of obstructive SDB. In patients with a high clinical suspicion of OSA, but without concern for other sleep-related breathing disorders or other non-respiratory sleep disorders, home portable sleep testing (HST) offers a more cost-effective, accessible, convenient, and reliable assessment of OSA severity.

F If the HST confirms OSA, a medical and/or surgical treatment plan can be initiated (*see* Chapters 79 and 80). If the HST was an adequate quality study but negative for OSA, management can be directed toward nonapneic snoring if clinically indicated (*see* Chapter 78). If the HST was inadequate or nondiagnostic, and a strong clinical concern for OSA remains based on the history and examination, consideration should be given for repeat testing with a full-montage in-lab polysomnography (PSG).

G Polysomnography should also considered for first-line diagnostic sleep testing when (1) significant cardiopulmonary disease, neuromuscular disease, or other conditions are present that confer high risk of central sleep apnea or sleep-related hypoventilation syndrome, or (2) periodic limb movement disorder, narcolepsy, or other nonrespiratory sleep disorders are suspected. The American Academy of Sleep Medicine (AASM) practice parameters provide more detailed guidance on the indications of PSG.

H In situations where PSG and/or other clinical workup confirms non-OSA sleep pathology, consultation with a sleep medicine specialist may be indicated. The International Classification of Sleep Disorders, 3rd edition (ICSD-3) classifies ~80 other sleep disorders that are divided into sleep-related breathing disorders, insomnia, parasomnia, central disorders of hypersomnolence, circadian rhythm disorders, and movement disorders. Additional evaluation, depending on the disorder, may include sleep log, bloodwork, actigraphy, a multiple sleep latency test, or other testing. A detailed discussion of the evaluation and management of all sleep medicine disorders is beyond the scope of this chapter but the reader is encouraged to begin with the ICSD-3.

DISCLOSURES

Dr Soose is an investigator in the Inspire STAR Trial and consultant for Inspire Medical Systems. Dr Kent has no conflicts of interest to disclose.

SUGGESTED READING

Collop NA, Anderson WM, Boehlecke B, et al. Clinical guidelines for the use of unattended portable monitors in the diagnosis of obstructive sleep apnea adult patients. J Clin Sleep Med. 2007;3:737-747.

Dempsey JA, Veasey SC, Morgan BJ, et al. Pathophysiology of sleep apnea. Physiol Rev. 2010;90:47-112.

International Classification of Sleep Disorders, 3rd edition. Darien, IL: American Academy of Sleep Medicine; 2014.

Kushida CA, Littner MR, Morgenthaler T, et al. Practice parameters for the indications for polysomnography and related procedures. Sleep. 2005;28:499-521.

Marin JM, Carrizo SJ, Vicente E, et al. Long-term cardiovascular outcomes in men with obstructive sleep apnoea-hypopnoea with or without treatment with continuous positive airway pressure: an observational study. Lancet. 2005;65:1046-1053.

Scharf AM, Tubman A, Smale P. Prevalence of concomitant sleep disorders in patients with obstructive sleep apnea. Sleep Breath. 2005;9:50-56.

White DP. Pathogenesis of obstructive and central sleep apnea. Am J Resp Crit Care Med. 2005;172:1363-1370.

Young T, Finn L, Peppard PE, et al. Sleep-disordered breathing and mortality: eighteen year follow-up of the Wisconsin Sleep Cohort. Sleep. 2008;31:1071-1078.

CHAPTER 78

Non-apneic Snoring

David T Kent, Ryan J Soose

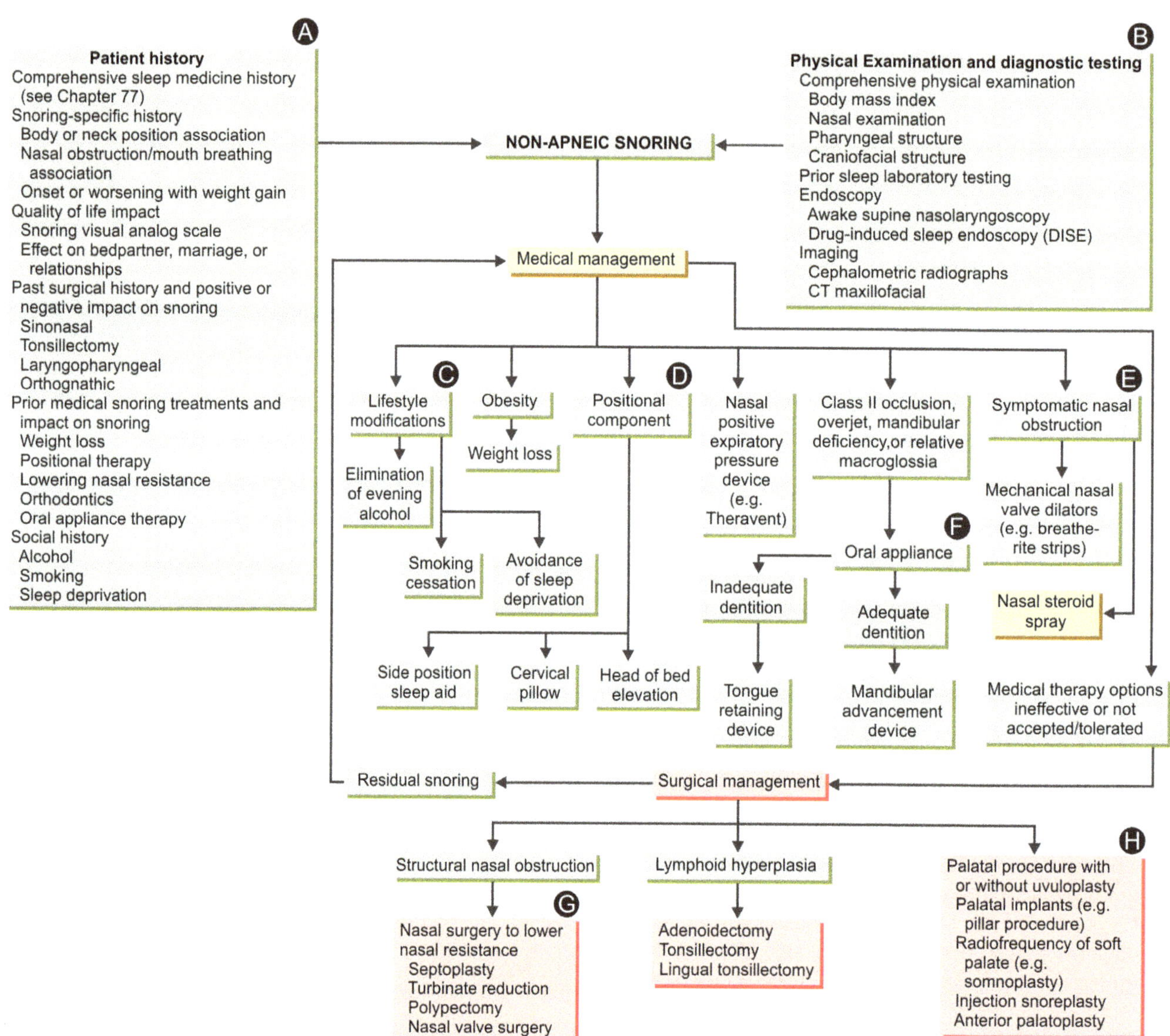

The most common, and the most bothersome, symptom that drives sleep-disordered breathing patients to a physician is loud disruptive snoring. Snoring results from vibrational flutter of the tissues of the upper airway, most commonly from flutter of the soft palate. Even in the absence of more clinically significant obstructive sleep apnea (OSA), snoring may negatively affect the patient's sleep and quality of life, as well as that of the bedpartner. Recent evidence also suggests that non-apneic snoring may even be an independent contributor to vascular risk. At this juncture, a validated and consensus objective measure of snoring does not exist. Outcome assessment is therefore based on the patient's or bedpartner's report. After clinical workup and diagnostic sleep testing has ruled-out OSA, treatment may be directed at the non-apneic snoring. Both medical and surgical treatment options are available to improve airflow, reduce upper airway collapsibility, and subsequently reduce the volume of and negative consequences of snoring.

A In addition to a standard comprehensive sleep medicine history, several historical factors may help guide management including the association of snoring with certain positions, behaviors, nasal congestion, or weight gain. The effect of prior medical or surgical interventions, either positive or negative, on the volume and frequency of snoring may also help guide future management.

Ⓑ Physical examination, upper airway endoscopy, and/ or imaging may assist in phenotyping the anatomical structures of the upper airway that are contributing to the collapse and flutter during sleep.

Ⓒ If present, several modifiable risk factors may provide useful targets for low-risk intervention. Obesity, alcohol, smoking, and sleep deprivation each may contribute to upper airway collapsibility.

Ⓓ Position of the body and neck may also affect upper airway patency in some patients. In selected patients, there is limited evidence that side positioning, elevation of the head of the bed, or neck extension with a cervical pillow can reduce upper airway collapsibility.

Ⓔ Increased nasal resistance has been shown to be an independent risk factor for snoring. Furthermore, treatment to lower nasal resistance may reduce snoring in selected patients. Medical therapy options include mechanical dilators, nasal decongestants, and topical intranasal steroid sprays. Combining and implementing these nasal medical therapy options for a few nights can also serve as a useful test to determine the potential impact of treating the nose on the volume of snoring.

Ⓕ For patients without an easily modifiable target, oral appliance therapy has substantial data on effectively reducing snoring and providing multilevel stabilization of the upper airway. Mandibular repositioning appliances are the most widely used and most successful as long as adequate dentition and adequate adherence are present. Devices range from over-the-counter thermoplastic appliances to custom devices fitted by a specially trained sleep dentist. Potential side effects that may limit the use include drooling, dry mouth, jaw or temporomandibular joint discomfort, tooth discomfort, and occlusal change.

Ⓖ For those patients who have failed medical management or who have clear evidence of modifiable structural abnormalities of the upper airway, minimally invasive surgical options may be considered. Surgical treatments to lower nasal resistance or remove obstructing adenotonsillar hypertrophy can provide substantial improvement in snoring.

Ⓗ Palatal stiffening procedures have been demonstrated to successfully manage non-apneic snoring, as it is estimated that at least 80% of snoring originates in the flutter of the soft palate. Each palatal surgery approach has unique advantages, disadvantages, costs, risks, and benefits that must be assessed in and tailored to each individual patient.

DISCLOSURES

Dr Soose is an investigator in the Inspire STAR Trial and consultant for Inspire Medical Systems. Dr Kent has no conflicts of interest to disclose.

SUGGESTED READING

Chen WC, Lee LA, Chen NH, et al. Treatment of snoring with positional therapy in patients with positional obstructive sleep apnea syndrome. Sci Rep. 2015;5:181-188.

Choi JH, Kim SN, Cho JH. Efficacy of the pillar implant in the treatment of snoring and mild-to-moderate obstructive sleep apnea: a meta-analysis. Laryngoscope. 2013;123:269-276.

Koutsourelakis I, Keliris A, Minaritzoglou A, et al. Nasal steroids in snorers can decrease snoring frequency: a randomized placebo-controlled crossover trial. J Sleep Res. 2015;24:160-166.

Kushida CA, Rao S, Guilleminault C, et al. Cervical positional effects on snoring and apneas. Sleep Res Online. 1999;2:7-10.

Li HY, Lee LA, Wang PC, et al. Nasal surgery for snoring in patients with obstructive sleep apnea. Laryngoscope. 2008;118:354-359.

Li Y, Liu J, Wang W, et al. Association of self-reported snoring with carotid artery intima-media thickness and plaque. J Sleep Res. 2012;21:87-93.

Ramar K, Dort LC, Katz SG, et al. Clinical practice guideline for the treatment of obstructive sleep apnea and snoring with oral appliance therapy: an update for 2015. J Clin Sleep Med. 2015;11:773-827.

Woodson BT, Han JK. Relationship of snoring and sleepiness as presenting symptoms in a sleep clinic population. Ann Otol Rhinol Laryngol. 2005;114:762-767.

Medical Management of Obstructive Sleep Apnea

David T Kent, Ryan J Soose

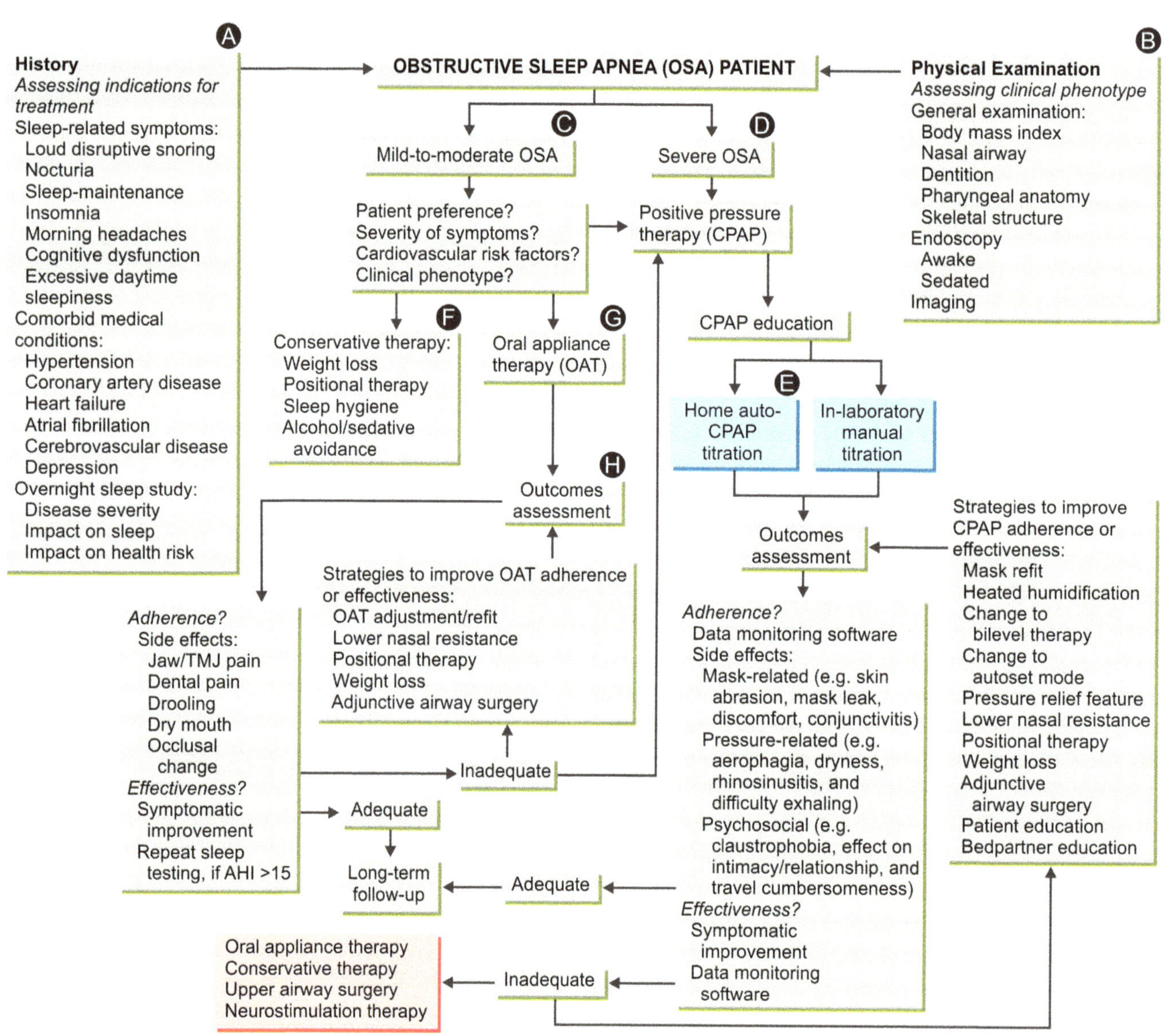

Obstructive sleep apnea (OSA) is a chronic condition that requires management across the life span. For most OSA patients, the goals of treatment include (1) symptom and quality of life improvement and (2) reduction of cardiovascular and general health risk. Obstructive sleep apnea treatment should be customized to the unique clinical presentation of each patient, airway anatomy phenotype, body mass index, disease severity, and presence of other medical and sleep comorbidities. For many patients, particularly with more severe disease, combination therapy may provide optimum results over single-modality therapy.

Positive airway pressure (PAP) therapy and oral appliances are the foundation of OSA medical management in the majority of adult patients. Nevertheless, there are many other medical and surgical management tools that can be employed to optimize results with these medical device therapies. An individualized approach considering all available treatment options and a longitudinal care model with continued reassessment of adherence and effectiveness are essential to an effective long-term management strategy.

A The decision to treat and the initial approach to treatment depend upon the patient's symptoms and quality-of-life impact, the presence of related medical comorbidities, and the results of overnight diagnostic sleep testing, either in the sleep laboratory or in the home environment.

B Anatomic and pathophysiologic phenotyping with physical examination, endoscopy, and/or imaging can further direct appropriate treatment decision making. For example, in patients with significant obesity, continuous positive airway pressure (CPAP) and weight loss would be most appropriate regardless of disease severity. Similarly, patients lacking adequate dentition would not be good candidates for oral appliance therapy while patients with massive adenotonsillar hypertrophy would have low likelihood of success with any medical device and may benefit from first-line surgical therapy.

C In patients with mild-to-moderate OSA, CPAP, oral appliances, and weight loss or other conservative measures may be considered as first-line treatment strategies. Factors driving the decision-making process include patient preference, clinical presentation and symptoms, the presence of cardiovascular risk or comorbid medical conditions, and the anatomic phenotype. For example, an oral appliance may provide effective first-line therapy for an otherwise healthy, nonobese, symptomatic patient with moderate OSA, a report of mouthbreathing at night, mandibular deficiency on examination, and good dentition.

D In severe OSA, CPAP is considered the standard first-line therapy with all other medical and surgical options most commonly reserved for a salvage, adjunctive, or second-line role. Continuous PAP has the most robust data on improving symptoms and lowering cardiovascular risk. Proper education and close clinical follow-up are essential in optimizing treatment results.

E Depending on the clinical presentation, CPAP can be initiated either in the sleep laboratory with an overnight manual titration or in the home setting with an auto-CPAP setup. Practice parameters have been published for each. Patients with severe hypoxemia, significant cardiopulmonary disease, morbid obesity, concern for central apnea, or other comorbid sleep disorders should be considered for in-laboratory manual titration to ensure adequate clinical response. Otherwise, the average uncomplicated OSA patient may do just as well, if not better, in the home environment.

F In selected patients, particularly with milder disease, the conservative measures listed may provide benefit with very little downside or risk; however, evidence is limited on the long-term effectiveness of many conservative strategies.

G Oral appliances are indicated for first-line treatment of mild-to-moderate OSA (when dictated by the clinical presentation and/or the patient preference) or as second-line treatment of severe OSA after failure of CPAP. Clinical practice guidelines have been published for the indications, patient selection, device fabrication and fitting, and long-term management. Successful management is determined by assessing (1) adherence (by self-report at the current time although objective adherence monitoring is on the horizon) and (2) effectiveness. Effectiveness is determined by improvement in patient-reported outcome measures and, in moderate or severe OSA, repeat sleep testing to ensure adequate clinical response on health risk reduction.

H For patients with side effects, discomfort, or other factors limiting adherence or for patients with incomplete clinical response, oral appliance adjustment, lowering nasal resistance, positional therapy, weight loss, or adjunctive surgical therapy have the potential to improve adherence and further augment the effectiveness. For patients who fail to achieve adequate clinical response despite these measures, consideration should be given to either revisit positive pressure therapy or explore alternative treatment options.

As with oral appliances, the success of CPAP is also assessed by evaluating adherence to the device and both subjective and objective measures of effectiveness. Data card monitoring software currently provides the standard objective measure of adherence as well as pressure effectiveness. A number of device-related side effects may limit adherence. For most of the mask-related, pressure-related, and psychosocial adverse events, troubleshooting strategies can be implemented to overcome these obstacles. Proper patient education and close clinical follow-up remain the cornerstone of effective long-term management. For patients who are intolerant and unable to achieve benefit with positive pressure therapy, second-line treatment options such as oral appliance therapy, pharyngeal surgery, skeletal surgery, and neurostimulation therapy may be considered.

DISCLOSURE

Dr Soose is an investigator in the Inspire STAR Trial and consultant for Inspire Medical Systems. Dr Kent has no conflicts of interest to disclose.

SUGGESTED READING

Epstein LJ, Kristo D, Strollo PJ, et al. Clinical guideline for the evaluation, management and long-term care of obstructive sleep apnea in adults. J Clin Sleep Med. 2009;5:263-276.

Kushida CA, Littner MR, Hirshkowitz M, et al. Practice parameters for the use of continuous and bilevel positive airway pressure devices to treat adult patients with sleep-related breathing disorders. Sleep. 2006;29:375-380.

Morgenthaler TI, Aurora N, Brown T, et al. Practice parameters for the use of autotitrating continuous positive airway pressure devices for titrating pressures and treating adult patients with obstructive sleep apnea syndrome. Sleep. 2008;31:141-147.

Phillips CL, Grunstein RR, Darendeliler MA, et al. Health outcomes of continuous positive airway pressure versus oral appliance treatment for obstructive sleep apnea: a randomized controlled trial. Am J Respir Crit Care Med. 2013;187:879-887.

Pliska BT, Nam H, Chen H, et al. Obstructive sleep apnea and mandibular advancement splints: occlusal effects and progression of changes associated with a decade of treatment. J Clin Sleep Med. 2014;10:1285-1291.

Ramar K, Dort LC, Katz SG, et al. Clinical practice guideline for the treatment of obstructive sleep apnea and snoring with oral appliance therapy: an update for 2015. J Clin Sleep Med. 2015;11:773-827.

Soose RJ, Strollo PJ. Medical Therapy for obstructive sleep apnea. In: Johnson JT, Rosen CR (Eds). Bailey's Head and Neck Surgery: Otolaryngology, 5th edition. Philadelphia, PA: Lippincott Williams & Wilkins; 2013.

Sutherland K, Vanderveken OM, Hiroko T, et al. Oral appliance treatment for obstructive sleep apnea: an update. J Clin Sleep Med. 2014;10:215-227.

Veasey SC, Guillemineault C, Strohl KP, et al. Medical therapy for obstructive sleep apnea: a review by the Medical Therapy for Obstructive Sleep Apnea Task Force of the Standards of Practice Committee of the American Academy of Sleep Medicine. Sleep. 2006;29:1036-1044.

Surgical Management of Obstructive Sleep Apnea

David T Kent, Ryan J Soose

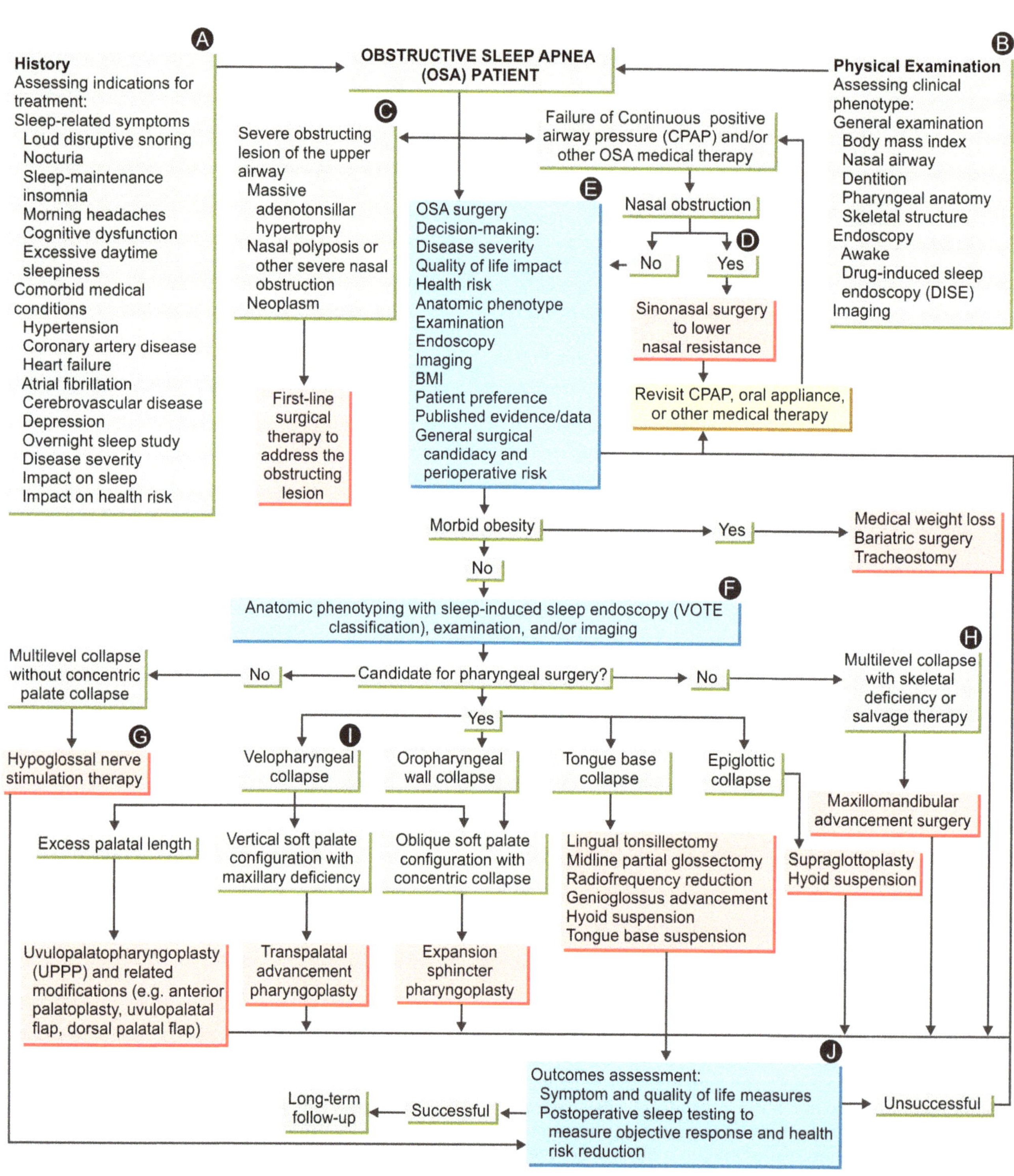

The approach to the evaluation and management of obstructive sleep apnea (OSA) is constantly evolving. Although continuous positive airway pressure (CPAP) therapy remains the standard first-line therapy with the most robust data on effectiveness, suboptimal adherence and acceptance rates necessitate consideration of alternative treatment strategies for many patients.

A As with medical therapy, the goals of treatment must be established preoperatively and understood by both the patient and the physician. The sleep and medical history, in conjunction with diagnostic sleep testing, can determine the impact of the disease on sleep-related symptoms, quality-of-life measures, personal relationships, occupational safety, driving risk, neurocognitive function, and cardiovascular risk.

B Anatomic and pathophysiologic phenotyping with physical examination, endoscopy, and/or imaging is essential to surgical decision making.

C For patients with massive adenotonsillar hypertrophy or other severe obstructing intraluminal lesion of the upper airway, a first-line surgical treatment is likely most appropriate whereas CPAP and oral appliances may have lower effectiveness in these phenotypes.

D For patients without an obstructing lesion, who have failed to achieve adequate treatment response to CPAP or other OSA medical therapy, the status of the nasal airway should be assessed first. Increased nasal resistance has been shown to negatively affect CPAP and oral appliance results. Similarly, surgery to lower nasal resistance is a relatively low invasive method to improve the effectiveness of these medical devices, converting some CPAP failures into CPAP successes.

E For patients who are unable to achieve benefit with standard medical options and do not have a correctible nasal or intraluminal obstruction, the decision on when and how to proceed with more invasive OSA surgery procedures depends on multiple factors (listed in the box). Morbid obesity is associated with a more complex pathophysiologic phenotype that involves reduced lung volume, increased pharyngeal fat deposition, and sleep-related hypoventilation. Medical or surgical weight loss or even tracheostomy may be more appropriate in such cases rather than upper airway surgery.

F Drug-induced sleep endoscopy (DISE), physical examination, and/or imaging can be used to phenotype the skeletal structure, the pharyngeal muscle buttress system, and the patterns of upper airway collapse. The majority of patients have multilevel and multifactorial patterns of upper airway collapsibility which may be improved with multilevel pharyngeal surgery, maxillomandibular skeletal advancement surgery, or hypoglossal nerve stimulation (HNS) therapy.

G Hypoglossal nerve stimulation therapy has been shown to provide multilevel (retropalatal and retrolingual) upper airway improvement in properly selected patients with sustainable long-term improvements in both subjective and objective outcome measures. Hypoglossal nerve stimulation therapy differs from traditional upper airway surgery in that HNS is titratable and is nonanatomy altering—often resulting in substantially lower recovery and risk compared to traditional airway surgery. The therapy is currently indicated for patients with moderate-to-severe OSA, who are unable to adhere to CPAP, are not significantly obese, and do not have a concentric pattern of collapse at the palate.

H Maxillomandibular advancement surgery has some of the highest published success rates of any OSA surgery. This provides a very effective multilevel improvement in upper airway structure, but its potential risk and morbidity, and recovery preclude widespread use and limit its implementation to those patients with skeletal deficiency or as a salvage treatment after exhausting other medical and surgical options.

I A paradigm shift is underway toward the implementation of more reconstructive and physiologically sound palatal surgery techniques and away from the traditional excisional uvulopalatopharyngoplasty (UPPP). The length, width, depth, lateral wall component, sagittal configuration, and other anatomic factors of the soft palate anatomy determine the most appropriate palatal surgery technique.

J After undergoing any surgical intervention, both the subjective and objective OSA outcome measures (as well as complications or adverse side effects) must be assessed postoperatively to ensure adequate therapeutic response. If the goals of therapy have been successfully met, the patient may be transitioned to long-term follow-up. If symptoms or markers of health risk persist postoperatively, the patient should be reintroduced in the algorithm to revisit medical therapy options and/or to reevaluate for additional surgical options.

DISCLOSURES

Dr Soose is an investigator in the Inspire STAR Trial and consultant for Inspire Medical Systems. Dr Kent has no conflicts of interest to disclose.

SUGGESTED READING

Camacho M, Riaz M, Capasso R, et al. The effect of nasal surgery on continuous positive airway pressure device use and therapeutic treatment pressures: a systematic review and meta-analysis. Sleep. 2015;38:279-286.

DeVito A, Carrasco Llatas M, Vanni A, et al. European position paper on drug-induced sedation endoscopy (DISE). Sleep Breath. 2014;18:453-465.

Li HY, Lee LA, Wan PC, et al. Can nasal surgery improve obstructive sleep apnea: subjective or objective? Am J Rhinol Allergy. 2009;23:e51-55.

Pang KP, Pang EB, Win MT, et al. Expansion sphincter pharyngoplasty for the treatment of OSA: a systemic review and meta-analysis. Eur Arch Otorhinolaryngol. 2016;273(9):2329-2333.

Strollo PJ Jr, Soose RJ, Maurer JT, et al. Upper-airway stimulation for obstructive sleep apnea. N Engl J Med. 2014;370:139-149.

Woodson BT. A method to describe the pharyngeal airway. Laryngoscope. 2015;125(5):1233-1238.

Woodson BT, Sitton M, Jacobowitz O. Expansion sphincter pharyngoplasty and palatal advancement pharyngoplasty: airway evaluation and surgical techniques. Oper Techn Otolaryngol. 2012;23:3-10.

Woodson BT, Soose RJ, Gillespie MB, et al. Three-year outcomes of cranial nerve stimulation for obstructive sleep apnea: the STAR trial. Otolaryngol Head Neck Surg. 2016;154(1):181-188.

Zaghi S, Holty JE, Certal V, et al. Maxillomandibular advancement for treatment of obstructive sleep apnea: a meta-analysis. JAMA Otolaryngol Head Neck Surg. 2016;142:58-66.

CHAPTER 81

Obstructive Sleep Apnea in the Pediatric Population

Nira A Goldstein

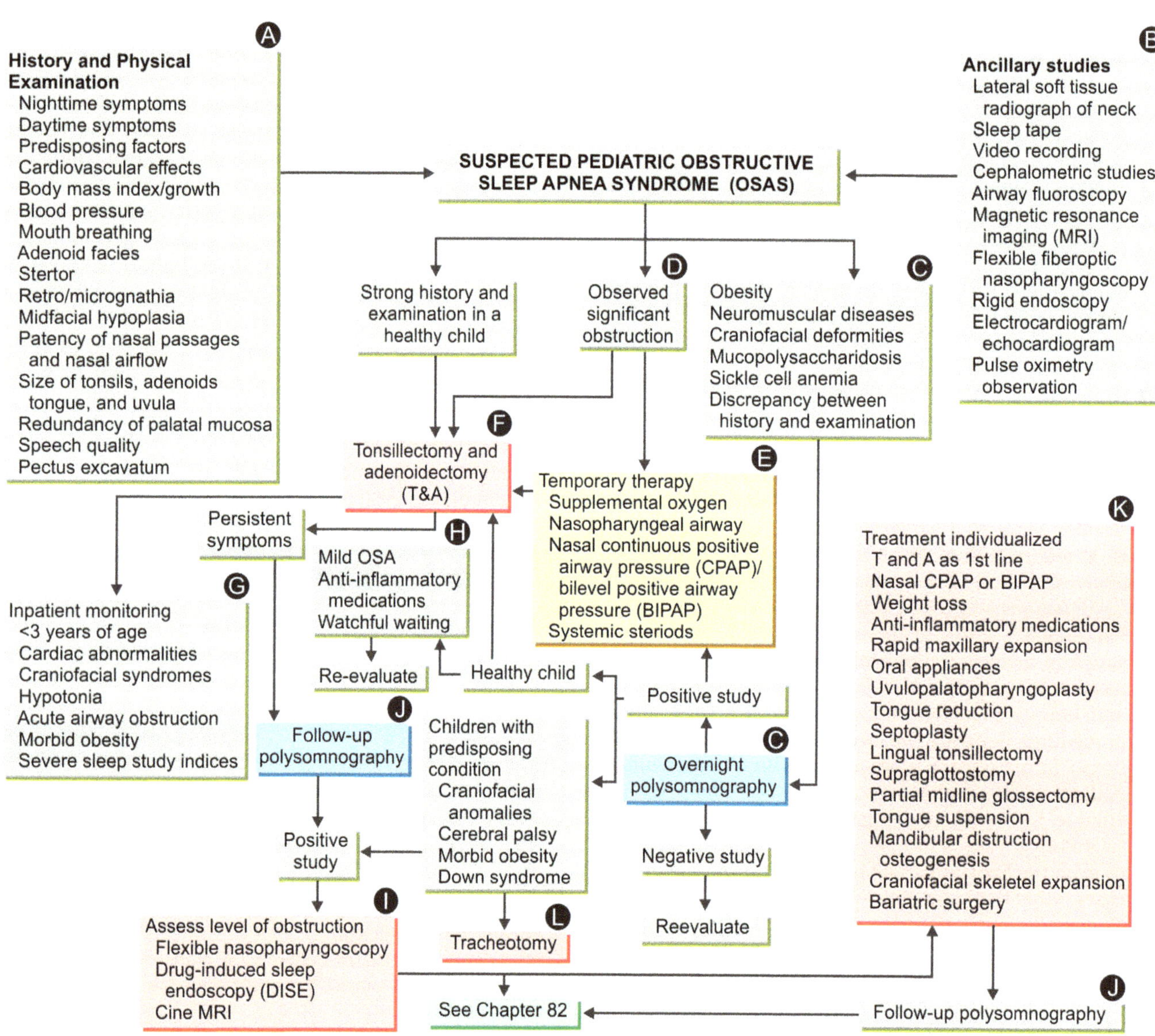

Pediatric sleep-disordered breathing (SDB) is viewed as a continuum of severity from partial obstruction of the upper airway producing snoring, to increased upper airway resistance to continuous episodes of complete upper airway obstruction or obstructive sleep apnea (OSA). SDB is an important cause of morbidity in children and may lead to growth failure, neurocognitive and behavioral abnormalities, and cardiovascular dysfunction. Early recognition and treatment are important in order to prevent or treat these complications.

A Snoring is the most common symptom of SDB. Other night-time symptoms include apneic pauses, snorting, gasping, restless sleep, frequent arousals, frequent awakenings, sleeping with the neck hyperextended, unusual sleeping positions, diaphoresis, enuresis, and other parasomnias. Hypertrophy of the tissues of Waldeyer's ring may lead to daytime obstructive symptoms including mouth breathing, hyponasality, chronic rhinorrhea, nasal obstruction, and dysphagia. Behavioral and neurocognitive difficulties have been found in 8.5–63% of children with SDB. Failure to thrive has been reported to occur in approximately 10% of children and 42–56% of infants with OSA. Ventricular dysfunction, pulmonary hypertension, cor pulmonale, systemic hypertension, and altered autonomic regulation have been reported in children with OSA, although many of these findings are subclinical and their long-term effects are still unknown. Predisposing conditions include obesity, Down syndrome, craniofacial anomalies, abnormalities of neuromuscular control, mucopolysaccharide storage disease, and iatrogenic causes such as pharyngeal flaps.

B Ancillary studies are optional and dictated by the clinical situation.

C There is much controversy as to whether an otherwise healthy child with a clinical assessment suggestive of OSA requires overnight polysomnography (PSG) before tonsillectomy and adenoidectomy (T&A) to confirm the diagnosis. On the basis of the published studies demonstrating poor predictive utility of clinical assessment in predicting a positive PSG, and because only 20–30% of snoring children have positive PSG, the 1996 American Thoracic Society Consensus Committee and the 2012 American Academy of Pediatrics (AAP) Clinical Practice Guidelines recommend that PSG be obtained prior to T&A to differentiate primary snoring from OSA. In contrast, the Clinical Practice Guideline of the American Academy of Otolaryngology–Head and Neck Surgery (AAOHNS) recommend PSG prior to tonsillectomy only for selected children with premorbid conditions and for otherwise healthy children for whom the need for surgery is uncertain and for whom there is a discordance between tonsil size and reported severity of SDB.

D The American Thoracic Society acknowledges that the sleep study may be deferred when obstructive apnea is observed by medical personnel directly or by audio and video recording "to proceed with therapy expeditiously."

E Severe OSA can be temporarily treated with supplemental oxygen, nasal continuous positive airway pressure (CPAP) or bilevel positive airway pressure (BIPAP) or a nasopharyngeal airway, and systemic corticosteroids.

F The first-line therapy for the treatment of OSA or significant SDB in otherwise healthy children is T&A. It may also be the first-line treatment in complex patients if the tonsils and adenoids are enlarged. Most studies find that T&A significantly improves respiratory indices; however, the published OSA "cure rates" vary widely, but are generally around 60%. Due to ethical concerns, there is only one randomized, controlled trial comparing T&A to no treatment at 7-month follow-up (Childhood Adenotonsillectomy Trial, CHAT). The study found improved symptoms, behavior, quality-of-life, and sleep study indices, but improvements in the primary endpoint, a measure of attention and executive function, did not occur.

G Children with OSA are at risk for postoperative respiratory complications. Risk factors are age under 3, pulmonary hypertension or other cardiac abnormalities, craniofacial syndromes, failure to thrive, hypotonia, acute airway obstruction, morbid obesity, and severe sleep study indices. Although the definition of "severe" OSA varies, the clinical practice guidelines published by the AAOHNS recommend admission for a child with an AHI of ≥10 or an oxygen saturation nadir of <80% or both, while the AAP guidelines use a cutoff of AHI of ≥24, an oxygen saturation nadir of <80% or peak end tidal CO_2 of ≥60 mm Hg. These high-risk children require in-patient monitoring of their cardiorespiratory status after T&A.

H Topical intranasal steroids with or without leukotriene modifiers may be considered for the treatment of mild OSA (AHI < 5), although the optimal duration of therapy is not known. Watchful waiting may also be considered for children with mild OSA as in the CHAT trial, 46% of the watchful waiting group no longer met PSG criteria for OSA at the 7-month follow-up.

I Successful treatment of OSAS in children with predisposing conditions and in otherwise healthy children with idiopathic sleep apnea after T&A requires accurate assessment of the level of obstruction. The site of obstruction can be determined by office physical examination including flexible fiberoptic laryngoscopy, but examination awake does not take into account the airway collapsibility that occurs during sleep. Drug-induced sleep endoscopy may be performed in the operating room under general anesthesia to evaluate dynamic collapse in the supine position during sleep. Cine magnetic resonance imaging, performed under mild sedation, provides a high-resolution examination of the dynamic airway and is particularly useful in identifying multiple sites of obstruction.

J Postoperative sleep studies are required to evaluate response to treatment in any otherwise healthy child with persistent symptoms after T&A and in all children with predisposing conditions after first-line surgical therapy. If the studies are positive, further treatment is individualized but involves the medical and surgical therapies described in Step K, either alone or in combination.

K CPAP or BIPAP may be used as the primary therapy, as an adjunct to surgical therapies, or after the failure of surgical therapies. Children with a constricted maxillary arch and associated narrowing of the nasal airway may benefit from rapid maxillary expansion. Lingual tonsillectomy alone or in combination with additional procedures has a reported success rate of 57–88% in normalizing PSG indices, whereas supraglottoplasty for treatment of occult laryngomalacia has a reported success rate of 58–72%. Craniofacial skeletal expansion procedures have been successful in children with craniofacial abnormalities and neurologic disorders. Bariatric surgery is increasingly being performed in adolescents for treatment of morbid obesity.

L Tracheotomy is the definitive procedure because it bypasses the site of obstruction. It may be temporary while future options are pursued, particularly in infants and young children. Permanent tracheostomy is sometimes necessary in children with craniofacial syndromes or morbid obesity or when other procedures fail.

SUGGESTED READING

American Thoracic Society. Standards and indications for cardiopulmonary sleep studies in children. Am J Respir Crit Care Med. 1996;153:866-878.

Friedman M, Wilson M, Lin HC, et al. Updated systematic review of tonsillectomy and adenoidectomy for treatment of pediatric obstructive sleep apnea/hypopnea syndrome. Otolaryngol Head Neck Surg. 2009;140:800-808.

Manickam PV, Shott SR, Boss EF, et al. Systematic review of site of obstruction identification and non-CPAP treatment options for children with persistent pediatric obstructive sleep apnea. Laryngoscope. 2016;126(2):491-500.

Marcus CL, Brooks LJ, Draper KA, et al. Clinical Practice Guideline: diagnosis and management of childhood obstructive sleep apnea syndrome. Pediatrics. 2012;130:576-584.

Marcus CL, Moore RH, Rosen CL, et al. A randomized trial of adenotonsillectomy for childhood sleep apnea. N Engl J Med. 2013; 368:2366-2376.

Roland PS, Rosenfeld RM, Brooks LJ, et al. Clinical practice guideline: polysomnography for sleep-disordered breathing prior to tonsillectomy in children. Otolaryngol Head Neck Surg. 2011; 145(Suppl 1):S1-15.

Persistent Pediatric Obstructive Sleep Apnea After Tonsillectomy and Adenoidectomy

Deepak Mehta, Noémie Rouillard-Bazinet

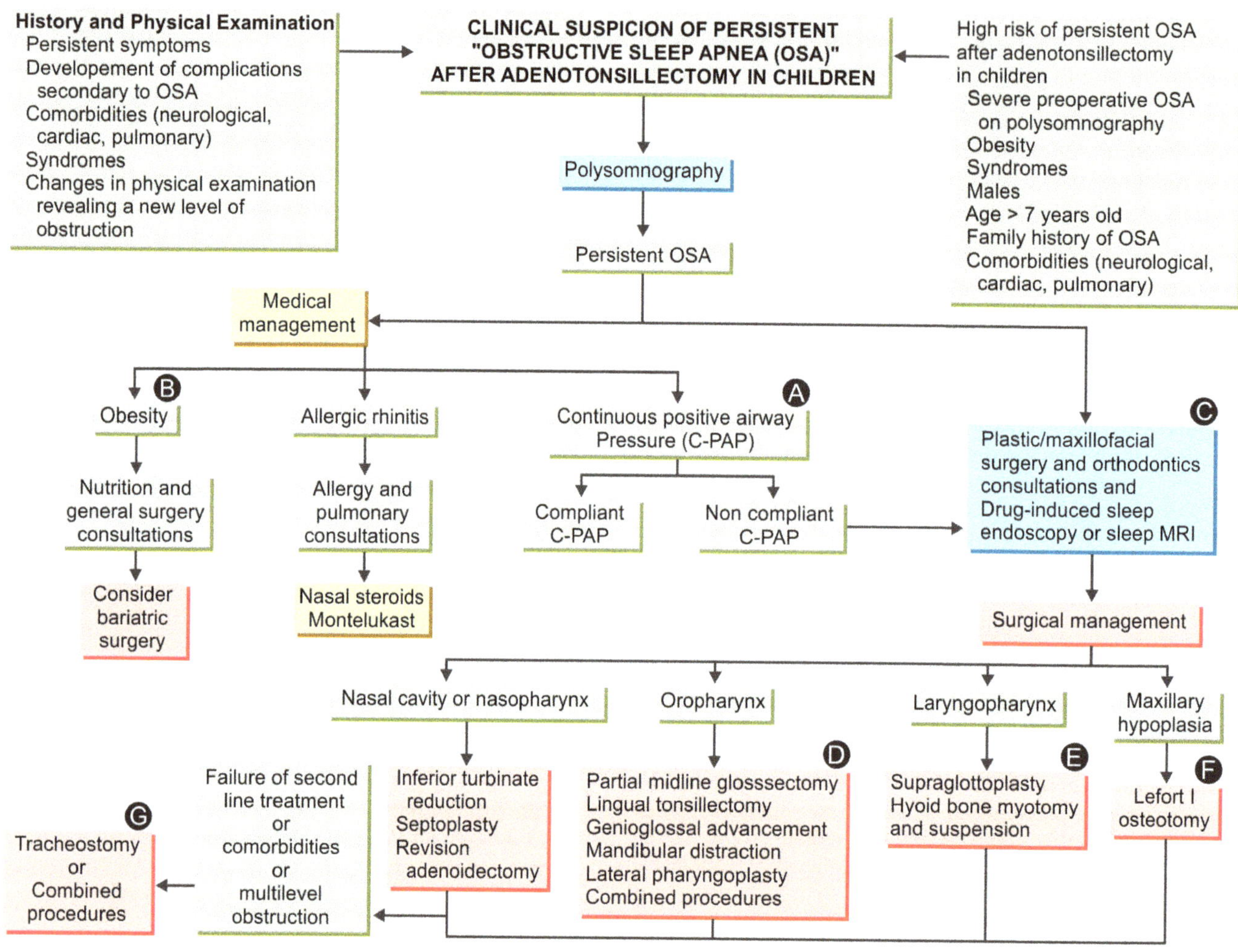

According to the American Academy of Pediatrics, the first-line treatment for pediatric obstructive sleep apnea (OSA) remains tonsillectomy and adenoidectomy. It results in complete normalization of the apnea–hypopnea index (AHI) in 60–85% of children. However, exceptions are seen within particular groups. For example, only 12% of obese children will be completely cured. This chapter is reviewing the medical and surgical options for the Otolaryngologist facing persistent pediatric OSA after adenotonsillectomy.

A For mild OSA, medical treatment is based on the cause of the OSA, as weight loss, nasal steroids therapy, oral Montelukast or rapid maxillary expansion and mandibular advancement devices. Furthermore, children with OSA can be successfully treated by continuous positive airway pressure (C-PAP). Continuous positive airway pressure has been reported superior to surgical treatment as the first-line therapy. About 75% of children will have AHI < 5 with C-PAP compared to 74% with surgery for uncomplicated children and 39% for children with comorbidities. However, the long-term compliance is a significant problem. Only 31% of patients will use it >6 hours per night. Also, the risk of midface hypoplasia and skin injury is concerning. The surgical management for persistent OSA represents an opportunity to achieve the same results of C-PAP without the above serious side effects.

B Bariatric surgery significantly reduces the comorbidities related to pediatric obesity, a finding that supports early intervention for children and adolescents. The American Society of Metabolic and Bariatric Surgery guidelines established a body mass index (BMI) > 35 kg/m^2 and AHI > 15, or a BMI > 40 kg/m^2 and AHI > 5 as selection criteria for bariatric surgery in obese patients with OSA. Resolution rates for sleep apnea following bariatric surgery are reported by the literature as 100%, with the resolution rates for hypertension ranging between 50% and 100%. Average BMI losses were about 17.8 and 22.3 units from the preoperative period.

C The decision as to the surgical management of OSA must be done by the identification of the anatomic level of obstruction. Drug-induced sleep endoscopy is the most studied assessment tool and consists of the evaluation of the level of airway obstruction by flexible endoscopy combined with a direct laryngoscopy and tracheobronchoscopy, usually described with anesthetic agents such as propofol, dexmedetomidine, midazolam, ketamine, desflurane, sevoflurane, or pentobarbital. The sleep magnetic resonance imaging (MRI) study and the sleep fluoroscopy have been reported also. Development of a scoring system by Chan et al. can help validate the obstruction and correlate it to the appropriate management. Furthermore, children with Down syndrome could represent a challenge for diagnosis and management as the reason of the obstruction may be multifactorial, and the rate of failure after a second-line surgical treatment is higher than the uncomplicated child. About 74% will present macroglossia with fatty infiltration and absence of a median sulcus. About 63% will have recurrence of tonsils and adenoids. As 63% will show glossoptosis, only 30% will have lingual tonsils hypertrophy and 22% will present a hypopharyngeal collapse. Finally, the multidisciplinary approach with sleep medicine and pulmonary, orthodontics, plastic, and maxillofacial surgery, and allergy is mandatory.

D The radiofrequency treatment of the base of the tongue was reported by several studies to be successful in 20–88% of patients. The genioglossal advancement presents success rate between 39% and 69%. The combination of radiofrequency ablation of the base of the tongue and genioglossal advancement has been reported to be successful in 58% of syndromic patients and 66% of uncomplicated patients. Additionally, the partial midline glossectomy presents success rate of 25–83%. The hyoid bone myotomy and suspension has also been proved to be effective in 17–78% of patients. Interestingly, the comparison of all oropharyngeal procedures shows that the tongue radiofrequency and the tongue stabilization had the worst outcomes. Moreover, subperiosteal release of the floor of the mouth is effective in children with microretrognathia and glossoptosis unresponsive to nasopharyngeal airway or ventral positioning. Finally, the lateral pharyngoplasty has not been commonly performed

in children. However, some studies demonstrated that it could benefit for children with comorbidities, such as obesity, neurologic impairment, or Down syndrome.

E Supraglottoplasty represents the second most common procedure after lingual tonsillectomy. Studies demonstrated resolution of OSA in 58–72% of the selected patients with occult laryngomalacia identified with sleep endoscopic studies.

F LeFort I osteotomy has been reported to reduce the AHI under 10 in the adult population and to significantly increase the retroglossal airway volume by 17.8%.

G Tracheostomy must be considered if children experience complications of OSA, such as cor pulmonale, hypertension, and cardiac failure. It remains important for the treatment of children with severe persistent OSA, craniofacial anomalies, syndromes, neuromuscular disorders, or failure of second-line surgical management.

SUGGESTED READING

Chan A, Chan CH, Ng DK. Validation of sleep-related breathing disorder scale in Hong Kong Chinese snoring children. Pediatr Pulmonol. 2012;47(8):795-800.

Costa DJ, Mitchell R. Adenotonsillectomy for obstructive sleep apnea in obese children: a meta-analysis, Otolaryngol Head Neck Surg. 2009;140:455-460.

Donnelly LF, Shott SR, Larose CR, et al. Causes of persistent obstructive sleep apnea despite previous tonsillectomy and adenoidectomy in children with Down syndrome as depicted on static and dynamic cine MRI. Am J Roentgenol. 2004;183(1):175-181.

Hochban W, Condradt R, Brandenburg U, et al. Surgical maxillofacial treatment of obstructive sleep apnea. Plast Reconstr Surg. 1997;99(3):619-626.

Ishman SL. Evidence-based practice pediatric obstructive sleep apnea. Otolaryngol Clin N Am. 2012;45:1055-1069.

Kezirian EJ, Goldberg AN. Hypopharyngeal surgery in obstructive sleep apnea. Arch Otolaryngol Head Neck Surg. 2006;132:206-213.

Manickam PV, Shott SR, Boss EF, et al. Systematic review of site of obstruction identification and non-CPAP treatment options for children with persistent pediatric obstructive sleep apnea. Laryngoscope. 2016;126(2):491-500.

Marcus CL, Brooks LJ, Draper KA, et al; American Academy of Pediatrics. Diagnosis and management of childhood obstructive sleep apnea syndrome. Pediatrics. 2012;130(3);576-584.

Pirelli P, Saponara M, Guilleminault C. Rapid maxillary expansion (RME) for pediatric obstructive sleep apnea: a 12-year follow-up. Sleep Med. 2015;16:933-935.

Treadwell JR, Sung F, Schoelles K. Systematic review and meta-analysis of bariatric surgery for pediatric obesity. Ann Surg. 2008; 248(5):763-776.

Woodson BT. Non-pressure therapies for obstructive sleep apnea: surgery and oral appliances. Respir Care. 2010;55(10):1314-1320.

Adenotonsillar Disease in Children

Glenn Isaacson

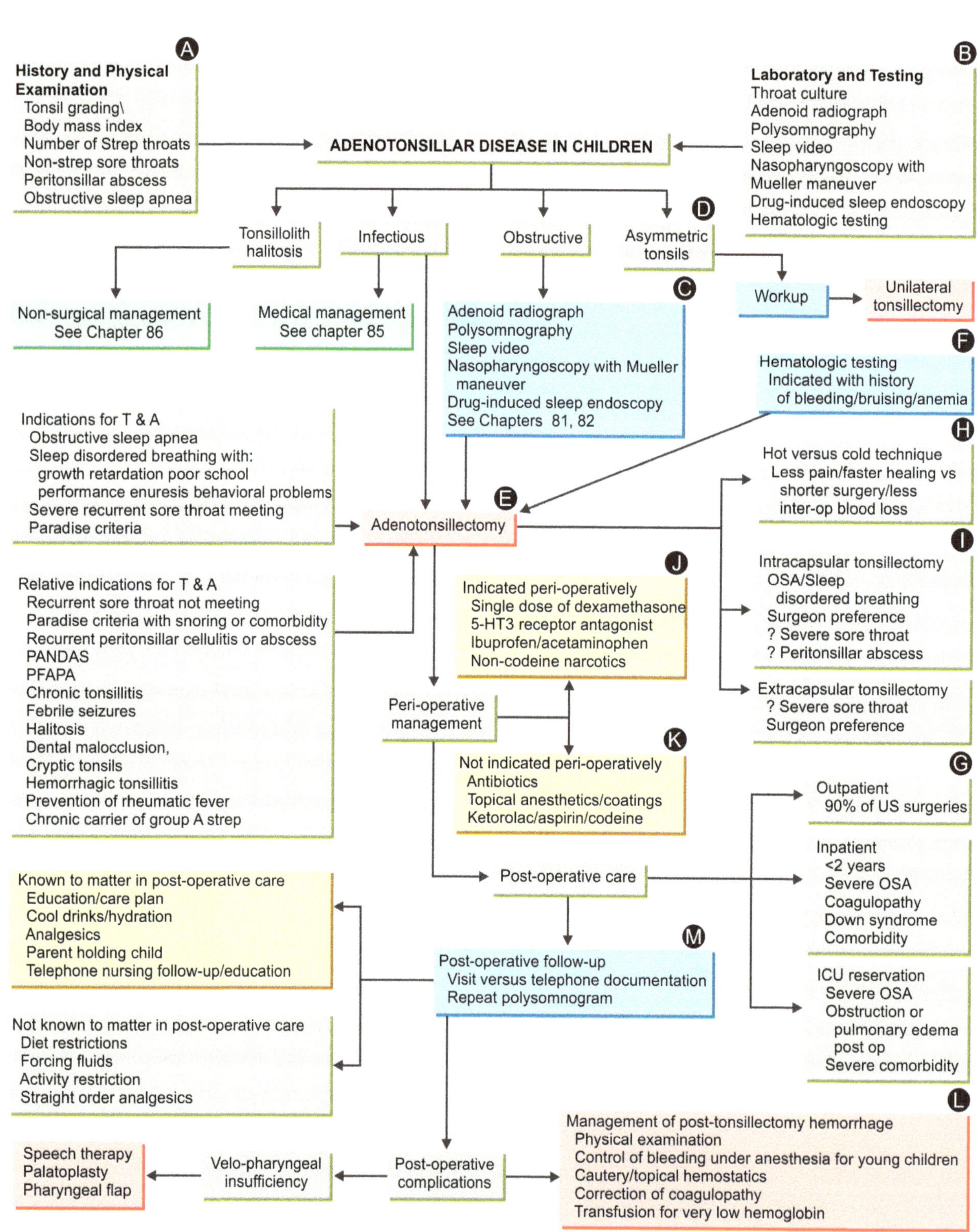

Children commonly present with problems related to tonsils and adenoids. While children may suffer from recurrent or chronic infections of these structures, they are also often evaluated for the infections of ears or sinuses due to possible association or causality. Adenotonsillar hypertrophy is commonly associated with upper airway obstruction or apnea and may be responsible for abnormal craniofacial development.

A History and physical examination are the first and most crucial steps in ascertaining the relative indications for tonsillectomy with or without adenoidectomy. History of snoring, disturbed sleep, problems with attention, and behavior should be elicited. Risk factors including bleeding history, comorbidities, and problems with anesthesia are documented. Physical examination should include anterior rhinoscopy and evaluation of tonsil size using a grading system.

B Radiographs of the adenoids, flexible nasopharyngoscopy with or without Mueller maneuver, and review of video recordings of sleep supplement the physical examination.

C In high-risk situations or when the diagnosis of obstructive sleep apnea is in doubt, formal polysomnography and/or drug-induced sleep endoscopy may provide valuable information.

D The vast majority of asymmetric tonsils in childhood are benign and hyperplastic. However, tonsillar asymmetry is a common physical sign of lymphoma of the tonsil. Unilateral tonsillectomy is indicated for children with asymmetry and other signs of malignancy (color alteration or visible lesion, cervical lymphadenopathy > 3 cm, dysphagia, snoring, recurrent fever, weight loss > 10%, immunosuppression, or prior radiotherapy).

E Adenotonsillectomy is very effective in nonobese children with obstructive sleep apnea and enlarged tonsils and adenoids. It is modestly effective in reducing the frequency of severe recurrent sore throat in children who satisfy the Paradise criteria. Its value in decreasing symptoms must be balanced against the morbidity of the procedure and its risks of bleeding (4–5%) and death (about 1/ 35,000) when considering its role in the treatment of sleep-disordered breathing and other relative indications. PANDAS = pediatric autoimmune neuropsychiatric disorder associated with streptococcal infection; PFAPA = periodic fever, aphthous stomatitis, pharyngitis, cervical adenitis.

F Routine hematologic testing before tonsillectomy is of little value in the absence of a personal or family history of abnormal bleeding, bruising, or anemia.

G More than 80% of tonsillectomies in the United States are performed in the outpatient setting. Inpatient surgery should be considered for very young children, those with moderate-severe obstructive sleep apnea by polysomnography, coagulopathies, and selected comorbidities. ICU observation may be necessary children with severe obstructive sleep apnea, major comorbities (e.g. Down syndrome), or respiratory problems after surgery.

H Cold dissection techniques are superior in terms of postoperative pain and rapid healing. Hot techniques including monopolar and bipolar electrosurgery, Coblation and laser cause greater tissue damage and slower healing but are preferred by many surgeons because of shorter operative time and less intraoperative bleeding.

I Intracapsular tonsillectomy causes less pain and postoperative bleeding than extracapsular (total) tonsillectomy. The two techniques are equivalent for the control of obstructive sleep apnea and sleep-disordered breathing. There is some evidence that they may be equivalent for recurrent sore throat and control of peritonsillar abscess.

J A single intraoperative dose of dexamethasone decreases postoperative pain and edema. Serotonin receptor antagonists are effective for preventing postoperative nausea. Ibuprofen and acetaminophen are safe and effective for pain control after pediatric tonsillectomy. Ketorolac, aspirin, and codeine should not be used.

K Analgesics, cool drinks, education, and a well-prescribed care plan decrease postoperative anxiety and pain. Children who are held by their parents are more comfortable. Restrictions on diet and activity have not been demonstrated to decrease pain or bleeding risk after tonsillectomy.

L Immediate or delayed hemorrhage after tonsillectomy can result in morbidity or death. Patients who bleed after tonsillectomy should be examined. Significant bleeding may require control under general anesthesia in young children. Suture, cautery, and topical hemostatics are commonly used. Correction of coagulopathy with blood products and transfusion are occasionally required.

M Follow-up may consist of a postoperative telephone questionnaire or office visit. Children with persistent symptoms of sleep-disordered breathing may benefit from repeat polysomnography.

SUGGESTED READING

Baugh RF, Archer SM, Mitchell RB, et al. American Academy of Otolaryngology-Head and Neck Surgery Foundation. Clinical practice guideline: tonsillectomy in children. Otolaryngol Head Neck Surg. 2011;144:S1-30.

Guimarães AC, de Carvalho GM, Correa CR, et al. Association between unilateral tonsillar enlargement and lymphoma in children: a systematic review and meta-analysis. Crit Rev Oncol Hematol. 2015;93(3):304-311.

Isaacson G. Pediatric tonsillectomy: an evidence-based approach. Otolaryngol Clin North Am. 2014;47(5):673-690.

Pinder DK, Wilson H, Hilton MP. Dissection versus diathermy for tonsillectomy. Cochrane Database Syst Rev. 2011;(3):CD002211.

Sutters KA, Isaacson G. Post-tonsillectomy pain in children. Am J Nurs. 2014;114(2):36-42; quiz 43.

Wang H, Fu Y, Feng Y, et al. Tonsillectomy versus tonsillotomy for sleep-disordered breathing in children: a meta-analysis. PLoS One. 2015;10(3):e0121500.

CHAPTER 84
Mucosal Diseases of the Mouth and Pharynx

Susan E Calderbank

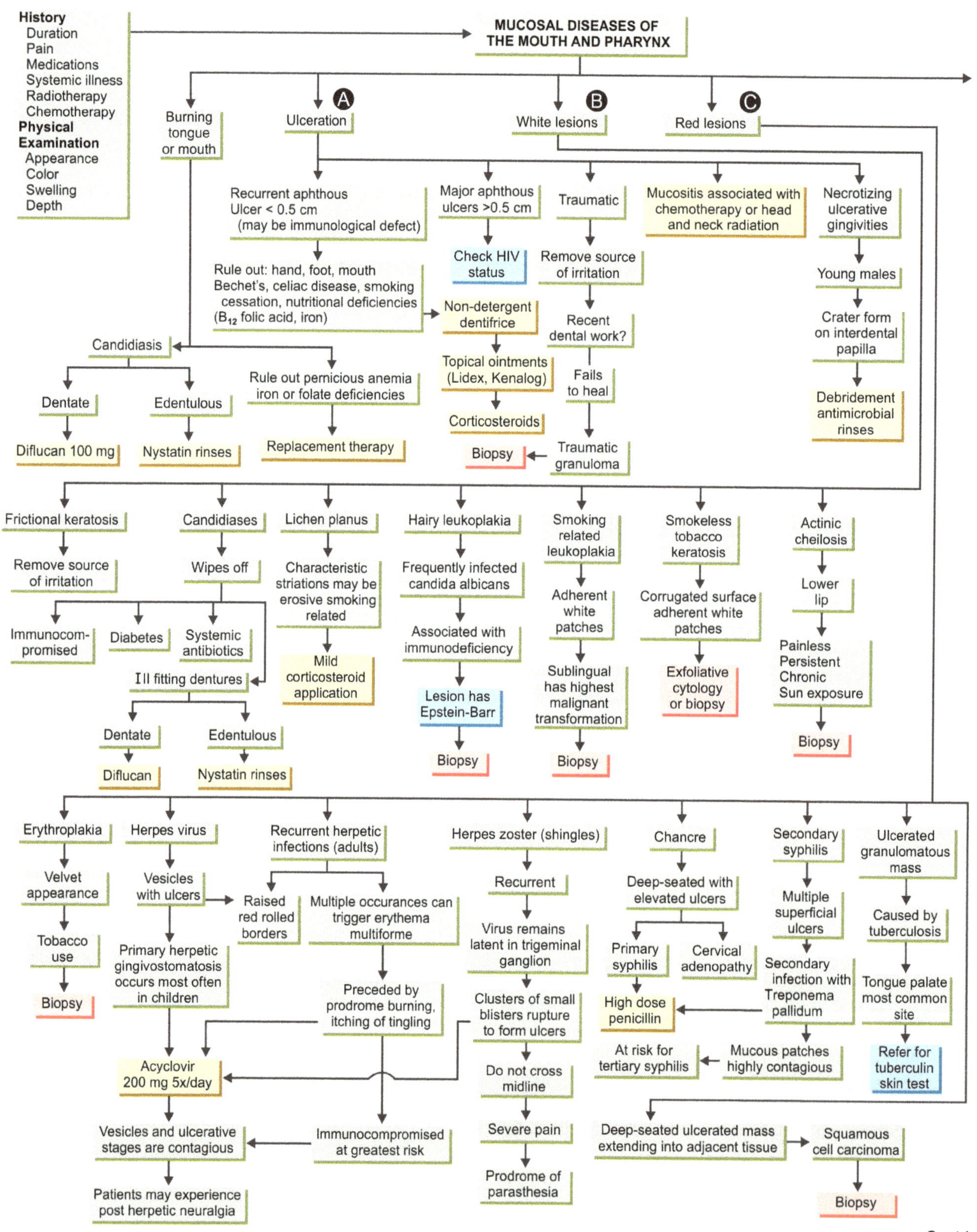

Contd...

Contd...

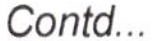

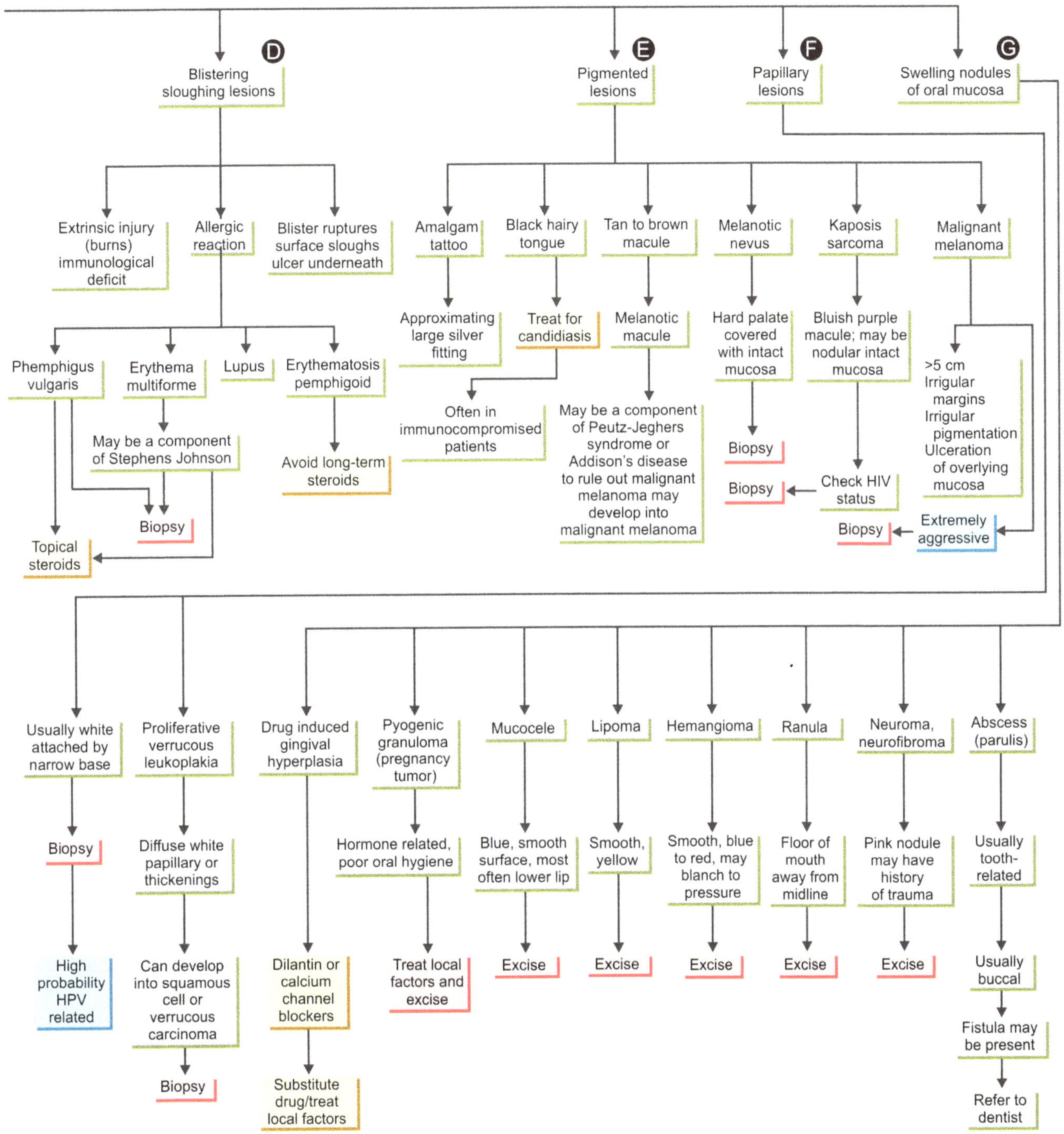

D — Blistering sloughing lesions

- Extrinsic injury (burns) immunological deficit
- Allergic reaction
- Blister ruptures surface sloughs ulcer underneath

- Phemphigus vulgaris
- Erythema multiforme
- Lupus
- Erythematosis pemphigoid

- May be a component of Stephens Johnson
- Avoid long-term steroids
- Biopsy
- Topical steroids

E — Pigmented lesions

- Amalgam tattoo → Approximating large silver fitting
- Black hairy tongue → Treat for candidiasis → Often in immunocompromised patients
- Tan to brown macule → Melanotic macule → May be a component of Peutz-Jeghers syndrome or Addison's disease to rule out malignant melanoma may develop into malignant melanoma
- Melanotic nevus → Hard palate covered with intact mucosa → Biopsy
- Kaposis sarcoma → Bluish purple macule; may be nodular intact mucosa → Check HIV status → Biopsy
- Malignant melanoma → >5 cm Irrigular margins Irrigular pigmentation Ulceration of overlying mucosa → Extremely aggressive → Biopsy

F — Papillary lesions

- Usually white attached by narrow base → Biopsy → High probability HPV related
- Proliferative verrucous leukoplakia → Diffuse white papillary or thickenings → Can develop into squamous cell or verrucous carcinoma → Biopsy

G — Swelling nodules of oral mucosa

- Drug induced gingival hyperplasia → Dilantin or calcium channel blockers → Substitute drug/treat local factors
- Pyogenic granuloma (pregnancy tumor) → Hormone related, poor oral hygiene → Treat local factors and excise
- Mucocele → Blue, smooth surface, most often lower lip → Excise
- Lipoma → Smooth, yellow → Excise
- Hemangioma → Smooth, blue to red, may blanch to pressure → Excise
- Ranula → Floor of mouth away from midline → Excise
- Neuroma, neurofibroma → Pink nodule may have history of trauma → Excise
- Abscess (parulis) → Usually tooth-related → Usually buccal → Fistula may be present → Refer to dentist

Oral health is a key component of total body health. Many systemic diseases and conditions have oral manifestations. This chapter is designed to be a guide to the swift and accurate diagnosis of oral soft tissue lesions and disease. It is divided into sections related to the appearance of the tissue.

Oral soft tissue is both a delicate and sensitive tissue. It can be greatly affected by poly-pharmacy. Thirty-four of the top hundred medicines prescribed can dry out these tissues. This can result in the complaint of dry mouth and a burning sensation. Systemic chemotherapy and radiation treatment of the head and neck can also have deleterious effects on the oral mucosa. The side effect of chemotherapy will disappear following the cessation of chemotherapy, while the effects of radiation of the head and neck can last a lifetime.

A Ulcerative lesions are classified as superficial (aphthous ulcers) or deep-seated (squamous cell carcinoma). This classification is based on the extent of their extension into underlying tissue. As a rule an ulceration lasting 2 weeks following appropriate treatment should be biopsied. Oral ulcers are associated with a wide variety of systemic conditions and in some cases can be the first clinical manifestation of the condition. Due to their contagious nature, some ulcerations pose a risk to health-care workers.

B When the oral epithelium becomes thicker or produces more keratin, the tissue will have a white appearance. In addition a white color may be associated with accumulations of surface microorganisms as in the case of an infection with Candida albicans. This will be characterized as pseudomembranous. White oral lesions can also be associated with human papillomavirus (HPV) infections. In general, white lesions are routinely biopsied due to their high degree of premalignant and malignant tendencies.

C Red lesions appear so due to the oral epithelium becoming thinner (atrophic), a proliferation of blood vessels, or due to submucosal bleeding. An oral burning sensation is often associated with atrophic tissue. These lesions, especially leukoplakias associated with tobacco usage, can be premalignant.

D Oral blister formation results from damage to some component of the oral mucosa. Blisters >0.5 cm are termed bulba. Those <0.5 cm are referred to as vesicles. When the blister ruptures and the surface layer is lost or sloughs, the lesion is classified as ulcerated. This can result in severe local pain. This tissue can become so painful that routine oral care is not possible.

E A primary concern when attempting to diagnose a pigmented lesion is to rule out malignancy. The color of these lesions can range from yellow to white and from blue to reddish brown. Some oral pigmentations are associated with systemic diseases such as Addison's disease. Other pigmentation occurs naturally as is seen in the darkening of gingival tissue in the black and Indian populations.

F Papillary lesions are epithelial in nature, are predominately white, and are avascular or have diminished vascularity. Oral papillary lesions are commonly associated with the HPV. When the term verrucous is used, it refers to a wart-like appearance.

G Oral soft tissue swellings can be the result of infection, reactive proliferations, trauma, and neoplastic activity. The surface may be smooth, hyperkeratotic, or ulcerated. They are also the category most likely affected by local factors such as poor oral hygiene.

Oral mucosa can also be affected by poly-pharmacy exhibited by many patients, especially geriatric patients. This can result in complaints of dry mouth and burning oral tissues. Systemic chemotherapy and radiation treatment of the head and neck can also have deleterious effects on oral tissue.

SUGGESTED READING

Kahn MA, Hall JM. The ADA Practical Guide to Soft Tissue Oral Disease. Wiley-Blackwell - Ames Lowa; 2014.

Lawson W. White oral lesions: how to distinguish the benign from the deadly. Consultant 360. 2012;52(4):311-317.

Newland R, Meiller TF, Wynn RL, et al. Oral Soft Tissue Diseases, 2nd edition. Lexicomp; 2002.

Regezi JA, Sciubba J, Jordan R. Oral Pathology. Elsevier - St. Lovis; 2016.

Sore Throat and Pharyngitis

Larry A Zieske

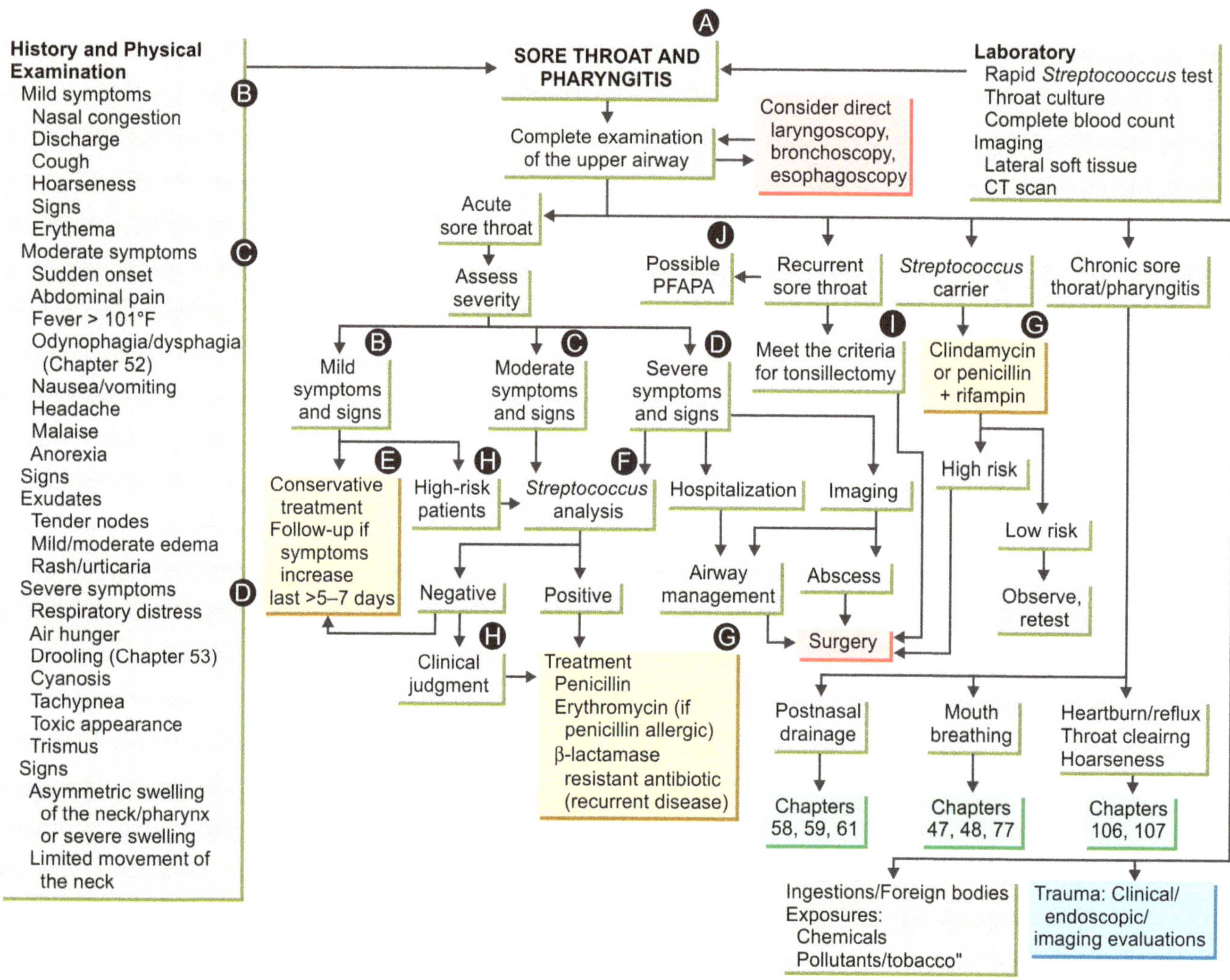

Differentiating between the various etiologies for sore throat and pharyngitis begins with associated historical factors. There have been infectious exposures, traumas, potential ingestions, or foreign bodies. Determining whether the symptoms are acute, chronic, or recurrent as well as the severity of symptoms and signs besides directing the urgency of evaluations assists in decisions about the need for imaging, hospitalization, and airway management. Complete evaluation of the upper airways is appropriate including potential endoscopy.

A Acute pharyngitis and sore throat are considered herein for patients older than 3 years. The primary differential is between a viral and bacterial cause, especially group A β-hemolytic Streptococcus (GABS). The severity of symptoms is considered with the potential for complications.

B These mild symptoms without other issues suggest a viral cause.

C Moderate symptoms with exudate, tender lymph nodes, and rash and urticaria are associated with Streptococcus infection. These symptoms can also occur with infectious mononucleosis.

D Severe symptoms with significant swelling warrant consideration of hospitalization and assessment of possible complications using imaging studies. Airway management should supersede all other considerations. Peritonsillar abscess can often be determined, allowing outpatient management. Level of care, monitoring, and intervention are guided by severity of symptoms, facilities available, and clinical judgment. Complications such as peritonsillar abscess, retropharyngeal abscess, and cellulitis must be ruled out with clinical examination and imaging studies (magnetic resonance imaging or computed tomography). Airway management may include intubation or tracheostomy. Ability and availability of personnel to perform an emergency tracheostomy should be considered when planning intubation. Intravenous antibiotics against β-lactamase-producing organisms should be given. Epiglottis, supraglottis, and uvulitis can be identified by examination, endoscopy, and imaging.

E Conservative management includes rinses with warm salt water (teaspoons per 6–8 oz); elevation of the back and head; room mist vaporizer; increasing oral fluids; administration of lozenges and hard candy, acetaminophen or ibuprofen, cool fluids, food, and popsicles; and bed rest.

F Identification and treatment of GABS is beneficial to prevent rheumatic fever (RF), suppurative complications, and secondary spread of cellulitis and to shorten the duration of the illness. Rapid Streptococcus test (RST) is a good screening measure with nearly 100% specificity and rapid result. In addition, the information facilitates rapid initiation of therapy. If negative, it should be backed by Streptococcus culture because of its relatively low sensitivity. Streptococcus culture has lower cost than RST, is easy to obtain, and is considered the gold standard. While awaiting culture results, empirical treatment with appropriate drugs should be considered if symptoms are significant.

G Penicillin (PCN) remains the drug of choice. Amoxicillin and ampicillin are also effective but have no advantage over PCN. Erythromycin should be given if PCN allergy is present cephalexin is also appropriate. Clindamycin or PCN with rifampin has been used to eliminate the carrier status. Patients should restrict unnecessary contacts until after 24 hours of treatment.

H Potentially high-risk patients include those with previous RF, those who are HIV positive, those undergoing chemotherapy, those who are immunosuppressed, diabetics, and pregnant women. The risks of untreated infection in these situations warrant Streptococcus analysis at minor symptom levels.

I Criteria for tonsillectomy (with or without adenoidectomy) include seven episodes in the 1st year, five episodes each year for 2 years, or three episodes each year for 3 years. History of peritonsillar abscess or other severe sequelae as well as amount of school or work missed by the patient are other factors to consider. Most Streptococcus carriers are believed to be at low risk and require no treatment. Adenotonsillectomy can be recommended, especially if a family history of RF exists, other family members are being affected, there is concern about spread in groups such as day care centers, and substantial family anxiety is present.

J Another subset is periodic fever, aphthous stomatitis, pharyngitis, and adenitis (PFAPA).

SUGGESTED READING

Berman S. Pediatric Decision Making, 2nd edition. Philadelphia: BC Decker; 1991. p. 50.

Bisno AL. Acute pharyngitis: etiology and diagnosis. Pediatrics. 1997;97(6 Pt 2):949-954.

Dajani A, Taubert K, Ferrieri P, et al. Treatment of acute streptococcal pharyngitis and prevention of rheumatic fever: a statement for health professionals. Pediatrics. 1995;96(4 Pt 1):758-764.

Kaplan EL. The group A streptococcal upper respiratory tract carrier state: an enigma. J Pediatr. 1980;97(3):337-345.

Markowitz M, Gerber MA, Kaplan EL, et al. Treatment of streptococcal pharyngotonsillitis: reports of penicillin's demise are premature. J Pediatr. 1993;123(5):679-685.

Paradise JL, Bluestone CD, Bachman RZ, et al. Efficacy of tonsillectomy for recurrent throat infection in severely affected children: results of parallel randomized and nonrandomized clinical trials. N Engl J Med. 1984;310(11):674-683.

Oral Fetor

Mariann C McElwain

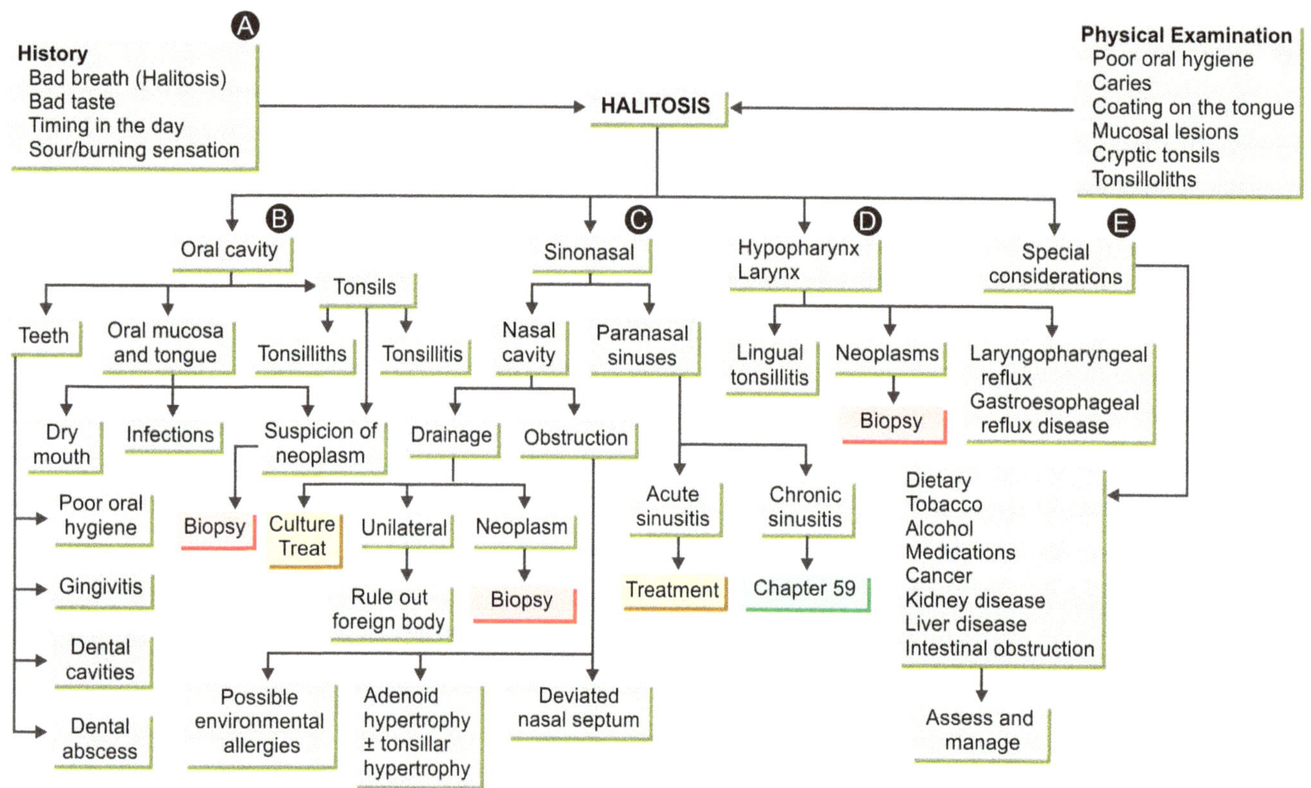

Halitosis is defined as when a bad or foul odor emanates from the mouth. Studies worldwide indicate a high prevalence of moderate halitosis, whereas severe cases are restricted to around 5% of the population. Halitosis relates to the odoriferous substances in exhaled air. The odor comes from the by-products of bacterial degradation. The high prevalence of halitosis is related to the fact that it affects both male and female patients and spans the entire population from very young to the generic population. Halitosis can arise from the entire aerodigestive tract. Specifically, the oral cavity is the most common origin. Clinical management includes oral approaches. However, the oral cavity is only one origin of halitosis. If an oral site is not identified, or if oral strategies are not successful, the clinician must look elsewhere. Successful management is dependent upon locating the system that is involved. The proper diagnosis and treatment of halitosis can involve many specialties. Many of those affected by halitosis suffer for a long time before seeking professional help. Using standardized strategies a high level of treatment success can be achieved.

A Typically the patient will present with complaints of bad breath. Associated complaints include bad taste in the mouth, typically worse in the morning. Occasionally, the patient complains of a sour or burning sensation in the mouth or throat. Typically, the symptoms are painless but can be associated with tooth pain or sore throat or difficulty swallowing. The cause of halitosis is best diagnosed with a careful history and detailed physical examination of the oral cavity, nose, and throat.

B The most common cause of halitosis arises from the oral cavity. Poor oral hygiene is the most likely cause. Dental cavities or abscesses usually present with swelling and/or pain. Gingivitis (periodontal disease) is also usually associated with poor dental hygiene. Treatment includes frequent and thorough tooth brushing along with flossing. Coating of the tongue may be treated with commercial tongue scrapers as well as oral rinses. A thorough examination of the oral cavity looking specifically for oral cavity lesions or infections including tonsillitis should be carried out. Tonsillitis or tonsil stones are commonly noted. These can be the causes of halitosis related to cryptic tonsils as well as posterior nasal drainage. Rarely do tonsil stones warrant a tonsillectomy. Patients should be reassured of their benign nature. Rarely are they completely resolved by irrigations. Any neoplasm of the oral cavity should be biopsied to rule out malignancy.

C Examination of the nasal cavity is best undertaken with rigid/flexible nasal endoscopy after adequate decongestion. Drainage found should be considered for culture and/or treatment. Obstruction such as a deviated nasal septum and adenoid hypertrophy can lead to chronic mouth breathing and xerostomia. A diagnosis of chronic sinusitis generally requires a thorough history and examination as well as imaging (a CT scan). Neoplasms in the nasal cavity/nasopharynx should be considered for biopsy to rule out malignancies.

D The hypopharynx and larynx is best examined by palpation and direct visualization usually with a flexible nasopharyngolaryngoscope. Conditions such as laryngopharyngeal reflux and lingual tonsillitis are commonly associated with halitosis. Neoplasms in this area should be biopsied to rule out malignancies.

E Special considerations should be given to diet. Pungent foods such as garlic, onions, and coffee can cause halitosis. Tobacco products and alcohol should be considered as well. Systemic diseases should be considered:

- *Cancer*: colon, oral cavity, nasal cavity, nasopharynx, hypopharynx, larynx, lung, and digestive tract
- *Diabetes*: fruity smell to breath associated with ketoacidosis
- Gastroesophageal reflux disease
  Kidney disease: can be associated with ammonia smell
- Liver disease
- *Intestinal obstruction*: fecal odor.

SUGGESTED READING

American Academy of Periodontology. Glossary of Periodontal Terms, 4th edition. Chicago: American Academy of Periodontology; 2001. p. 56.

Armstrong BL, Sensat ML, Stolternberg JL. Halitosis: a review of current literature. J Dent Hyg. 2010;84(2):65-74.

Bollen CM, Beikler T. Halitosis: the multidisciplinary approach. Int J Oral Sci. 2012;4(2):55-63.

Rosing CK, Loesche W. Halitosis: an overview of epidemiology, etiology and clinical management. Braz Oral Res. 2011;25(5): 466-471.

Oral Hard Tissue Diseases

Susan E Calderbank

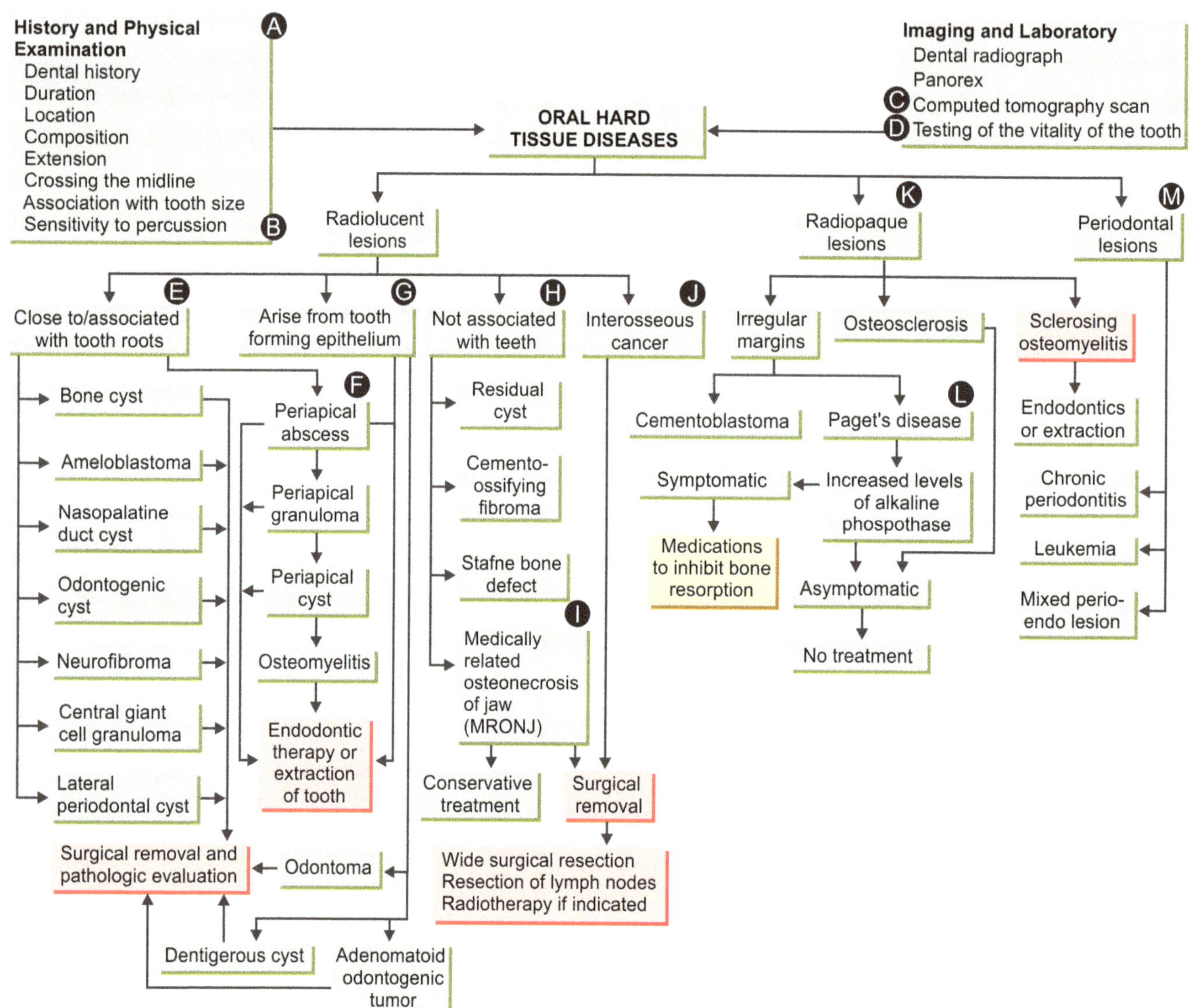

Oral hard tissue diseases are often more difficult to diagnose than those that form in other skeletal bones due to the presence of teeth. The majority of these hard tissue diseases are visible on radiographic studies. In the vast majority of cases, an appropriate referral should be made to the dentist or dental specialist.

A In the jaws, two types of disease states present themselves: those that destroy bone and appear as radiolucent lesions, and those that synthesize calcified materials and appear as radiopaque. The diagnostic phase should include a detailed patient health assessment, history of present illness, a dental history, and a review of symptoms. A complete examination of the head and neck and an intraoral examination must be performed.

B In lesions associated with a tooth, the tooth should be percussed. If the lesion is an abscess, the tooth will be sensitive to percussion. If the lesion is more chronic in nature the tooth may not be sensitive.

C Once radiographic studies are completed, several questions must be asked including location, composition, extension (does the lesion cross the midline), is the lesion associated with a tooth, and the size of the lesion. Lesions, radiolucent or radiopaque, with irregular margins can represent inflammatory processes, primary malignant neoplasms, or metastatic neoplasms.

D Testing of the vitality of the tooth is another diagnostic test that can be performed. Often, microscopic evaluation of the lesion is necessary to confirm an initial diagnosis.

When a tooth is involved in the lesion the choice must be made either to do an endodontic procedure or to extract the tooth.

E Bone cysts may appear as circumscribed lesions in the molar or premolar region. Ameloblastoma has a soap bubble appearance and may metastasize. A nasopalatine duct cyst is at the midline of the maxilla and may erode adjacent tooth roots. Neurofibroma is seen adjacent to the mandibular canal. Odontogenic cysts are seen in adults in the pre-molar area of the mandible. Central giant cell granuloma presents in anterior mandible. Lateral periodontal cysts are seen in the maxilla between lateral and canine teeth.

F Periapical abscess may have purulent exudate at the root apex, and may progress to periapical granuloma, periapical cyst, or osteomyelitis.

G Dentigerous cyst is well defined, benign, and contains mature teeth; more common in young adults. Adenomatoid odontogenic tumor is associated with nonerupted molars and seen in children. Odontoma is mixed radiopaque/radiolucent maxillary mass seen in children.

H Residual cyst is associated with an extracted tooth and may develop into squamous cell cancer. Cemento-ossifying fibroma may be unilocular or multilocular located in posterior mandible. Stafne bone defects are located below the inferior canal and contain an accessory lobe of the submandibular gland.

I MRONJ or medically related osteonecrosis of the jaw is defined as exposed bone in the maxillofacial region without resolution for >8 weeks in patients treated with antiresorptive and/or an antiangiogenic agents who have not received radiation to the jaws. Usually associated with dentoalveolar trauma. Conservative management with antimicrobial rinses and systemic antibiotic therapy. May require surgical debridement/resection.

J Interosseous cancer is associated with paresthesia of the lower lip, may perforate the cortex and fracture the posterior mandible. Breast, prostate, or colon cancer may metastasize and present with local discomfort and paresthesia of the lower lip. Osteogenic sarcoma may also be seen.

K Sclerosing osteomyelitis is a circumscribed radiopaque lesion associated with deep caries usually of the mandibular molar or premolar teeth. Treated with endodontics or extraction. Osteosclerosis forms between roots of the teeth and does not need treatment if asymptomatic. Cementoblastoma has radiolucent appearance that with time may exhibit a radiopaque center.

L Paget's disease has a "cotton wool" appearance, causes facial deformity, and has an increased risk of osteogenic sarcoma.

M Mixed perioendo lesion is radiolucent and surrounds the root of endodontically treated teeth. Leukemia presents with a radiolucent lesion where teeth appear to float. This is also present in Langerhans cell disease. Chronic periodontitis is seen in adults, with diminished level of bone surrounding the teeth, which may be mobile, and is often accompanied by odor associated with pathogenic bacteria.

SUGGESTED READING

Brad WN, Damm D, White D, et al. Color Atlas of Clinical and Oral Pathology. Philadelphia: Lea & Febiger; 1991.

Gardner DG. Some current concepts on the pathology of ameloblastomas. Oral Surg Oral Med Oral Pathol Oral Radiol Endod. 1996;82:600-609.

Newland JR. Oral Hard Tissue Diseases: A Reference Manual for Radiographic Diagnosis, 3rd edition. Lexi-Comp; Michigan. 2003.

Regezi JA, Sciubba JJ. Oral Pathology: Clinical–Pathological Correlations, 2nd edition. WB Saunders; Michigan. 1991.

Ruggiero SL, Dodson TB, Fantasia LA, et al. Medication-Related Osteonecrosis of the Jaws—2014 Update Position Paper American Association of Oral and Maxillofacial Surgeons.

Stockdale CR, Chandler NP. The nature of the periapical lesion—a review of 1108 cases. J Dent. 1988;16:123-129.

Xerostomia

Demetrios G Skedros

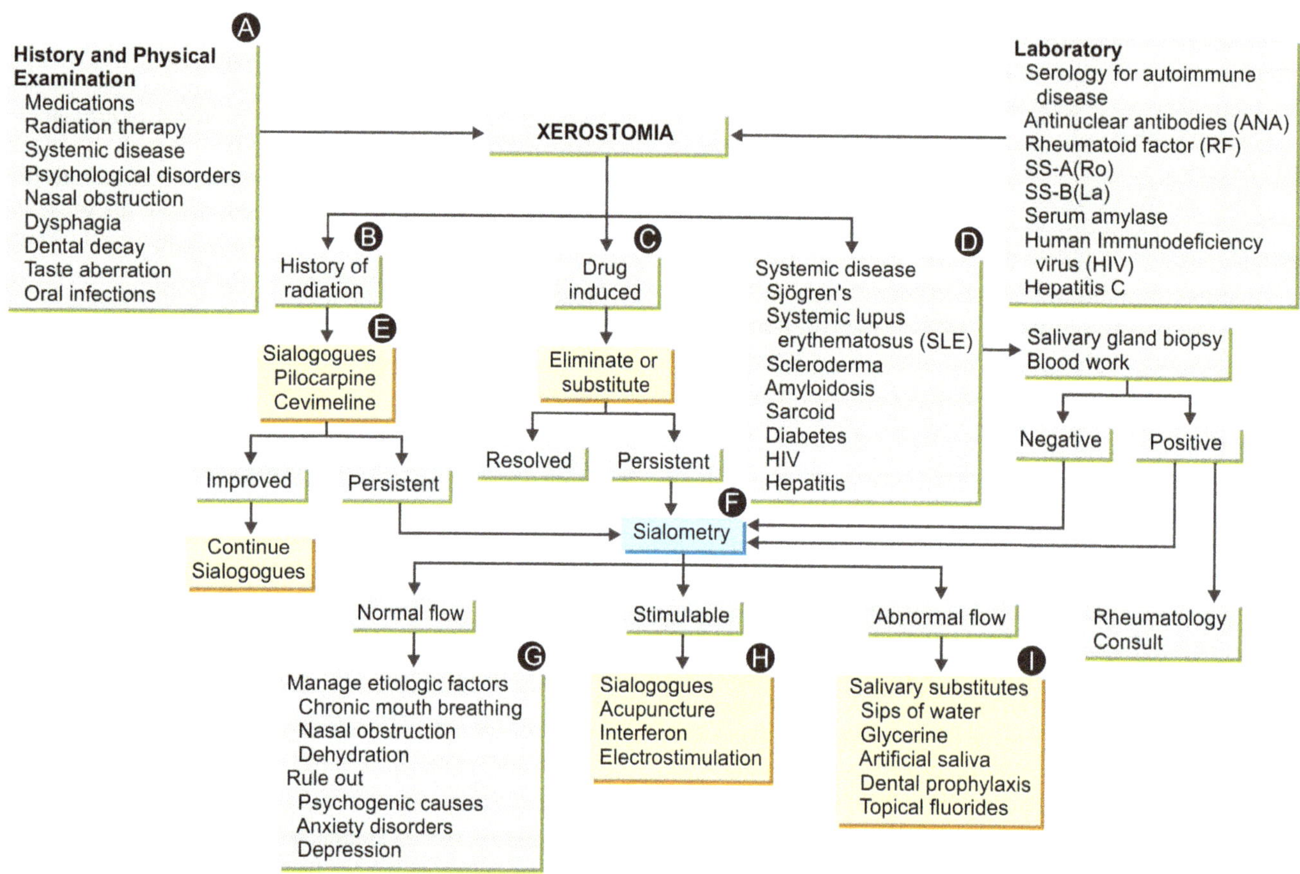

Xerostomia, or dry mouth, is a symptom that is related to salivary gland dysfunction. Xerostomia is a common problem, especially among the elderly, and can result in significant morbidity. Patients who suffer from decreased exocrine gland function typically have problems with voice production, dysphagia, oral pain, taste aberration, and oral infections. Decreased saliva also results in significant dental decay.

A The patient's history and physical findings are important in determining the underlying cause of xerostomia. Previous radiation therapy or the use of certain medications will lead to an immediate diagnosis. Other history may suggest underlying systemic disease, nasal problems, or psychological factors, and thereby direct further management. Patients with dysphagia due to xerostomia often complain initially of swallowing difficulties and further questioning leads to the symptoms of dry mouth.

B Radiation-induced xerostomia is seen in patients requiring this form of therapy for cancer of the head and neck. Radiation changes are irreversible and can lead to long-term disability. However, not all salivary tissue is affected, and some return of salivary function can be expected after the completion of radiation therapy. Cytoprotective agents may help to minimize tissue damage and decrease postradiation xerostomia. Despite this intervention, patients can still complain of dry mouth and require further intervention.

C Drug-related xerostomia is very common, especially in the elderly, where the use of multiple medications is common. More than 500 medications have been associated with oral dryness, including antidepressants, diuretics, antihistamines, antipsychotics, reflux medications, sedatives, and antihypertensives. Drug-induced xerostomia is usually reversible and treated by drug elimination or substitution.

D Many medical conditions are associated with dry mouth. The most common being Sjögren's syndrome. Sjögren's syndrome is characterized by exocrine gland dysfunction. Salivary gland biopsy demonstrates lymphocytic infiltration. Serologic identification of autoantibodies, including antinuclear antibodies, SS-A(Ro), SS-B(La), and serum amylase is also helpful in making the diagnosis.

E Sialogogues can increase salivary flow in conditions where functional glandular tissue is present. Pilocarpine and cevimeline are the two systemic medications approved by the Food and Drug Administration (FDA) for the treatment of xerostomia. Both medications increase saliva production by stimulating muscarinic receptors. Pilocarpine is administered at a dose of 5 mg three times a day (TID). Cevimeline is prescribed at 30 mg TID. Other stimulants include sugar free gum, sour lozenges, ascorbic acid, and malic acid.

F Sialometry is the measurement of salivary flow. A healthy adult produces 1.5 L of saliva every 24 hours or 0.4 mL/min. Stimulated saliva flow ranges from 1 to 2 mL/min. If unstimulated saliva flow is <0.1 mL/min the patient has salivary hypofunction. Paraffin wax and citric acid are the typical stimulants used. The determination of salivary flow in patients with xerostomia can be an essential step in further differentiating treatment options.

G Patients with xerostomia and normal salivary flow require further evaluation for other disorders. Chronic mouth breathing related to nasal obstruction, sinus disease, or even sleep apnea can result in xerostomia. Underlying psychiatric disease and anxiety disorders should be ruled out.

H Patients with salivary flow that can be stimulated have several options to manage their symptoms. Sialogogues are the mainstay of treatment. Other options include acupuncture, interferon-α (for severe Sjögren's disease), and electrostimulation.

I Salivary substitutes can provide relief of xerostomia in situations where abnormal flow exists. Small sips of water, glycerine preparations, or artificial saliva can be used to decrease symptoms. Many over-the-counter preparations exist including sprays, lozenges, gels, toothpastes, rinses, and gums. The prevention of dental decay is also important and can be aided by adequate dental hygiene and topical fluoride application.

SUGGESTED READING

Blom M, Davidson I, Fernberg JO, et al. Acupuncture treatment of patients with radiation-induced xerostomia. Eur J Cancer. 1996;32:182-190.

Cummins MJ, Papas A, Kammer GM, et al. Treatment of primary Sjögren's syndrome with low-dose human interferon alfa administered by the oromucosal route: combined phase III results. Arthritis Rheum. 2003;49(4):585-593.

Plemons JM, Ibtisam A, Marek CL. Managing xerostomia and salivary gland hypofunction. Executive summary of a report from the American Dental Association Council on Scientific Affairs. JADA. 2014;145(8):867-873.

Reike JW, Hafermann MD, Johnson JT, et al. Oral pilocarpine for radiation-induced xerostomia: integrated efficacy and safety results from two prospective randomized clinical trial. Int J Radiation Oncol Biol Phys. 1995;31:661-669.

Sreebny LM, Schwartz SS. A reference guide to drugs and dry mouth, 2nd edition. Gerodontology. 1997;14:33-47.

Villa A, Connell CL, Abati S. Diagnosis and management of xerostomia and hyposalivation. Ther Clin Risk Manag. 2015;11:45-51.

Wolff A, Fox PC, Porter S, et al. Established and novel approaches for the management of hyposalivation and xerostomia. Curr Pharm Des. 2012;18(34):5515-5521.

CHAPTER 89

Orthodontic Problems in Children and Adults

John M Burnheimer

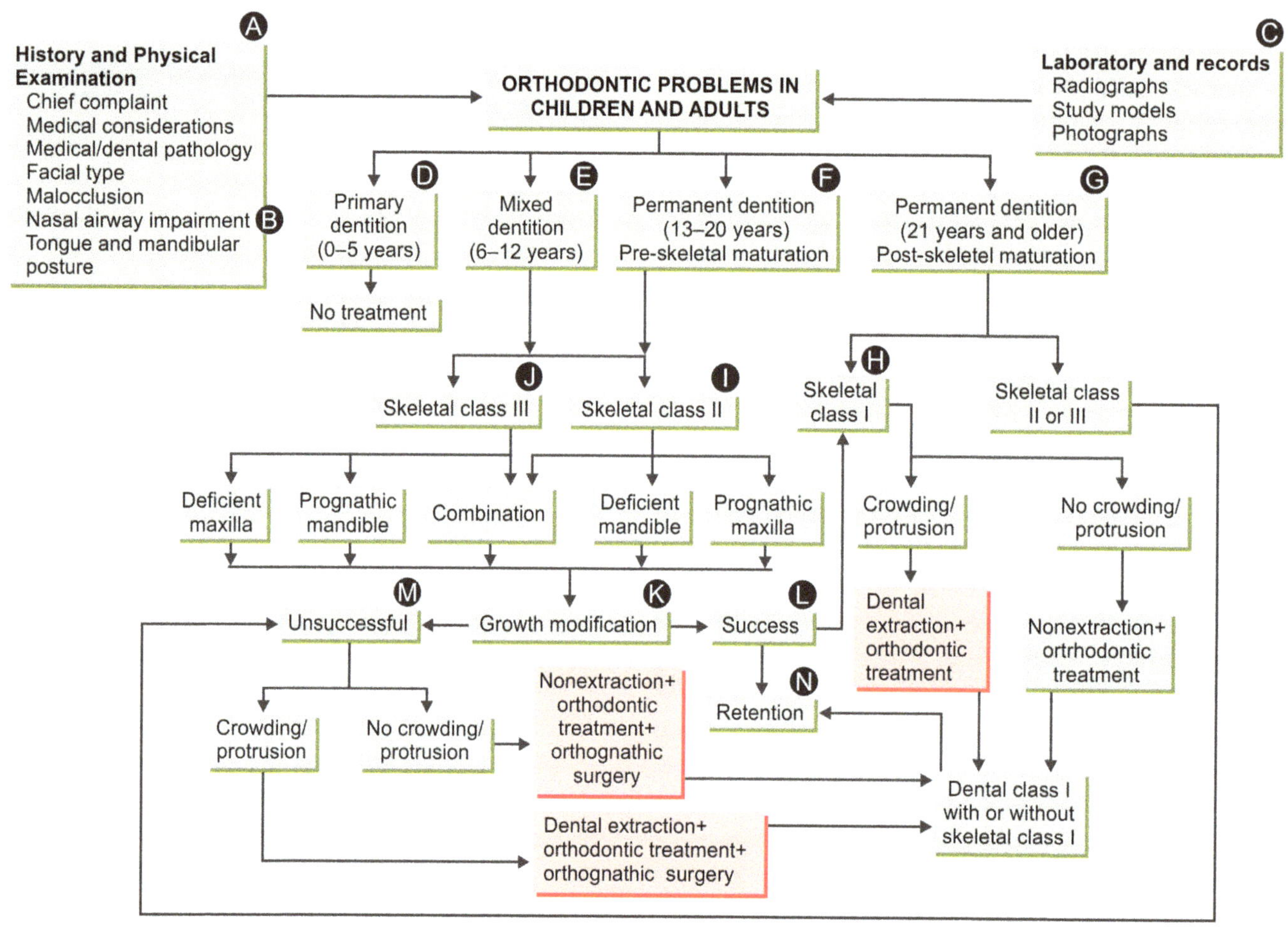

In the modern orthodontic paradigm, health is no longer just the absence of disease (malocclusion), but rather orthodontic health concerns improving a person's quality of life through improved smile esthetics and facial appearance. Smile esthetics can usually (but not always) be improved through orthodontic treatment alone; however, facial appearance often needs adjunctive therapy including surgery, collagen replacement and botulinum toxin type A (Botox).

A Certainly, a thorough history and physical examination is critical. An assessment of facial form, anterior tooth display, and orientation of the aesthetic line of the dentition is essential. The type of malocclusion, arch form and symmetry, as well as vertical and transverse relationships, is analyzed. Recognition of the patient's chief complaint is vital to post-treatment patient satisfaction and a successful orthodontic result. In addition, certain medical considerations may affect orthodontic treatment (e.g. osteoporosis requiring prostaglandin inhibitors and epilepsy requiring phenytoin, which may influence tooth movement).

B Nasal airway impairment is a potential factor that may influence dentofacial growth and development.

C Diagnostic records provide additional information on the type and severity of malocclusion. The skeletal relationship of the maxilla to the mandible as portrayed on standardized cephalometric films aids in treatment planning. Additional specialized radiographic techniques such as cone beam computed tomography (CBCT) may be required. In conjunction with the skeletal classification is the dental or Angle's classification, which is based on the relative position of the maxillary and mandibular canines and molars.

D The primary dentition (baby teeth) is usually seen between the ages of 0 and 5 years old. During this period of growth, the soft tissue generally masks any underlying skeletal discrepancy and, orthodontically, no treatment is indicated.

E The mixed dentition is seen between the ages of 6 and 12 years old and involves a combination of primary (baby) and permanent teeth. Both maxillary and mandibular jawbones are skeletally immature (preskeletal maturation) and are open to growth modification.

F The next age group of 13–20 years old has a permanent dentition, yet both maxillary and mandibular jawbones are, skeletally, not fully mature. This group is still amenable to growth modification (preskeletal maturation).

G This group, over the age of 21 years old, has a permanent dentition and fully mature maxillary and mandibular jawbones. These are considered postskeletal maturation.

H Skeletal class I has a "normal" jaw proportion between the maxilla and mandible in that both jaws approximate each other when seen from the profile view. In skeletal class I, there may be crowding of the dentition or protrusion of the anterior dentition. Either of these may be best treated with tooth extraction.

I In skeletal class II, the jaw disproportion is characterized by maxillary protrusion, mandibular retrusion, of a combination of both, relative to the cranial base.

J In skeletal class III, the jaw disproportion is characterized by mandibular protrusion, maxillary retrusion, or a combination of both, relative to the cranial base.

K Growth modification may be a treatment option for preskeletal maturation patients with both skeletal class II and class III malocclusions; however, it is most successful in skeletal class II cases.

L If growth modification is successful, then treat the patient as skeletal class I.

M If growth modification is unsuccessful or the patient is postskeletal maturation, then tooth extraction to treat any crowding and dentoalveolar protrusion must be considered along with orthognathic surgery to achieve an acceptable result.

N At the end of treatment, retention is important to hold the dentition in the corrected position.

SUGGESTED READING

Graber LW, Vanarsdall RL, Vig KWL. Orthodontics Current Principles and Techniques, 5th edition. St. Louis, MO: CV Mosby; 2012.

Hupp JR, Ellis E, Tucker MR. Contemporary Oral and Maxillofacial Surgery, 5th edition. St. Louis, MO: CV Mosby; 2008.

Nanda R. Esthetics and Biomechanics in Orthodontics, 2nd edition. St. Louis, MO: CV Mosby; 2015.

Proffit WR, Fields HW Jr, Sarver DM. Contemporary Orthodontics, 5th edition. St. Louis, MO: CV Mosby; 2013.

Warren DW. Breathing behavior and posture. In: McNamara JA Jr (Ed). The Enigma of the Vertical Dimension. Craniofacial Growth series, Vol. 36. Ann Arbor, MI: Center for Human Growth and Development, University of Michigan; 2000.

Masticatory Pain and Dysfunction

Justine S Moe, Shelly Abramowicz

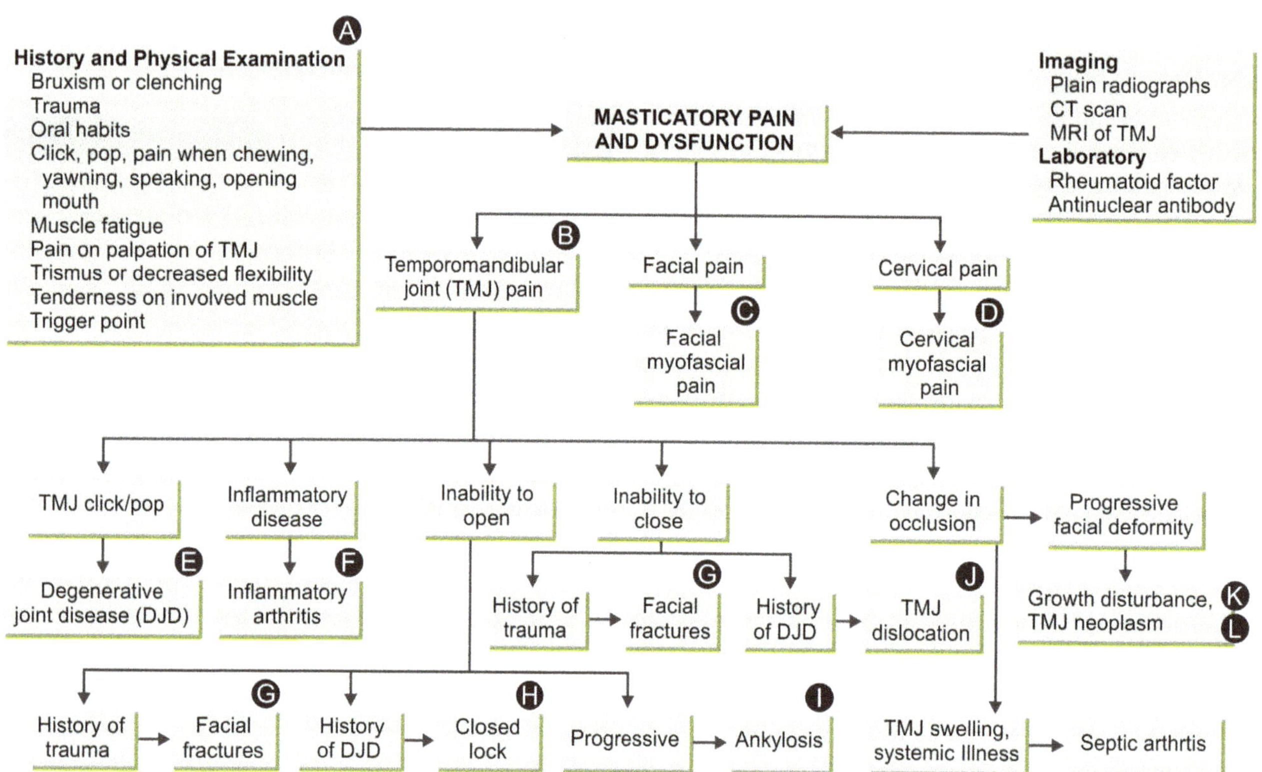

Any patient with a complaint of temporomandibular joint (TMJ) pain, otalgia, bilateral facial or cervical pain should be evaluated for *masticatory dysfunction*.

A Common complaints include TMJ click/pop, pain when chewing, yawning, speaking, or opening the mouth wide. Patients should be questioned for a history of parafunction (bruxism and clenching), oral habits and previous trauma.

B The *TMJ-associated pain* is suspected if the patient complains of pain directly over the TMJ, usually localized with a single finger anterior to the tragus where the mandibular condyle and articular eminence of the temporal bone are palpated. Other causes of pain should be excluded (i.e. otitis media, sinusitis, tonsillitis, malignancy, dermatologic conditions, and odontogenic infection).

C *Facial myofascial pain* manifests as poorly localized pain over large areas of the temples and cheeks. Patients may complain of muscle fatigue, worsening pain with continued jaw activation and restricted mouth opening. Examination shows tenderness of the masseter and temporalis, symptomatic trigger points and decreased flexibility on passive stretch. Other causes of poorly localized facial pain should be excluded (i.e. otalgia, odontogenic infection, parotiditis, sinusitis, headache,

temporal arteritis, hemicrania, trigeminal neuralgia, and carotid artery dissection). Management includes jaw rest, massage, cold or heat therapy, muscle relaxants, occlusal splint, botox and/or trigger point injection.

D *Cervical myofascial pain* is suspected with tenderness of the sternocleidomastoid and trapezius muscles and decreased cervical range of motion. Other causes of pain should be ruled out including odontogenic infection, lymphadenitis, sialadenitis, occipital neuralgia, and cervical spondylosis. Cervical myofascial pain is commonly seen with TMJ and facial myofascial pain. Treatment is similar to facial myofascial pain.

E Patients with a history of TMJ click or pop should be evaluated for *degenerative joint disease* (DJD) of the TMJ. Worsening pain and frequency of TMJ click or pop and a decrease in mouth opening correlate with progressive change in the joint. Examination reveals TMJ tenderness, a palpable or audible click with mouth opening and/or closing, deviation on opening and decreased mandibular range of motion. End-stage DJD is associated with joint crepitus, variable pain and mouth opening. Evaluation includes TMJ-dedicated magnetic resonance imaging (MRI) with open and closed mouth views. Management includes joint unloading (i.e. soft diet and occlusal splint), arthrocentesis, arthroscopy, arthroplasty, or joint replacement.

F Patients with a history of joint pain and swelling, constitutional symptoms and/or extra-articular complaints (i.e. fever, fatigue, weight loss, and skin changes) should be evaluated for *inflammatory arthritis*. Examination shows TMJ tenderness, decreased mandibular range of motion, asymmetric mouth opening, and/or retrognathia. Evaluation includes plain films, TMJ-specific MRI and hematologic studies (i.e. rheumatoid factor and antinuclear antibody). Management may include medications by a rheumatologist, analgesics, TMJ lysis and lavage, arthroplasty, or TMJ replacement in cases of significant joint destruction.

G *Facial fractures* can cause either restricted mouth opening or an anterior open bite. Fracture patterns associated with restricted opening include subcondylar, zygomatic arch and zygomaticomaxillary complex fractures as they can mechanically obstruct mandibular movement. Fracture patterns associated with anterior open bite include bilateral subcondylar and Le Fort fractures. Examination shows point tenderness over the fractured bony processes and step deformities. Evaluation includes plain radiography or computed tomography (CT). Management includes maxillomandibular fixation and/or surgical reduction with or without internal fixation.

H Patients with limited mouth opening with a history of previous TMJ clicking or popping should be evaluated for *TMJ closed lock*. Examination reveals tenderness over the TMJ, deviation on opening to the ipsilateral side and decreased mandibular range of motion. Diagnosis is based on clinical findings. Temporomandibular joint-specific MRI may only be necessary in chronic cases. Management includes pain control and reduction of the articular disc via arthrocentesis or arthroscopy with jaw manipulation.

I Patients with a progressive decrease in mouth opening without a TMJ click or pop should be evaluated for *TMJ hypomobility* (i.e. fibrous or bony TMJ ankylosis, coronoid hyperplasia, or intraoral scar band). Depending on the extent and location of ankylosis, management consists of arthroplasty or joint replacement. Coronoid hyperplasia is managed with coronoidotomy or coronoidectomy. Intraoral scar bands are treated with surgical release, *Z*-plasty, or skin grafting. Postoperative physical therapy is imperative to prevent reankylosis.

J Patients with a history of DJD and an inability to close the mouth should be evaluated for *TMJ dislocation* or *open lock*. Examination shows a depression at the glenoid fossa with the condyle palpated anteriorly to the TMJ and variable mandibular mobility. Evaluation includes plain radiographs and noncontrast CT. Acute management is manual reduction. Recurrent dislocation is managed by intra-articular sclerosing agents, capsulorrhaphy, lateral pterygoid botox injection and/or temporary maxillomandibular fixation. Surgical management includes eminectomy, Leclerc procedure, or TMJ replacement.

K Patients with progressive change in occlusion should be evaluated for *TMJ growth disturbance*. Paucity of growth is seen in condylar hypoplasia and aplasia. Excessive growth is seen in mandibular hyperplasia (i.e. prognathism and crossbite) and condylar hyperplasia (associated with progressive facial asymmetry, unilateral posterior open bite, and deviation of the mandibular midline). Idiopathic condylar resorption presents with worsening mandibular retrognathia and anterior open bite. Evaluation includes serial plain radiographs to monitor changes in growth over time or facial CT. Bone scintigraphy evaluates condylar growth in condylar hyperplasia. Management may include partial or total condylectomy, joint replacement, and/or orthognathic surgery.

L *Temporomandibular joint neoplasms* can cause TMJ swelling, pain, dysfunction, and change in occlusion. Most neoplasms of the TMJ are benign (i.e. chondroma, osteoma, and osteochondroma). Malignant TMJ neoplasms are most commonly metastatic while primary malignant TMJ neoplasms are rare. Osteoclastic neoplasms should be suspected when a patient presents with a pathologic fracture of the condyle without a history of trauma. Evaluation includes CT or MRI, biopsy and additional tests in cases of malignant disease (i.e. positron emission tomography). Management depends on the tissue diagnosis and may include surgical resection, reconstruction, radiation, and/or chemotherapy.

SUGGESTED READING

Kaban LB, Troulis MJ. Pediatric Oral and Maxillofacial Surgery. St Louis, MO: Elsevier; 2004.

Miloro M, Ghali GE, Larsen P. Peterson's Principles of Oral and Maxillofacial Surgery, 3rd edition. Shelton, CT/Philadelphia, PA: Lippincott Williams and Wilkins; 2011.

Okeson JP. Management of Temporomandibular Disorders and Occlusion, 7th edition. St Louis, MO: Elsevier; 2013.

Wilkes CH. Internal derangements of the temporomandibular joint: pathological variation. Arch Otolaryngol Head Neck Surg. 1989;115:469-477.

Taste Disturbance

Andrea M Hebert, Carl H Snyderman

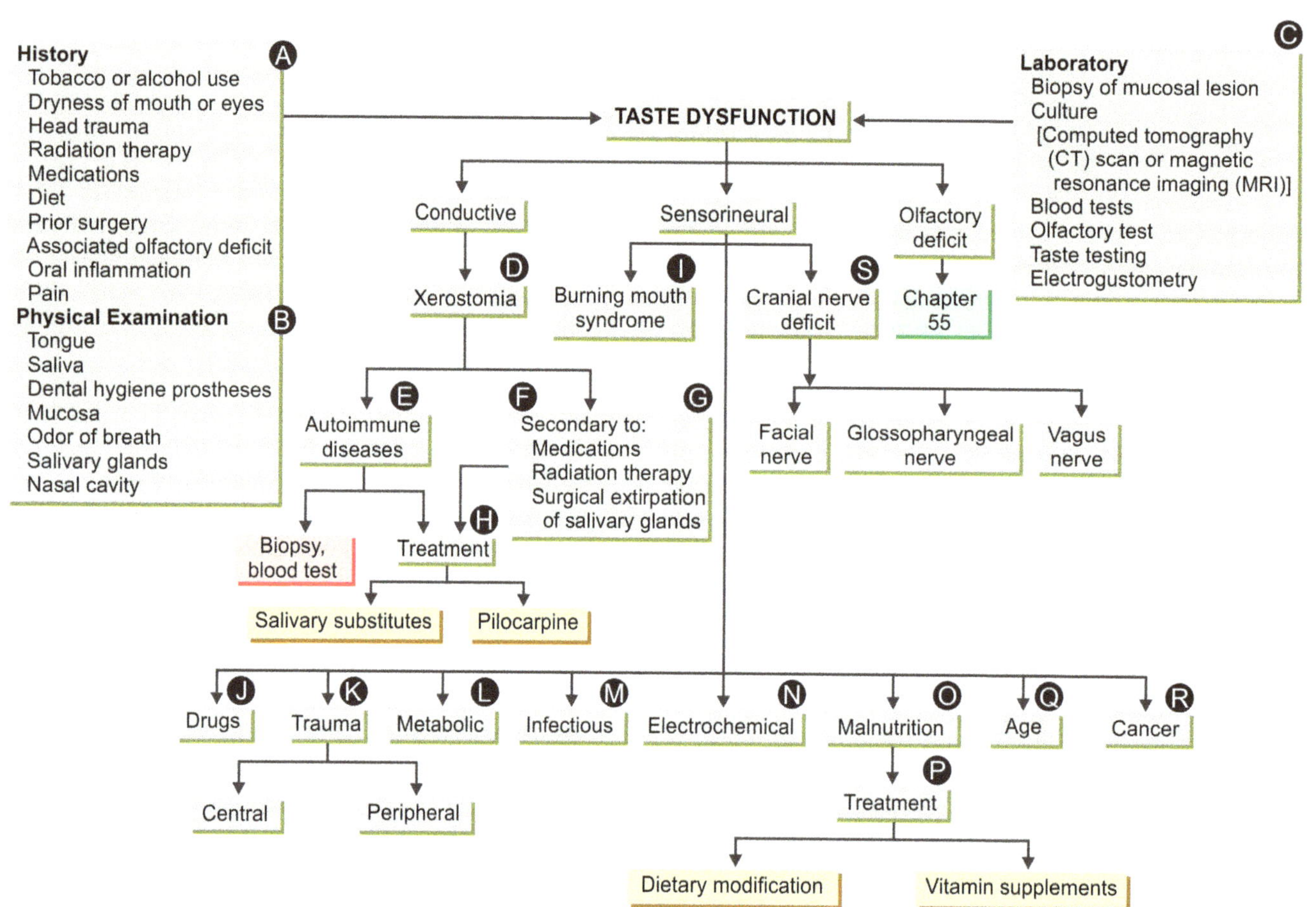

Isolated disorders of taste function are rare. Most complaints of decreased taste are due to associated olfactory dysfunction. Similar to olfactory disorders, taste dysfunction may be categorized as conductive or sensorineural disorders.

A A thorough history should be obtained, as clues to the etiology of the patient's taste disturbance will often be found. Patients should be questioned not only about taste, but also about associated olfactory symptoms and antecedent events as well as inflammatory or ulcerative conditions of the oral mucosa. Localization of the taste disturbance to one region may indicate involvement of a peripheral nerve (chorda tympani, glossopharyngeal, vagus).

B Particular attention is paid to the tongue (glossitis, ulceration, taste papillae, atrophy, tumors), oral mucosa, quantity and quality of saliva, and dental condition. Methylene blue will stain the pores of normally functioning taste buds. Absence of staining as a result of deafferentation (loss of sensory input) allows the clinician to distinguish central from peripheral gustatory loss. Assessment of cranial nerves may allow localization of the taste deficit to

a particular nerve. Sinonasal conditions should not be overlooked.

C Biopsy of suspicious lesions (neoplasia, pemphigus or pemphigoid, granulomatous disease, lichen planus, and amyloidosis) should be performed. Measurement of salivary flow can be performed to document xerostomia. Cultures, especially for actinomycosis and candida, may be indicated. Olfactory function should be assessed in all patients because it is often overlooked by patients. Patients should be screened for general medical conditions that may affect taste (diabetes, hypothyroidism, kidney failure, and liver disease). Imaging is indicated for evaluation of suspected cranial nerve lesions.

Specific taste testing is performed using suprathreshold stimuli, which represent the major taste groups (caffeine or quinine for bitter, citric acid for sour, sucrose for sweet, and sodium chloride for salty). Monosodium glutamate has recently been used for testing umami. Electrogustometry, which involves the stimulation of fields of taste buds with anodal or cathodal current, may be useful but provides an incomplete picture of taste function. Gustatory-evoked potentials and functional magnetic resonance imaging (MRI) have also been investigated as methods of objectively identifying taste disturbances.

D In addition to providing a medium for the distribution of tastants, saliva has homeostatic effects on the mucosal epithelium and taste buds. Xerostomia is frequently encountered and has multiple causes.

E Several autoimmune disorders can cause xerostomia and related-taste disturbance, including systemic lupus erythematosus, scleroderma, sarcoidosis, and rheumatoid arthritis. Keratoconjunctivitis sicca, xerostomia with or without salivary gland enlargement characterizes Sjögren's syndrome, an autoimmune disease of the exocrine glands. The diagnosis may be established by salivary gland biopsy and laboratory testing for autoantibodies (SS-A, SS-B).

F Numerous medications may cause xerostomia and affect taste sensation, including diuretics, antihistamines, antidepressants, antipsychotics, anxiolytics, analgesics, antihypertensives, anti-Parkinsonism drugs, and decongestants.

G Radiation therapy of the head and neck has both immediate and delayed effects due to inflammation and fibrosis, respectively. Direct damage to the mucosa and salivary glands causes xerostomia which contributes to taste dysfunction. Surgical removal of a single salivary gland, does not cause xerostomia.

H The treatment of xerostomia includes treatment of underlying causes as well as the discontinuation of offending medications and alcohol consumption, if possible. The use of commercially available saliva substitutes can provide temporary relief, but acceptance by patients is poor. Pilocarpine administration has been effective in some patients, though side effects can be prohibitive.

I Burning mouth syndrome is a pain disorder that affects the oral cavity. The cause is not known in most cases. Other symptoms frequently include dry mouth and parageusia (abnormal, usually offensive taste).

J Medications may cause a sensorineural modification that directly affects taste function (antirheumatic and antiproliferative agents). Drugs that are distributed to saliva or eye drops that drain via the nasolacrimal duct may be tasted in some cases.

K Post-traumatic ageusia after blunt head trauma is usually due to loss of olfaction; however, injury to the thalamus, brain stem or the ventral temporal lobes can cause an isolated taste disturbance. Unilateral ageusia is generally caused by peripheral nerve injury. A temporal bone fracture can cause a unilateral ageusia secondary to injury to the facial nerve.

L Endocrine disorders such as Addison's disease, diabetes mellitus, and hypothyroidism can affect taste but are usually diagnosed as a result of other symptoms or physical findings.

M Viral infection of the chorda tympani nerve (idiopathic facial paralysis) results in a temporary alteration of taste. Activation of herpes zoster within the geniculate ganglion may also affect gustation. Infections of the middle ear may involve the chorda tympani nerve. Mucositis resulting from fungi, such as *Candida albicans,* may be seen in immunosuppressed patients or after antibiotic therapy.

N Galvanic currents from metals in dental restorations or appliances may cause parageusia but is difficult to confirm.

O Severe malnutrition impairs mucosal regeneration and resistance to infection. Vitamin B_1 and zinc are necessary nutrients for normal taste bud function.

P Beyond treatment of underlying nutritional disorders and specific vitamin deficiencies, there is little evidence to support the use of nutritional supplements such as zinc in the majority of patients. The addition of seasonings and flavor enhancers and alteration of food temperature, texture, and consistency may improve the palatability of food.

Q Taste acuity and olfactory function decline with age and may contribute to malnutrition in the elderly.

R In patients with neoplasia of the upper aerodigestive tract, alteration of taste function may result from destruction of receptor cells and neural pathways, malnutrition, effects of chemotherapy and radiotherapy, and possibly paraneoplastic syndromes.

S Lesions of the facial, chorda tympani, lingual, glossopharyngeal, and vagus nerves may affect taste. Lesions can be primary in nature or a result of iatrogenic injury. Examples of iatrogenic causes include injury to the chorda tympani in middle ear surgery, sacrifice of the lingual nerve in head and neck cancer resections, and injury to the glossopharyngeal nerve during tonsillectomy. Localization of the lesion may be suggested by the constellation of cranial nerve deficits.

SUGGESTED READING

Getchell TV, Doty RL, Bartoshuk LM, Snow JB Jr. Smell and Taste in Health and Diseases. New York, NY, USA: Raven Press; 1991.

Heckmann JG, Lang CJ. Neurological causes of taste disorders. Adv Otorhinolaryngol. 2006;63:255-264.

Hummel T, Landis BN, Hüttenbrink KB, et al. Smell and taste disorders. GMS Curr Top Otorhinolaryngol Head Neck Surg. 2011;10:Doc04.

Kimmelman CP. Disorders of Taste and Smell, SIPAC Self-Instructional Package. Alexandria, VA, USA: American Academy of Otolaryngology-Head and Neck Surgery Foundation; 1996.

Mortazavi H, Baharvand M, Movahhedian A, et al. Xerostomia due to systemic disease: a review of 20 conditions and mechanisms. Ann Med Health Sci Res. 2014;4(4):503-510.

Seiden AM. Rhinology and Sinusology—Diagnosis, Medical Management, Surgical Approaches: Taste and Smell Disorders. New York, NY, USA: Thieme Medical Publishers; 1997.

Shoji N, Riwada SS, Sasano T. Clinical significance of umami taste and umami-related gene expression analysis for the objective assessment of umami taste loss. Curr Pharm Des. 2016; 22(15):2238-2244.

Stathas T, Mallis A, Naxakis S, et al. Taste function evaluation after tonsillectomy: a prospective study of 60 patients. Eur Arch Otorhinolaryngol. 2010;267(9):1403-1407.

Welge-Lüssen A, Dörig P, Wolfensberger M, et al. A study about the frequency of taste disorders. J Neurol. 2011;258(3):386-392.

Neoplasms of the Lip

Christopher H Rassekh

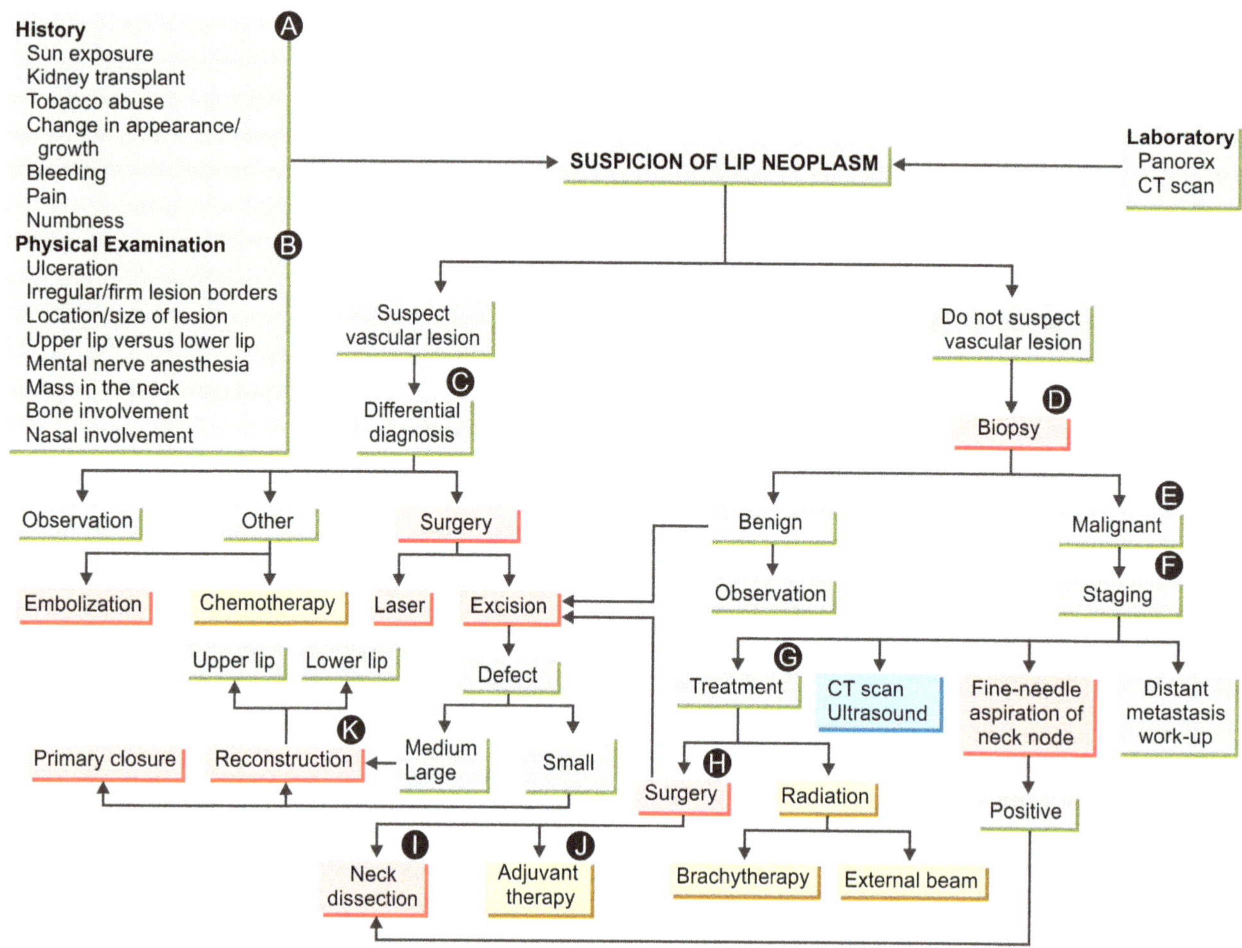

Neoplasms of the lip originate on the lower lip much more commonly than on the upper lip or oral commissure. A variety of pathologic entities may present on the lip. A diagnostic and therapeutic algorithm is valuable in the management of lip cancers. Surgery and radiotherapy play a role in the treatment of these lesions.

A A history of solar exposure or tobacco abuse increases the likelihood that a lip lesion is a cancer. Other risk factors include fair complexion, tobacco use, and immunosuppression. Change in appearance or growth, bleeding, pain, or numbness is important to note.

B Physical examination revealing ulceration, irregular or firm borders, or crusting should alert the physician to the possibility of cancer of the lip. The examination should include assessment of the oral sphincter function, palpation for cervical or facial adenopathy or masses, and assessment of the location and size of the lesion and its apparent growth characteristics. Anesthesia of the mental nerve, bone invasion, and nasal involvement are best detected clinically. The dentition should be evaluated.

C The differential diagnosis of lip lesions that may be vascular includes hemangioma, vascular malformation, thrombosed vessels, and pyogenic granuloma and other rare vascular tumors. Treatment might involve excision, but some lesions are treated by laser, others may be embolized (arteriovenous malformation), and some are treated with prednisone, interferon, or other chemotherapy or biological response modifiers.

D Most lesions of the lip require a biopsy to establish a diagnosis. In many instances, a shave biopsy is sufficient to allow treatment planning. If the lesion is benign, excision or observation may be recommended. Minor salivary gland cysts and tumors, fibrous tumors, and papillomas are included in the differential diagnosis.

E Malignant lesions include basal cell carcinoma, squamous cell carcinoma, salivary gland cancers, melanoma, sarcomas, and miscellaneous rare tumors. These are also varying degrees of actinic solar damage that may be considered premalignant change.

F Staging includes computed tomography (CT) scan of the neck and mandible and fine-needle aspiration (FNA) of any suspicious nodes. Ultrasonography or CT may be useful for image-guided FNA. Reactive lymph nodes are common and ultrasound may distinguish suspicious from less suspicious nodes.

G Treatment of lip cancers is usually surgical. However, radiation can be delivered for cure by both external beam and brachytherapy in selected patients. Radiation is also an option for patients who have distant metastatic disease or who are medically unfit for surgery.

H Surgery for most lip lesions requires excision with adequate margins. For carcinomas, a gross margin of 5 mm is preferred and a microscopic margin of at least 2 mm is considered adequate. Procedures available range from wedge (and shield) excision to resection of the entire lip. Lip shave (vermilionectomy) is useful for superficial lesions that involve large surface areas and can be combined with additional resection of any deeper lesions.

I Neck dissection should be performed if there is suspicion of cervical metastasis by examination, CT, and FNA. Elective neck dissection or elective neck radiation may be offered for the N0 neck when the neck is considered at high risk. Features that increase risk include large size of the primary tumor, involvement of the oral commissure or upper lip by squamous cell carcinoma, muscle invasion, bone invasion, and lymphatic invasion. An alternative strategy for T1 and T2 N0 cancers is sentinel lymph node biopsy. The first echelon nodes are generally level IB.

J Postoperative radiation is also advised for patients with T4 cancers and those with N2 or N3 neck metastases. Radiation and/or neck dissection may be considered for patients with perineural invasion. Reresection should be performed for positive margins followed by radiation.

K Reconstruction of the lip is a major challenge. Defects can be divided into small (less than half of the lip), medium (one-half to two-thirds) and large (more than two-thirds). Vermilionectomy can usually be adequately reconstructed by advancement of the mucosa from the gingival sulcus. Small defects on the upper lip can be closed primarily, perialar crescentic advancement, or small nasolabial transposition flaps. Small defects of the lower lip can usually be closed primarily. For medium-sized defects that do not involve the commissure, options are the Abbe flap (lip switch) or the Karapandzic flap. The Karapandzic flap is advantageous in that it preserves oral sphincter function and is performed in a single stage. However, it produces a rounded commissure. For involvement of the commissure, the Estlander modification of the Abbe flap can be used. For larger defects, full-thickness nasolabial flaps or cheek advancement techniques are required. If adjacent cheek tissue is inadequate, pedicled or free tissue transfer may be considered. If the mandible is invaded, a mandibulectomy is necessary using a free flap containing bone for reconstruction.

SUGGESTED READING

Bailey BJ, Calhoun KH, Coffey AR, et al. Lip Section, Atlas of Head and Neck Surgery-Otolaryngology. Philadelphia, PA: Lippincott-Raven; 1998. p. 42.

de Visscher JG, van den Elsaker K, Grond AJ, et al. Surgical treatment of squamous cell carcinoma of the lower lip: evaluation of long-term results and prognostic factors—a retrospective analysis of 184 patients. J Oral Maxillofac Surg. 1998;56:814-820.

Karapandzic M. Reconstruction of lip defects by local arterial flaps. Br J Plast Surg. 1974;27:93-97.

Onerci M, Yilmaz T, Gedikoglu G. Tumor thickness as a predictor of cervical lymph node metastasis in squamous cell carcinoma of the lower lip. Otolaryngol Head Neck Surg. 2000;122:139-142.

Renner GJ, Zitsch RP III. Cancer of the lip. In: Myers EN, Suen JY, Myers JN, et al (Eds.). Cancer of the Head and Neck, 4th edition. Philadelphia: WB Saunders; 2003. pp. 251-277.

Sollamo EM, Ilmonen SK, Virolainen MS, et al. Sentinel lymph node biopsy in cN0 squamous cell carcinoma of the lip. Head Neck. 2016;38(Suppl 1):E1375-1380.

Weber RS, Palmar JM, Edel E, et al. Minor salivary gland tumors of lip and buccal mucosa. Laryngoscope. 1989;99:6-9.

Zitsch RP III, Lee BW, Smith RB. Cervical lymph node metastases and squamous cell carcinoma of the lip. Head Neck. 1999;21:447-453.

CHAPTER 93

Neoplasms of the Tongue

David M Cognetti, Joseph M Curry

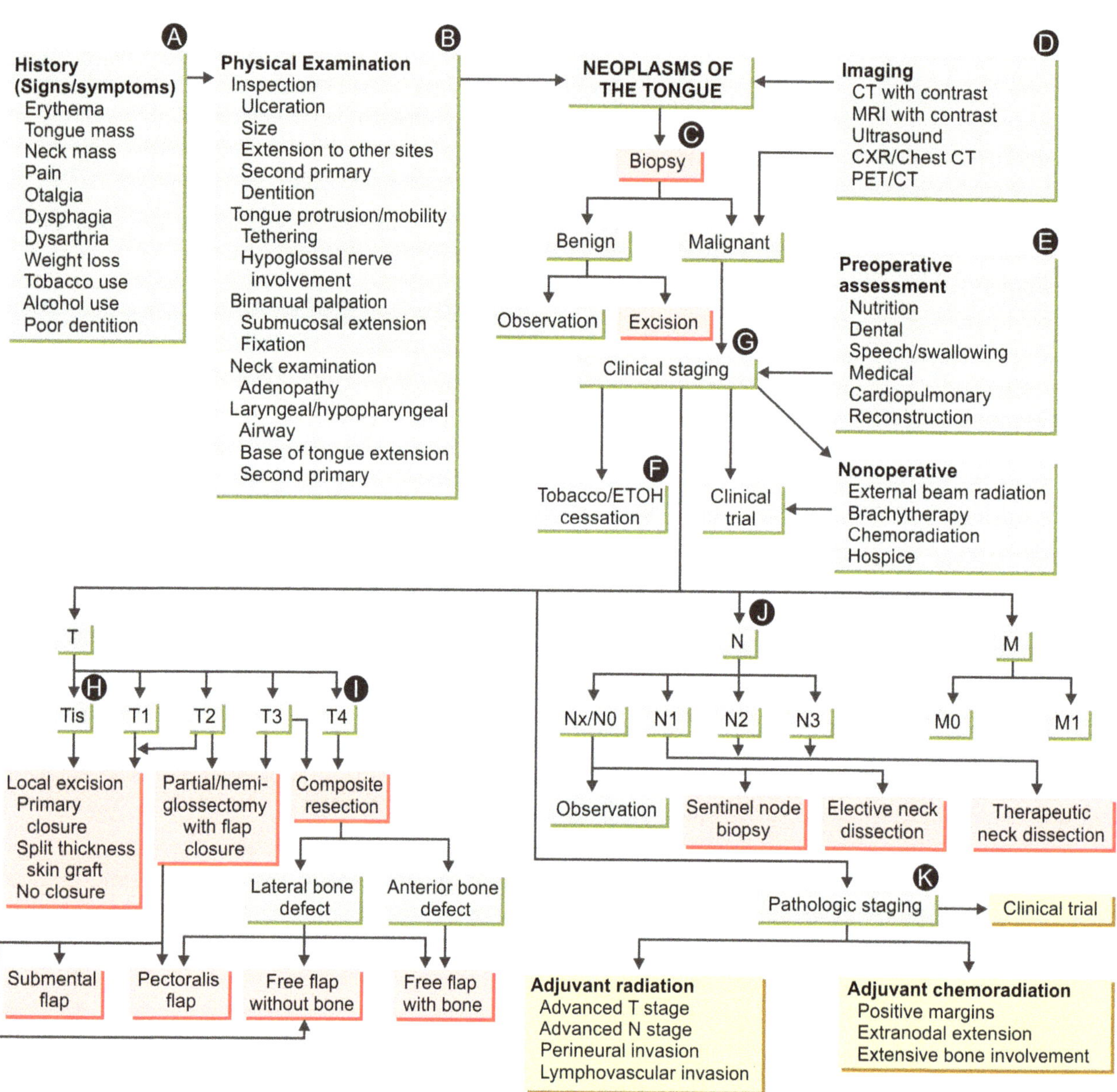

The oral tongue is the site of both benign and malignant neoplasms. Typically, these can be differentiated on the basis of a thorough history and physical examination. Squamous cell carcinoma is the most common malignancy of the tongue and is caused by the use of tobacco and alcohol.

A Benign neoplasms, such as fibroma, are smooth and painless. Erythema, ulceration, and pain should raise suspicion for malignancy. Referred otalgia is a common complaint in patients with cancer of the tongue. Cancer of the tongue can lead to dysphagia, dysarthria, and weight loss. A history of tobacco use and heavy alcohol use should further raise the index of suspicion for malignancy. There is an increasing incidence of cancer of the base of the tongue in younger, nonsmoking individuals related to the human papilloma virus (HPV).

B Physical examination is essential in the evaluation of tongue neoplasms. In cases of malignancy, physical examination must be directed to guide treatment planning. Extension to the floor of mouth, base of the tongue, deep tongue musculature, and mandible has important implications for staging and reconstruction. Careful examination of cervical lymph nodes should be performed as tongue cancer often metastasizes to the neck. Mirror examination or flexible laryngoscopy allows evaluation of the airway and surveillance for second primary tumors.

C Biopsy should be performed in any patient with suspected malignancy. This can typically be performed in the office setting. A cup forceps sample of the lesion is preferred over excisional biopsy to minimize the compromise of subsequent oncologic resection.

D Imaging is important for staging and surgical planning. Computed tomography (CT) scans provide better assessment of bone involvement while magnetic resonance imaging (MRI) provides better delineation of deep muscle involvement. Both allow evaluation of neck adenopathy and both can be limited by dental amalgam. Ultrasound can be used to evaluate the depth of tumors and cervical lymph nodes. In cases of malignancy, imaging of the chest is indicated to evaluate for a second primary lung cancer or metastases. In advanced malignancy, positron emission tomography/computed tomography (PET/CT) may be useful for staging.

E The treatment of cancer of the tongue is primarily surgical. Preoperative assessment should evaluate nutrition, dentition, and swallowing function. Appropriate medical, cardiac, and pulmonary evaluation should be pursued prior to surgical intervention. Reconstructive needs should be anticipated preoperatively to allow for appropriate counseling and single-stage repair. Dental extractions, as indicated should be pursued in patients who will require radiation therapy.

F Tobacco and alcohol abuse are high-risk factors for squamous cell carcinoma of the tongue. Abstinence of both is critical to treatment success. Cessation counseling must be incorporated into the treatment plans of all active users of tobacco and alcohol.

G The treatment of cancer of the tongue is determined by the clinical staging. Primary surgery is the treatment of choice for all stages. Adjuvant radiation or chemoradiation may be added for advanced disease. All patients should be evaluated for available clinical trials. In cases in which patients are medically unfit or refuse surgery, nonsurgical approaches such as external beam radiation, brachytherapy, and chemotherapy can be pursued. These should be rare exceptions. Nonoperative management is offered for palliation in patients with unresectable local cancer or distant metastases. For these patients, clinical trials should be considered and early referral to hospice is beneficial.

H Early-stage primary cancer can be managed using a transoral excision. Typically, the surgical defect can be closed primarily or left open to granulate and remucosalize. When the defect involves the floor of mouth, reconstruction using a split thickness skin graft is recommended.

I Advance-staged cancer will require at least a hemiglossectomy. Large cancers may require transcervical or transmandibular access. For larger tongue defects, flap reconstruction is recommended with free tissue transfer preferred. When the mandible is involved, a segmental resection is indicated. Reconstruction using osteocutaneous free flaps is mandatory for anterior mandibular defects and preferred but optional for lateral mandibular defects.

J Due to a high rate of cervical metastases, treatment of the neck is mandated in all but the earliest stage cancer of the tongue. For T1 tumors, depth of invasion is a determinant for risk of occult metastases. Patients with cancer with a histologic depth <4 mm and without adenopathy on imaging are candidates for close observation of the neck. All other patients require treatment of the neck. Levels 1–4 are included in neck dissections. Sentinel node biopsy has been shown to be effective in patients with a clinically negative neck. A small cancer on the lateral aspect of the tongue can be treated with ipsilateral neck dissection. Large cancer approaching or crossing the midline require bilateral neck dissection.

K Adjuvant therapy is based on pathologic staging. Only the earliest stage cancer (T1–T2 and N0–N1) is treated with surgery alone. Patients with advanced cancer or high-risk pathologic features (perineural invasion and lymphovascular invasion) should be offered adjuvant radiation. Adjuvant chemoradiation is indicated in patients with positive surgical margins, extranodal extension, and extensive bone involvement.

SUGGESTED READING

Cognetti D, Ferris R. Mass in the oral cavity. In: Stewart M, Selesnick S (Eds). Differential Diagnosis in Otolaryngology—Head and Neck Surgery. New York: Thieme; 2011. p. 196.

Deshler DG, Erman AB. Oral cavity cancer. In: Johnson JT, Rosen CA (Eds). Bailey's Head and Neck Surgery—Otolaryngology, 5th edition. Baltimore, MD: Lippincott Williams and Wilkins; 2014. p. 1849.

Myers EN, Myers JN. Cancer of the anterior tongue. In: Gates GA (Ed). Current Therapy in Otolaryngology—Head and Neck Surgery. St Louis, MO: Mosby–Year Book; 1998. p. 262.

Neoplasms of the Floor of the Mouth

Miriam N Lango

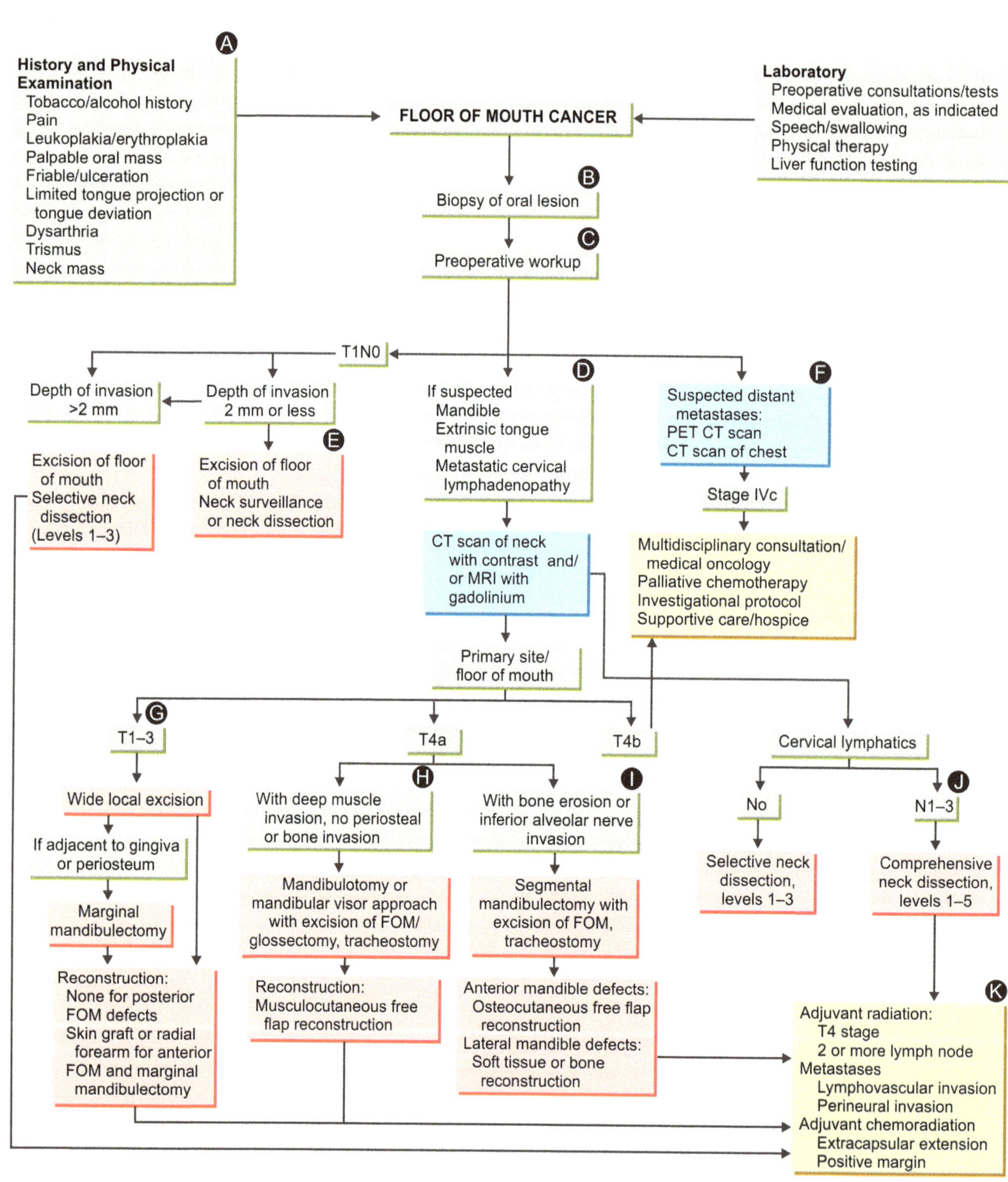

A persistent lesion or mass of the floor of the mouth (FOM) should be evaluated for cancer. Minor salivary gland tumors and cancers are more likely to manifest as nontender submucosal masses, while tender ulcerated mucosal lesions are more often squamous cell carcinomas.

(A) *History and physical examination*: Tobacco and alcohol are known risk factors for cancer of the floor of the mouth. A lesion associated with changes in tongue mobility (limitations in tongue protrusion, tongue deviation), trismus, and the presence of palpable cervical lymphadenopathy should be considered a cancer until proven otherwise.

(B) *Tissue diagnosis*: A biopsy performed in the office will establish the diagnosis and facilitate initial clinical staging. A punch biopsy is effective in diagnosing submucosal masses.

(C) *Preoperative consultation and testing*: A preoperative speech and swallowing and physical therapy evaluation will document the pretreatment function and facilitate postoperative rehabilitation.

(D) *Preoperative imaging*: Imaging such as a computed tomography (CT) scan is indicated if mandible, extrinsic tongue muscle invasion, or metastatic cervical lymphadenopathy is suspected. A CT scan of the neck will assess both invasion of the mandible and the presence of abnormal cervical lymphadenopathy. The radiologic criterion for pathologic lymphadenopathy depends on size (>1.0 cm) or central necrosis. Involved nodes are usually in levels 1 and 2 (submental, submandibular, and upper jugulodigastric regions). Negative imaging does not rule out microscopic metastatic disease. The extent of tongue muscle involvement may be better demonstrated with a magnetic resonance imaging (MRI) with gadolinium than a CT scan. Chest radiograph or CT of the chest is recommended for smokers who may have second primary lung cancers or patients with oral cancers suspected of metastasis to the lungs.

(E) *Stage I and dysplasia/carcinoma in situ*: The frequency of micrometastatic disease for T1N0 FOM cancers with depth of invasion ≤2 mm is low; surveillance rather than elective neck dissection may be entertained. However, FOM cancers >2 mm deep should be managed with a selective neck dissection, or possibly a sentinel lymph node biopsy.

(F) *Stage IVc*: Metastases to the lungs are usually indicative of incurable disease; however, metastases must be distinguished from second primary lung cancers, which may be curable. If a second primary cancer is found in the lung and is resectable, debate exists as to which lesion should be treated first (*see* Chapter 177).

(G) *Transoral resection*: Lesions limited to the floor of the mouth, ventral tongue, or alveolus may be resected transorally. If the tumor is adherent to the gingiva or the mandibular periosteum, marginal mandibulectomy should be performed. Small posterior FOM defects may potentially be allowed to granulate in; however, larger defects and those in the anterior FOM will yield better long-term function if they are reconstructed with a skin graft or a radial forearm free flap.

(H) *Extended primary resection without mandibulectomy*: Transoral exposure will be inadequate for deeply invasive cancers that involve the extrinsic tongue musculature. A mandibulotomy or mandibular visor approach that releases the FOM and tongue into the neck will facilitate a complete extirpation. Care must be taken to preserve at least one lingual artery to preserve the blood supply of the residual tongue. Reconstruction usually requires laryngeal resuspension and free tissue transfer with a musculocutaneous flap such as an anterolateral thigh flap.

(I) *Segmental mandibulectomy*: Extirpation of a cancer that erodes the alveolar or cortical bone should include a segmental mandibulectomy. An anterior segmental mandibular resection requires a bone reconstruction with microvascular reconstruction such as a fibula free flap. Lateral mandible defects do not necessarily require bony reconstruction for adequate functional rehabilitation.

(J) *Management of the neck*: An elective selective neck dissection of levels 1–3 should be performed in the absence of metastatic disease. In the presence of lymph node metastasis, a comprehensive neck dissection with removal of lymph nodes in levels 1–5 is indicated.

(K) *Adjuvant treatment*: The indications for adjuvant treatment with radiation or chemoradiation have been well defined in the literature.

SUGGESTED READING

Cunningham MJ, Johnson JT, Myers EN, et al. Cervical lymph node metastasis after local excision of early squamous cell carcinoma of the oral cavity. Am J Surg. 1986;152:361-366.

D'Cruz AK, Vaish R, Kapre N, et al. Elective versus therapeutic neck dissection in node-negative oral cancer. N Engl J Med. 2015;373(6):521-529.

Ganly I, Goldstein D, Carlson DL, et al. Long-term regional control and survival in patients with "low-risk," early stage oral tongue cancer managed by partial glossectomy and neck dissection without postoperative radiation: the importance of tumor thickness. Cancer. 2013;119(6):1168-1176.

Hidalgo D. Fibula free flap: a new method of mandible reconstruction. Plast Reconstr Surg. 1989;1:71-79.

Hubert Low TH, Gao K, Elliott M, et al. Tumor classification for early oral cancer: re-evaluate the current TNM classification. Head Neck. 2015;37(2):223-228.

Tumors of the Base of the Tongue

Umamaheswar Duvvuri, David E Eibling

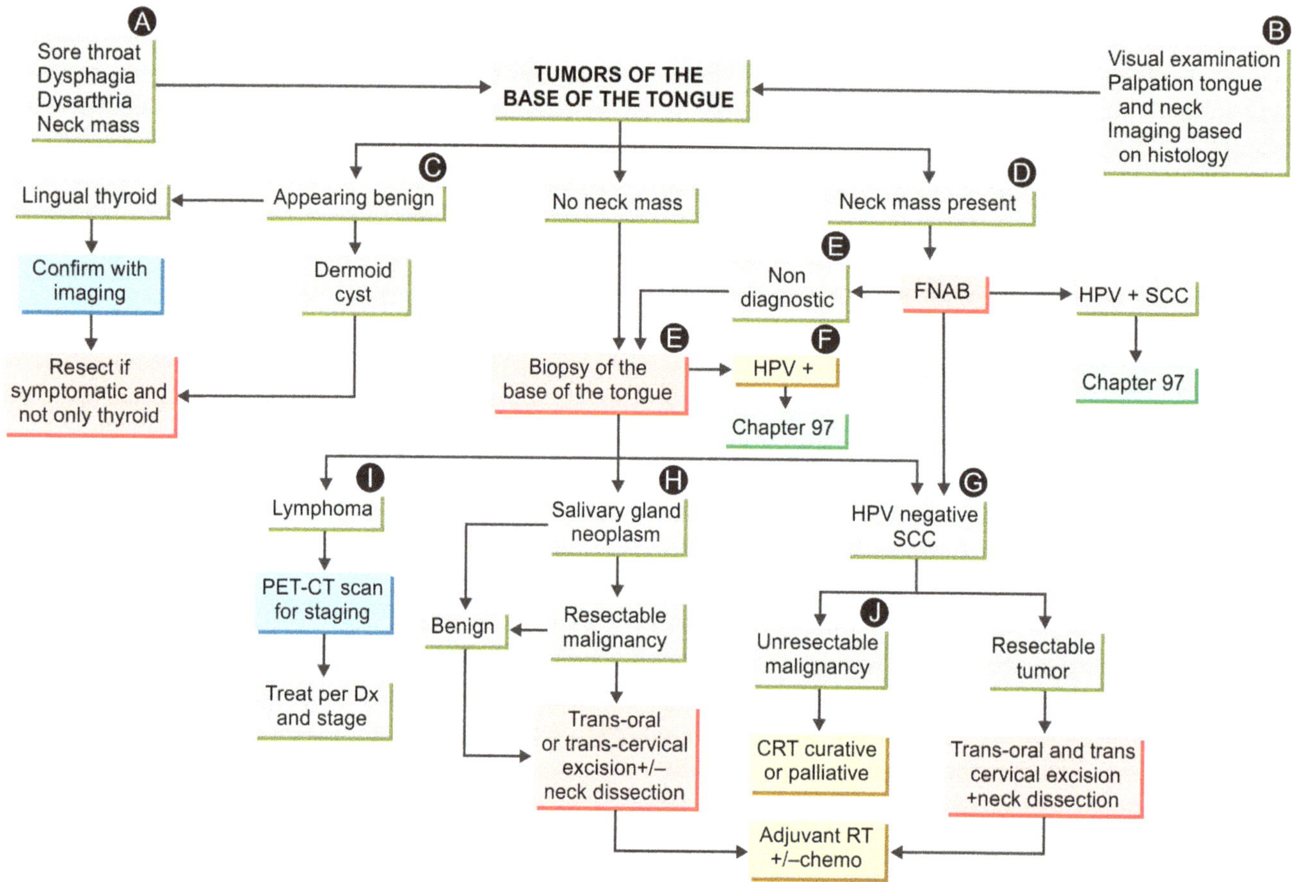

The upsurge in the incidence of human papillomavirus (HPV)-related oropharyngeal cancer (tumors) of the oropharynx over the past decade has dramatically changed the predominant malignant tumor of the head and neck. The incidence of squamous cell carcinoma (SCC) of the oropharynx is now more common than either cancers of the larynx or oral cavity. HPV positive (+) oropharyngeal squamous cell carcinoma is a unique disease with different prognostic markers, treatment algorithms, and treatment outcomes, and now a different staging system has been introduced to begin in 2018. Hence, decision-making for HPV+ tonsil and tongue base cancers has been combined into one algorithm in this edition of this book (Chapter 97). Although HPV related SCC is now the most common malignancy of the base of the tongue, other malignant and benign tumors are found in this region, with the evaluation and treatment dictated by the specific tumor type.

A Patients with a tumor of the base of the tongue may be asymptomatic, or may present with symptoms such as sore throat with odynophagia, dysphagia, globus sensation, or referred otalgia. Occasionally, bleeding can be a presenting symptom with large friable tumors. Many patients will present with a metastatic neck mass, with the base of tongue cancer identified only in the search for the primary site.

B The basic evaluation mandates visualization of the base of the tongue, along with palpation to assess size and extent. Bimanual examination may be beneficial for deeply invasive tumors. Examination of the neck, and assessment of the dental status should be routine.

C If examination suggests that the mass is clearly benign, such as lingual thyroid or dermoid cyst, biopsy is not required. Resection is performed if the mass is symptomatic. If physical examination suggests lingual thyroid, ultrasound assessment of the thyroid should be performed to determine whether the lingual thyroid is the patient's only thyroid prior to undertaking excision.

D The presence or absence of enlarged cervical node(s) should be noted on initial examination. If present, fine-needle aspiration biopsy (FNAB) of the neck node is often the most expeditious strategy to make the diagnosis. If sufficient material is collected, often stains for p16 can confirm the presence of HPV-related SCC.

E If no palpable nodes are apparent or if FNAB is non-diagnostic, then direct biopsy of the base of the tongue will be required. Occasionally, this can be performed as an outpatient, but typically biopsy must be done under general anesthesia.

F Once the histology has been ascertained, further evaluation and management is driven by the diagnosis and stage. If HPV + SCC, refer to Chapter 97.

G Treatment of HPV negative (−) SCC may consist of surgery, radiation, chemotherapy, or a combination of modalities. Positron emission tomography-computed tomography (PET-CT) is required to assess the extent of the tumor as well as to identify local and distant metastases. Surgery may include robotic or other form of transoral resection, or open transcervical extirpation. Postoperative adjuvant radiation or chemoradiation therapy (CRT) is typically required due to tumor stage.

H Tumors of minor salivary gland origin are resected if feasible, possibly with robotic resection. Adjuvant radiation is used based on histology.

I Lymphomas are evaluated and managed per specific lymphoma subtype. Surgery is reserved for diagnosis and control of symptoms.

J Advanced salivary gland and HPV negative cancers that are unresectable may be treated with chemoradiation for palliative intent. Treatment outcomes for these cancers are less favorable than with HPV + cancers (Chapter 97).

SUGGESTED READING

Barnes L. Surgical Pathology of the Head and Neck. New York: CRC Press; 2001.

de Almeida JR, Li R, Magnuson JS, et al. Oncologic outcomes after trans-oral robotic surgery: a multi-institutional study. JAMA Otolaryngol Head Neck Surg. 2015;141:1043-1051.

Dolezal J, Vizda J, Horacek J, et al. Lingual thyroid: diagnosis using a hybrid of single photon emission computed tomography and standard computed tomography. J Laryngol Otol. 2013;127: 432-434.

Iyer NG1, Kim L, Nixon IJ, et al. Factors predicting outcome in malignant minor salivary gland tumors of the oropharynx. Arch Otolaryngol Head Neck Surg. 2010;136:1240-1247.

Kirke DN, Chitguppi C, Rubin SJ, et al. Adenoid cystic carcinoma of the base of tongue: A population-based study. Am J Otolaryngol. 2017;38(3):279-284.

Saul SH, Kapadia SB. Primary lymphoma of Waldeyer's ring. Clinico-pathologic study of 68 cases. Cancer. 1985;56:157-166.

CHAPTER 96

Neoplasms of the Tonsil and Retromolar Trigone

Umamaheswar Duvvuri, David E Eibling

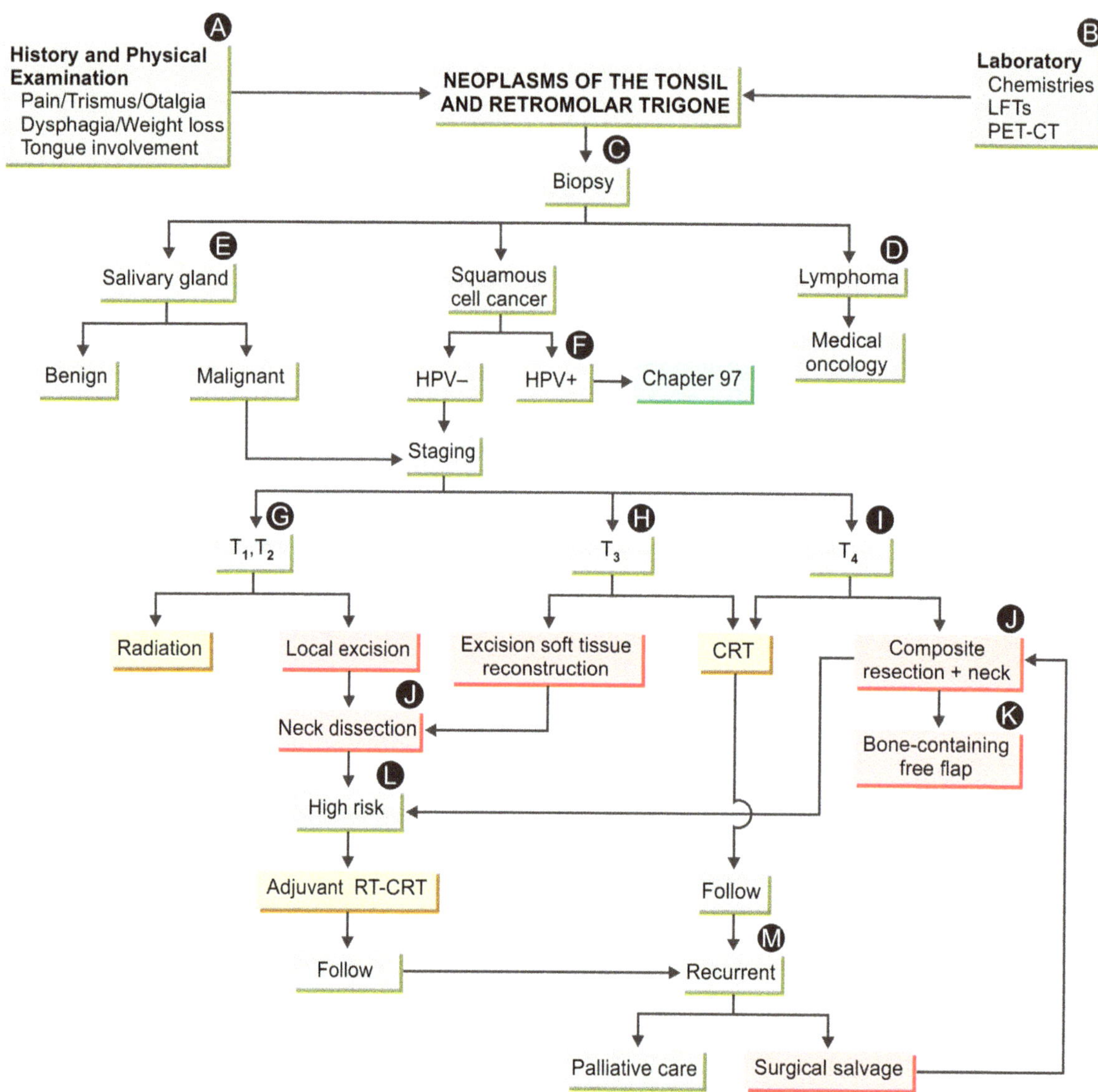

Cancers arising in the oropharynx often present in late stages due to their position posterior to the oral cavity. Examination is often challenging due to strong gagging, and their presence is unsuspected until the tumor has grown to large size or the patient presents with neck metastasis. HPV positive (+) tumors of the tonsil are addressed in Chapter 97, and not discussed in this chapter. HPV negative oropharyngeal tumors arising in the base of the tongue are addressed in Chapter 95.

A Patients with cancer of the tonsil, palate, and retromolar trigone (RMT) typically have a history of smoking and excessive alcohol consumption. The recent epidemic of HPV+ tonsil cancer is a different cancer and often occurs in nonsmoking, younger, usually male patients, and is

addressed in Chapter 97. A social history with focus on substance use may help predict patients at risk for alcohol withdrawal during treatment. The mass in the neck is often the presenting sign of carcinoma of the tonsil; these metastases are often cystic and can be mistaken for branchial cleft cysts. The diagnosis of cancer should be considered in any adult patient with a mass of the neck. Numbness of the teeth and lower lip signifies of the mandible with invasion and involvement of the mandibular nerve.

B Imaging is used to assess the extent of the cancer and nodal metastases. Positron emission tomography (PET) adds metabolic information and is helpful in identifying regional and distant metastases as well as second primary cancers, and is now used routinely in most centers. Magnetic resonance imaging (MRI) can also be useful in assessing invasion of the mandible. It is best to obtain imaging before extensive biopsies are performed to avoid artifact as a result of edema or hematoma from the biopsy.

C Biopsy of the tonsil or RMT may be performed in the office, with panendoscopy delayed until definitive surgery, if performed. Very small or submucosal cancer of the tonsil may require tonsillectomy for biopsy, which must be performed in the operating room. If lymphoma is suspected, the specimen must be sent fresh (not fixed in formalin) to the pathology laboratory.

D Patients diagnosed with lymphoma are referred to medical oncology for staging and treatment. Radiation is used if the tonsil is the only site of involvement; chemotherapy is used for disseminated disease.

E Malignant tumors arising from minor salivary glands occur infrequently in the oral cavity and oropharynx; however, RMT and tonsil are unusual sites. Benign tumors of salivary gland origin, which account for 25–50% of minor salivary gland tumors, may be excised via a transoral route. Malignant tumors usually require the same approach as HPV– squamous cell carcinoma.

F Squamous cell carcinoma tissue should be tested for the presence of human papillomavirus, utilizing its surrogate marker p16. HPV oropharyngeal cancer is biologically distinct from HPV cancer with different outcomes and behavior. HPV+ cancers have a distinct staging system, and treatment algorithms are different than HPV–squamous cell cancer. See Chapter 97.

G Radiation is used to treat many patients with T_1 or T_2 tumors of the oral cavity and oropharynx. However, nearly 30% of these patients will acquire a new primary tumor and may need radiation therapy in the future, and radiation effects of fibrosis and xerostomia result in long-term morbidity. Surgery takes much less time and often results in minimal morbidity. Neck dissection is not necessary in patients with superficial T_1 RMT cancers and no evidence of adenopathy on PET-CT scan. All patients who have cancer of the tonsil or deeply invasive RMT cancers should have the neck treated even if adenopathy is not present preoperatively.

H Surgical extirpation of more advanced cancer, especially those involving the walls of the oropharynx or base of the tongue, requires wide-field exposure, usually via

mandibulotomy. Reconstruction is often easily achieved with a skin graft or local tissue flaps. Patients require a tracheostomy for clearance of secretions and airway maintenance. Advanced cancers often respond poorly to chemoradiation therapy (CRT), but the modality is often used in patients who are poor surgical candidates.

I Composite resection is required if bone is involved, typically as a segmental mandibulectomy. Free flap reconstruction with bone is considered standard of care. In carefully chosen cases, a marginal mandibulectomy may permit adequate tumor clearance.

J Neck dissection for N0 necks includes zones I, II, and III for oral cavity cancers (retromolar trigone) and II, III, and IV for oropharyngeal cancers (tonsil). Palpable lymphadenopathy (N_1 to N_3) requires modified radical or radical neck dissection.

K Dentulous patients who are able to tolerate extensive surgery are offered reconstruction with bone-containing free flaps. Edentulous patients may be reconstructed with soft tissue only.

L The presence of perineural invasion, multiple (>3) positive nodes, extracapsular spread, or large primary cancers (T_3 or larger) mandate postoperative adjuvant radiation therapy. Many centers also use concomitant chemotherapy in patients who have extracapsular nodal metastases. The contralateral neck should be included in radiation treatment in all HPV– tonsil cancers that are T_3, T_4, or N+ due to the incidence of contralateral neck metastases.

M Decisions regarding management of treatment failure are difficult; often the choice is between palliative care and aggressive surgery with limited chance of success. Involvement of the palliative care team is often invaluable.

SUGGESTED READING

Bernier J, Domenge C, Ozsahin M, et al. Postoperative irradiation with or without concomitant chemotherapy for locally advanced head and neck cancer. N Engl J Med. 2004;350:1937-1944.

Bolzoni A, Cappiello HJ, Piazza C, et al. Diagnostic accuracy of magnetic resonance imaging in the assessment of mandibular involvement in oral-oropharyngeal squamous carcinoma. A prospective study. Arch Otolaryngol Head Neck Surg. 2004;130: 837-843.

Petruzzeli GJ, Knight FK, Vandevender D, et al. Posterior marginal mandibulectomy in the management of cancer of the oral cavity and oropharynx. Otolaryngol Head Neck Surg. 2003;129:713-719.

Management of Squamous Cell Carcinoma of the Oropharynx

Mathew Geltzeiler, Robert L Ferris

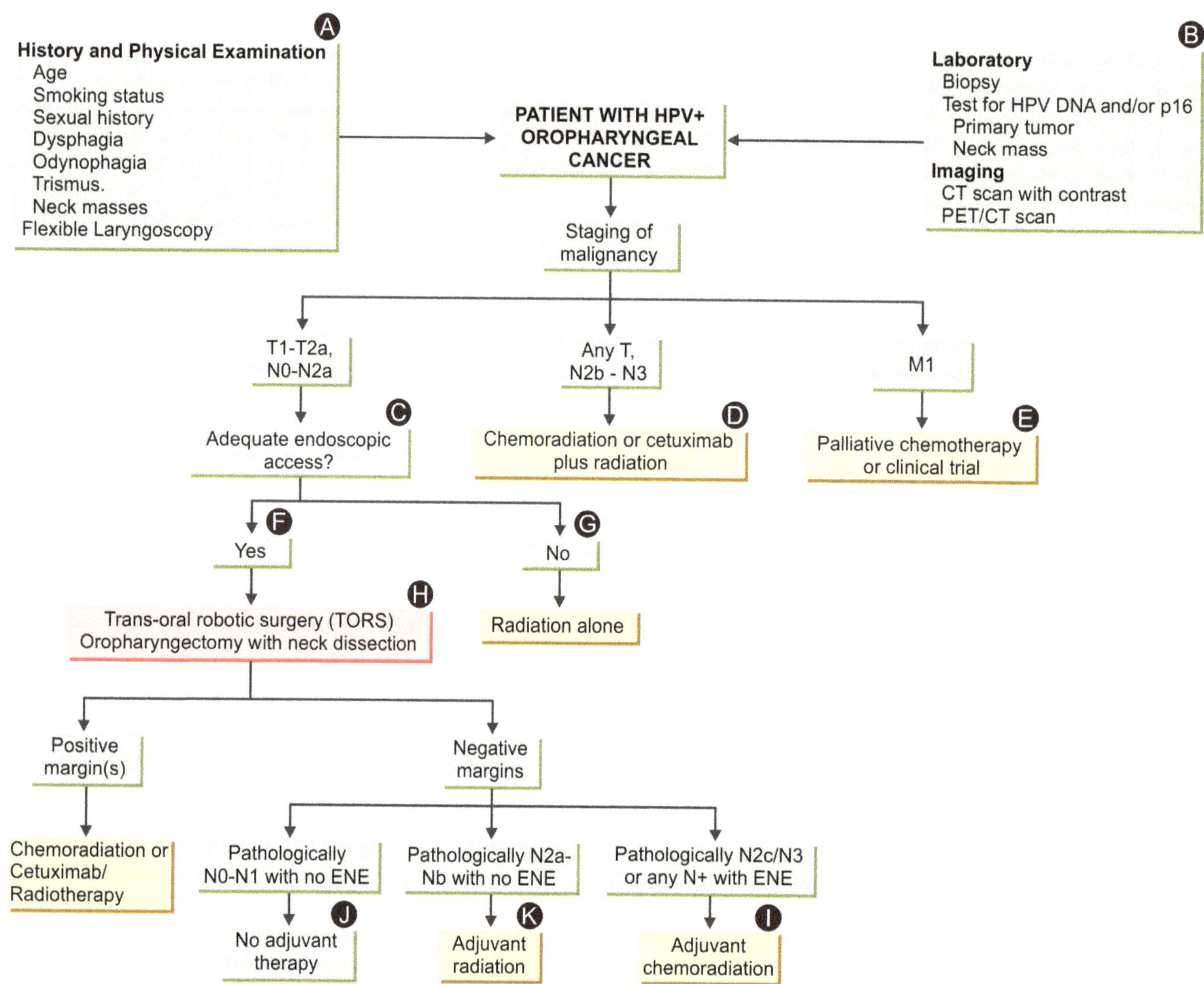

The incidence of oropharyngeal squamous cell carcinoma (OPSCC) has been rising dramatically in the setting of the human papillomavirus (HPV) epidemic. Patients presenting with HPV-related cancer are typically younger with a less extensive history of tobacco abuse. The HPV-related cancer carries a better prognosis at all stages than HPV-negative cancers. Patients with HPV-related OPSCC with>20 pack years of smoking have intermediate risk cancers. Transoral surgery has substantially improved the surgeon's ability to access the oropharynx with minimal morbidity and remove the cancers with a negative margin. Transoral robotic surgery (TORS) with the da Vinci Surgical System and transoral laser microsurgery are equally efficacious.

A Any patient with a cancer of the oropharynx should undergo a complete examination of the head and neck including flexible laryngoscopy. The diagnosis of SCC can be made by a biopsy of the pharyngeal mass itself or from a fine needle aspiration of the neck mass if present. Other benign and malignant tumors can present in the oropharynx. The discussion of their management is beyond the scope of this chapter.

B Complete staging of the cancer patient should include a computed tomography (CT) scan of the neck and chest or a positron emission tomography/CT. If surgical intervention is being considered, a CT scan of the neck is always obtained to evaluate the resectability of the tumor.

C Transoral surgery is currently indicated for low-volume cancer (T1–T2) with clinically minimal neck metastasis (N0–N1). Patients with T3–T4 cancers are more challenging to remove with negative margins due to their size and long-term results from TORS on these patients are still under investigation. At this point, TORS should not be considered for patients with a CT scan concerning for N2a or worse neck disease. These patients are at higher risk for extranodal extension (ENE) and have an ~50% rate of requiring chemotherapy in addition to adjuvant radiation. If operated upon, half of these HPV-related OPSCC patients would end up requiring triple modality therapy and be subject to the acute morbidity of surgery plus chronic toxicity of chemoradiation. In the future, trials such as Eastern Cooperative Oncology Group (ECOG) 3311 can help us to better understand the role of TORS in this patient population.

D Primary radiation therapy for OPSCC is typically delivered at a dose of 66–74 Gy while adjuvant dosing is lower at 50–60 Gy. Radiation therapy to the head and neck is commonly delivered with intensity-modulated radiation therapy (IMRT). Systemic therapy is typically platinum based, usually with cisplatin. Cetuximab, an epidermal growth factor receptor inhibitor, is another US Food and Drug Administration approved therapy that can be combined with radiation as primary or recurrent treatment. When both chemotherapy and radiation are required, they are most commonly dosed concurrently. The use of induction chemotherapy is typically reserved for advanced cancer.

E Patients with distant metastasis are candidates for palliative chemotherapy or a clinical trial.

F The patient who has a T1–T2 cancer with a neck that is clinically N0–N2a, should be evaluated for TORS. Adequate oral accessibility is critical for successful surgical exposure. Rich et al. have described the "eight Ts" of endoscopic access that should be examined prior to considering TORS. These are as follows: teeth, trismus, transverse dimensions (mandibular), mandibular tori, tongue, tilt (atlanto-occipital extension), treatment (prior radiotherapy) and tumor.

G If adequate exposure cannot be achieved, the patient with T1–T2 cancer with an N0–N1 neck can undergo RT alone.

H If adequate exposure can be achieved, a TORS oropharyngectomy with ipsilateral neck dissection should be performed. The oropharyngectomy involves resection of both tonsil pillars and part of the posterior pharyngeal wall. Medially, the pharyngeal constrictor muscle is taken as the deep margin, which involves exposing parapharyngeal adipose tissue. If an additional deep margin is required, the stylohyoid muscle can also be resected. This usually involves sacrifice of the glossopharyngeal nerve. The medial margin is at least 1 cm from the tumor along the lingual tonsil. Intrinsic tongue muscle must be taken as a deep tumor margin in this area. Selective neck dissection is performed ipsilateral to the tumor. Levels 2a and 3 should be resected in all cases with level 4 being included if the patient is N1. After the neck dissection, ligation of the facial, lingual and ascending pharyngeal arteries is performed. Similarly, one may also ligate the external carotid artery. These strategies do not reduce the rate of minor postoperative oropharyngeal bleeding, but they do decrease the rate of catastrophic, life-threatening hemorrhage.

If a fistula is created between the oropharynx and neck, the defect should be closed primarily, if possible, with local tissue flaps being rotated in to bolster the repair. This can be accomplished with the digastric and/or sternocleidomastoid muscles in the neck and the buccal adipose tissue transorally. Most patients do not require a feeding tube. We typically allow the patients to advance their diet as tolerated. If the patient fails to have adequate oral intake over the first several postoperative days, we will then place a nasogastric feeding tube.

The specimen should be removed en bloc and taken to pathology. Frozen sections should be taken preferentially off the primary specimen; however, additional margins can also be taken circumferentially and deep if necessary after the cancer has been removed. The surgeon is encouraged to bring the specimen to the pathology laboratory to help orient the specimen for the pathologists. As these are complex, three-dimensional specimens, a face-to-face conversation can facilitate accurate pathologic analysis.

I The two accepted indications for adjuvant systemic therapy plus radiation are positive margins or ENE, although there is controversy given that this was derived from a retrospective subset analysis of Radiation Therapy Oncology Group (RTOG) 9501 trial, and because HPV+ patients are only of "intermediate" risk, even with these pathologic features. At present, any patient with either of these features generally receives both additional modalities and, subsequently, thus usually receives triple modality therapy. This is being addressed in ECOG 3311, a randomized prospective trial, to avoid chemotherapy and offer reduced dose RT (50 vs 60 Gy) for close (<1 mm) margins and/or ≤1 mm ENE.

J Upon final pathologic analysis, if the patient has negative margins and is N0–N1 with no ENE, additional therapy has no proven benefit. This is the ideal outcome to achieve for TORS patients. We believe that these patients will have the least long-term morbidity from therapy.

K If the patient has N2a or greater neck metastasis on final pathology, then he/she requires adjuvant RT.

SUGGESTED READING

Huang SH, Xu W, Waldron J, et al. Refining American Joint Committee on Cancer/Union for International Cancer Control TNM stage and prognostic groups for human papillomavirus-related oropharyngeal carcinomas. J Clin Oncol. 2015;33(8):836-845. [online] Available from: http://www.ncbi.nlm.nih.gov/pubmed/25667292 [Accessed on 2/10/2016].

Maxwell JH, Ferris RL, Gooding W, et al. Extracapsular spread in head and neck carcinoma: impact of site and human papillomavirus status. Cancer. 2013;119(18):3302-3308.

Rich JT, Milov S, Lewis JS, et al. Transoral laser microsurgery (TLM) ± adjuvant therapy for advanced stage oropharyngeal cancer: outcomes and prognostic factors. Laryngoscope. 2009;119(9):1709-1719.

Shaw RJ, Holsinger FC, Paleri V, et al. Surgical trials in head and neck oncology: Renaissance and revolution? Head Neck. 2015;37(7):927-930. [online] Available from: http://www.ncbi.nlm.nih.gov/pubmed/25043823 [Accessed on 2/10/2016].

Neoplasms of the Hypopharynx

Alec Vaezi

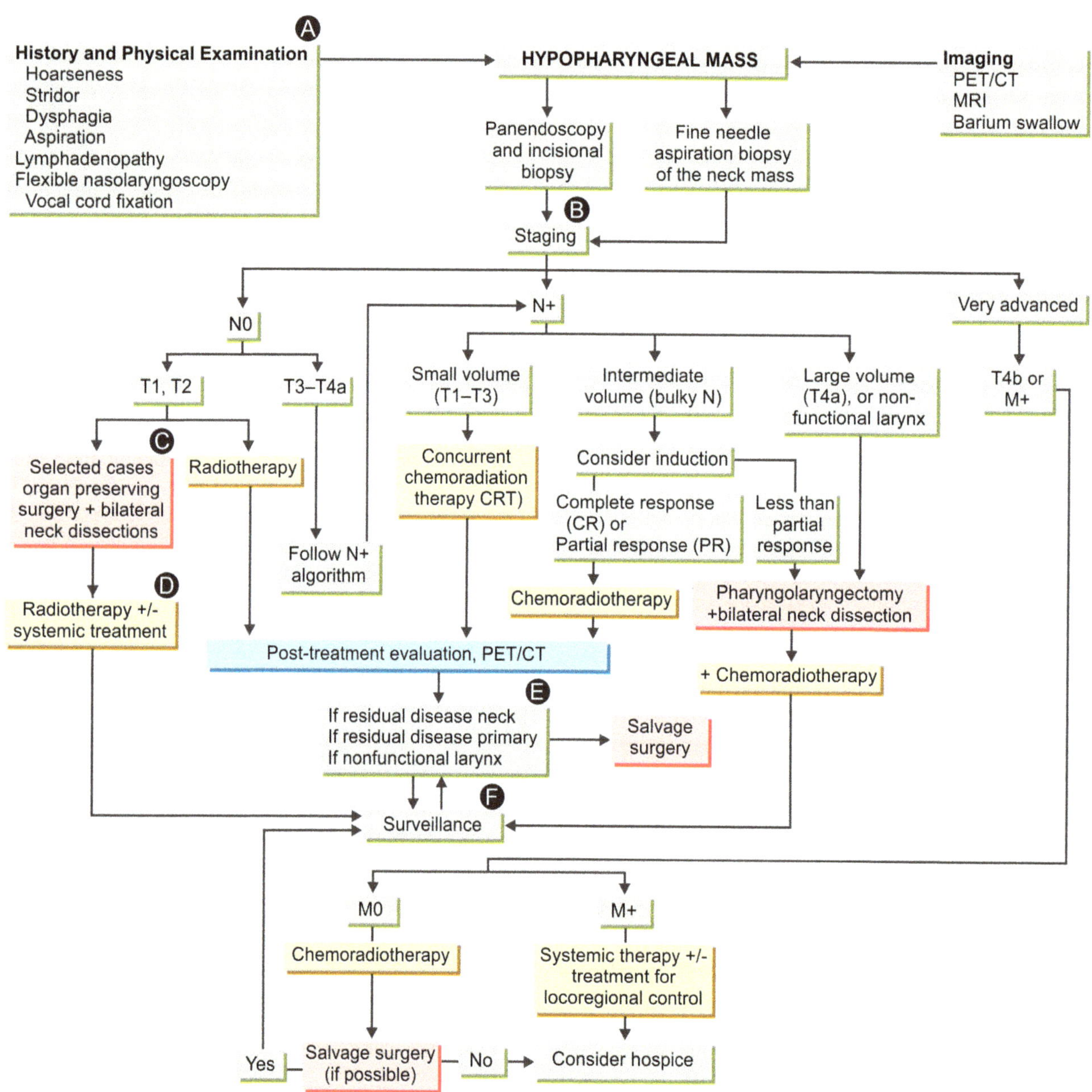

Cancers of the hypopharynx represent only 5% of cancers of the head and neck, but usually present at an advanced stage (80% present with AJCC stage III of IV), in part because of paucity of symptoms. The disease often affects heavy alcohol drinkers, who have several other comorbidities. Because of the late presentation, the proximity of the cancer to the larynx, the tendency for submucosal spread, and the characteristics of the affected population, hypopharyngeal cancers have a far worse prognosis compared to other cancers of the head and neck with a 5-year overall survival of only 15–45%.

A Evaluation of a hypopharyngeal mass includes history with emphasis on laryngeal function (voice, dysphagia, aspiration), physical examination with evaluation of laryngeal fixation and lymphadenopathy, flexible laryngoscopy to delineate the extent of the cancer and vocal cord motion, computed tomography (CT) of the neck with contrast to characterize the extent of the cancer, laryngeal framework involvement and metastasis to the neck including retropharyngeal. Tissue diagnosis is obtained either by fine-needle aspiration of a mass in the neck or through an incisional biopsy during panendoscopy. Staging is completed with a Positron Emission Tomography/Computed Tomography (PET/CT). Additional examinations that may be considered are magnetic resonance imaging with attention to laryngeal framework invasion and prevertebral fascia involvement using a modified barium swallow may help to evaluate the sliding motion of the posterior pharyngeal wall suggesting resectability.

B Cancer size staging is as follows: (T1) cancer affecting one subsite and <2 cm; (T2) cancer affects more than one subsite, or measures >2 cm but <4 cm; (T3) fixation of larynx or tumor >4 cm; (T4a) cancer invading cricoid/thyroid cartilage, or hyoid bone, or esophagus, or thyroid gland, or central soft tissue invasion; (T4b) tumor invading the prevertebral fascia, the mediastinum, or encasing the carotid artery. The three subsites of the hypopharynx are the pyriform sinus, posterior pharyngeal wall, and postcricoid area. *For lymph node staging* (N0) indicates no pathologic lymphadenopathy; (N1) one pathologic lymph node <3 cm; (N2a) one pathologic lymph node >3 cm; (N2b) two or more ipsilateral pathologic lymph nodes; (N2c) any contralateral pathological lymph node (N2c); (N3) any node >6 cm.

C Types of laryngeal preserving surgeries to consider include transoral laser and transoral robotic microsurgery. These techniques may be used for resection of cancers affecting the medial or superior portion of the pyriform sinus, for small cancers of the posterior pharyngeal wall for resection of one arytenoid, or cancer affecting the soft tissue covering the arytenoid, or for resection of selected superficial cancers of the postcricoid area. Open surgery is also possible using supracricoid hemilaryngopharyngectomy, supraglottic hemilaryngopharyngectomy, or partial pharyngectomy techniques. Because of frequent contralateral lymphatic drainage, hypopharyngeal cancers are often treated with bilateral neck dissection.

D Pathological risk factors indicating the need for adjuvant radiotherapy (RT) are lymphatics or vascular invasion, perineural invasion, close margins (<3 mm), T3–T4, and N2–N3 disease. Pathological risk factors indicating need for adjuvant chemoradiation therapy (CRT) for survival benefit include positive margins and extracapsular spread.

E If the recurrent cancer involves the primary site, salvage surgery should address both the primary site and bilateral neck dissections; If the recurrence is limited to the neck, bilateral neck dissection without surgery to the primary site is sufficient.

F The frequency of follow-up visits and imaging varies depending on the institutions. Usually, the patient is seen once every 1–3 months for the first year, once every 2–4 months for the second year, once every 4–8 months for year 3–5 and yearly thereafter. The surveillance involves physical examination and flexible laryngoscopy. In addition, baseline imaging is done at the completion of the treatment usually PET/CT done 2.5–3 months post-treatment. A follow-up PET/CT may be necessary if equivocal response is seen on the initial post-treatment PET/CT. Positron Emission Tomography/Computed Tomography performed earlier than 2.5 months post-treatment yields an unacceptably high-false-positive rate. Additional imaging is recommended for worrisome signs or symptoms, or if the site of the cancer is not easily visualized. Since deep recurrences are not easily visualized, I recommend CT of neck and chest every 6 months for the first 3 years, as the majority of recurrences are expected during this time frame. Finally, thyroid-stimulating hormone levels should be checked every 6–12 months if the patient has been irradiated.

SUGGESTED READINGS

Hall SF, Groome PA, Irish J, et al. The natural history of patients with squamous cell carcinoma of the hypopharynx. Laryngoscope. 2008;118(8):1362-1371.

Newman JR, Connolly TM, Illing EA, et al. Survival trends in hypopharyngeal cancers: a population-based review. Laryngoscope. 2015;125(3):624-629.

Pfister DG, Ang KK, Brizel DM, et al. Head and neck cancer. Clinical guidelines in oncology. J Natl Compr Canc Netw. 2011;9:596-650.

Takes RP, Strojan P, Silver CE, et al.; International Head and Neck Scientific Group. Current trends in initial management of hypopharyngeal cancer: the decline of open surgery. Head Neck. 2012;(2):270-281.

CHAPTER 99

Salivary Gland Enlargement

Jason Trahan, Rohan R Walvekar

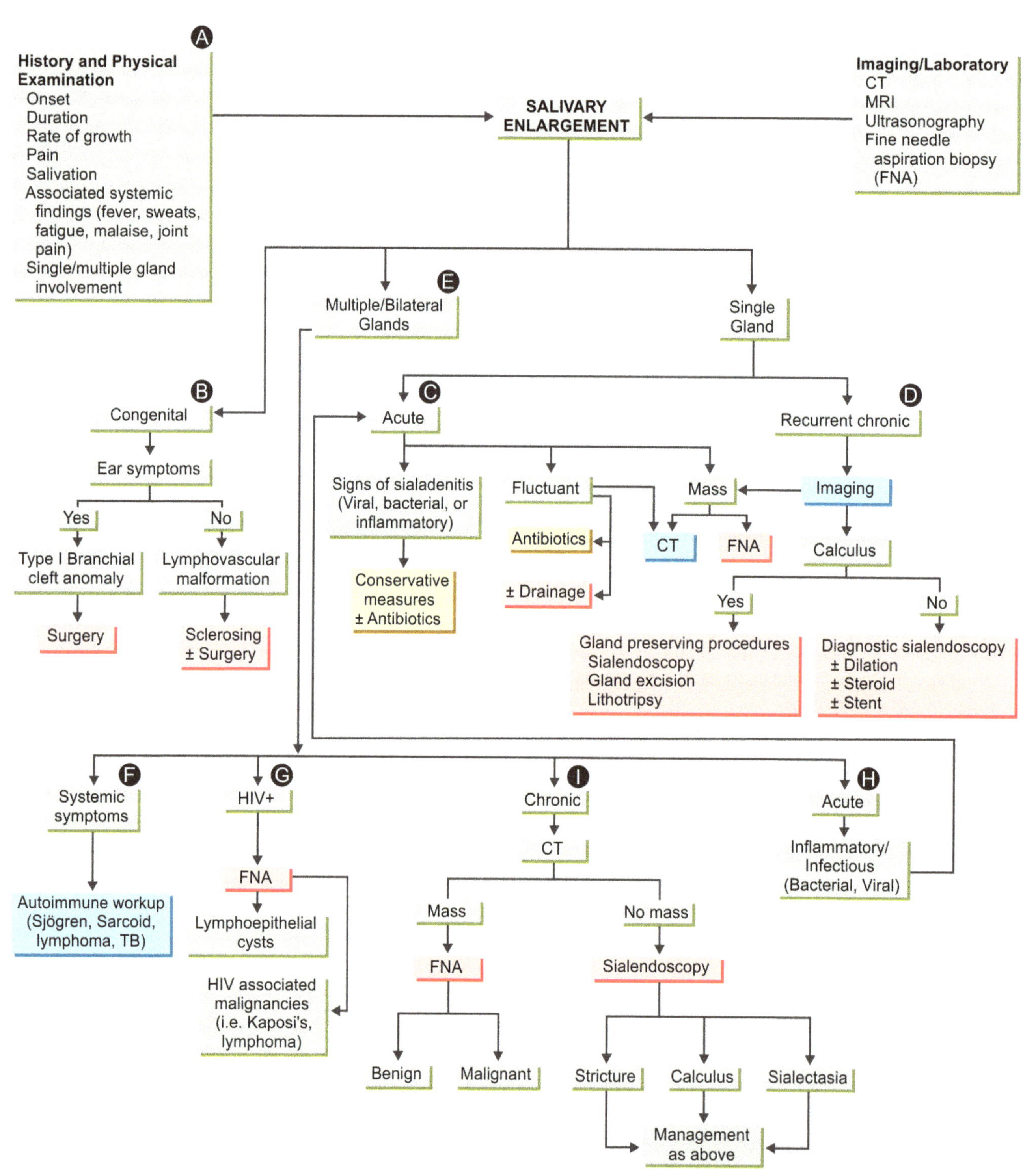

Salivary gland enlargement is a fairly uncommon condition in the general population; however, it can be encountered regularly in the general otolaryngology practice. Salivary gland enlargement can be caused by a variety of etiologies including viral and bacterial infections, salivary duct obstruction, benign and malignant neoplasms, or a result of autoimmune or other systemic illnesses. A concise and reliable stepwise approach is essential in the evaluation diagnosis, and treatment of these problems.

A A thorough history including onset, duration, rate of growth, pain, salivation, associated systemic findings and a complete examination of the head and neck are critical in helping to establish a working differential diagnosis. Determining, if the problem is related to one or more glands can help the clinician begin to formulate a working diagnosis.

B In single-gland disease, congenital manifestations tend to arise early in life and can be attributed to lymphovascular malformations or rarely Type I branchial cleft anomalies.

C Acute unilateral enlargement can often be attributed to viral, bacterial, or obstructive processes. Palpable masses or fluctuance should prompt the clinician to obtain imaging and proceed with biopsy or drainage as indicated. Acute sialadenitis typically responds well to conservative measures including hydration, gland massage, sialagogues, and ± antibiotics.

D Chronic or recurrent unilateral problems may be indicative of an inflammatory, structural, or obstructive problem. Ultrasonography, computed tomography (CT) and magnetic resonance imaging (MRI) can help assess for neoplasm or sialolithiasis. Ultimately, therapeutic or diagnostic duct evaluation (sialendoscopy) may be warranted.

E Bilateral or multigland enlargement can be attributed to infection/inflammatory issues, neoplasms (e.g. Warthin's tumor), but also should alert the clinician to the possibility of systemic or autoimmune pathology.

F Patients exhibiting other systemic symptoms including but not limited to arthralgia, recurrent fevers, and night sweats, should undergo evaluation for possible salivary manifestations of autoimmune/systemic illnesses (i.e. Sjögren's syndrome, sarcoid, and tuberculosis).

G Human immunodeficiency virus (HIV)-positive patients have a high incidence of benign lymphoepithelial cysts of the parotid glands. Human immunodeficiency virus-associated malignancies such as lymphoma and Kaposi's sarcoma have been reported as well. Fine-needle aspiration (FNA) biopsy may be warranted in these patients. Repeated FNA for treatment of a benign lymphoepithelial cyst is highly ineffective with a near 100% recurrence rate. If more definitive treatment is desired for cosmetic reasons, sclerotherapy or surgery (i.e. parotidectomy) has been shown to be more effective.

H Acute onset of bilateral disease can be a manifestation of inflammatory (i.e. postradiation) or infectious sialadenitis (viral or bacterial). Symptoms may affect an individual gland or multiple glands.

I Prolonged or recurrent sialadenitis/salivary gland swelling will usually require CT imaging. Findings consistent with neoplasm will require fine-needle or core-needle biopsy followed by definitive management usually surgical. Imaging or examination positive for sialolithiasis will require treatment that can include observation/conservative therapy, gland preserving techniques, i.e. sialendoscopy and combined endoscopic and open techniques, and gland resection. With a negative CT scan, a diagnostic sialendoscopy is indicated, especially with symptoms that persist in spite of conservative management.

SUGGESTED READING

Bowen MA, Tauzin M, Kluka EA, et al. Diagnostic and interventional sialendoscopy: a preliminary experience. Laryngoscope. 2011;121(2):299-303.

Rogers J, McCaffrey TV. Inflammatory disorders of the salivary glands. In: Flint PW, Haughey BH, Lund VJ, et al. (Eds). Cummings Otolaryngology Head and Neck Surgery, 5th edition. Philadelphia, PA: Mosby Elsevier; 2010. pp. 1151-1161.

Schiødt M, Dodd CL, Greenspan D, et al. Natural history of HIV-associated salivary gland disease. Oral Surg Oral Med Oral Pathol. 1992;74(3):326-331.

Shivhare P, Shankarnarayan L, Jambunath U, et al. Benign lymphoepithelial cysts of parotid and submandibular glands in a HIV-positive patient. J Oral Maxillofac Pathol. 2015;19(1):107.

Simental A, Carrau RL. Malignant neoplasms of the salivary glands. In: Cummings CW, Flint PW, Harker LA, et al. (Eds). Cummings Otolaryngology Head and Neck Surgery, 4th edition. Philadelphia, PA: Mosby; 2004. pp. 1378-1405.

Steehler MK, Steehler MW, Davison SP. Benign lymphoepithelial cysts of the parotid: long-term surgical results. HIV AIDS (Auckl). 2012;4:81-86.

Su CH, Lee KS, Tseng TM, et al. Endoscopic holmium:YAG laser-assisted lithotripsy: a preliminary report. B-ENT. 2015;11(1): 57-61.

Neoplasms of the Parotid Gland

Nicole C Schmitt, Seungwon Kim

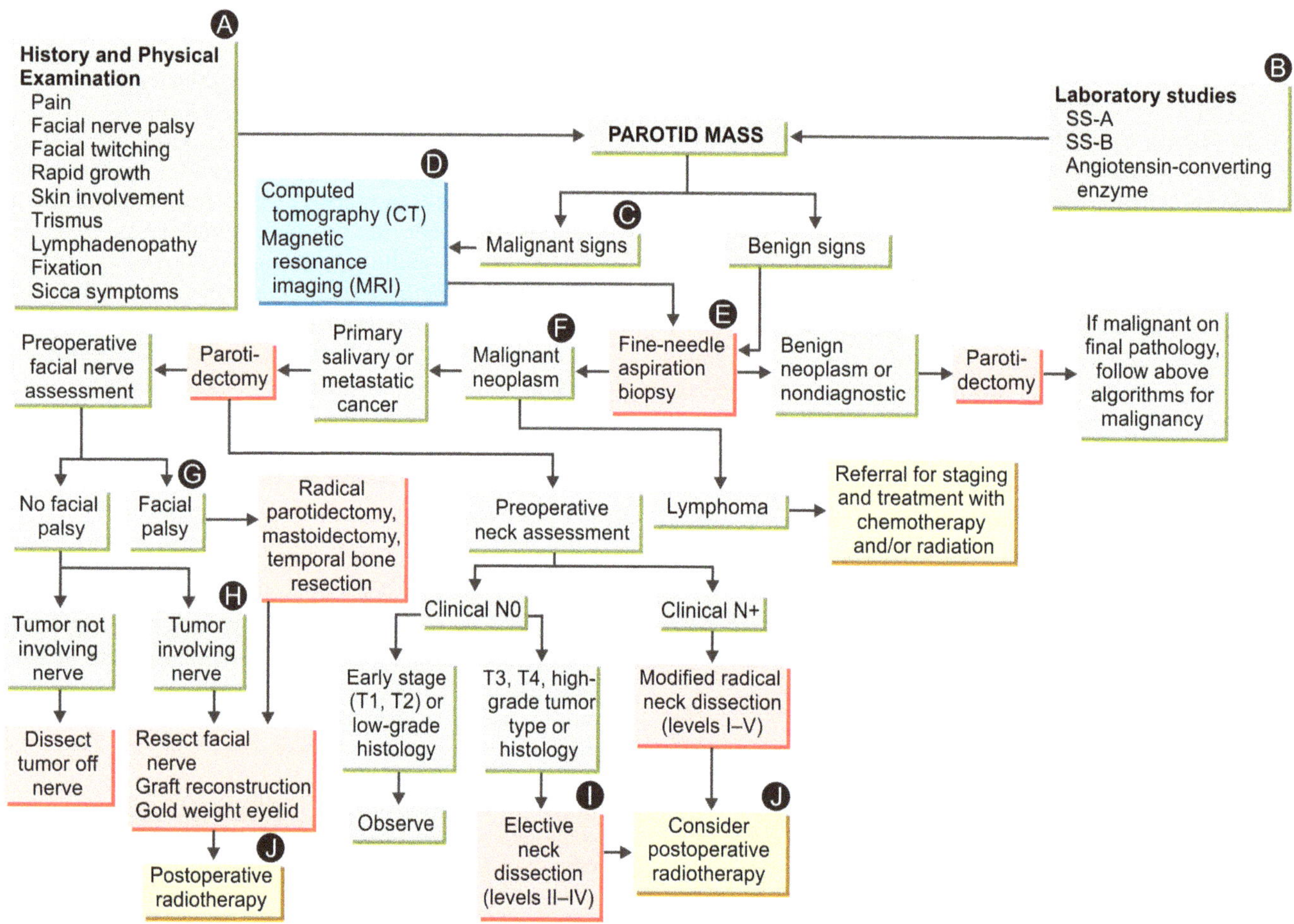

Tumors of the parotid gland are relatively uncommon. The majority of these tumors are benign including pleomorphic adenoma and Warthin's tumors. Parotid neoplasms most commonly present as a painless preauricular mass. Malignant tumors of the parotid gland include relatively indolent tumors such as low-grade mucoepidermoid or acinic cell carcinoma, or aggressive tumors such as high-grade mucoepidermoid, adenoid cystic, and salivary duct carcinoma. Lymphoma and metastatic tumors from the skin and other sites can also present as a mass in the parotid gland.

A A mass in the parotid has a broad differential diagnosis. A careful history and physical examination are required. Advanced age, smoking, and bilateral lesions are frequently associated with Warthin's tumors.

B Laboratory studies are ordered when Sjögren's syndrome, sarcoidosis, or other systemic disorders are suspected.

C Signs concerning for malignancy include facial palsy or twitching, fixation of the mass or involvement of overlying skin, pain, cervical lymphadenopathy, and rapid growth.

D Computed tomography or magnetic resonance imaging can be useful in assessing the location (superficial lobe, deep lobe, parapharyngeal space, proximity to the facial nerve), extent (extraparotid extension), resectability, and the presence of enlarged cervical lymph nodes.

E Fine-needle aspiration (FNA) biopsy does not determine whether parotidectomy is offered, as parotidectomy is recommended in most cases. However, suggestion of malignancy on FNA may guide preoperative patient counseling regarding the possible need for facial nerve sacrifice and neck dissection. In patients with a benign-appearing parotid mass, FNA prior to parotidectomy may not be necessary. Fine-needle aspiration may also be indicated when observation is chosen over surgery (i.e. patient does not wish to undergo surgery or is a poor medical candidate for surgery). If there is concern for malignancy and FNA is diagnostic, an intraoperative frozen section can be done.

F Fine-needle aspiration suggestive of squamous cell carcinoma or other metastatic cancers warrants further evaluation to search for the site of the primary cancer, including a thorough examination of the head and neck, nasopharyngoscopy, and laryngoscopy. Cancers can also metastasize to the parotid from gastrointestinal or urogenital sites.

G Facial palsy strongly suggests direct involvement of the nerve and aggressive behavior of the cancer. Mastoidectomy and temporal bone resection should be considered based on the extent and location of the cancer. Frozen section of the proximal facial nerve stump is recommended to assess for tumor clearance, and the facial nerve should be reconstructed with a nerve graft when possible.

H Facial nerve resection is not recommended unless the tumor is invading the nerve.

I In patients with high-grade cancers or advanced T stage, there is a high incidence of occult metastases in the clinically N0 neck. Levels II–IV appear to be involved most commonly in this situation. In contrast, there is a lower incidence of occult metastases when the primary parotid cancer is T1, T2, or low-grade mucoepidermoid carcinoma.

J In patients with advanced T stage, N+ stage, or other high-risk factors (perineural invasion, positive margins), postoperative radiotherapy improves locoregional control and may improve survival.

SUGGESTED READING

Ali S, Palmer FL, DiLorenzo M, et al. Treatment of the neck in carcinoma of the parotid gland. Ann Surg Oncol. 2014;21: 3042-3048.

Chisholm EJ, Elmiyeh B, Dwivedi RC, et al. Anatomic distribution of cervical lymph node spread in parotid carcinoma. Head Neck. 2011;33:513-515.

Lim CM, Gilbert M, Johnson JT, et al. Is level V neck dissection necessary in primary parotid cancer? Laryngoscope. 2014;125: 118-121.

Mercante G, Marchese C, Giannarelli D, et al. Oncological outcome and prognostic factors in malignant parotid tumors. J Cranio-Maxillo-Fac Surg. 2014;42:59-65.

Nobis CP, Rohleder NH, Wolff KD, et al. Head and neck salivary gland carcinomas—elective neck dissection, yes or no? J Oral Maxillofac Surg. 2014;72:205-210.

Richter SM, Friedmann P, Mourad WF, et al. Postoperative radiation therapy for small, low-/intermediate-grade parotid tumors with close and/or positive surgical margins. Head Neck. 2012;34: 953-955.

Walvekar RR, Andrade Filho PA, Seethala RR, et al. Clinicopathologic features are stronger prognostic factors than histology or grade in risk stratification of primary parotid malignancies. Head Neck. 2011;33:225-231.

Neoplasms of the Submandibular Gland

Anna M Pou

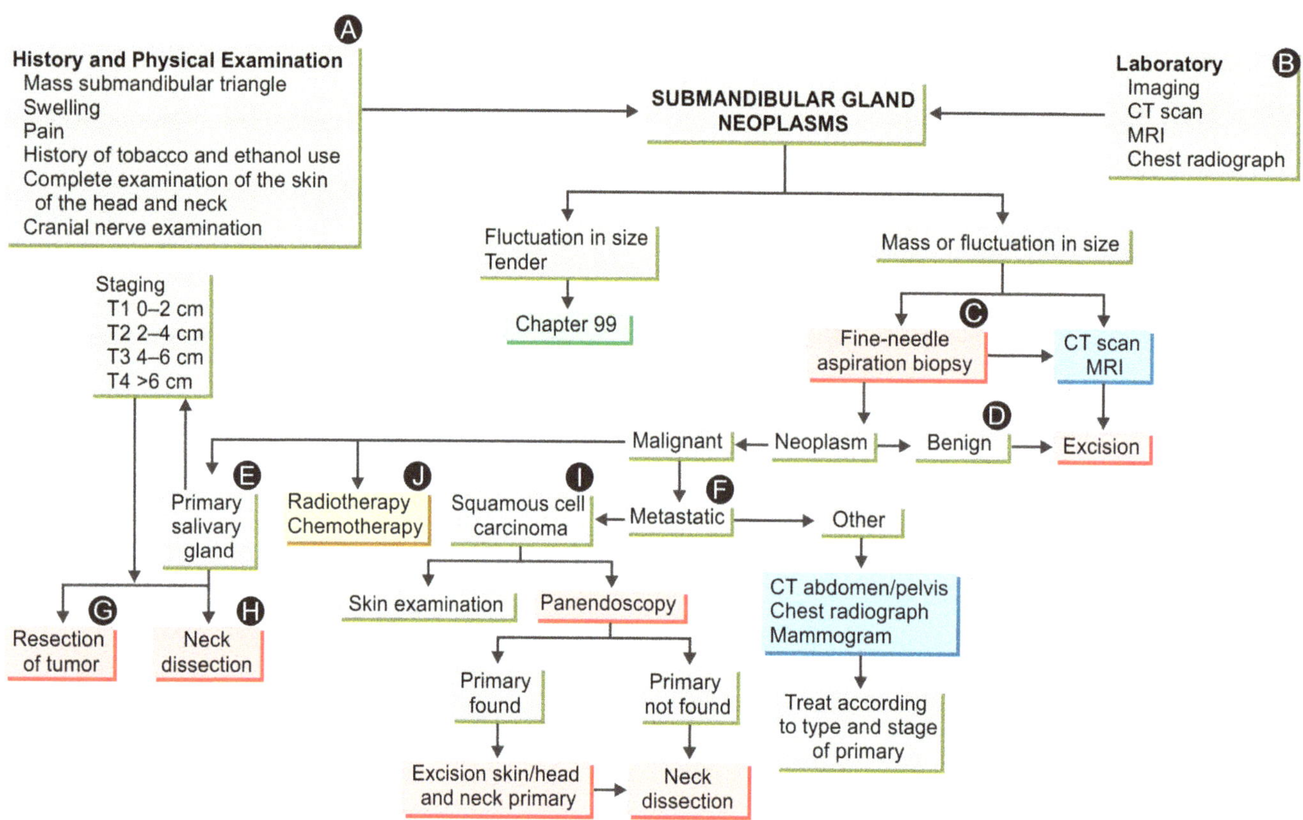

Neoplasms of the submandibular glands are rare, and the majority are malignant. Primary surgery is the treatment of choice.

A A neoplasm in the submandibular gland is typically malignant and usually presents as a slow-growing, painless mass. However, patients can present with symptoms of pain and numbness in the face/tongue, which can suggest malignancy. A complete history should include risk factors such as HIV infection and/or Epstein-Barr virus, exposure to radiation of the head and neck, as well as environmental exposure to nickel, rubber, asbestos, and other chemicals. A complete examination of the head and neck, including bimanual examination of the gland, cranial nerves, and skin, should be performed to evaluate the extent of the mass, involvement of cranial nerves, and the presence of other lesions in the upper aerodigestive tract or skin suggesting metastatic cancer to the submandibular triangle. The presence or absence of purulent material or a calculus in Wharton's duct should also be determined to exclude this as a benign cause.

B Tumors arising from the submandibular gland have a high rate of malignancy, and, therefore, imaging is recommended. Computed tomography (CT) scans can characterize a mass and identify calculi but often cannot distinguish inflammation from tumor. Magnetic resonance imaging (MRI), provides superior soft-tissue detail, including the detection of perineural invasion. Patients with high-grade cancers have a high incidence of metastasis to the lung. A chest radiograph should be obtained when staging the disease and at regular follow-up intervals.

C An ultrasound-guided fine-needle aspiration (FNA) is obtained if a neoplasm is suspected, if presumed inflammatory process persists or recurs, or if diagnosis is uncertain. Aspirates should be examined by a cytologist who is expert in salivary gland histopathology. Ultrasound-guided FNA was found in one study to be 75.7% sensitive, 100% specific, and 95.8% sensitive in distinguishing between benign and malignant neoplasms. Only 59.6% of malignant tumors could be identified preoperatively due to the challenges in diagnosing these tumors. If a neoplasm is confirmed or suspected, a CT scan or MRI is obtained.

D If the FNA is consistent with a benign neoplasm of the salivary gland, excision of the gland is the treatment of choice. This can be performed transcervical or transoral +/– the use of a robot.

E Approximately 75% of submandibular gland neoplasms are malignant; these cancers include primary salivary gland malignancies or metastases from other sites. If the diagnosis is squamous cell carcinoma (SCCA), the gland is most likely involved through direct extension from an adjacent site (i.e. oral cavity) or from a lymph node in the submandibular triangle. Primary SCCA of the submandibular gland is extremely rare; high-grade mucoepidermoid carcinoma must be ruled out. Also, non-Hodgkin's lymphoma is the predominant lymphoma found to arise from lymph nodes adjacent to the salivary gland.

F Resection of the primary cancer includes excisional biopsy with regional lymphadenectomy (submandibular triangle). Surrounding tissue (floor of mouth, tongue, mandible, and cranial nerves) is also resected if involved with tumor. Because of the predilection for perineural invasion in adenoid cystic carcinoma, special attention should be given to the submandibular ganglion, lingual, hypoglossal and marginal nerves, and the nerve to the mylohyoid. Frozen section can help to determine involvement.

G A neck dissection is recommended when the cancer is intermediate or high grade and when large or palpable nodes are present.

H If the FNA suggests metastatic cancer, a search for the primary is undertaken. Primary cancers that metastasize to lymph nodes around the submandibular gland include SCCA of the upper aerodigestive tract and skin, and cancer of the lung, breast, and kidney. A positron emission tomography CT scan can be very helpful in finding the primary cancer.

I A search for SCCA in the head and neck region is undertaken to find the primary cancer.

J Adjuvant radiation therapy is recommended for primary submandibular malignancies in cases of recurrent or advanced disease, extraglandular extension, positive surgical margins when re-resection is not possible, perineural invasion, and metastasis to the regional lymph nodes. Chemotherapy has not been found to be efficacious in treating cancer of salivary origin. In the case of metastatic cancer to the submandibular gland, radiation with or without chemotherapy is recommended according to the type, stage, and histopathologic characteristics of the primary cancer.

SUGGESTED READING

Cho HN, Kim J, Choi J, et al. Sonographically guided fine-needle aspiration biopsy of major salivary gland masses: a review of 245 cases. AJR Am J Roentgenol. 2011;196:1160-1163.

Hanna EYN, Suen JY. Malignant tumors of the salivary glands. In: Myers EN, Suen JY, Myers JN, Hanna EYN (Eds). Cancer of the Head and Neck, 4th edition. Philadelphia, PA: Elsevier Science; 2003. p. 475.

Oh, YS, Russell MS, Eisle DW. Salivary gland neoplasms. In: Johnson JT, Rosen CA (Eds). Head and Neck Surgery—Otolaryngology, 5th edition. Philadelphia, PA: Wolters/Lippincott Williams & Wilkins; 2014. p. 1760-1787.

Spiegel JH, Brys AK, Bhakti A, et al. Metastasis to the submandibular gland in head and neck carcinomas. Head Neck. 2004; 26(12):1064-1068.

Congenital Malformations of the Esophagus

Joseph C Fusco, George K Gittes

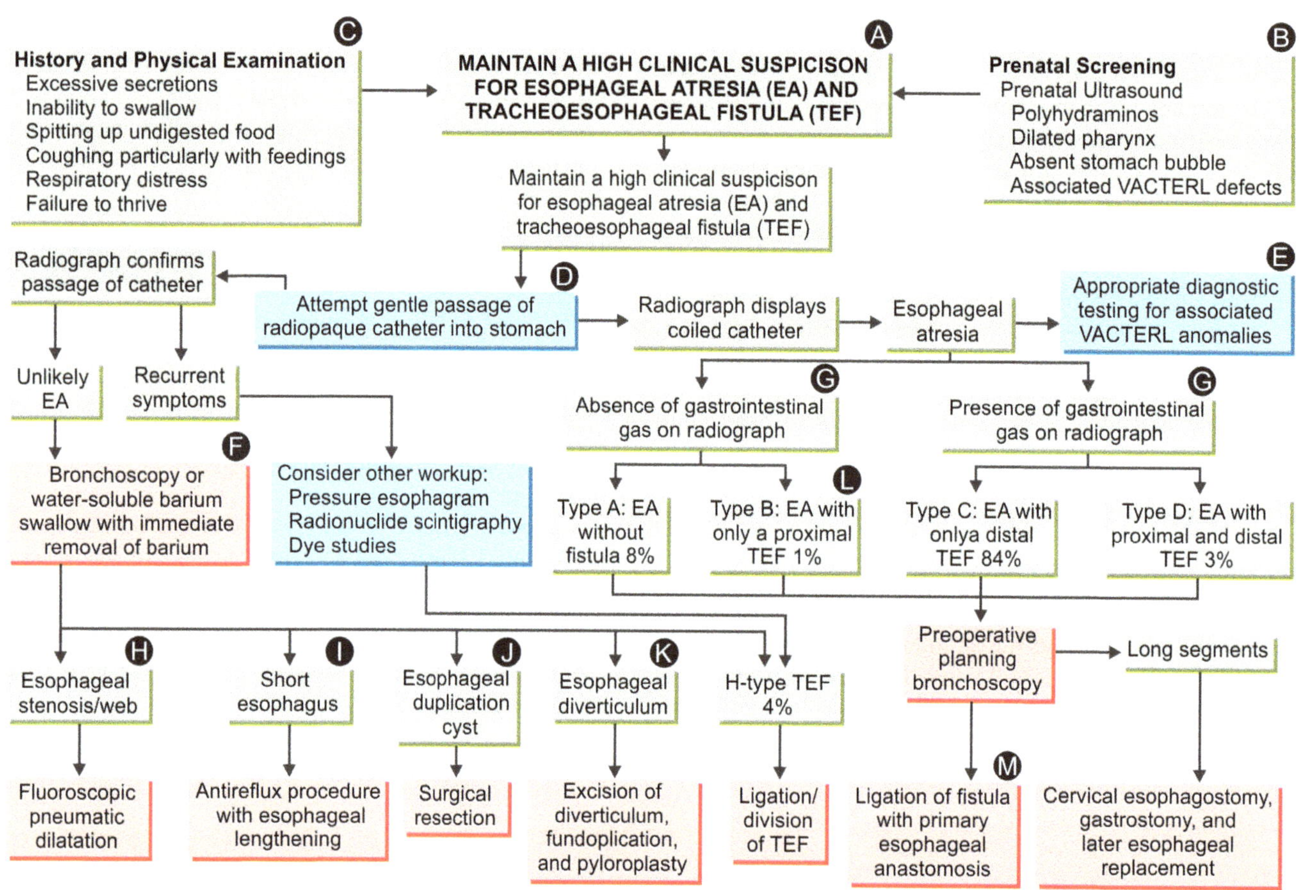

The esophagus, which is derived from the Greek word oisophagos meaning "entrance for eating", is part of the alimentary tract that connects the pharynx to the stomach. It is an endodermally derived muscular tube that represents the only communication between the oral cavity and the stomach to facilitate food transit via peristalsis. Thus, diseases of the esophagus, whether congenital or acquired, lead to significant morbidity. This chapter provides a brief algorithmic overview for management of the commonly encountered congenital malformations of the esophagus.

Ⓐ Congenital malformations of the esophagus can present significant clinical challenges. Often, these malformations are found in conjunction with tracheal anomalies, and up to half of the cases are a part of either the CHARGE [coloboma, heart defects, atresia choanae (also known as choanal atresia), growth retardation, genital abnormalities, and ear abnormalities] or VACTERL (vertebral defects, anal atresia, cardiac defects, tracheoesophageal fistula, renal anomalies and limb abnormalities) associations. Other subtle associated anomalies have been described including absent or abnormal vagus nerves, abnormal intrinsic innervation, and malformed tracheobronchial tree or lung.

Ⓑ Both the esophagus and the trachea are derived from a single anterior foregut tube. The key mechanism is a failure of the dorsal esophageal and ventral tracheal foregut to separate properly during embryologic development. When esophageal atresia (EA) is present polyhydramnios occurs in two-thirds of pregnancies. A dilated pharynx or an absent stomach bubble can also be noted.

Ⓒ Infants typically become symptomatic immediately after birth. The symptoms that should produce a high index of suspicion include excessive secretions causing drooling, choking, respiratory distress, and an inability to feed. Gastric distention and reflux can lead to aspiration pneumonia further adding to the morbidity. Small H-type tracheoesophageal fistulas (TEFs), however, can go unnoticed for years.

Ⓓ The diagnosis of EA is made by the inability to pass a catheter into the stomach. Radiographs will instead demonstrate proximal coiling of the catheter in a blind pouch.

E The VACTERL association is commonly seen in EA patients, thus necessitating investigation for the other anomalies. An echocardiogram can display a cardiac anomaly, most commonly a ventricular septal defect. The echocardiogram is also useful in planning the operative approach in that it aids in the determination of the location of the aortic arch. The abdominal radiograph is an important adjunct, as it can reveal vertebral abnormalities, along with spinal ultrasound, renal ultrasound, and upper extremity examination for radial anomalies.

F With recurrent symptoms and an uncertain diagnosis, or if a proximal TEF is suspected, a small amount of water-soluble contrast material can be instilled under fluoroscopic guidance to confirm the EA. It is important for this procedure to be done using continuous fluoroscopy to allow rapid removal of contrast to prevent aspiration. Isolated fistulas without atresia may be seen with upper gastrointestinal series using thickened contrast. However, bronchoscopy and esophagoscopy may be necessary to delineate the anatomy. Additional studies such as cine contrast swallow studies with pressure, or dye studies during bronchoscopy may also be used.

G The abdominal radiograph will hint as to the presence of a TEF. The EA with distal TEF will show a normal gastrointestinal gas pattern, whereas those with only a proximal fistula or those without a fistula will show an absence of gastrointestinal gas.

H Strictures of the esophagus may be congenital in the distal esophagus, lined by normal mucosa, and unrelated to reflux. Patients often present with similar symptoms to those of a TEF including aspiration and pneumonia. Dysphagia and regurgitation are more pronounced with solid food. Strictures can also be a product of esophageal webs. Pneumatic dilatation or balloon dilation under fluoroscopy can be diagnostic and therapeutic.

I Congenital short esophagus is associated with a hiatal hernia and an intrathoracic stomach. Infants usually present with significant reflux and failure to thrive. Surgical intervention includes an antireflux procedure in combination with an esophageal lengthening procedure.

J Esophageal duplications cysts include esophageal cystic/tubular duplications and bronchogenic cysts. The cysts are characterized by well-developed smooth muscle, an epithelial lining, and an attachment to the alimentary tract or bronchial tree. Large duplications can result in cardiac or respiratory symptoms. Chest radiographs show a soft-tissue mass, possibly with mediastinal shift, and ultrasound will further distinguish between a solid and cystic mass, whereas computed tomography can show the exact location prior to definitive resection.

K A diverticulum of the esophagus is a true diverticulum. Symptoms include emesis, regurgitation, and recurrent lung infections. Treatment consists of surgical excision of the diverticulum, fundoplication, and pyloroplasty.

L The most common EA classification scheme is based on the presence and location of the fistula. Those systems with the corresponding percent of cases are type A, atresia without TEF (7%); type B, atresia with proximal TEF (2%); type C, atresia with distal TEF (86% most common); type D, atresia with both proximal and distal TEF (1%); and type E, TEF without EA, H-type (4%).

M Definitive management consists of surgical division and ligation of the fistula. Bronchoscopy is an important step in preoperative planning for localization of the fistula or identifying an occult fistula. Isolated TEFs are typically amenable to a cervical approach. In cases with EA, primary anastomosis is preferred. When the distance is too large between segments, other options are available including a staged procedure, elongation of the esophagus, interposition of the colon, or gastric pull-up. The prognosis is generally good when the EA is isolated, but associated anomalies can make the prognosis more guarded. Early complications include leak, stricture, and recurrence. Late complications include motility disorders and respiratory dysfunction. Barrett's esophagus is increased four fold compared to the general population.

SUGGESTED READING

El-Gohary Y, Gittes GK, Tovar JA. Congenital anomalies of the esophagus. Semin Pediatr Surg. 2010;19(3):186-193.

Goyal A, Jones MO, Couriel JM, et al. Oesophageal atresia and tracheo-oesophageal fistula. Arch Dis Child Fetal Neonatal Ed. 2006; 91(5):F381-F384.

Haight C. Congenital atresia of the esophagus with tracheoesophageal fistula: reconstruction of esophageal continuity by primary anastomosis. Ann Surg. 1944;120(4):623-652.

Konkin DE, O'hali WA, Webber EM, et al. Outcomes in esophageal atresia and tracheoesophageal fistula. J Pediatr Surg. 2003;38(12):1726-1729.

Shaw-Smith C. Oesophageal atresia, tracheo-oesophageal fistula, and the VACTERL association: review of genetics and epidemiology. J Med Genet. 2006;43(7):545-554.

Spitz L. Oesophageal atresia treatment: a 21st-century perspective. J Pediatr Gastroenterol Nutr. 2011;52(Suppl 1):S12.

Cricopharyngeal Achalasia

Bridget Hathaway

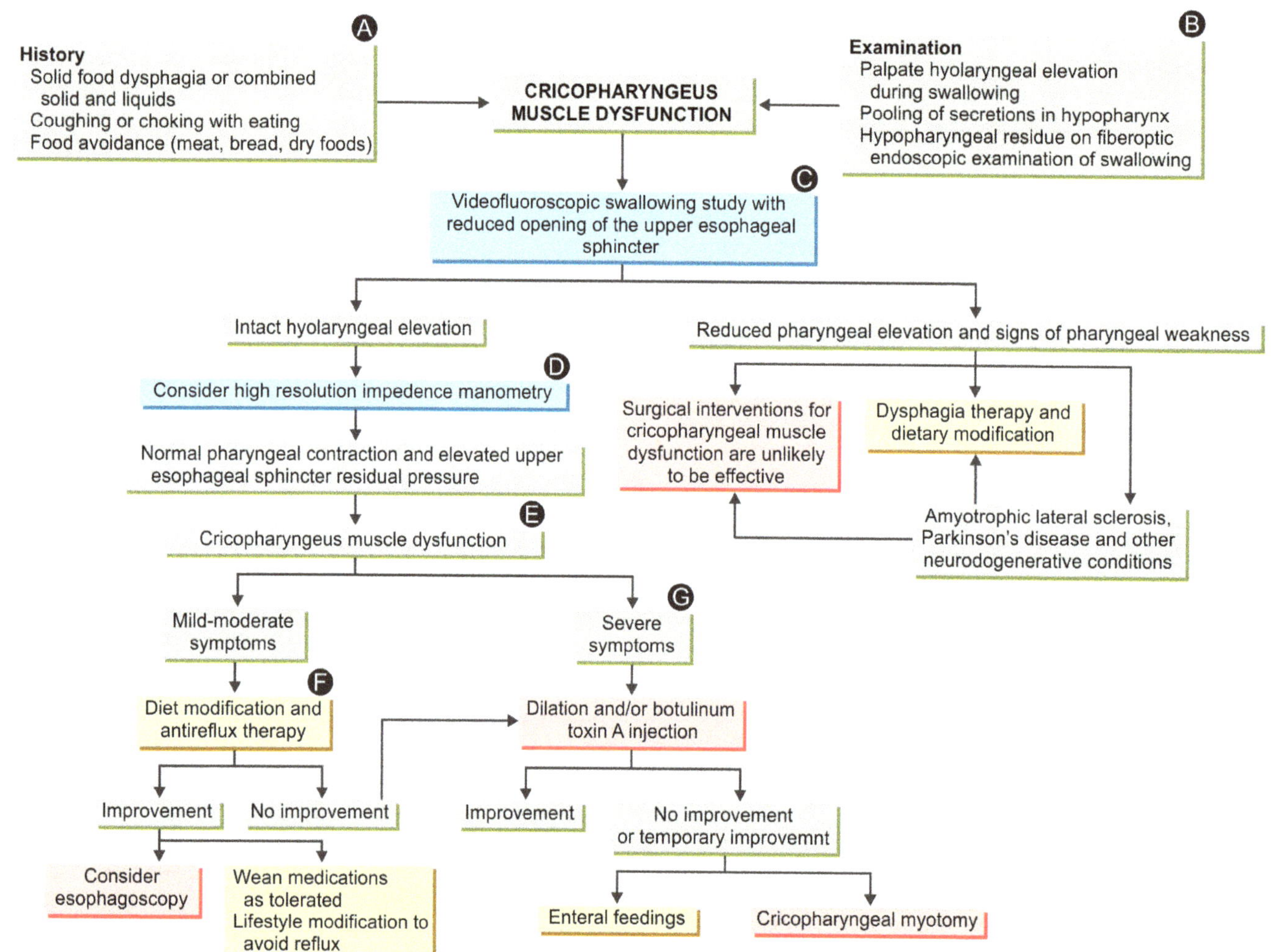

The cricopharyngeus muscle (CPM) is a 1–2 cm C-shaped muscle that originates from the lateral portions of the cricoid cartilage. The upper esophageal sphincter (UES) is a 2.5–4.5 cm high pressure zone that includes the distal inferior pharyngeal constrictor, CPM, and proximal cervical esophageal musculature. The UES is tonically contracted at rest and relaxes during deglutition. Cricopharyngeus muscle dysfunction (CPD) occurs as a result of impaired or uncoordinated UES relaxation. There are a variety of causes for CPD. Some of the common etiologies include neoplasm, neurodegenerative conditions, cerebrovascular accident, radiation therapy, and laryngopharyngeal reflux.

A Accurate diagnosis of CPD is essential in developing an effective management strategy. A history of dysphagia to solids or combined solids and liquids is usually present but further evaluation is necessary to differentiate CPD from pharyngeal or esophageal dysphagia. Symptoms may also include coughing and choking with eating and drinking and patients will often localize symptoms to the cervical region. Failure of active hyolaryngeal elevation (HLE) may mimic failure of UES relaxation leading to miss-diagnosis of CPD.

B Flexible endoscopic evaluation of swallowing (FEES) is often beneficial in evaluating the laryngopharyngeal anatomy and ruling out other pathology such as neoplasms. Pooling of secretions in the hypopharynx and hypopharyngeal residue are suggestive of CPD but UES opening is not directly assessed with FEES.

C A videofluoroscopic swallow study (VFSS) allows for objective measurements of UES opening with respect to opening size and duration. Assessments of HLE and pharyngeal strength are also essential. Decreased HLE and pharyngeal strength in the setting of decreased UES opening suggests that the problem is more than isolated CPD and interventions directed at the CPM are likely to be ineffective. Cricopharyngeal bars (CPBs) are often observed incidentally during VFSS and may not cause symptoms. The UES opening is often adequate in those with radiographically evident CPBs.

D High-resolution impedance manometry can be a useful tool in the diagnostic evaluation of CPD as it allows for measurement of pharyngeal strength, UES relaxation, and intrabolus pressures. During swallowing, normal pharyngeal contraction with elevated UES residual pressure is suggestive of CPD. Elevated resting pressure of the UES may be seen in gastroesophageal reflux disease which is not necessarily indicative of CPD.

E Multiple factors should be considered when devising a treatment plan for CPD including the severity of symptoms, the underlying condition causing CPD, and the overall health of the patient.

F A trial of antireflux therapy may be considered prior to other interventions. Dietary modifications with softer foods should also be recommended as first-line therapy.

G For patients with more severe symptoms (weight loss, severe dietary restriction, aspiration-related complications) or those who have failed conservative therapy, surgical intervention should be offered. Procedures for CPD include dilation, CPM botulinum toxin (BTx) injection, and CPM myotomy. Dilation and/or BTx injection are often done prior to myotomy, as they are less invasive and have the potential to result in long-term relief for some patients.

SUGGESTED READING

Jones CA, Ciucci MR, Hammer MJ, et al. A multisensor approach to improve manometric analysis of the upper esophageal sphincter. Laryngoscope. 2016;126(3):657-664.

Kuhn MA, Belafsky PC. Management of cricopharyngeus muscle dysfunction. Otolaryngol Clin N Am. 2013;46:1087-1099.

Leonard R, Kendall K, McKenzie S. UES opening and cricopharyngeal bar in nondysphagic elderly and nonelderly adults. Dysphagia. 2004;19(3):182-191.

Leonard R, Rees CJ, Belafsky P, et al. Fluoroscopic surrogate for pharyngeal strength: the pharyngeal constriction ratio (PCR). Dysphagia. 2011;1:13-17.

Murry T, Wasserman T, Carrau RL, et al. Injection of botulinum toxin A for the treatment of dysfunction of the upper esophageal sphincter. Am J Otolaryngol. 2005;26(3):157-162.

Esophageal Diverticula

Jonathan B Overdevest, Andrew N Goldberg

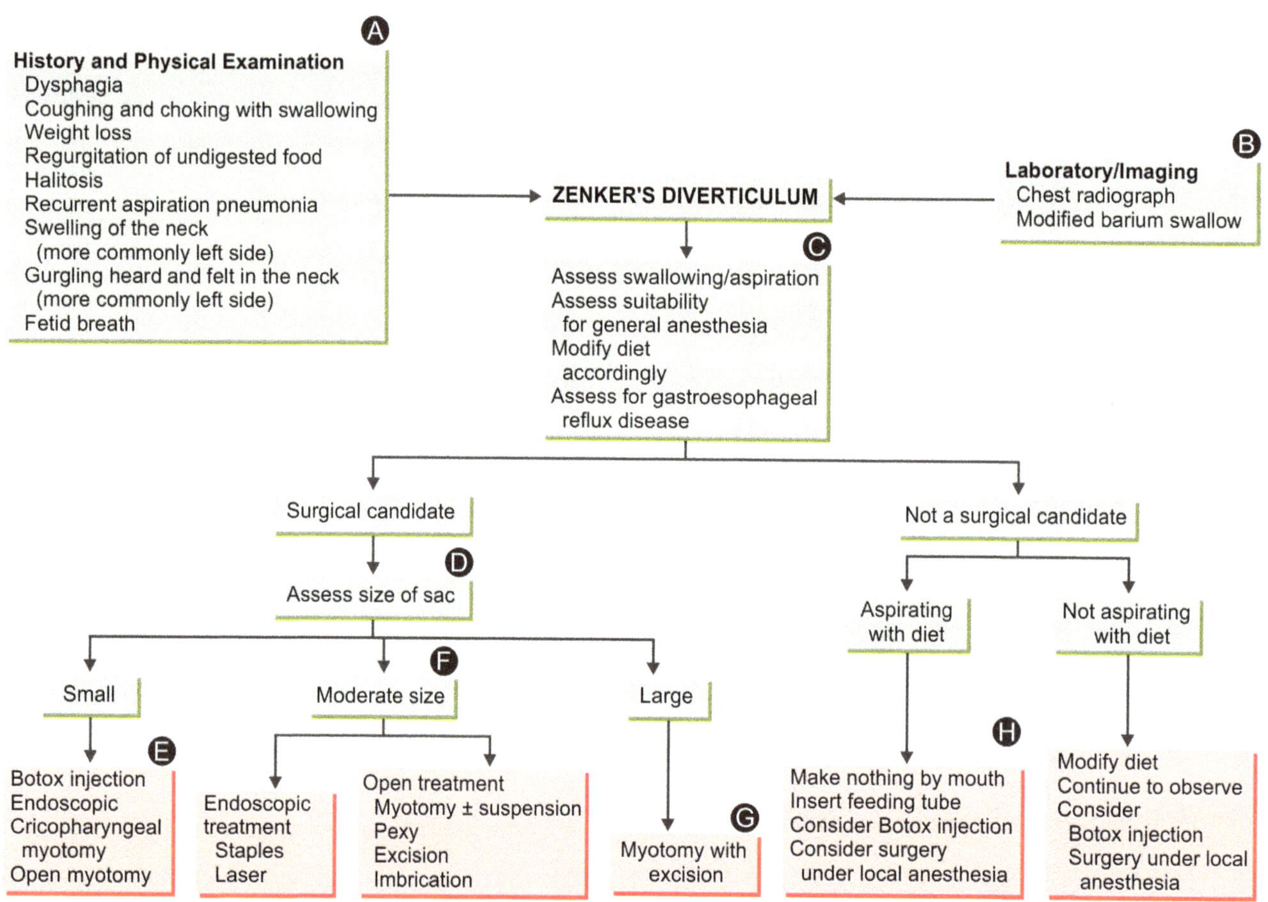

Esophageal diverticula include pharyngoesophageal diverticula, commonly known as Zenker's diverticulum (ZD), which occurs above the cricopharyngeus (CP) muscle. Others at the esophageal inlet include the Killian-Jamieson or Laimer's diverticula located below the CP muscle. The annual incidence of ZD is believed to be quite low, 2 per 100,000 patients, occurring three times more likely in males. Affected patients are often elderly with multiple medical comorbidities, and report progressive dysphagia, halitosis, and regurgitation of undigested food. Recurrent aspiration pneumonia occurs in 20% or more of patients. With progression weight loss may occur due to inability or unwillingness to ingest solid foods. The exact pathophysiology remains debated; however, esophageal dysmotility, CP dysfunction, and gastric reflux may be contributing factors.

A Although Killian's triangle is midline, patients often present with a left-sided ZD possibly due to the path of the esophagus. Large diverticula may be palpable or visible on the left side of the neck. Other diagnostic signs are fetid odor or dysgeusia due to decomposing food retained in the sac.

B Flexible fiberoptic laryngoscopy rarely permits visualization of the diverticular sac, since the opening is usually distal to the postcricoid region. Flexible endoscopic evaluation of swallowing examination may show by regurgitation of the bolus it passes from view. This has been termed the "sign of the rising tide" and is a sensitive indicator for ZD. Although chest radiograph will occasionally show a cervical air-fluid level or other evidence of a ZD, modified barium swallow (MBS) is the diagnostic study of choice. In addition to demonstrating the diverticulum, MBS can show incomplete relaxation of the CP muscle and evidence of reflux. Retained food in the diverticulum can create filling defects that may be confused with carcinomas. Carcinoma arising in the ZD is exceedingly rare, with only 60 cases of diverticular-based carcinoma reported in the English language. Nevertheless, some authors recommend excision of the pouch in all cases. Additional studies that are occasionally performed, but are not critical to the diagnosis, include esophageal manometry, ambulatory pH monitoring, and esophagogastroduodenoscopy (EGD). Studies usually reveal elevated pharyngeal pressures, incomplete relaxation of the upper esophageal sphincter, and evidence of reflux.

C Decision-making is difficult as many patients are elderly with multiple medical comorbidities. Dangerous symptoms include recurrent aspiration pneumonia or unintentional weight loss that may be attributable to dysphagia or cibophobia (Fear of food). Close consultation with the patients' medical physicians is essential, as is accurate assessment of their swallowing risk. Sometimes dietary modifications (soft or liquid diet) and therapy for gastroesophageal reflux disease are sufficient to control symptoms and allow adequate oral intake. Severely debilitated patients may benefit from an initial strategy of nonoperative management followed by surgical intervention after weight gain and medical improvement. Healthy, symptomatic patients should be offered elective surgery.

D Multiple methods exist to determine the size of the diverticulum. Because most patients will undergo MBS for definitive diagnosis of their diverticulum, this is the easiest method to determine the size of the sac. Another common method is to deploy a measurement wire during EGD. Finally, direct measurement is possible with surgical neck exploration. Although size is an important criterion in surgical planning, other factors are also important. For instance, a dentulous patient with a hypoplastic mandible and limited neck flexion is not an ideal candidate for an endoscopic approach because of difficulty accessing the pouch.

E Conservative management with observation alone may be pursued for small diverticula (<2 cm); however, simple CP myotomy often results in complete resolution. Cricopharyngeus myotomy is the key maneuver in any surgical procedure for ZD to reverse the underlying disease and to help decrease the incidence of recurrence. When performing open CP myotomy, the incision should include a segment of hypopharyngeal muscle and ~2 cm of circular esophageal fibers. To prevent scarring and reformation of a constricting band, a strip of muscle (~1 cm) can be removed instead of a single vertical myotomy. A minimally invasive alternative procedure is injection of the CP muscle with botulinum toxin (Botox). Although the injections must be repeated several times per year, this can often palliate symptoms in patients who are too ill for operative interventions. Botox can also be used as a diagnostic aid before performing myotomy. If symptoms improve after Botox, CP myotomy should offer permanent relief. Histopathologic examination of myotomy specimens has shown a significant degree of CP fibrosis in some patients with ZD, indicating that not all patients will improve with chemical denervation. Small diverticula are not well treated by endoscopic diverticulotomy because the CP muscle is not completely transected by division of the party wall. Endoscopic CO_2 laser CP myotomy can offer a less invasive approach in carefully selected patients.

F Medium size (2–10 cm) diverticula are ideally managed endoscopically. All endoscopic procedures for ZD are similar in that they divide the party wall between the diverticulum and the esophagus. By dividing the party wall, the CP muscle is also divided, helping to prevent recurrence. Many different means of division have been reported, including electrocautery (Dohlman procedure), carbon dioxide and other lasers, and endoscopic stapling devices. Endoscopic stapling is currently the favored endoscopic technique because it seals the mucosal edges together during division, decreasing the possibility of salivary leaks. Although the procedure offers advantages over laser or electrocautery, exposure can be difficult due to the bulkiness of the Weerda diverticuloscope and the large stapler. In some patients the diverticulum cannot be adequately exposed and mucosal tears and perforations do occur occasionally. Endoscopic procedures require general anesthesia but are performed very quickly. Large diverticula often have residual dependent pouches that may continue to cause symptoms. Patients not considered candidates for endoscopic treatment for anatomic or other reasons can undergo open treatment as described next.

G A large (>10 cm) ZD is best approached via a left cervical incision. The pouch is dissected free of the surrounding structures and can then be excised, surgically fixated (diverticulopexy), or inverted and imbricated. No procedure has been proven superior, although pexis and imbrication have the theoretical advantage of maintaining mucosal integrity. Massive diverticula should be excised. In all these procedures, a CP myotomy should also be performed. Risks of open surgery include pharyngocutaneous fistula, recurrent laryngeal nerve injury, and mediastinitis.

H Patients deemed unsuitable for general anesthesia can be managed in several ways. If aspirating, they should be kept on nothing by mouth orders and have a feeding tube placed. Botox injection into the cricopharyngeal muscle can be performed in the office with no sedation and may offer some relief. Finally, open diverticulectomy under local anesthesia can be performed in cooperative patients, but most patients will require general anesthesia.

ACKNOWLDGMENT

We would like to acknowledge the contributions of Dr Timothy D Anderson for his review and edits to the manuscript.

SUGGESTED READING

Bizzotto A, Iacopini F. Zenker's diverticulum: exploring treatment options. Acta Otorhinolaryngol Ital. 2013;33:219-229.

Greene CL, Mcfadden PM, Oh DS, et al. Long-term outcome of the treatment of Zenker's diverticulum. Ann Thorac Surg. 2015;100:975-978.

Khan AS, Dwivedi RC, Sheikh Z, et al. Systematic review of carcinoma arising in pharyngeal diverticula: a 112-year analysis. Head Neck. 2014;36(9):1368-1375.

Papaspyrou G, Schick B, Papaspyrou S, et al. Laser surgery for Zenker's diverticulum: European combined study. Eur Arch Otorhinolaryngol. 2016;273(1):183-188.

Scher RL. Cummings Otolaryngology—Head and Neck Surgery. In: Flint PW, et al. (Eds), 5th edition. Philadelphia, PA; Mosby Elsevier; 2010. pp. 986-997.

Westrin KM, Ergün S, Carlsöö B. Zenker's diverticulum—a historical review and trends in therapy. Acta Otolaryngol. 1996;116: 351(3):351-360.

Wilken R, Whited C, Scher RL. Endoscopic staple diverticulostomy for Zenker's diverticulum: review of experience in 337 cases. Ann Otol Rhinol Laryngol. 2015;124:21-29.

Zaninotto G, Portale G, Costantini M, et al. Therapeutic strategies for epiphrenic diverticula: systematic review. World J Surg. 2011;35:1447-1453.

Foreign Body Injury to the Esophagus

Andrew C Urquhart

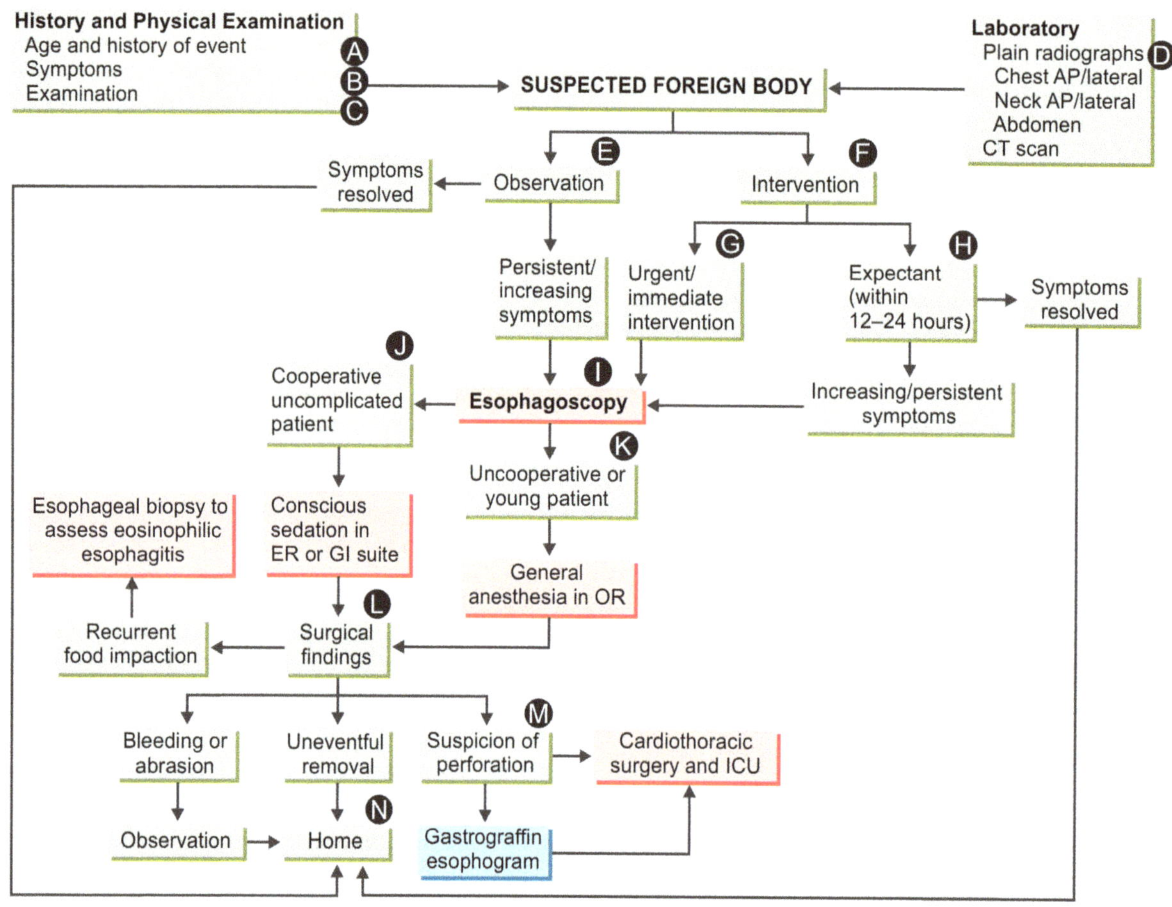

Foreign body or food bolus impaction usually occurs in children or mentally impaired and edentulous adults. Coins are most common in children and food impaction above a stricture in adults. Most foreign bodies pass without the need for intervention.

A The circumstances in which the ingestion occurred may suggest a certain type of object or food type. Younger children or impaired adults may give no history and should be evaluated with the assumption that a foreign body is present. Adults and older children generally give a history of ingestion and point to a specific area of discomfort in the neck or chest.

B Symptoms usually include acute onset of dysphagia and difficulty swallowing saliva. Other symptoms may consist of drooling, retrosternal fullness, choking, refusal to eat, and regurgitation of undigested food. Occasionally wheezing, respiratory distress, and blood-tinged mucus may occur.

C Examination usually reveals an afebrile patient in discomfort and occasionally distress. There may be tenderness in the neck and increased salivation. In the rare event of esophageal perforation, symptoms will be more severe and include severe chest pain, tachycardia, fever, and shock.

D Plain radiographs consisting of anteroposterior and lateral chest and neck and flat plate of the abdomen. If it is obvious that there is symptomatic simple food impaction, radiographs may not be necessary. Computed tomography (CT) scan may be helpful (multidetector CT) if radiographs are negative. In cases of sharp objects with negative clinical examination, CT scan should be the initial study. Barium swallow should not be performed as the contrast material will compromise subsequent endoscopy.

E Most patients can be managed conservatively, as the majority of objects will pass spontaneously.

F Symptomatic patients and those with positive imaging studies require intervention. If patients have an identified foreign body radiologically or persistent symptoms despite negative radiology, intervention is required.

G Immediate/emergent intervention with endoscopy is indicated in complete obstruction of the esophagus, disk batteries, sharp objects, perforating foreign bodies, high-powered magnets, and signs of airway compromise.

H Expectant management in patients without complete obstruction of food, blunt esophageal foreign bodies, sharp objects in stomach or duodenum, larger objects in the duodenum, and normal magnets. Surgery is required within 12–24 hours if no improvement.

I Flexible endoscopes are used in most centers as the instrument of choice usually with conscious sedation. Rigid esophagoscopy may be needed for upper esophageal and pharyngeal lesions as well as sharp objects. In institutions where pediatric otolaryngologists manage esophageal foreign bodies, rigid endoscopy is usually performed and should be considered standard of care.

J Cooperative, uncomplicated adults can be operated under conscious sedation in the Emergency Room or Gastro-enterology suite.

K Children, uncooperative adults, patients with multiple foreign bodies and those requiring rigid esophagoscopy will require intubation and general anesthesia in the operating room. Uncomplicated simple foreign bodies (most coins) can be removed under general anesthesia without intubation.

L With uneventful endoscopic removal, observe and discharge in 2–4 hours. If bleeding and abrasion is noted with removal, observe for 24 hours. When food impaction occurs, especially with recurrent impaction in the absence of a stricture, biopsy should be done at the time of the food impaction removal to exclude eosinophilic esophagitis.

M If a perforation is noted, place a nasogastric tube under direct visualization. Consult cardiothoracic surgery to consider open exploration via thoracotomy with irrigation and repair as indicated. Intensive care unit (ICU) care is required. In most cases, a perforation may not be apparent at the time of surgery, and postoperatively, there may be a need for contrast esophagram with Gastrografin.

N Discharge home depending on surgical findings, subsequent barium swallow, and repeat endoscopy if stricture or other causes such as eosinophilic esophagitis is suspected.

SUGGESTED READING

Biancari F, D'Andrea V, Paone R, et al. Current treatment and outcome of esophageal perforations in adults: systematic review and meta-analysis of 75 studies. World J Surg. 2013; 37(5):1051-1059.

Lam HC, Woo JK, van Hasselt CA. Management of ingested foreign bodies: a retrospective review of 5240 patients.J Laryngol Otol. 2001;115(12):954-957.

Stool SE, Manning SC. Foreign bodies of the pharynx and esophagus. In: Bluestone CD, Stool SE (Eds). Pediatric Otolaryngology. Philadelphia, PA: WB Saunders; 1996; pp. 1169-1180.

Sung SH, Jeon SW, Son HS, et al. Factors predictive of risk for complications in patients with oesophageal foreign bodies. Dig Liver Dis. 2011;43(8):632-635.

Wu WT, Chiu CT, Kuo CJ, et al. Endoscopic management of suspected esophageal foreign body in adults. Dis Esophagus. 2011; 24(3):131-137.

Gastroesophageal Reflux Disease

Bridget Hathaway

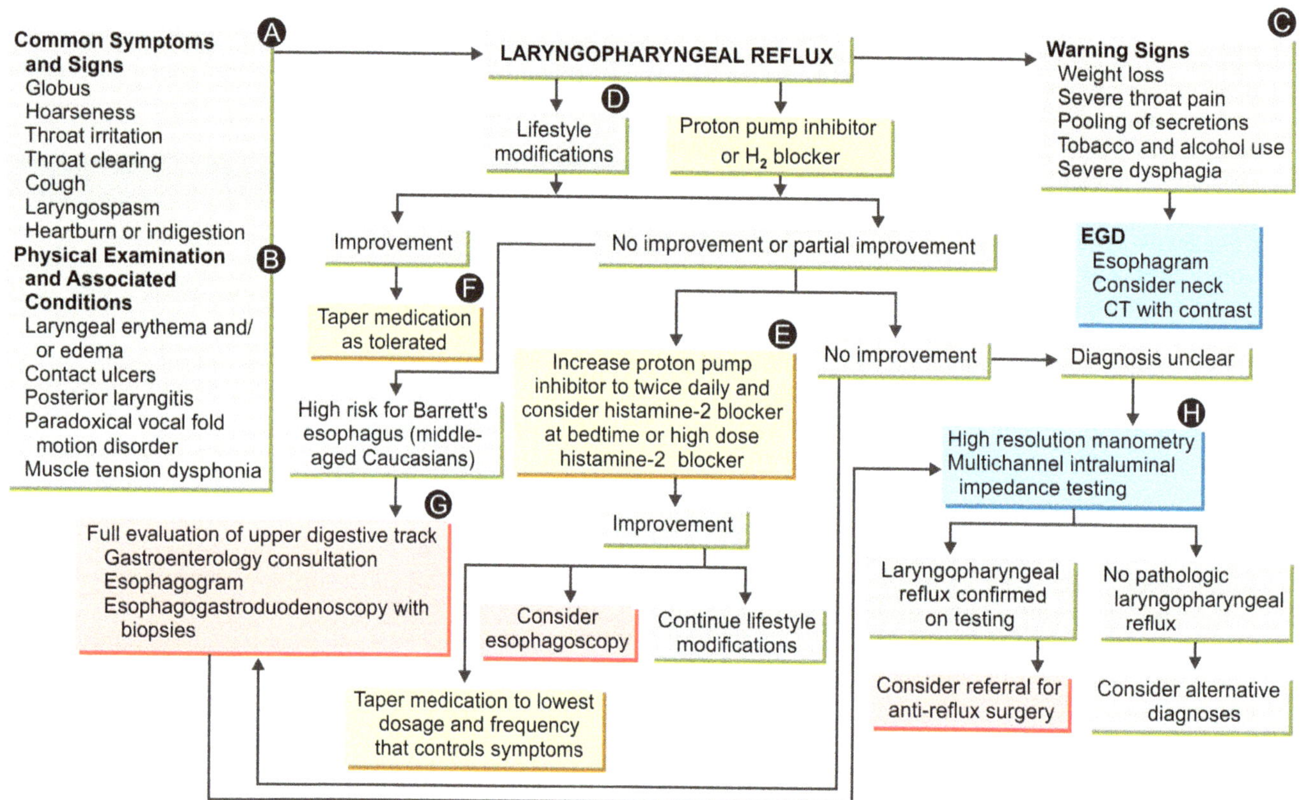

Laryngopharyngeal reflux disease (LPRD) has been increasingly recognized as a clinical entity distinct from gastroesophageal reflux disease (GERD). Less than half of patients presenting with LPRD have "typical" GERD symptoms of heartburn or dyspepsia. The LPRD can be a diagnostic challenge for the Otolaryngologist as the signs and symptoms are not specific and can be attributed to a variety of causes including allergy, asthma, or postviral processes. The role of diagnostic tests for LPRD, including pH testing and high resolution manometry, continues to evolve.

Ⓐ Symptoms of LPRD include hoarseness, sore throat, dysphagia, globus, throat clearing, postnasal drip, cough, and laryngospasm.

Ⓑ Examination with flexible laryngoscopy is essential to rule out other pathologies such as malignancy or infection. It is also helpful to identify inflammatory changes of the laryngopharynx and other pathologic conditions associated with LPRD including muscle tension dysphonia and paradoxical vocal fold motion disorder.

Ⓒ Clinicians should have a low threshold for initiating a more extensive evaluation for patients presenting with weight loss, moderate or severe dysphagia, or severe throat pain. These patients may require evaluation with imaging or esophagoscopy. Patients with a history of tobacco or alcohol use should be considered a high-risk population for malignancy.

Ⓓ Lifestyle modifications should be emphasized at every step in the treatment algorithm of LPRD. These include avoidance of triggers such as nicotine exposure, caffeine, alcohol, carbonated soft drinks, acidic foods, and lying down after eating (minimum of 3 hours). Weight loss can also be beneficial for overweight or obese patients.

Ⓔ Empiric therapy with a proton pump inhibitor (PPI) or H_2 blocker can provide further evidence for the diagnosis of LPRD if it is effective. For patients with persistent symptoms on antireflux medication, escalation of therapy includes BID PPI dosing or the addition of an H_2 blocker at bedtime. High-dose H_2 blocker therapy is an alternative strategy.

Ⓕ Patients who have complete resolution of their symptoms can be weaned from medication with the goal of controlling symptoms with lifestyle modifications. If medication is still necessary, the patient is instructed to titrate the medication to the lowest effective dose and frequency.

G Patients who continue to be symptomatic despite maximal medical therapy should have a full evaluation of the upper digestive tract. This includes a Gastroenterologist consultation with a esophagram, and esophagogastroduodenoscopy (EGD) with biopsies. Transnasal esophagoscopy is an alternative to EGD for endoscopists experienced with this technique. In addition, patients at high risk for Barrett's esophagus (i.e. middle-aged Caucasians) and those who require high-dose PPI for control of their symptoms should also undergo a full evaluation of the upper digestive tract.

H If the diagnosis of LPRD is still unclear in a patient with persistent symptoms, high-resolution manometry and multichannel intraluminal pH impedance testing may be useful for diagnosis and further management.

SUGGESTED READING

Altman KW, Prufer N, Vaezi MF. The challenge of protocols for reflux disease: a review and development of a critical pathway. Otolaryngol Head Neck Surg. 2011;145(1):7-14.

Hom C, Vaezi MF. Extraesophageal manifestations of gastroesophageal reflux disease. Gastroenterol Clin N Am. 2013;42:71-91.

Hoppo T, Sanz AF, Nason KS, et al. How much pharyngeal exposure is "normal"? Normative data for laryngopharyngeal reflux events using hypopharyngeal multichannel intraluminal impedance. J Gastrointest Surg. 2012;16:16-25.

Otolaryngologic Manifestations of Gastroesophageal Reflux Disease in the Pediatric Age Group

Todd Otteson

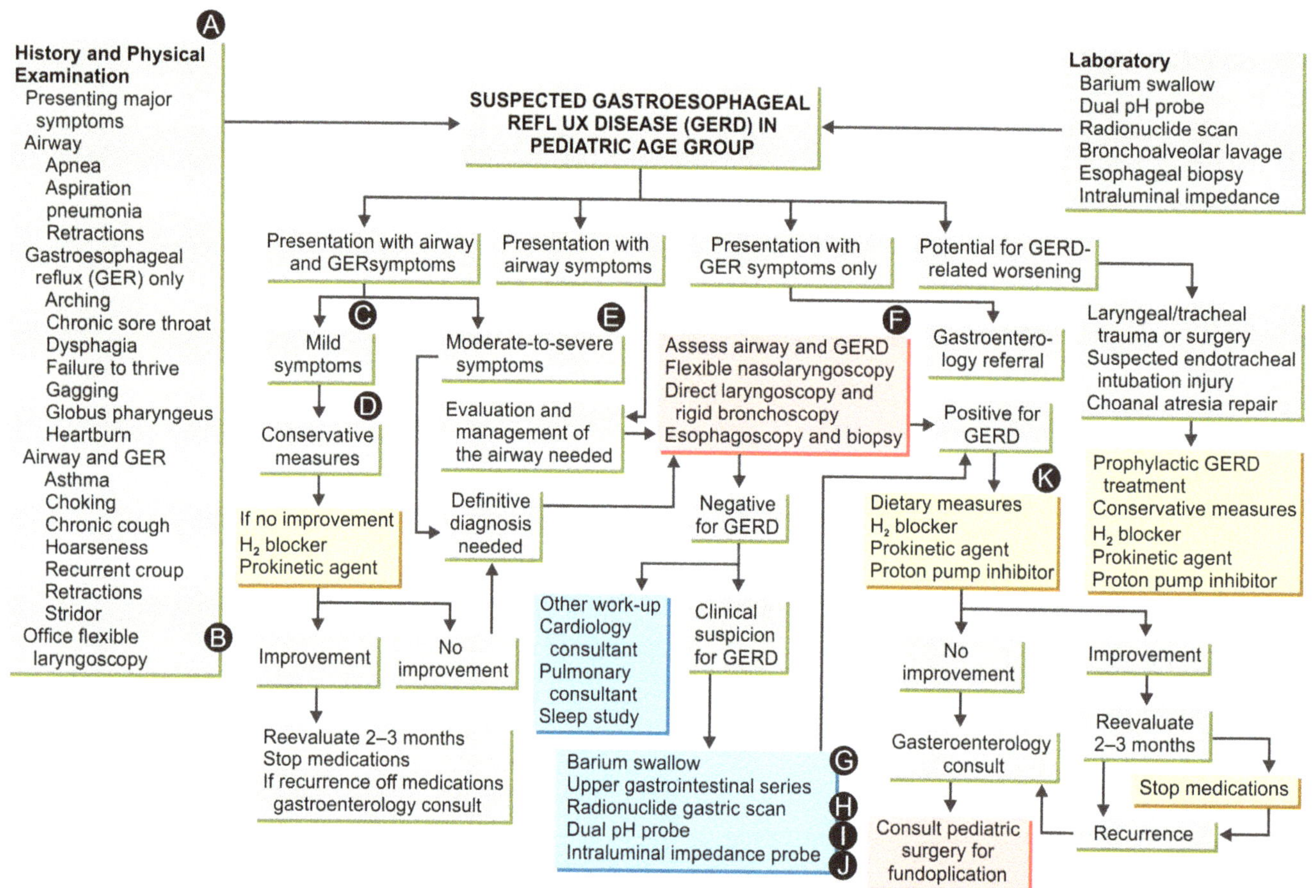

Pathologic gastroesophageal reflux disease (GERD) occurs in all age groups, including children. The presentation of GERD in children may differ from adults, so a high index of suspicion is required to identify affected children. The GERD may present in different ways at different ages; a degree of vomiting may be normal in neonates and infants after feedings.

A History and physical findings suggestive of GERD include apnea, arching, aspiration, aspiration pneumonia, asthma, choking, chronic cough, chronic sore throat, dysphagia, emesis, failure to thrive, gagging, globus pharyngeus, heartburn, hoarseness, recurrent croup, retractions, stridor, and throat clearing.

B Selected cooperative patients with little or no airway problem may undergo flexible laryngoscopy in the office. Erythema or edema of the posterior glottis or arytenoids, obliteration of the laryngeal ventricles, or vocal cord nodules may be associated with GERD.

C Mild problems associated with GERD include asthma, chronic cough, dysphagia, globus pharyngeus, hoarseness, posterior laryngitis, minimal stridor, throat clearing, and vocal cord nodules.

D Conservative measures include thickening of liquid nutrition; and avoidance of overeating and consumption of coffee, chocolate, high-fat and spicy foods; and elevation of the head of the bed. For Otolaryngologists without an extensive experience treating infants and children with GERD, a consultation with a Gastroenterologist should be considered.

E Moderate-to-severe problems that may be associated with GERD include apnea, cyanosis, failure to thrive, and airway problems (including laryngomalacia, tracheomalacia, or subglottic stenosis), even if GERD signs and symptoms are not obvious.

F It is useful for children who are undergoing flexible and direct laryngoscopy and rigid bronchoscopy for diagnosis of airway problems to undergo esophagoscopy and biopsy of the distal one-third of the esophagus, particularly if GERD is suspected. The advantages are speed and safety. A potential disadvantage is that reflux may affect the airway mucosa more than the esophageal mucosa that is more resistant to gastric juice and may yield a negative biopsy even with airway findings. Esophagoscopy and biopsy should not be performed in a child with a very tenuous airway to avoid edema and further airway obstruction. Combined endoscopic evaluation of airway and esophagus with Pediatric Gastroenterologist, Pediatric Otolaryngology, and Pediatric Pulmonology can be very helpful in the diagnosis and management of these patients.

G Barium swallow with upper gastrointestinal series is useful to rule out problems such as hiatal hernia, webs, achalasia, swallowing dysfunction, and intestinal malrotation, which may mimic GERD. Barium swallow may demonstrate GERD. However, if negative for GERD, it is possible that the patient still has GERD that was not seen during the study's narrow window of time.

H A radionuclide gastric scan will demonstrate acid and nonacid reflux, delayed gastric emptying, and reflux with aspiration and is generally well tolerated in children. The length of time of the scan is generally shorter than a 24-hour pH probe; thus, the sensitivity to detect GERD is lower.

I The 24-hour dual pH probe is considered the definitive study for the diagnosis of GERD. However, it will not demonstrate nonacid reflux, may not be readily available, and may not be well tolerated in children. The dual 24-hour pH probe with pH electrodes in the distal esophagus, proximal esophagus, or pharynx is better for demonstration of gastropharyngoesophageal (extraesophageal or laryngopharyngeal) reflux. A 24-hour pH probe may be performed simultaneously with a sleep study to detect GERD-induced apnea.

J Multichannel esophageal intraluminal impedance testing with pH monitoring is a very accurate way of diagnosing GERD, in particular the numbers of reflux events, and correlates well with endoscopic findings of reflux esophagitis.

K A consultation with a Gastroenterologist should be considered when it is necessary to start a proton pump inhibitor in an infant or child.

SUGGESTED READING

Cash H, Trosman S, Abelson T, et al. Chronic cough in children. JAMA Otolaryngol Head Neck Surg. 2015;141(5):417-423.

Gooi Z, Ishman SL, Bock JM, et al. Changing patterns in reflux care: 10-year comparison of ABEA members. Ann Otol Rhinol Laryngol. 2015;124(12):940-946.

Liu YW, Wu JF, Chen HL, et al. The correlation between endoscopic reflux esophagitis and combined multichannel intraluminal impedance-pH monitoring in children. Pediatr Neonatol. 2015; 23:183-187.

Venkatesan NN, Pine HS, Underbrink M. Laryngopharyngeal reflux disease in children. Pediatr Clin North Am. 2013;60(4):865-878.

Yellon RF, Goyal A. What is the best test for pediatric gastroesophageal reflux? Laryngoscope. 2013;123:2925-2927.

CHAPTER 108

Management of Caustic Ingestion in Children

Jeffrey P Simons, Cuneyt M Alper

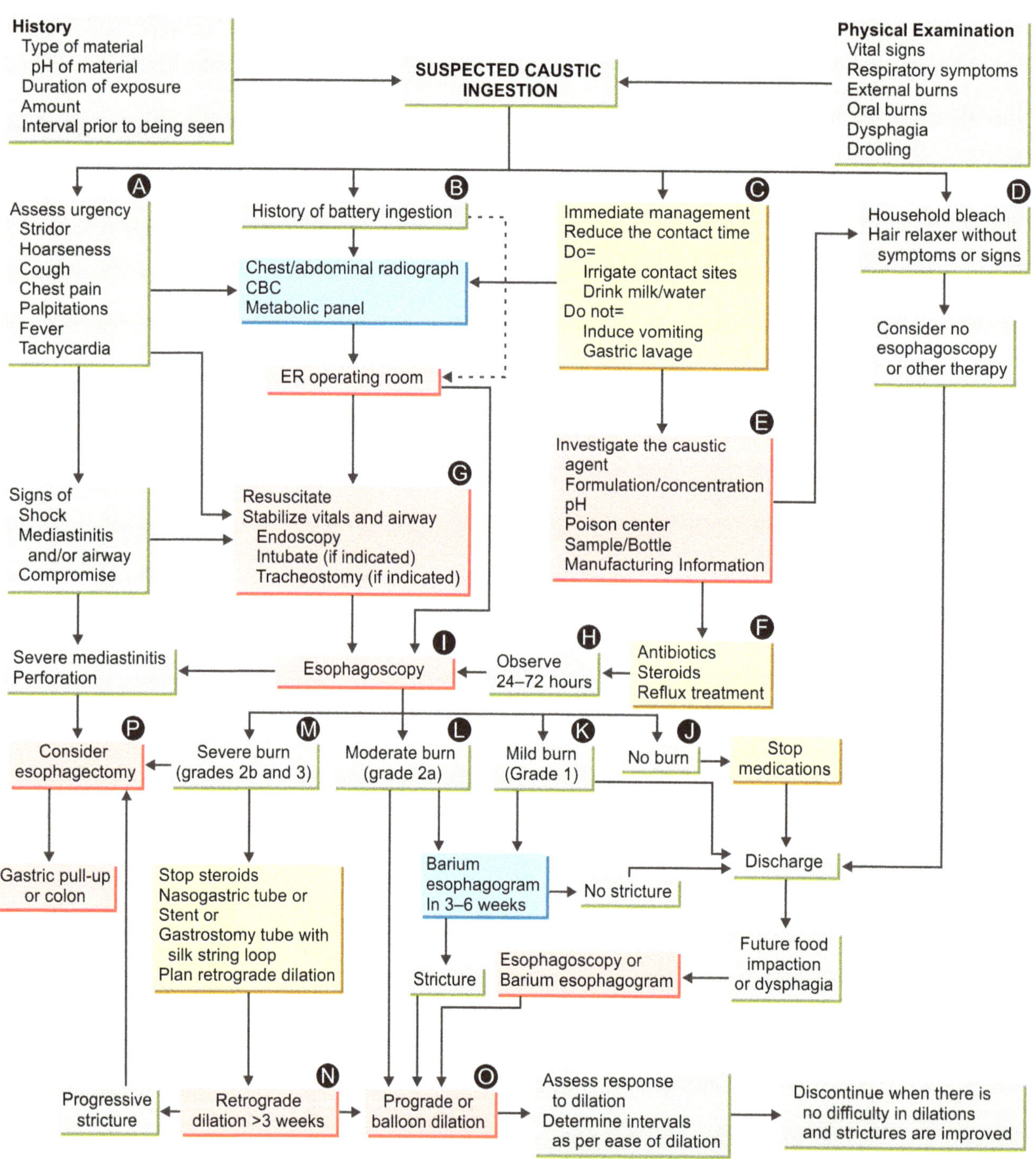

Caustic ingestions in children and their resultant esophageal injuries can cause significant morbidity and mortality. There are about 26,000 caustic injuries per year in the United States. Most cases of caustic ingestion occur in children under age 5, although adolescents attempting suicide form another group with this problem. Caustic injuries to the esophagus can result from ingestion of various products, including alkali substances, acidic substances, button batteries, and bleach. A systematic approach to the management of caustic ingestions in children can help to reduce morbidity and improve outcomes.

A A careful history and physical examination should be performed and the urgency of the situation should be assessed. It is important to look for stridor, hoarseness, cough, dysphagia, and fever. The child should be examined for burns on the lips, chin, face, hands, and chest and in the mouth. However, the presence of oral cavity or oropharyngeal burns is not a reliable index of esophageal damage. The upper airway and lungs should be auscultated. The chest and abdomen should be examined for signs of mediastinitis or peritonitis. Radiographs of the chest and abdomen are obtained. A complete blood count (CBC) and metabolic panel should also be obtained. It must be a priority to resuscitate the patient and stabilize the vital signs and the airway in those patients who have signs of shock, mediastinitis, peritonitis, or airway compromise.

B Button battery ingestions represent a true medical emergency. Mucosal injury can occur in <1 hour after impaction of the battery. An electrolytic current is created and hydroxide ions are generated at the battery's negative pole (anode), leading to significant caustic injury. Some batteries (nonlithium) can also contain concentrated sodium hydroxide or potassium hydroxide, which can leak out and contribute to caustic injury. Pressure necrosis at the site of the battery ingestion can also contribute to tissue damage. Larger batteries (e.g. 20 mm lithium ion battery) are less likely to pass into the stomach. Caustic injury from button batteries can result in severe mucosal injury, stricture formation, esophageal perforation, mediastinitis and death. Button batteries typically have a classic double contour or halo appearance on PA radiograph and a "step-off" on lateral view. Rapid removal of the foreign body is crucial. If the battery passes into the stomach, attempts at retrieval are typically not recommended unless the battery remains in the stomach for >2–4 days. Once a button battery is removed from the esophagus, management of the patient follows the same principles of other caustic ingestions.

C Initial steps after ingestion may impact the outcome. It is important to reduce the contact time of the concentrated caustic substance. Irrigating the contact sites and having the child drink water or milk can be considered. However, inducing vomiting and the use of gastric lavage can increase the degree of esophageal injury and should be avoided.

D Household bleach (hypochlorous acid, HClO) is usually available in a low concentration salt (5.25% sodium hypochlorite) and almost neutral pH. Household bleach (i.e. Chlorox) ingestion rarely results in esophageal injury and in the absence of signs or symptoms may not require esophagoscopy or other treatment. More concentrated formations of hypochlorous acid may cause esophageal injury and should be treated like other caustic ingestions. Hair relaxing agents are typically sold in nonchild-proof containers as an alkali cream with a pH of 11–13.

Despite their high pH, hair relaxer ingestions rarely result in significant esophageal injury; therefore, asymptomatic patients with a hair relaxer ingestion who can tolerate oral intake can likely be managed conservatively with clinical observation; esophagoscopy may not be necessary in this population.

E The specific substance should be determined by history if possible. An attempt should be made to estimate the amount ingested. However, even small amounts of ingested caustic substances can cause significant esophageal damage. It is helpful if parents/caregivers have the bottle or a sample of the substance. The nearest poison center can be contacted to help obtain information on the formulation, concentration, pH, and any other recommendations on the specific substance.

F Typically, antibiotics, corticosteroids, and reflux medication are given. Although there have been no prospective randomized clinical studies evaluating the benefits of antibiotics in caustic ingestion patients, the thought is that reducing the bacterial load in the burned tissue may decrease granulation tissue formation, improve healing, and help prevent stricture formation. The most common antibiotics used are ampicillin/sulbactam or amoxicillin/clavulanate. Acid exposure to the injured esophageal mucosa may also impair wound healing. Aggressive antireflux treatment with H_2-receptor blockers or proton pump inhibitors should be started as soon as possible and continued throughout the observation and treatment period. Steroids may help decrease stricture formation in patients with grade 2 esophageal injury. To be effective, steroids must be given within the first 8 hours of the injury. The equivalent of prednisone, 2 mg/kg per day to a maximum of 60 mg/day, is recommended to be given intravenously initially, then orally after a few days as the ability to swallow returns.

G Patients with signs of shock, mediastinitis, peritonitis, or airway compromise need to be managed in an intensive care unit setting. Vital signs should be monitored closely. Acute chemical laryngitis can lead to significant edema and airway obstruction. Mediastinitis secondary to esophageal perforation can lead to shock and hemodynamic instability. Emergent rigid endoscopy, intubation, and/or tracheostomy may be necessary to manage airway obstruction. Shock and metabolic acid-base disturbances are managed by standard critical care principles, including fluid resuscitation, electrolyte replacement, and correction of acid–base balance. In addition to potential surgical management of the airway, patients may also require other emergency surgery, such as laparotomy (if there is peritonitis or ruptured stomach with free air in the abdomen), esophagectomy (if there is severe transmural necrosis and mediastinitis), and/or possible gastrostomy tube placement. Involvement of a General Surgeon or a Cardiothoracic Surgeon early in the clinical course of these more unstable and severely injured patients is critical.

H Most physicians recommend performing an esophago-scopy 24–72 hours after the caustic ingestion. If esophago-scopy is performed within the first 24 hours, the full extent of injury may be underestimated. Esophagoscopy per-formed later than 72 hours after the event may result in unnecessary medical treatment and hospitalization if no significant burns of the esophagus are found. Esophago-scopy should ideally be avoided between 5 and 15 days after caustic ingestion to reduce the risk of perforation of the esophagus when it is most susceptible to injury.

I Direct visualization via esophagoscopy is the only accu-rate way to diagnose caustic esophageal injury. The grad-ing scale developed by Zargar et al. can be used to describe the degree of esophageal injury. Grade 0 is defined as a normal-appearing esophagus. Grade 1 lesions reveal mucosal edema and hyperemia. Grade 2a lesions have friable mucosa, hemorrhages, erosions, blisters, whitish membranes, exudates, and superficial ulcerations. When these grade 2a findings include deep or circumferen-tial ulceration they are called grade 2b. Grade 3a lesions include small areas of necrosis, whereas grade 3b lesions include extensive necrosis.

Esophagoscopy should be performed in all symp-tomatic children. Whether esophagoscopy should be performed in asymptomatic children is more controver-sial, but because it is possible for some children without obvious symptoms to have significant esophageal injury (grades 2 and 3), we recommend having a low threshold for performing esophagoscopy in these children as well.

J If no burn is seen on esophagoscopy (grade 0), medica-tions are discontinued and the child can be discharged. If any symptoms of dysphagia develop, an esophagram can be considered.

K Patients with mild esophageal injury (grade 1) can remain on antireflux therapy for 3–6 weeks and possibly a course of antibiotics. The patient can be seen back in the clinic in 3–6 weeks and consideration can be given to obtaining an esophagram at that point, particularly if the patient has any symptoms of dysphagia or difficulty feeding. If the patient is asymptomatic, the decision to obtain a follow-up esophagram in this group with grade 1 injury is more controversial and the esophagram may be unnecessary. If there is evidence of stricture formation on esopha-gram, the patient can proceed to a dilation protocol. If the esophagram is normal or the patient is asymptomatic and the decision is made not to obtain an esophagram, the antireflux medication can be discontinued and the patient can be discharged from the Otolaryngologist's care, with follow-up on an as needed basis.

L Patients with moderate esophageal injury (grade 2a) should remain on antireflux therapy, antibiotics, and ste-roids. The steroids can be tapered after 2–3 weeks, so that the total time on the steroids including the taper is 3–4 weeks. This group of patients should be seen back in clinic with a repeat esophagram 3–6 weeks after the injury. If there is evidence of stricture formation on esophagram,

the patient can proceed to a dilation protocol. If the esophagram is normal, without evidence of stricture for-mation, antibiotics can be discontinued. The antireflux medication may be continued for several months. The patients should be seen every 3 months for 1 year and may have one more repeat esophagram 3–6 months after the injury. If the patient remains asymptomatic after 1 year and the esophagram has been normal, the patient can then be discharged from the otolaryngologist's care, with follow-up on an as needed basis.

M Patients with severe esophageal injury (grades 2b and 3) will have the steroids discontinued, as to continue ste-roids in this group has little benefit and may increase the risk of esophageal perforation. Antibiotics and antireflux medications are continued. There is a significant risk of stricture formation in patients with severe burns. A nasogastric tube or stent can be attempted to be placed beyond the area of the esophageal burn under endo-scopic guidance to help prevent stricture formation and to facilitate dilation. In many severe burns, esophageal rest is important to promote healing and a gastrostomy or gastrojejunostomy tube can be placed. A string loop can be placed from the nose/mouth through the esophagus using the gastrostomy site in order to facilitate retrograde dilation. Repeat esophagoscopy procedures will be neces-sary to assess the progress of healing response to dilation procedures. Retrograde dilation can be started after 3–6 weeks, after the first esophagram, once the gastro-stomy stoma is mature and there is less risk of esophageal perforation.

N The technique of retrograde dilation with Tucker dilators using a gastrostomy tube site and string loop allows for a greater degree of safety and decreased risk of esophageal perforation for dilation of severe strictures in comparison to prograde or balloon dilation. The dilation procedures can be performed once or twice a week at first and then less frequently as it becomes easier to reach the target size. Once the interval can be spread to every 2 weeks and the stricture becomes less severe, it may be possible to progress to prograde dilation, either with balloon dilation or esophageal bougies.

O Prograde balloon dilatation is the procedure of choice for the management of most esophageal strictures in chil-dren. The advantage of using this form of dilatation is that the catheter can be passed through a narrow stricture, and the balloon, when inflated, dilates in a radial direc-tion. Balloon dilation is optimal for shorter strictures as opposed to longer-segment strictures. The procedure can be done under direct endoscopic visualization. Hurst or Maloney dilators can also be used for prograde dilation. Several dilatations may be necessary, depending on the return of symptoms of obstruction and the length and density of the stricture. The intervals between dilation procedures can be determined by the return of symptoms and the ease of dilation. It is important to note that there is a risk of esophageal perforation from all esophageal dilation techniques.

Esophagectomy with reconstruction can be considered in two situations in the management of caustic ingestions. (1) Acutely, when there is a severely perforated esophagus with mediastinitis, an immediate esophagectomy is sometimes recommended, leaving the patient with a cervical esophagostomy and a gastrostomy. In these cases, reconstruction with a gastric pull-up or colonic interposition would be reserved for a later date once the patient has stabilized and the infection has resolved. (2) For chronic esophageal strictures, if repeated dilatation fails, esophagectomy with esophageal replacement may be the alternative. In most cases, every effort should be made to maintain esophageal function for as long as possible. Reconstruction can be performed with gastic pull-up or colonic interposition. There is a significantly increased risk of developing esophageal carcinoma after severe esophageal burns (1,000-fold increased risk) and

long-term follow-up and surveillance is necessary. Therefore, in some cases, esophagectomy with reconstruction may be a reasonable alternative to long-term stricture dilation.

SUGGESTED READING

Colman KL, Simons JP, Alper CM. Caustic injuries and acquired strictures of the esophagus. In: Bluestone CD, Simons JP, Healy GB (Eds). Bluestone and Stool's Pediatric Otolaryngology, 5th edition. Shelton, CT: PMPH-USA; 2014. pp. 1365-1380.

Contini S, Scarpignato C. Caustic injury of the upper gastrointestinal tract: a comprehensive review. World J Gastroenterol. 2013;19(25):3918-3930.

Zargar SA, Kochhar R, Mehta S, et al. The role of fiberoptic endoscopy in the management of corrosive ingestion and modified endoscopic classification of burns. Gastrointest Endosc. 1991;37:165-169.

Hematemesis

Andrew J Hotaling, Zachary C Fridirici

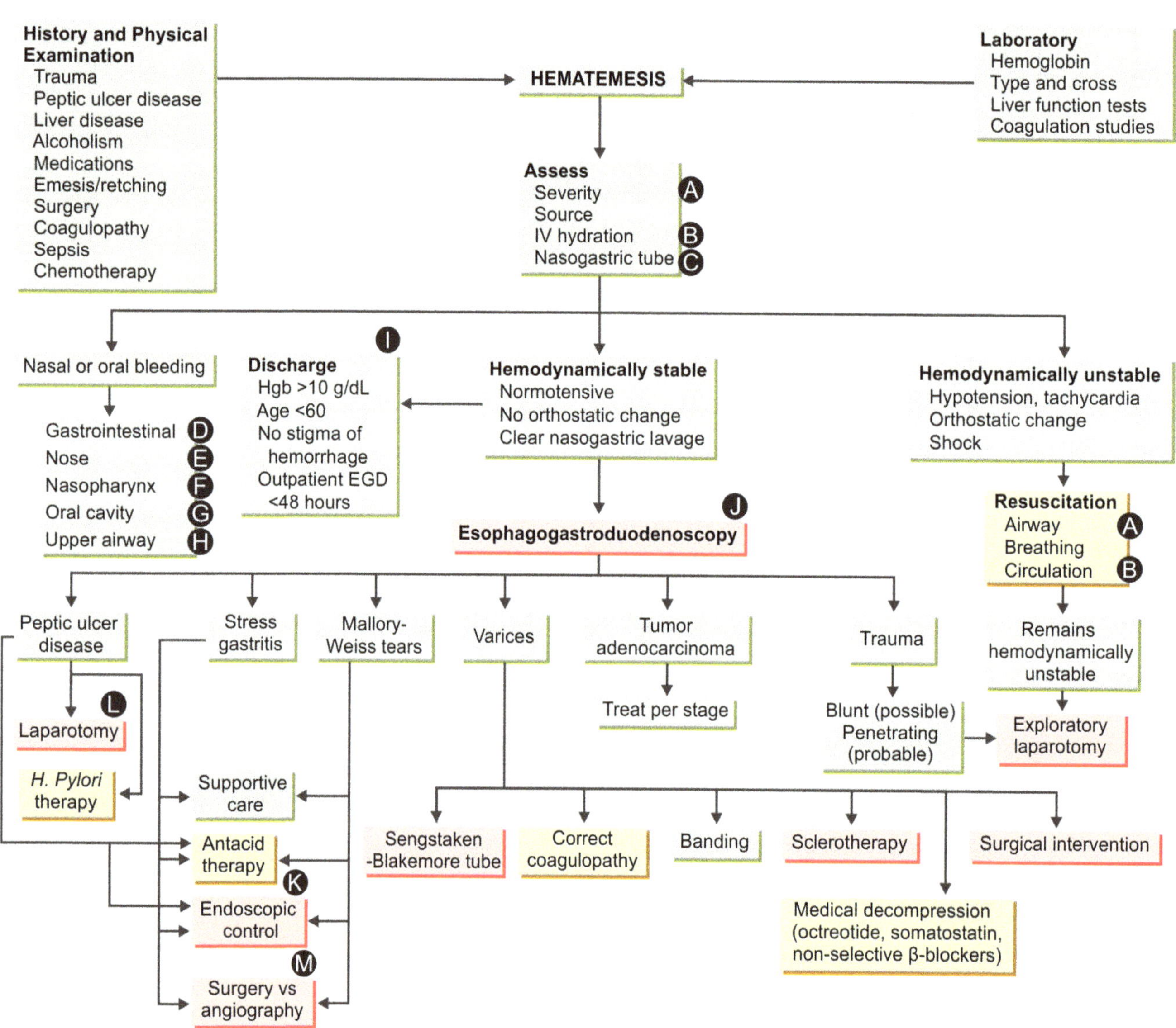

Otolaryngologists are commonly consulted when patients vomit blood. Hematemesis is a potentially life-threatening emergency with an overall mortality of 6–10%. The initial diagnosis, evaluation and treatment are critical. Otolaryngologists offer upper aerodigestive tract expertise, the ability to perform bedside nasopharyngoscopy, and intervention when appropriate.

A The amount of bleeding should be ascertained. If the patient has significant bleeding, the ABCs of resuscitation (*a*irway, *b*reathing, *c*irculation) should be initiated. Most critically, the airway must be controlled and protected. Once the airway is secure, attention is directed to making sure that breathing is satisfactory. The circulatory volume must be maintained to ensure that perfusion is adequate.

B Crystalloid fluid resuscitation, if needed, is initiated via two large bore intravenous (IVs) lines or a central line. Blood transfusion, if needed, should be administered.

C The bleeding must be further localized within the upper digestive tract. The history and physical examination will direct treatment to the appropriate area. Frequently, flexible nasopharyngoscopy and nasogastric tube placement with suctioning are required to ascertain the level of bleeding within the upper aerodigestive tract.

D Peptic ulcer and liver disease account for 50–80% of hematemesis. Specific medications such as aspirin and nonsteroidal anti-inflammatory drugs can cause stress ulcers that present with hematemesis or significantly increase the risk of hematemesis, if another underlying disease process is present. Recent severe vomiting or retching is indicative of Mallory-Weiss tears. In addition, trauma, sepsis, malignancy, and recent gastric surgery may cause hematemesis.

E Bleeding from the nose could be from a site in the nose or nasopharynx. A history of recurrent anterior or posterior epistaxis, recent sinus surgery, or recent adenoidectomy may suggest the cause. There are many methods and materials utilized to control epistaxis. If needed, we recommend Afrin soaked Gelfoam, Surgicel, and/or merocels covered in bacitracin.

F Most commonly, bleeding from the nasopharynx suggests recent adenoidectomy, sinus surgery, or a tumor such as a juvenile nasoangiofibroma.

G Frequently, the cause will be a recent tonsillectomy. In addition, pharyngeal tumors or foreign bodies can present with oral bleeding.

H Common causes of nonmassive hemoptysis include bronchitis, bronchiectasis, malignancy, cystic fibrosis, foreign body, pulmonary hemosiderosis, and tuberculosis.

I Patients can be risk stratified using the Rockall or Blatchford score. If the patient is competent, reliable, younger than 60 years, hemodynamically stable, has a hemoglobin level > 10 g/dL, no stigmata of hemorrhage, and no comorbidities, they may be discharged after a period of observation.

J Esophagogastroduodenoscopy is diagnostic and therapeutic. Inpatients should have it performed within 24 hours and outpatients within 48 hours.

K Endoscopic control of bleeding can be performed using injection, heat energy, or mechanical devices.

L If peptic ulcer disease is significant and endoscopic control is inadequate, a laparotomy is indicated. Depending on the site of bleeding and the patient's surgical risk, procedures include pyloroplasty, partial gastrectomy, oversewing the bleeder, and vagotomy [largely replaced by proton pump inhibitor (PPI) therapy].

M If endoscopic control of bleeding is inadequate for stress gastritis or Mallory-Weiss tear, angiography can be considered with arterial embolization. If angiography does not control bleeding, partial gastrectomy or oversewing the bleeder is indicated.

SUGGESTED READING

Clark M, Bunting D, Smart N. The surgical management of acute upper gastrointestinal bleeding: a 12-year experience. Int J Surg. 2010;8:377-380.

Conlong PJ. Practical advice on treating hematemesis. Hosp Med. 2002;59:851-855.

Katchinkski B, Logan R, Davies J, et al. Prognostic factors in upper gastrointestinal bleeding. Dig Dis Sci. 1994;39:706-712.

Kim J, Sheibani S, Park S. Causes of bleeding and outcomes in patients hospitalized with upper gastrointestinal bleeding. J Clin Gastroenterol. 2014;48:113-118.

Norton LW, Steele G Jr, Eiseman B (Eds). Upper gastrointestinal bleeding. In: Surgical Decision Making, 3rd edition. Philadelphia, PA: WB Saunders; 1993. p. 116.

Palmer K. Management of haematemesis and melaena. Postgrad Med J. 2004;80:399-404.

Poultsides G, Kim C, Rocco O. Angiographic embolization for gastroduodenal hemorrhage. Arch Surg. 2008;143:457-461.

Stanley, A. Update on risk scoring systems for patients with upper gastrointestinal hemorrhage. World J Gastroenterol. 2012;18:2739-2744.

Wrenn KD, Thompson LD. Hemodynamically stable upper GI bleeding. AM J Emerg Med. 1991;9:309-312.

SECTION

4

Larynx, Trachea and Bronchi

Hoarseness and Dysphonia

Shaum S Sridharan, Clark A Rosen

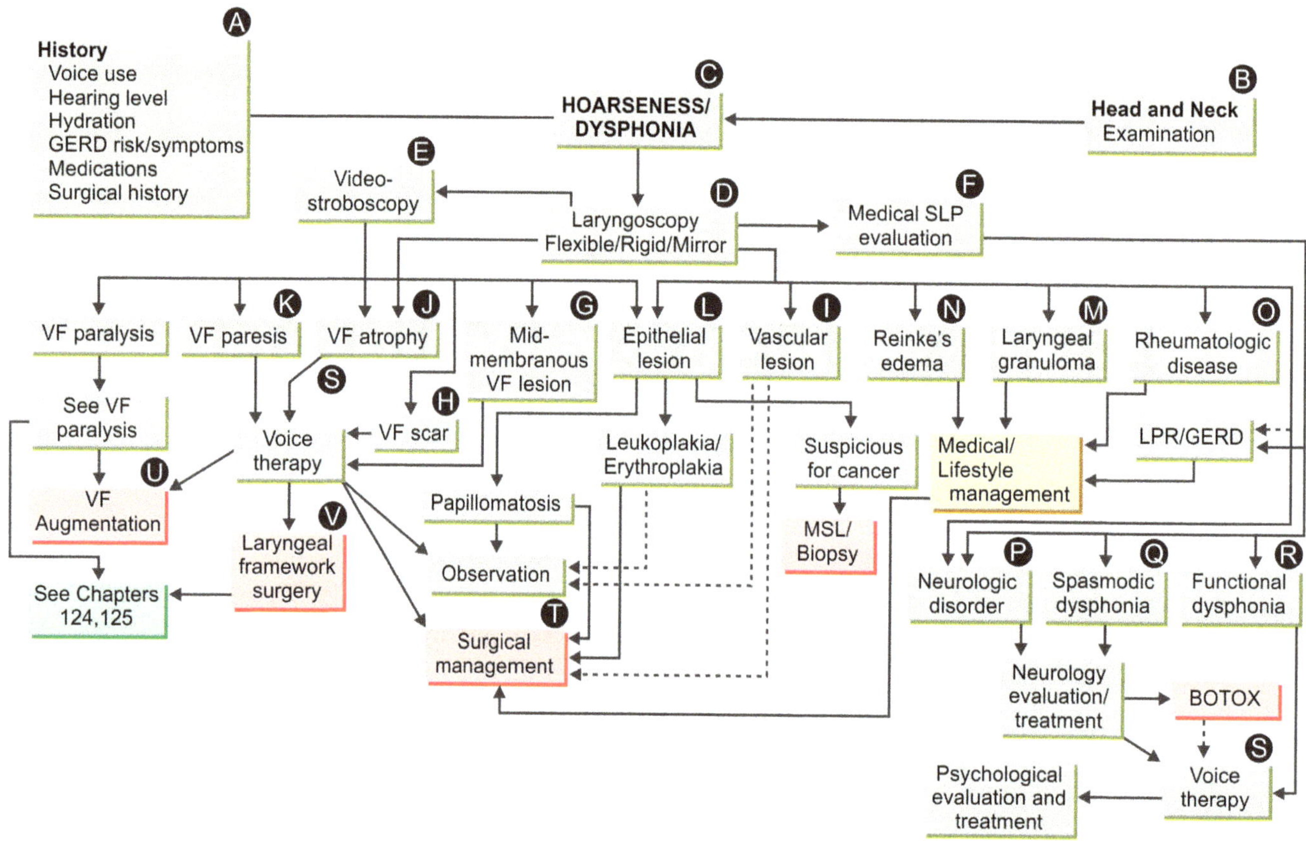

Hoarseness (dysphonia) is a one of the more common complaints of patients seeking medical treatment by otolaryngologists. Dysphonia can be acute such as after an acute upper respiratory tract infection and can be self-limited. For those who have persistent hoarseness, a thorough head and neck examination is warranted. The evaluation and treatment algorithm for hoarseness will be discussed in this chapter.

A A history of dysphonia should include inquiries regarding onset and duration of the hoarseness, specifically a medical and personal history of voice problems and singing limitations resulting from the hoarseness. Often, a standardized, patient-based self-perception outcome measure such as the Voice Handicap Index-10 (VHI-10) is helpful to assess the patient's perception of the severity of the voice disorder.

B A complete examination of the head and neck is mandatory for all patients who present with hoarseness. This includes a thorough otologic and rhinologic examination as well as an examination of the mucosa of the upper airway and digestive tract.

C Dysphonia is defined by an abnormal voice quality. Hoarseness is a poorly defined term used by the patient that must be further elaborated on by the clinician. Common complaints that fall into the category of hoarseness include loss of volume, lack of pitch range, globus sensation, vocal fatigue, and intermittent loss of the voice.

D Examination of the larynx is paramount for the evaluation of dysphonia. This can be done by indirect mirror laryngoscopy, indirect rigid laryngoscopy, or transnasal flexible laryngoscopy. The latter is of utmost importance for disorders related to function of the larynx and is the method that allows examination of the larynx in the most natural, in vivo setting.

E Laryngovideostroboscopy allows for high-quality, detailed imaging of vocal fold (VF) vibration during sustained phonation. This examination can be done via the rigid or flexible laryngoscope. This examination gives information regarding glottal closure pattern, lamina propria disease, VF bulk, and mucosal wave activity. Stroboscopic evaluation is an essential diagnostic tool without which many voice disorders cannot be assessed properly.

F Medical speech evaluation is often a crucial component in the evaluation of dysphonia, particularly when an obvious lesion cannot be identified on laryngoscopy and stroboscopy. This examination is performed by a speech-language pathologist (SLP) experienced in the evaluation and care of voice disorders. It typically includes both perceptual and objective (instrumental) assessment of the patient's speech and voice production. In addition, SLPs may perform "stimulability" testing to clarify if a patient is a suitable candidate for voice therapy.

G Benign midmembranous VF lesions are caused by repeated trauma to the VF causing injury to the underlying lamina propria. The membranous VF refers to the anterior two-thirds of the VFs from the anterior commissure to the vocal process. Lesions present most often at the midway point of the membranous VFs. A nomenclature paradigm was introduced in the hopes of standardizing lesion terminology that would improve patient counseling, facilitate VF treatment, and research. This classification scheme defines nine distinct benign mid-VF lesions: (a) VF nodules; (b) VF polyp; (c) VF cyst-sub epithelial; (d) VF cyst-ligament; (e) fibrous mass-sub epithelial; (f) fibrous mass-ligament; (g) reactive VF lesion; (h) nonspecific VF lesion and (i) pseudocyst. Differentiating these lesions and planning therapy usually requires stroboscopy. In brief, these lesions are benign and initially treated with voice therapy. If the lesions do not respond to voice therapy and the patient's symptoms are persistent, they may need phonomicrosurgical intervention.

H Vocal fold scar and sulcus vocalis (acquired) are thought to occur due to repeated injury to the VF possibly combined with repeated vocal hemorrhage. Theoretically, both VF scar and sulcus vocalis involve this detrimental cyclic wound-healing, but differ in the ultimate fate of the lamina propria. Vocal fold scar represents the replacement of the lamina propria layer with fibrous tissue that will maintain or slightly enlarge this space. Sulcus vocalis, on the other hand, represents loss of a portion of the lamina propria and leaves vocal epithelium directly adherent to the vocal ligament, thereby reducing the overall bulk of the VF and negatively impacting the vibratory characteristics. Both VF scar and sulcus vocalis will cause vibratory changes, but sulcus will also likely result in glottal insufficiency. Stroboscopy is required for evaluation of the effect on the mucosal wave. Treatment modalities include voice therapy, phonomicrosurgery surgery, or correction of the glottic gap.

I Vascular lesions of the VF arise from blood vessels encountered in the subepithelial layer of the VF. Normally, the vessels run parallel to the longitudinal axis of the VF. In contrast, anomalous vascular lesions will often run in a transverse nature perpendicular to the VF. These lesions can be visually subdivided into ectasia, telangiectasia, or varix. Varices are characterized as enlarged veins or tortuous vessels, while ectasias have the appear on a coalescent hemangiomas. Telangiectasias can resemble a fine network of blood vessels. They can be stand alone or associated with benign or malignant lesions of the VF. Most lesions are self-limiting but on occasion they can cause mucosal vibratory changes, visible on stroboscopy. On occasion, with trauma, these lesions may be sheared open and cause VF hemorrhage. Surgical management of these lesions is only necessary when the patient has a documented history of VF hemorrhage or the lesion is causing voice disturbances.

J Vocal fold atrophy represents primarily a loss of muscle bulk of the VF. This is often associated with advanced age but also can be found after VF paralysis or paresis. It is most easily diagnosed by noting a drop-off at the junction of the membranous VF and vocal process and glottal incompetence. This condition is treated with voice therapy unless it is quite severe or unresponsive to voice therapy, in which case it is treated with VF augmentation (lipoinjection) or medialization laryngoplasty.

K Vocal fold paresis represents a VF with purposeful, gross motion, but it not normal in terms of motion, range of motion, and/or speed. Paresis is caused by injury to the central or peripheral nervous system responsible for innervation of the VF(s). Neurogenic injury can be associated with iatrogenic injury, mass effect/invasion by tumor, or idiopathic causes. The diagnosis can be confirmed with laryngeal electromyography if the cause of injury is not obviated by history, clinical examination, or radiologic studies. Treatment initially most often involves voice therapy with VF augmentation reserved for refractory dysphonia. Vocal fold paralysis represents a VF with no purposeful motion. *See* Chapters 124 and 125.

L Lesions arising from the epithelium of the VFs typically are keratosis, malignancy, or papillomatosis. Concern for malignancy warrants direct laryngoscopy with biopsy. Treatment for keratosis and recurrent respiratory papillomatosis is often surgical especially in cases where patients have significant symptoms (i.e. dysphonia and dyspnea) or when there are concerns for malignant degeneration.

M Granulomas of the larynx usually arise as a result of trauma to the vocal process of the arytenoid cartilage causing a local inflammation reaction, namely perichondritis of the arytenoid cartilage. Lesions can be associated with ulcerations and/or exophytic masses that arise from the vocal process of the arytenoid cartilage. Granulomas can be further subdivided as intubation-related versus nonintubation-related masses. Nonintubation-related vocal process granulomas are more difficult to successfully treat and are associated with laryngopharyngeal reflux and voice abuse. Though most lesions, regardless of etiology, will resolve with conservative management, some will require surgical management. Granulomas can also occur at an operative site of the membranous VF but are less common and conservative treatment is usually successful.

N Reinke's edema is a diffuse accumulation of submucosal, gelatinous material in the superficial layer of the lamina propria, usually associated with tobacco abuse, vocal abuse, and laryngopharyngeal reflux disease (LPRD) or gastroesophageal reflux disease (GERD). Unless impending airway limitation is present, the treatment should be reduction or elimination of the causative factors followed by phonomicrosurgery on an as-needed basis.

O Rheumatologic diseases have many manifestations in the head and neck, with some causing laryngeal pathology. Thorough history taking can focus the differential diagnosis when treating a patient with laryngeal complaints while minimizing unnecessary surgical and medical treatments. Rheumatologic disease can create laryngeal pathology such as cricoarytenoid joint arthritis or VF lesions. Conditions such as Wegener's granulomatosis, sarcoidosis, amyloidosis, and rheumatoid arthritis can often involve the larynx. Collaboration with the patient's rheumatologist is essential to provide optimal care for these conditions. Surgical therapy should only be considered after the patient has been maximally treated for the rheumatologic condition.

P A variety of neurologic diseases can cause hoarseness and can be identified on laryngeal examination with or without a medical speech and language pathology evaluation. The most common neurologic diseases include Parkinson's disease, amyotrophic lateral sclerosis, essential tremor, and myasthenia gravis. Suspicion of a neurologic cause of dysphonia warrants a neurology consultation. Often the associated hoarseness can be successfully treated with voice therapy.

Q Spasmodic dysphonia represents a focal dystonia which involves the laryngeal musculature triggered with phonation. Spasmodic dysphonia is most common of the adductor nature when the voice is characterized as strained or strangled. Spasmodic dysphonia may involve the posterior cricoarytenoid muscles, abductor spasmodic dysphonia, which is characterized by a weak, breathy dysphonia during connected speech. Botulinum toxin (Botox) injection to the affected muscles is the primary treatment for both types of spasmodic dysphonia.

R Functional dysphonia/aphonia, also termed muscle tension dysphonia/aphonia, is an inappropriate coordination of the respiratory and laryngeal apparatus to produce normal phonation. The condition can have a variety of etiologies including post-upper respiratory infection, LPRD, postenvironmental exposure, idiopathic and stress reactivity.

This can also be associated with a conversion disorder or underlying psychopathology. When there is a mental health disturbance associated with the voice disorder, treatment involves voice therapy and psychological evaluation and treatment.

S Voice therapy is a specialized form of speech therapy that involves the behavioral management and modification of voice use and production. This is optimally performed by an SLP with specialized training and an interest in the evaluation and care of voice disorders. A variety of methods of voice therapy are used depending on the nature of the dysphonia, patient factors, and the experience of the voice therapist. Voice therapy typically involves 6–8 sessions as sole or combined treatment for dysphonia. Voice therapy is rarely warranted on a "chronic" basis and rarely go past 3 months of duration.

Singing voice therapy is a specialized form of vocal rehabilitation designed to restore and maximize singing voice function after an injury or phonomicrosurgery. This treatment is usually performed by a voice teacher with a voice disorders background/training or SLP with vocal pedagogy knowledge. This type of treatment does not have to be limited to use for singers only.

T Surgical Management involves direct treatment of the VF either in the operating room or office. Surgical procedures in the operating room can involve phonomicrosurgery, laser treatment, or a combination of both. Phonomicrosurgery is specialized, elective microsurgery of the larynx for benign lesions of the VFs, such as a VF polyp or cyst and usually performed by voice specialists with special equipment.

U Vocal fold augmentation can be performed with various injection materials that have different properties. Injection procedures can be performed in the office setting or in the operating room based on surgeon preference, patient tolerance, and injection material (i.e. adipose tissue injection cannot be done in the office). The aim of VF augmentation, regardless of underlying pathology, is to decrease the glottal gap. Autologous injection of adipose tissue can be an attractive and reliable choice for long-term augmentation.

V The most common laryngeal framework surgery is medialization laryngoplasty (thyroplasty). This procedure involves the placement of an implant (Gortex or silastic) in the paraglottic space in order to medialize the VF(s). In addition to thyroplasty, other surgeries for the treatment of unilateral VF paralysis include arytenoid adduction and cricothyroid subluxation.

See Chapter 124.

SUGGESTED READING

Akbulut S, Gartner-Schmidt JL, Gillespie AI, et al. Voice outcomes following treatment of benign midmembranous vocal fold lesions using a nomenclature paradigm. Laryngoscope. 2016;126(2):415-420.

Hochman I, Sataloff RT, Hillman RE, et al. Ectasias and varices of the vocal fold: clearing the striking zone. Ann Otol Rhinol Laryngol. 1999;108:10-16.

Loehrl TA, Smith TL. Inflammatory and granulomatous lesions of the larynx and pharynx. Am J Med. 2001;111(Suppl 8A):113S-7S.

Rosen CA, Gartner-Schmidt J, Hathaway B, et al. A nomenclature paradigm for benign midmembranous vocal fold lesions. Laryngoscope. 2012;122:1335-1341.

Rosen CA, Johnson JT. Chapter 70: Neurologic disorders of the larynx. In: Johnson JT, Rosen CA (Eds). Bailey's head and neck surgery—Otolaryngology, Vol. 1, 5th edition. Wolters Kluwer; 2014. pp. 1026-1047.

Rosen CA, Johnson JT. Chapter 71: Voice therapy for the treatment of voice disorders. In: Johnson JT, Rosen CA (Eds). Bailey's head and neck surgery—Otolaryngology, Vol. 1, 5th edition. Wolters Kluwer; 2014. pp. 1048-1058.

Rosen CA, Johnson JT. Chapter 72: Treatment of the professional voice. In: Johnson JT, Rosen CA (Eds). Bailey's head and neck surgery—Otolaryngology, Vol. 1, 5th edition. Wolters Kluwer; 2014. pp. 1059-1077.

Rosen CA, Mau T, Remacle M, et al. Nomenclature proposal to describe vocal fold motion impairment. Eur Arch Otorhinolaryngol. 2016;273(8):1995-1999.

Ylitalo R, Hammarberg B. Voice characteristics, effects of voice therapy, and long-term follow-up of contact granuloma patients. J Voice. 2000;14:557-566.

Ylitalo R, Ramel S. Extraesophageal reflux in patients with contact granuloma: a prospective controlled study. Ann Otol Rhinol Laryngol. 2002;111:441-446.

Dyspnea

Shannon Fraser

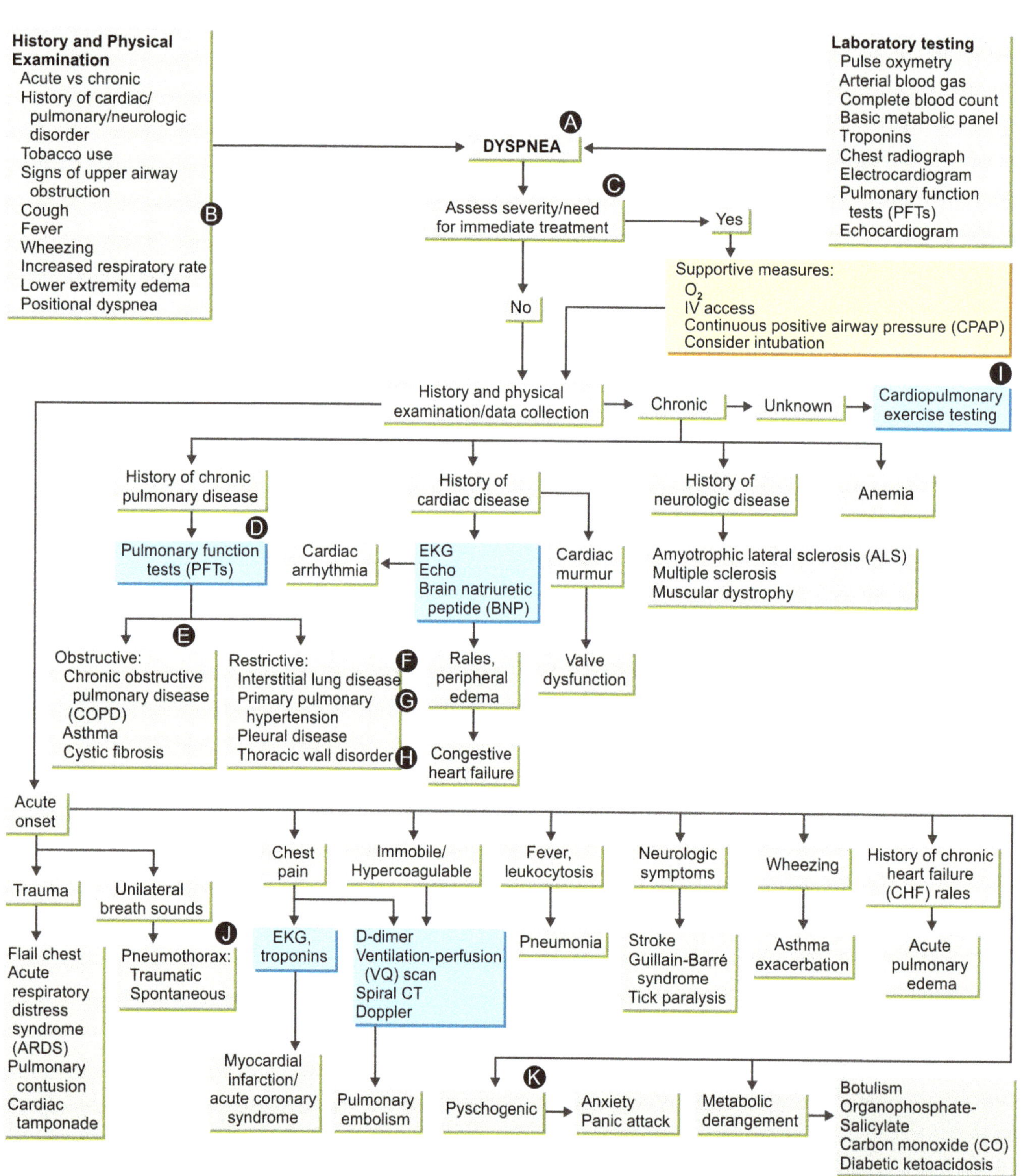

Dyspnea, or shortness of breath, is one of the most common reasons that individuals seek medical attention. The evaluation and management of dyspnea can be quite complex due to the potential contributions and interaction of pulmonary, cardiac, neurologic, and otolaryngologic pathologies. Efficient diagnosis and treatment is essential, particularly in acute and rapidly progressing dyspnea, which can quickly evolve into a life-threatening situation.

Ⓐ Dyspnea is a subjective complaint of breathlessness or shortness of breath. It is usually best evaluated and managed in conjunction with the patient's primary care physician, pulmonologist, and/or cardiologist.

Ⓑ For acute upper airway obstruction and neonatal respiratory distress, *see* chapters 113 to 116.

Ⓒ Accurate assessment of the patient's clinical status is essential. Signs and symptoms of severe dyspnea requiring immediate treatment include cyanosis, tachypnea, tachycardia, increased respiratory effort, altered mental status, and worsening hypoxemia as measured by pulse oximetry or arterial blood gas. Patients in severe distress may require immediate intervention including intubation and mechanical ventilation prior to performing diagnostic workup.

Ⓓ Pulmonary function testing should include forced expiratory volume in 1 second (FEV_1), forced vital capacity (FVC), total lung capacity, flow volume loops, maximum minute ventilation, determination of forced expiratory flow after 50% of vital capacity has been expelled, and forced inspiratory flow at 50% of vital capacity.

Ⓔ A reduced FEV_1 or a ratio of FEF_1/FVC of <70% indicates obstructive disease. In asthma, FEV_1/FVC may be <50%.

Ⓕ Restrictive lung diseases are characterized by a decrease in total lung capacity (reduced FVC). The FEV_1/FVC ratio may be normal or increased.

Ⓖ Chronic interstitial diseases can include chronic pneumoconiosis from inhalational injury, damage from radiation therapy, systemic diseases (e.g. sarcoidosis, amyloidosis, and scleroderma). Medication-induced pulmonary fibrosis is a known side effect of bleomycin, amiodarone, nitrofurantoin, and methotrexate among others.

Ⓗ Thoracic wall diseases include kyphoscoliosis, obesity, and increased abdominal pressure (e.g. ascites and pregnancy).

Ⓘ Cardiopulmonary testing should be performed when the cause of dyspnea (especially when exertional) is unclear and when pulmonary as well as cardiac disease may be present.

Ⓙ Tension pneumothorax should be suspected in trauma patients who present with unstable hemodynamic status. Tension pneumothorax requires emergency decompression of the pleural space with a chest-tube or a large bore needle.

Ⓚ Psychogenic dyspnea is a diagnosis of exclusion. It is essential to rule out organic causes of dyspnea in all patients.

SUGGESTED READING

Braithwaite SA, Perina D Dyspnea. In: Marx JA, Hockberger RS, Walls RM, et al, (Eds) Rosen's Emergency Medicine: Concepts and Clinical Practice. 8th ed. Philadelphia, PA: Elsevier Saunders; 2014: chap 25.

Morgan WC, Hodge HL. Diagnostic evaluation of dyspnea. Am Fam Physician. 1998;57(4):711-716.

Pratter MR, Abouzgheib W, Akers S, et al. An algorithmic approach to chronic dyspnea. Respir Med. 2011;105:1014-1021.

Wahls SA. Causes and evaluation of chronic dyspnea. Am Fam Physician. 2012;86(2):173-180.

Zoorob RJ, Campbell JS. Acute dyspnea in the office. Am Fam Physician. 2003;68(9):1803-1810.

Prenatal Suspicion of Airway Obstruction

David L Mandell

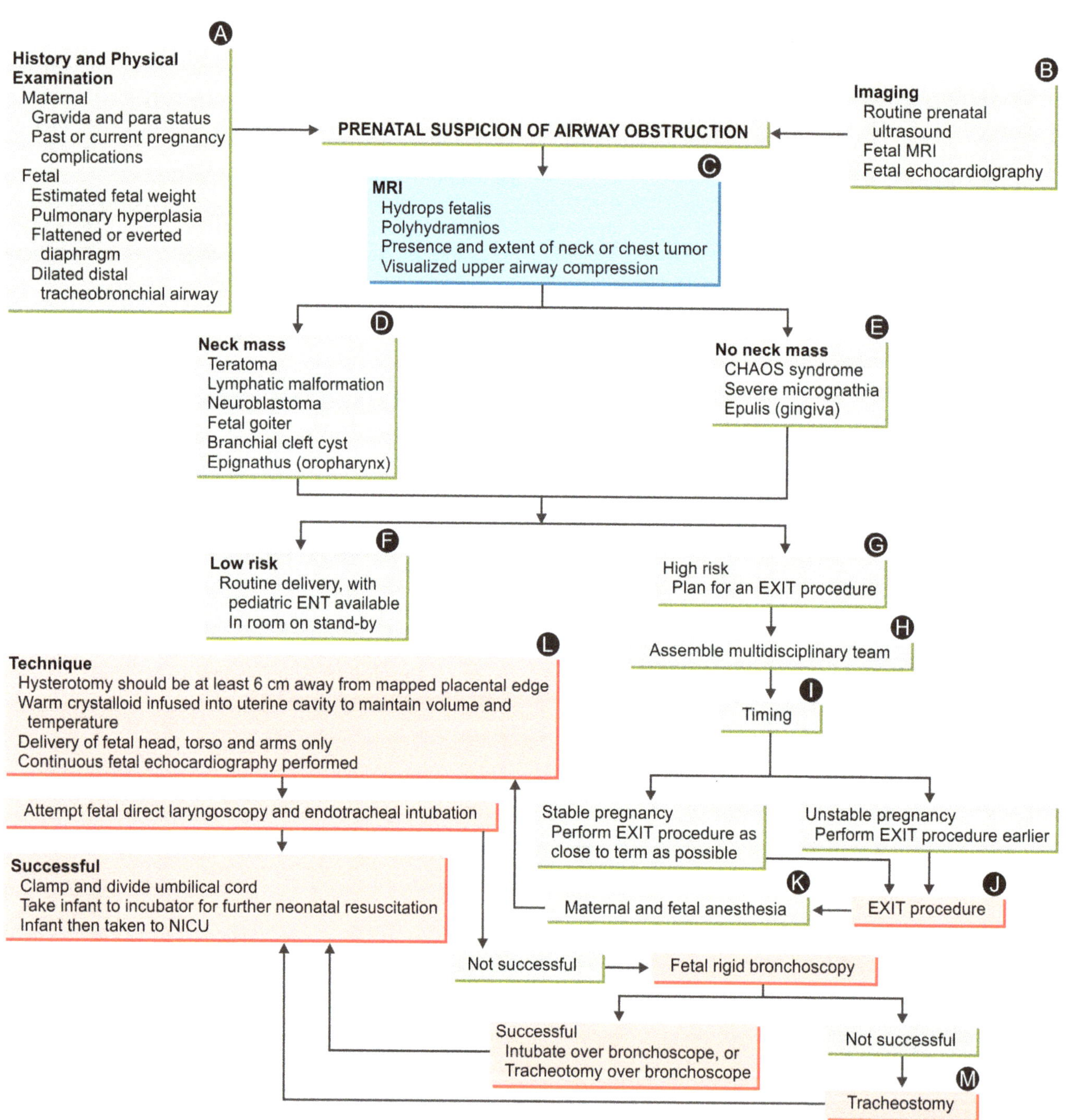

If prenatal imaging demonstrates fetal upper airway obstruction that will not be compatible with infant life after delivery, an ex utero intrapartum treatment (EXIT) procedure can be planned to improve fetal outcomes. At the time of delivery, uteroplacental gas exchange is maintained while the fetus is partially delivered, allowing time to establish the fetal airway, only after which the umbilical cord can be clamped. Maintenance of uteroplacental support requires cesarean (C) section with inhibition of uterine contractility and can be sustained for approximately 60 minutes before placental separation occurs.

A Fetal ultrasound is often operformed routinely between weeks 18 and 20 of gestation as a screening test for structural fetal anomalies. Sonographic findings suspicious for fetal airway obstruction include bilateral expanded lungs, flattened or everted diaphragms, and/or a dilated tracheobronchial airway. Fetal lungs produce amniotic fluid. Upper airway obstruction prevents the natural egress of this fluid, leading to distention of the tracheobronchial tree and lungs; this distension is often indirectly the first sign of fetal upper airway obstruction.

B Unrelated to upper airway obstruction, there are other cardiopulmonary conditions seen on fetal imaging that could lead to respiratory/ventilatory crisis after delivery include pulmonary agenesis, pleural effusion, congenital diaphragmatic hernia, aortic stenosis, and hypoplastic left heart syndrome. EXIT procedure may be planned with placement of ECMO catheters while the fetus is still on placental support.

C More detailed imaging is subsequently obtained with fetal magnetic resonance imaging (MRI) which can show signs of upper airway obstruction such as hydrops fetalis and polyhydramnios, and more direct findings such as neck or chest tumor causing airway compression. Hydrops occurs when upper airway obstruction prevents egress of amniotic fluid from the lungs, leading to a distended respiratory tree which then directly compresses the vena cava, leading to venous congestion and accumulation of excess fluid in multiple body compartments.

D Neck masses that can lead to fetal airway obstruction include teratoma and lymphatic malformation (these are the most common), followed by neuroblastoma, goiter, branchial cleft cyst, and epignathus (a rare form of teratoma arising from the oropharynx).

E Anomalies other than a neck mass that can lead to fetal upper airway obstruction include congenital high airway obstruction syndrome (CHAOS), severe micrognathia, and epulis. With CHAOS, the actual lesion is not always seen, but the associated findings of hydrops fetalis suggest severe upper airway obstruction due to an intrinsic laryngeal obstruction, most commonly a laryngeal web, congenital subglottic stenosis, or laryngeal atresia. The intrinsic laryngeal obstruction leads to distention of the distal respiratory tree from prevention of the natural egress of pulmonary secretions, which then compresses the vena cava leading to ascites and hydrops. Epulis is a rare benign gingival tumor; the etiology of the cell of origin is not known.

F A situation of relatively "low risk" would occur when an anomaly has been identified on prenatal imaging that is expected to lead to some degree of airway obstruction, but the consensus decision is that most likely the newborn will be able to maintain an airway initially with relatively routine support. In cases such as this, an argument can be made to perform routine delivery (either vaginally or via C-section, at the obstetricians' discretion), with a Pediatric Otolaryngologist available in the delivery room, in the unlikely event that there is a need for urgent airway intervention.

G A situation of "high risk" regarding the fetal airway would be a case in which the infants prenatal imaging demonstrates fetal airway obstruction that simply will not be compatible with life after delivery. In this case, an EXIT procedure should be planned. The EXIT procedure involves a modified C-section in which as minimal an amount of the fetus is delivered as possible to allow access to establish the airway while maintaining fetal oxygenation on uteroplacental support.

H A multidisciplinary team should be assembled (including a Pediatric and Obstetric Anesthesiologist, Obstetrician, Radiologist, Pediatric Surgeon, Pediatric Otolaryngologist, Neonatologist, Maternal-Fetal Medicine Specialist, and dedicated nursing staff). Regularly scheduled team meetings should be planned well ahead of the scheduled procedure, to map out a precise plan for the procedure. It is recommended that the patient's family meet with the team.

I An EXIT procedure would preferably be performed as close to term as possible, to increase the likelihood of fetal lung maturity and fetal viability. However, if there is significant worsening of polyhydramnios or increased risk of preterm labor, the EXIT procedure may have to be performed earlier.

J The operating room should be set up ahead of time, with equipment for maternal general anesthesia, sterile operating equipment for C-section, sterile table with neonatal intubating, bronchoscopic, and tracheostomy equipment with associated dedicated nursing staff, incubator with neonatology team for neonatal resuscitation, and separate operating room table with head and neck surgical equipment and separate team to be used in the event that further neonatal surgery is needed after delivery. Maternal cross-matched blood should be available, and warm O-negative blood should be available for the fetus.

K Unlike a typical C-section, deep general maternal anesthesia is required to allow for complete uterine relaxation, to prolong the duration of uteroplacental circulation.

L If a mass in the neck compresses the trachea too much to prevent endotracheal intubation, or impedes access to tracheostomy, partial resection of the mass on placental support is performed. If the mass is cyst, it can be decompressed.

M Neonatal tracheostomy access to the performed using standard techniques.

SUGGESTED READING

Doubilet PM. Should a first trimester dating scan be routine for all pregnancies? Semin Perinatol. 2013;37(5):307-309.

Laje P, Howell LJ, Johnson MP, et al. Perinatal management of congenital oropharyngeal tumors: the ex utero intrapartum treatment (EXIT) approach. J Pediatr Surg. 2013;48:2005-2010.

Lin EE, Tran KM. Anesthesia for fetal surgery. Semin Pediatr Surg. 2013;22:50-55.

Makhlouf M, Saade G. Should second trimester ultrasound be routine for all pregnancies? Semin Perinatol. 2013;37(5):323-326.

Moldenhauer JS. Ex utero intrapartum therapy. Semin Pediatr Surg. 2013;22:44-49.

Otteson TD, Hackam DJ, Mandell DL. The ex utero intrapartum treatment (EXIT) procedure: new challenges. Arch Otolaryngol Head Neck Surg. 2006;132:686-689.

Taghavi K, Beasley S. The ex utero intrapartum treatment (EXIT) procedure: application of a new therapeutic paradigm. J Paediatr Child Health. 2013;49(9):E420-427.

Neonatal Respiratory Distress

Wade McClain, Carlton J Zdanski

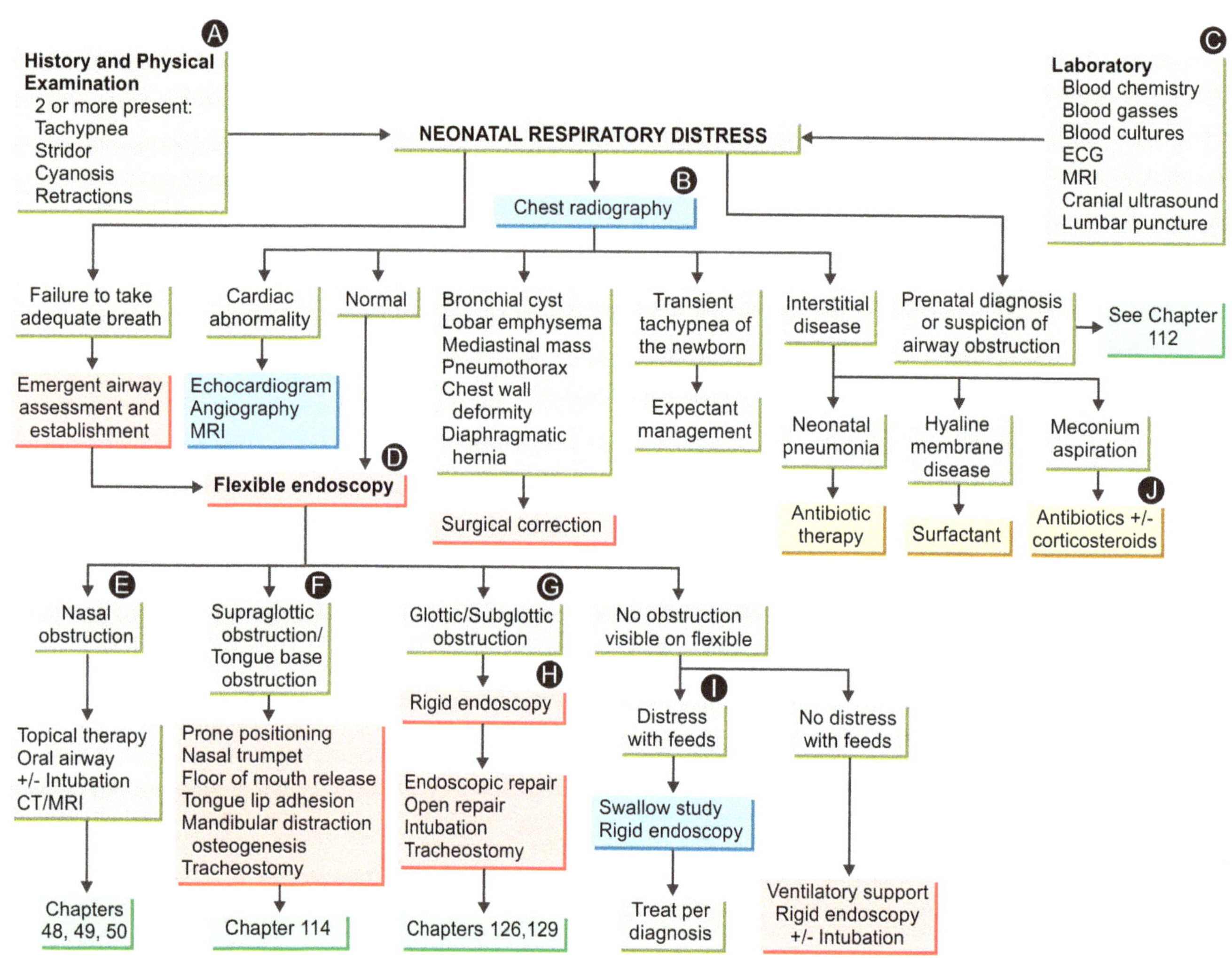

Neonatal respiratory distress can present immediately upon delivery or later in life. Many cases of distress present on delivery, i.e. those due to anatomic factors visible on ultrasound or pulmonary insufficiency related to prematurity, can be anticipated and prepared for prenatally. Many cases cannot be predicted and a well thought-out stepwise approach to the diagnosis and treatment of these is vital to successful management.

Ⓐ Neonatal respiratory distress may present with tachypnea (>60 breaths per minute), expiratory grunting or stridor, cyanosis, and retraction of the chest wall. Clinical diagnosis of neonatal respiratory distress is made when two or more of these signs are present. Individually, they are not necessarily diagnostic and may occur transiently in normal infants.

Ⓑ A chest radiograph may be diagnostic in patients with neonatal respiratory distress. Hyaline membrane disease may demonstrate a diffuse, fine reticulogranular pattern on air bronchograms. In meconium aspiration, the chest is hyperexpanded; there are mottled densities throughout the lungs with increased radiolucencies; pneumothorax and pneumomediastinum are common. Neonatal pneumonia may present with a varied pattern, with diffuse opacification or coarse or lobar/segmental consolidation. Transient tachypnea of the newborn presents with a chest radiograph demonstrating prominent linear densities radiating from the hilum and thickening of the fissures and pleural margins. Pneumomediastinum, pneumothorax, and pulmonary interstitial emphysema are usually secondary to other lung disease or to active resuscitation.

Ⓒ Hypoglycemia and acidosis are common findings associated with respiratory distress in the neonate.

Ⓓ Bedside flexible fiberoptic endoscopy can be quickly performed and help guide subsequent management by identifying the site(s) of upper airway obstruction, if any, that exists. Additionally, it can be a therapeutic tool, allowing transnasal intubation in cases where the anatomy precludes orotracheal intubation. In many cases, flexible laryngoscopy and bronchoscopy can be performed at the bedside under sedation and topical anesthesia. In most cases, formal rigid and/or flexible laryngoscopy and bronchoscopy under general anesthesia may be necessary to evaluate the airway safely and definitively.

E The degree to which healthy term neonates are obligate nasal breathers is debatable. Premature infants, however, are likely to experience respiratory distress associated with nasal obstruction. The bedside examination should include examination of the patency of both nasal passages. Conditions associated with nasal obstruction include neonatal rhinitis, septal deflection, hemangioma, encephalocele, glioma, dacryocystocele/nasolacrimal duct cyst, pyriform aperture stenosis, and choanal atresia. A magnetic resonance imaging (MRI) can aid in the diagnosis and management of nasal masses; a fine cut computed tomography (CT) can aid in surgical planning.

F Laryngomalacia is the most common cause of inspiratory stridor in the neonate. The majority of infants can be treated conservatively but many require surgical intervention. Endoscopic supraglottoplasty is usually effective and well tolerated.

Tongue-based and supraglottic airway obstruction is common in children with Pierre Robin sequence (PRS) and micrognathia. A significant number of these can be managed with positioning. Placement of a nasopharyngeal airway can serve as a temporizing measure and some neonates can be successfully managed entirely with this intervention. Laryngeal mask airway (LMA) placement can be successful for emergent airway management if oroendotracheal intubation is impossible. Growing evidence supports the idea that mandibular distraction osteogenesis can help avoid tracheostomy placement in carefully selected patients with PRS. Other causes of macroglossia and supraglottic obstruction are trisomy 21, lymphatic malformations, hemangioma, lingual thyroid, mucopolysaccharidoses, and Beckwith-Wiedemann syndrome.

G Biphasic stridor may be due to glottic or subglottic pathology. Idiopathic bilateral vocal cord paralysis requires imaging such as MRI to rule out Chiari malformation. Even transient intubation in the neonatal period can lead to subglottic stenosis and cyst formation. The recent identification of propranolol as a safe and effective treatment for airway hemangioma has revolutionized treatment of these lesions so they can often be managed medically.

H Direct laryngoscopy and bronchoscopy are necessary to identify glottic, subglottic, and tracheal pathology that can be difficult or impossible to assess on bedside flexible endoscopy. Bronchoscopy is necessary to reveal distal obstruction such as tracheal stenosis, aorto-innominate compression, complete tracheal rings, vascular rings and slings, and tracheobronchomalacia. A bronchogram can be a useful adjunct to bronchoscopy, particularly if complete tracheal rings are suspected. It has a low sensitivity in evaluation of neonatal stridor in general and so serves as a poor screening examination without a high index of suspicion. Vascular compression of the trachea can be further characterized with MRI or ultrasound. Complete tracheal rings are frequently associated with cardiac abnormalities and a complete cardiac evaluation is warranted.

I Distress associated with feeding is commonly due to neuromuscular and developmental problems but may also be secondary to laryngomalacia, tracheoesophageal fistula, and laryngotracheoesophageal clefts (LTECs). Laryngeal lesions, especially LTECs, can prove elusive; a high degree of clinical suspicion and direct laryngoscopy are important to avoid any delay in diagnosis.

J Limited studies show some benefit from corticosteroid treatment in severe meconium aspiration syndrome. Prophylactic antibiotic therapy has not been shown to be of benefit.

SUGGESTED READING

Bergeson PS, Shaw JC. Are infants really obligatory nasal breathers? Clin Pediatr (Phila). 2001;40:567-569.

Marques, IL, de Sousa TV, Carneiro AF, et al. Clinical experience with infants with Robin sequence: a prospective study. Cleft Palate Craniofac J. 2001;38:171-178.

Meyer AC, Lidsky ME, Sampson DE, et al. Airway interventions in children with Pierre Robin sequence. Otolaryngol Head Neck Surg. 2008;138:782-787.

Phelan PD, Olinsky A, Robertson CF. Respiratory Illness in Children, 4th edition. Cambridge, MA: Blackwell Scientific; 1994.

Tomasi SM, Zalzal GH, Saal HM. Airway obstruction in the Pierre Robin sequence. Laryngoscope. 1995;105:111-114.

Stridor in the Pediatric Age Group

Renee E Park

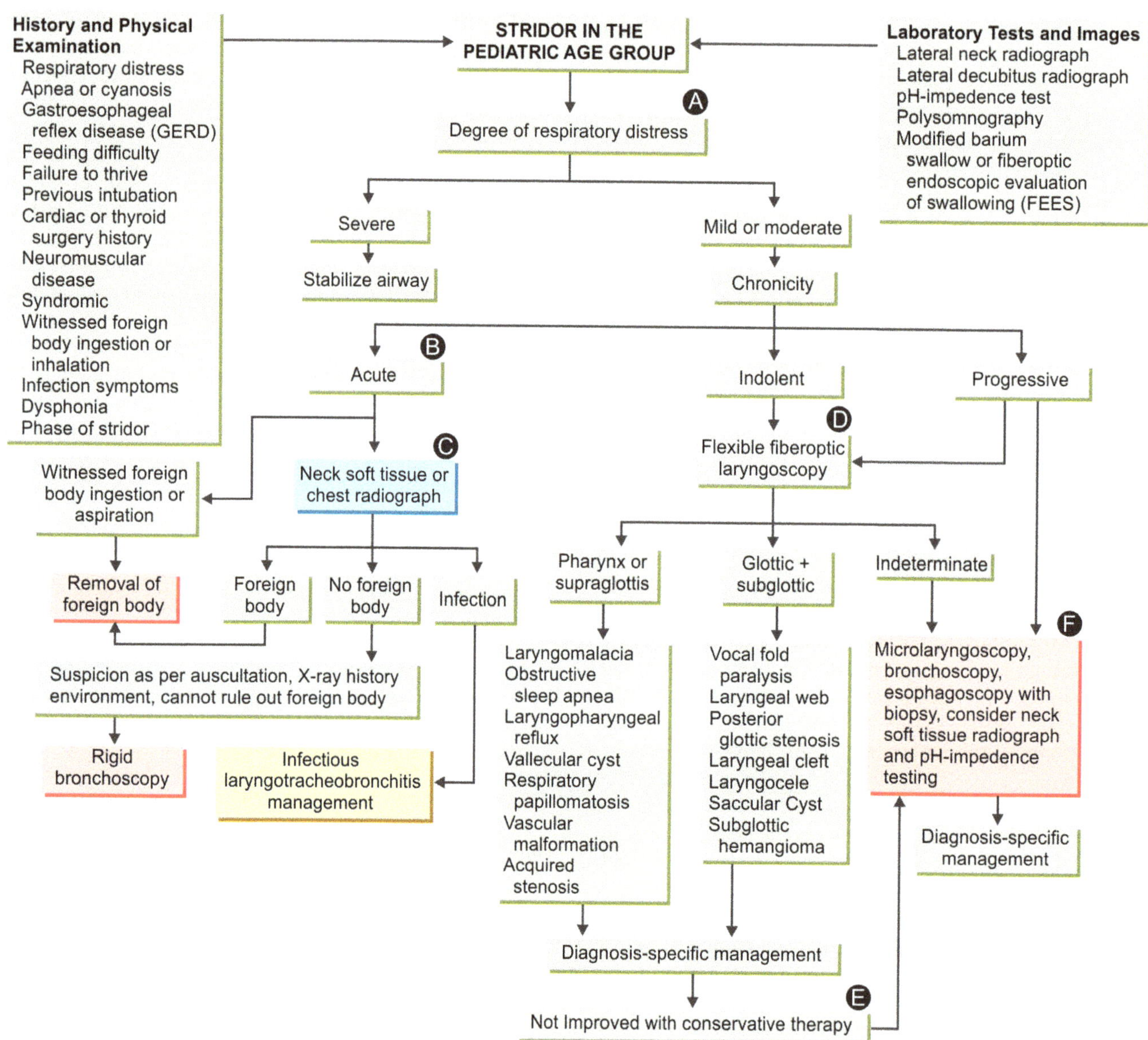

Noisy breathing is a reflection of turbulent airflow, and indicates possible airway obstruction. Stridor, or *Stridere* (*Latin*: to make a harsh or shrill noise), is used to describe laryngeal or tracheal sounds, which are characterized as high-pitched or musical. The phase of stridor can help to localize the site of obstruction. Inspiratory stridor is indicative of a supraglottic or glottic lesion. Biphasic stridor is associated with glottic or subglottic pathology, while expiratory stridor suggests, intrinsic or extrinsic, tracheal or bronchial obstruction. A thorough history and physical examination are important in order to ensure a safe-airway, as well as to determine the site of pathology.

Ⓐ The degree of respiratory distress must be assessed on initial presentation. Loudness of stridor is not indicative of the severity of airway obstruction. A history of posturing, severe retractions, cyanosis or hypoxia would indicate an unstable airway, potentially requiring immediate stabilization with supplemental oxygen, bag masking, intubation or tracheostomy tube placement.

Ⓑ Chronicity of symptoms provides insight into the etiology of stridor. Acute-onset stridor is primarily related to infection or foreign body aspiration or ingestion.

Ⓒ Croup is the most common noncongenital cause of pediatric stridor, and can be diagnosed by history, examination, and radiograph. Other infections may include supraglottitis or membranous laryngotracheobronchitis. Classically, a foreign body in the airway is suspected with a history of choking or coughing, unilateral diminished breath sounds, and chest radiograph demonstrating air trapping. However, only 10–20% of aspirated foreign bodies are radiopaque, and more than 50% of patients can have a normal chest radiograph. Therefore, history and physical examination are critical in the evaluation of a suspected foreign body aspiration. Although uncommon, esophageal foreign bodies can also present with stridor.

(D) In a stridulous patient with a stable airway, flexible fiberoptic laryngoscopy allows for evaluation of anatomy and vocal-fold mobility, and is often diagnostic. This allows for dynamic evaluation of the upper airway, including the oropharynx, hypopharynx, supraglottis, glottis and occasionally the subglottis. The most common cause of infantile stridor is laryngomalacia.

(E) Microlaryngoscopy and bronchoscopy under general anesthesia is recommended if conservative therapy does not improve symptoms. A complete and thorough examination of the anatomy of the airway can be performed in the sedated patient. Synchronous airway lesions have been reported in 8–58% of laryngomalacia cases. Patients with an unwitnessed, radiolucent foreign body aspiration may present with persistent stridor as their only symptoms. Further, a recent study found that eosinophilic esophagitis was identified in 3.7% of patients with persistent airway symptoms. The diagnosis of eosinophilic esophagitis requires esophageal biopsies after reflux has been adequately treated, or has been excluded as a comorbid diagnosis.

(F) The subglottis and trachea require sedation for a complete tracheobronchoscopy. Subglottic lesions such as a hemangioma, subglottic stenosis or subglottic cyst may occasionally be visualized on soft tissue radiograph. However, endoscopic evaluation with rigid telescopes is important for diagnosis. Tracheal lesions may include vascular compression, complete tracheal rings, tracheobronchomalacia, tracheoesophageal fistula, or rarely neoplasm.

SUGGESTED READING

Darras KE, Roston AT, Yewchuk LK. Imaging acute airway obstruction in infants and children. Radiographics. 2015;35(7): 2064-2079.

Haegen TW, Wojtczak HA, Tomita SS. Chronic inspiratory stridor secondary to a retained penetrating radiolucent esophageal foreign body. J Pediatr Surg. 2003;38(2):1-3.

Hill CA, Ramakrishna J, Fracchia MS, et al. Prevalence of eosinophilic esophagitis in children with refractory aerodigestive symptoms. JAMA Otolaryngol Head Neck Surg. 2013;139(9): 903-906.

Mortellaro VE, Iqbal C, Fu R, et al. Predictors of radiolucent foreign body aspiration. J Pediatr Surg. 2013;48(9):1867-1870.

Schroeder JW Jr, Bhandarkar ND, Holinger LD. Synchronous airway lesions and outcomes in infants with severe laryngomalacia requiring supraglottoplasty. Arch Otolaryngol Head Neck Surg. 2009;135(7):647-651.

Acute Airway Obstruction

Gregory L McHugh, Andrew Herlich

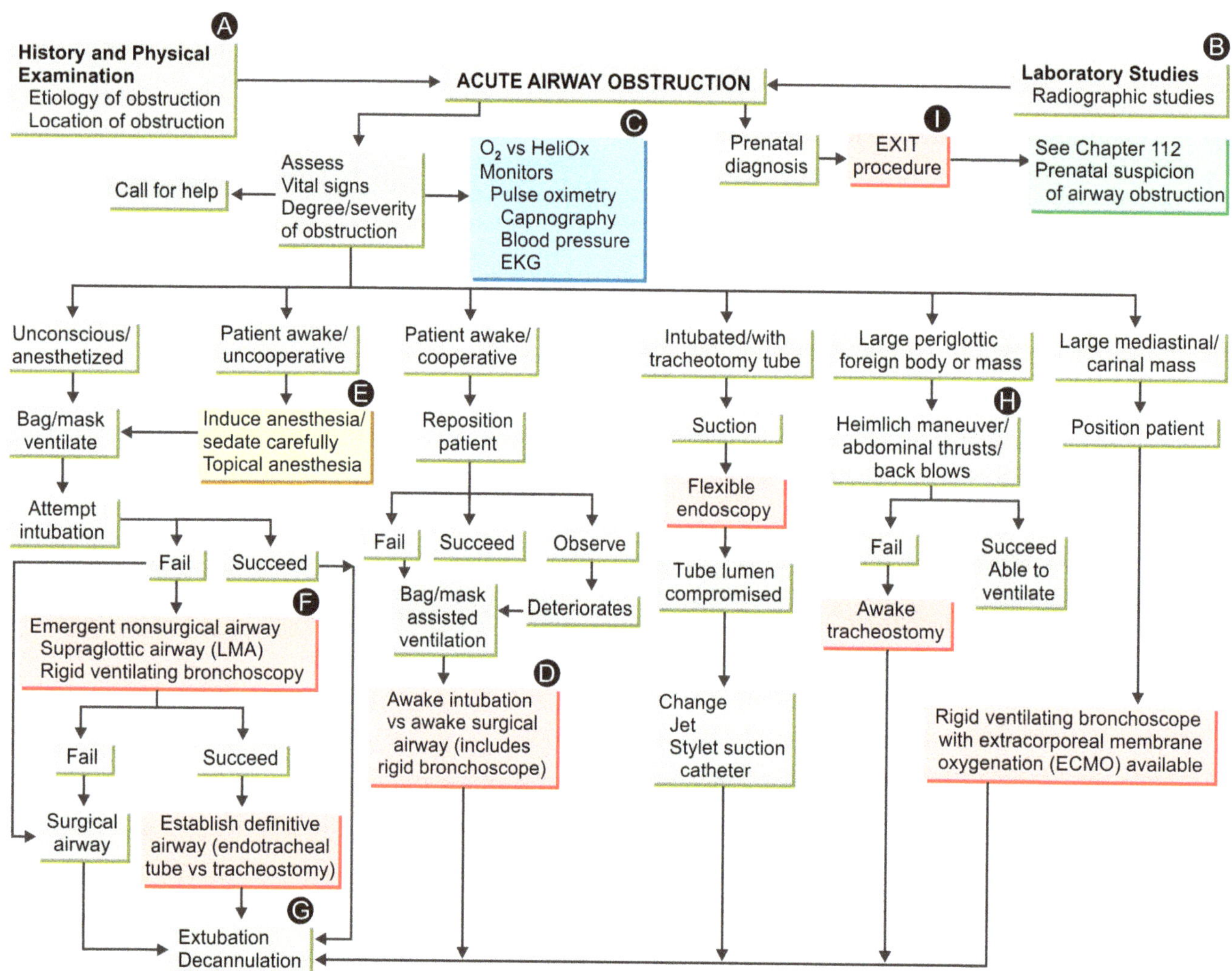

Acute airway obstruction is a life-threatening emergency requiring close communication and joint decision making between Anesthesiology, Critical Care, and Otolaryngology colleagues. An algorithmic approach to decision making can facilitate and expedite diagnosis and treatment, and result in the best possible outcome for the patient. Changes in practice and technology require constant review and, if necessary, modification of this algorithmic approach.

A History and physical examination of the patient are essential. Determination of partial versus complete airway obstruction will direct the immediate plan of action. Known tumors, infections, trauma, as well as the location and nature of a foreign body will also help determine management strategies. Objects lodged at the glottic inlet suggest awake tracheostomy. A large mediastinal or carinal mass may require the use of a rigid ventilating bronchoscope or institution of extracorporeal membrane oxygenation (ECMO) awake via the femoral vessels.

B Due to the acuity of airway management, rarely is there time for computed tomography or magnetic resonance imaging. However, if patient safety allows and there is time, these studies may provide valuable information. Portable radiographs of the head, neck, and chest may be valuable in identifying the level and extent of obstruction. Portable ultrasonography may also be quite helpful, especially with foreign bodies or obstruction, which may create an air-fluid level or air trapping.

C It is imperative to call for help as soon as possible in managing the patient. Apply pulse oximetry, capnography, electrocardiography, and blood pressure cuff. Additionally, the use of supplemental oxygen and, when appropriate with a constricted airway, heliox in 70/30 concentration may also be helpful in stabilizing the patient. The confirmation of expired carbon dioxide is always helpful in determining the success of overcoming an obstructed airway.

D Any time during the decision-making process when the patient acutely deteriorates and the Otolaryngologist is concerned that nonsurgical modalities will lead to adverse outcomes, it is wise to proceed to a surgical intervention such as an emergent tracheostomy or cricothyrotomy with transtracheal ventilation. In hospitals where cardiopulmonary bypass is available, certain distal tracheobronchial obstruction may warrant immediate institution of ECMO via the femoral vessels.

E The use of sedation, general anesthesia, or neuromuscular blocking drugs at this point is controversial. They may be very helpful in facilitating tracheal intubation. However, their use must be balanced with the strong possibility of rendering a patient unconscious and apneic who may not be able to be subsequently ventilated. Additionally, particularly in the case of anterior mediastinal masses, this class of drugs may eliminate normal transpulmonary and transvenous pressure gradients found in awake patients, resulting in airway and vascular collapse.

F Otolaryngologists may be unfamiliar with the use of the supraglottic airway (King airway, LMA) for rescue in the case of the emergent nonsurgical airway. These have an excellent record of success in such situations and should be part of the airway management armamentarium in addition to the rigid ventilating bronchoscope.

G Decannulation or extubation requires the same decision algorithm as intubation. Frequently, it is advisable to decannulate or extubate over a fiberoptic scope or jet stylet in the awake, spontaneously ventilating patient so that a protected airway may be safely re-established.

H Depending on the patient's age, the use of the Heimlich maneuver, abdominal thrusts, or back blows may be helpful in dislodging a suspected foreign body. If the obstruction is not relieved or the patient loses consciousness, a surgical airway is necessary at this junction. For further details, see Chapter 137.

I For fetal airway obstruction diagnosed in the prenatal period, ex utero intrapartum treatment (EXIT procedure) may be considered, while fetal oxygenation and ventilation remains independent of airway patency.

SUGGESTED READING

American Society of Anesthesiologists. Practice guidelines for management of the difficult airway. An updated report by the American Society of Anesthesiologist's Task Force on Management of the Difficult Airway. Anesthesiology. 2013;118(2):251-270.

Crosby ET, Cooper RM, Douglas MJ, et al. The unanticipated difficult airway with recommendations for management. Can J Anesth. 1998;45:757-776.

Gonzalez RM, Herlich A, Boerner T, et al. Recent advances in airway management in anesthesiology: an update for otolaryngologists. Am J Otolaryngol. 1996;17:145-160.

Gurkowski MA. Upper airway obstruction. In: Bready LL, Mullins RM, Noorily SH, et al. (Eds) Decision Making in Anesthesiology, 3rd edition. S. Louis, CV Mosby, 2000, p. 520.

Helfer DC, Clivatti J, Yamashita AM, et al. Anesthesia for ex utero intrapartum treatment (EXIT procedure) in fetus with prenatal diagnosis of oral and cervical malformations: case reports. Rev Bras Anesthesiol. 2012;62(3):411-423.

Herlich A. Complications from securing the difficult airway. Int Anesthesiol Clin. 1997;35:13-30.

Herlich A. Fiberoptics for head and neck patients. Anesth Clin North Am. 1991;9:111-127.

Mason RA, Fielder CP. The obstructed airway in head and neck surgery. Anaesthesia. 1999;54:625-628.

Morneault L, Johnston A, Perreault T. Management of acute airway obstruction using extracorporeal membrane oxygenation. ASAIO J. 1996;42:321-323.

Petruzzelli GJ, deVries EJ, Johnson JT, et al. Extrinsic tracheal compression from an anterior mediastinal mass in an adult: the multidisciplinary management of the airway emergency. Otolaryngol Head Neck Surg. 1990;103:484-486.

Stridor of Suspected Inflammatory Etiology

Charles M Myer III, Niall D Jefferson

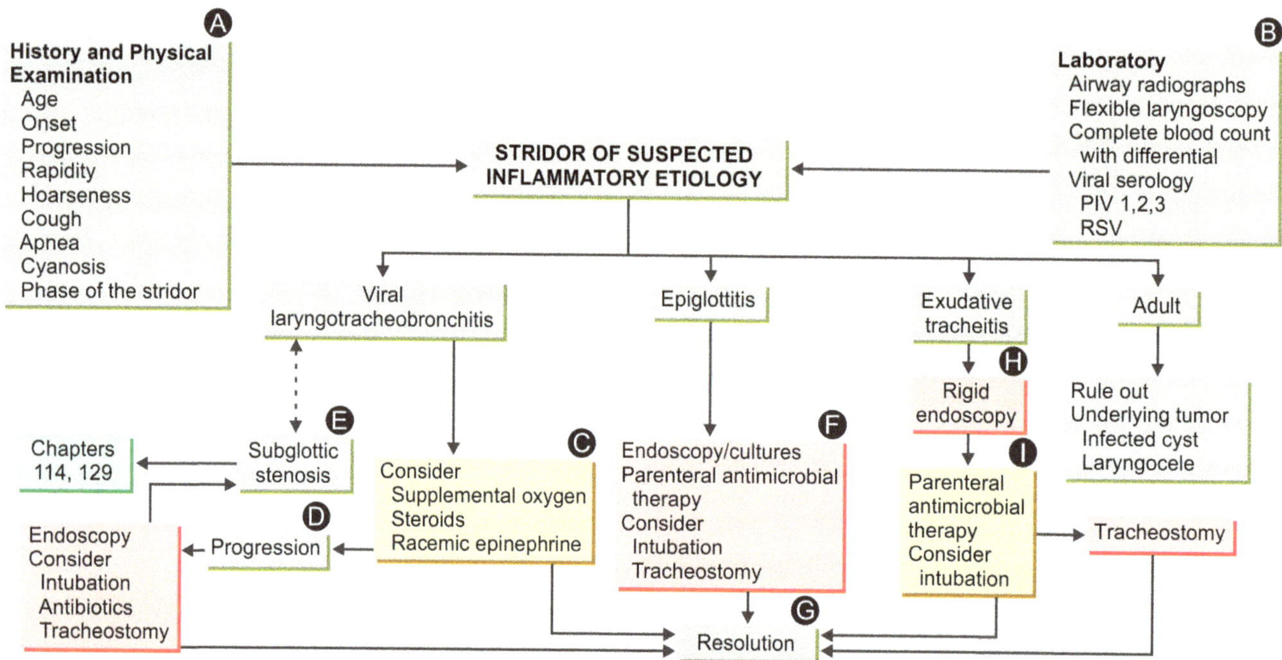

Airway inflammation can result in acute airway compromise and rapid deterioration. Recognizing the relevant signs and having a considered approach to the evaluation and management of this entity is essential. This summary aims to inform the reader of the current understanding of a number of common inflammatory airway conditions and provide a roadmap to their successful management.

A Regardless of the suspected cause of stridor in children, one should proceed with a standard method of evaluation. An inflammatory basis of stridor should be suspected in children when the stridor develops relatively acutely and is accompanied by signs and symptoms of a respiratory infection. Stridor in the adult is much less commonly inflammatory, and investigation should be directed to rule out an underlying malignancy. Although both viral laryngotracheobronchitis (croup) and epiglottitis are accompanied by inspiratory stridor, exudative tracheitis may include a component of expiratory stridor as well (biphasic stridor).

B If a child is in acute respiratory distress, one does not have the luxury of performing a comprehensive investigation. Rather, one should proceed to the operating room emergently to secure the airway. Microlaryngoscopy and bronchoscopy are diagnostic and, in some cases, therapeutic. If the cause of respiratory distress is not inflammatory, an alternative differential diagnosis can be developed and investigative studies obtained.

C Croup is the most common illness in children that causes acute stridor and is typically a clinical diagnosis. Up to 80% of viral laryngotracheobronchitis are caused by parainfluenza types 1, 2, and 3 and affect children between ages 6 months and 3 years. Children usually present with a low-grade fever, hoarseness, and a barking cough of 1–3 days duration. If the diagnosis is in question, radiographic confirmation can be of help, especially in older children in whom exudative tracheitis (membranous laryngotracheobronchitis) is a consideration. The cornerstones of treatment are corticosteroids and nebulized epinephrine; steroids have proven beneficial in severe, moderate, and even mild croup. Oral delivery of dexamethasone at a dose of 0.3 mg/kg for moderate croup and up to 0.6 mg/kg for severe croup as a single dose is helpful in decreasing symptoms at 6, 12, and 24 hours after treatment, decreasing the need to use nebulized epinephrine, reducing the length of stay in the emergency department, and resulting in fewer hospital admissions. Less than 1% of hospitalized children require intubation. The prognosis for croup is excellent, the majority of patients can be managed successfully as outpatients and recovery is almost always complete.

D If intubation is necessary, attempt extubation after a few days. If extubation fails, perform diagnostic rigid endoscopy. Lack of improvement or worsening symptoms may suggest a secondary bacterial infection and may warrant appropriate antimicrobial coverage. Some children may require tracheostomy for prolonged airway access or ventilation and to prevent the development of subglottic stenosis although this is rare.

E In children with recurrent episodes of croup (especially younger than 6 months), the possibility of undiagnosed congenital subglottic stenosis is important to consider. Likewise, after prolonged intubation iatrogenic subglottic stenosis can develop although this is a rare complication. Once the stenosis is mature, surgical reconstruction can take place (*see* Chapter 129).

F Because of the use of the *Haemophilus influenzae* type vaccine, the incidence of acute epiglottitis has diminished dramatically. One must however, remain cognizant of its presence and its potential to cause severe airway distress. In contradistinction to those with croup, these children are usually older, lack a viral prodrome, and generally present with a progressive sore throat, high temperature, and a toxic appearance. These patients often assume the "tripod" position for breathing and have a muffled voice with difficulty swallowing and drooling. Radiographs are being replaced by direct visualization of the epiglottis using nasopharyngoscopy/laryngoscopy and should be avoided in those patients who present in extremis.

G If the diagnosis of epiglottitis is suspected, endoscopy should take place in a secure environment. Blood cultures may be taken as they can be positive in up to 25% of cases where the patient is systemically unwell. Equipment for intubation, cricothyrotomy, or needle jet ventilation should be available at the bedside. Avoid sedation, inhalers, or racemic epinephrine as this may promote agitation. For patients in extremis, immediate airway management is required. When in doubt, securing the airway is the safest approach. Nasotracheal intubation and empiric parenteral antimicrobial therapy (preferably a third-generation cephalosporin given the increasing resistance to ampicillin) are important. Antibiotic therapy should ideally be started after blood and possibly epiglottic cultures have been obtained. Tracheostomy should be reserved for the patient who cannot be intubated. Resolution is expected within several days of onset of the disease process.

H Often called bacterial tracheitis or membranous laryngotracheobronchitis, the term exudative tracheitis is more accurate and descriptive. Although uncommon, it is now a more prevalent diagnosis than epiglottitis. With a clinical presentation similar to croup, this population is slightly older, more acutely ill, and does not respond to conventional croup treatments. Unlike croup and epiglottitis, microlaryngoscopy and bronchoscopy are essential for diagnostic confirmation and treatment, specifically débridement of tracheal membranes and crusts. This should be performed if there is any suspicion of the diagnosis based on the clinical history, radiographs of the neck (tracheal membrane), or a flexible endoscopy demonstrating purulent secretions within the airway. Pediatric-sized bronchoscopes and experts at pediatric airway management should be available.

I Material for culture should be obtained using a suction trap at endoscopy and broad-spectrum antimicrobial therapy instituted, including coverage for *Staphylococcus aureus*, *Moraxella catarrhalis*, *H. influenzae*, and *Streptococcus pneumoniae*. In susceptible communities clindamycin or vancomycin must be considered for *methicillin-resistant S. aureus*). If intubation is necessary, an endotracheal tube 0.5–1 size smaller than expected should be considered to avoid further damage to the tracheal mucosa. Frequent suctioning and humidification are recommended to deal with secretions and maintain tube patency. Approximately 50% of children will need to be intubated, usually for several days. Tracheostomy is rarely necessary because most patients are extubated successfully. Patients are continued on oral antimicrobial therapy after hospital discharge. Development of subglottic or tracheal stenosis is uncommon.

SUGGESTED READING

Bjornson C, Russell KF, Vandermeer B,Wet al. Nebulized epinephrine for croup in children. Cochrane Database Syst Rev. 2011. CD006619.

Chub-Uppakarn S, Sangsupawanich P. A randomized comparison of dexamethasone 0.15 mg/kg versus 0.6 mg/kg for the treatment of moderate to severe croup. Int J Pediatr Otorhinolaryngol. 2007; 71(3):473-477.

Delany DR, Johnston DR. Role of direct laryngoscopy and bronchoscopy in recurrent croup. Otolaryngol Head Neck Surg. 2015; 152(1):159-164.

Salamone FN, Bobbitt DB, Myer CM, et al. Bacterial tracheitis reexamined: is there a less severe manifestation? Otolaryngol Head Neck Surg. 2004;131(6):871-876.

Sobol SE, Zapata S. Epiglottitis and croup. Otolaryngol Clin North Am. 2008;41(3):551-566.

Tebruegge M, Pantazidou A, Thorburn K, et al. Bacterial tracheitis: a multi-centre perspective. Scand J Infect Dis. 2009;41(8):548-557.

Management of Speech and Language Disorders

Ali Lewandowski, Jackie L Gartner-Schmidt

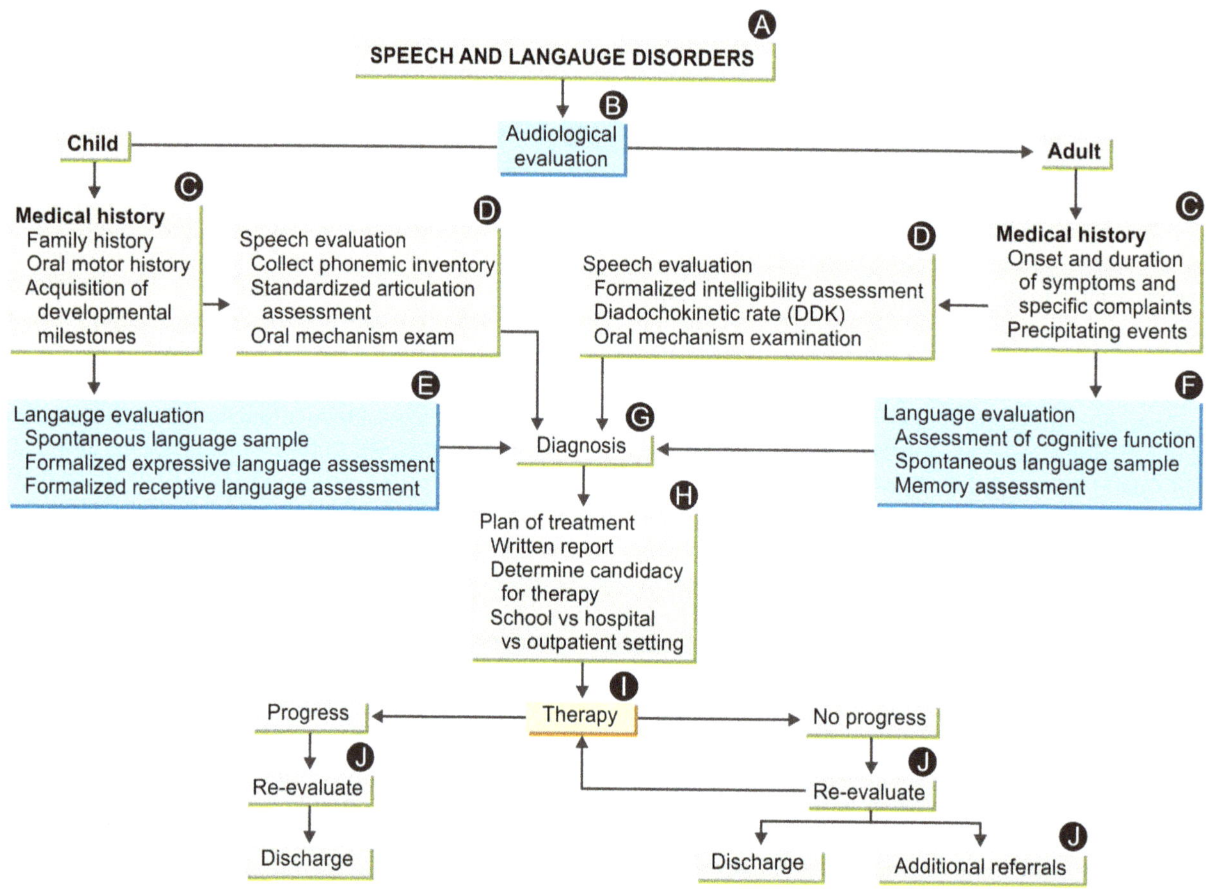

To date, there are ~142,000 practicing speech–language pathologists (SPLs) in the United States of America. Speech–language pathologists assess and treat speech and language disorders in both children and adults in a variety of settings. Approximately 5% of children have speech sound production disorders upon entrance into the first grade, and between 6 and 8 million people experience some form of language impairment in the United States (National Institute on Deafness and Other Communication Disorders). This chapter and the associated flowchart describe the processes included in evaluating and treating speech and language disorders.

A There are many factors that can contribute to the manifestation of a speech/language disorder. Within the pediatric population, genetic factors, birth defects, or early limited language exposure can all lead to communication deficits. Speech and language problems in adulthood can be a result of a progressive neurologic disease (i.e. Alzheimer's disease, amyotrophic lateral sclerosis, and Parkinsonism), stroke, or residual deficits from childhood.

B If possible, the patient should receive an audiological evaluation prior to receiving a speech and language evaluation. Results of standardized testing may be compromised if any hearing loss is present.

C Before any formalized testing begins it is crucial to obtain a thorough medical history of the patient. Important elements of the history include, but are not limited to, the onset and duration of symptoms, precipitating events that are linked to the onset, chief complaints, previous illnesses and/or disorders, family history of diseases and/or disorders, and current prescribed medications. When evaluating a pediatric patient, the clinician should also inquire about acquisition of developmental milestones, oral motor history (i.e. feeding and pacifier usage) and other services the child is receiving.

D Formalized testing is the gold standard of care when evaluating an individual for a communication disorder. However, informal measurements are also essential in the process of differential diagnosis. During a pediatric assessment, the SLP should collect a phonemic inventory to establish which sounds the child does and does not produce in spontaneous utterances. Speech testing may include a formal articulation test such as the Goldman-Fristoe Test of Articulation [2nd edition (GFTA-2)] and the Fisher-Logemann Test of Articulation Competence for adults. The Kaufman Speech Praxis Test for Children allows the clinician to evaluate basic motor tasks and speech patterns should Childhood Apraxia of Speech exist as a potential working diagnosis. An oral mechanism examination should be administered to all patients to evaluate anatomical structures and function.

E Language test batteries should be selected based on the communication deficit (i.e. written language, spoken language, and cognition). For children, common language tests include the Expressive One Word Picture Vocabulary Test, the Test of Auditory Comprehension of Language, or the Clinical Evaluation of Language Fundamentals which includes a number of language subtests. When young children are unable to participate in direct standardized assessment, parent questionnaires can assist in the formation of the child's communicative profile. The Receptive-Expressive Emergent Language Test-Third Edition and the MacArthur–Bates Communicative Development Inventory are widely used. Collecting a spontaneous language sample allows for analysis of mean length of utterance and complexity of language for all patients.

F Speech/language disorders in adults are usually a result of a cerebrovascular accident (CVA), traumatic brain injury, or a progressive neurologic disease. Common test batteries used for language assessment are the Western Aphasia Battery or the Boston Diagnostic Test. The Assessment of Intelligibility for Dysarthria is an appropriate tool to assess intelligibility of speech for those patients experiencing articulation changes due to progressive neuromuscular conditions. To further assess patients with dementia, the Arizona Battery for Communication Disorders of Dementia is appropriate to determine the patient's communicative profile, and the Cognitive Linguistic Quick Test can be used to evaluate cognitive function. A referral for a neuropsychological evaluation may be appropriate to further assess memory function for patients with progressive diseases.

G After the evaluation is complete, a written summary is created to interpret the test results and diagnosis. For adult patients, a medical diagnosis has most likely already been assigned. Results of the speech and language evaluation further determine severity, and the type of disability.

H After a diagnosis has been determined, a plan of treatment is formed. For children, treatment can be provided in an outpatient setting or private practice, a school setting, or in the home through Early Intervention. For school settings, children with ages 3–21 will have an Individualized Education Plan (IEP) that ultimately establishes the child's goals, length of treatment, and frequency of services within the school. If a child is under the age of 3, an Individualized Family Service Plan (IFSP) will determine the treatment plan in a similar manner. It is important that children who are found to have a speech or language disorder receive treatment as soon as possible, due to the high correlation between reading impairments and early language deficits.

Language treatment for adults often involves numerous therapy sessions in an inpatient or outpatient hospital setting, private practice, nursing home, or assisted living facility. Treatment can target language production, language comprehension, and/or reading and writing. The SLP may work with a vocational specialist to help the person return to work or school, if appropriate.

For motor speech disorders (loss of speech intelligibility as seen in apraxia or dysarthria), a training program that enhances planning, sequencing, pacing, and coordination of the muscles of speech is warranted. Often, compensatory strategies are taught to improve overall communication and sometimes augmentative and alternative communication is needed.

I The number of recommended sessions varies based on the severity of diagnosis, treatment facility, and patient compliance and motivation. Typically, an initial allotment of 3 months (anywhere between 12 and 24 sessions) is considered to be an appropriate duration to determine progress. Individual sessions allow the therapist to facilitate structured, specific tasks to directly target the patient's goals. On the contrary, group settings allow for generalization of skills, social communication, and peer support. However, each scenario does pose challenges. Individual sessions do not allow for immediate feedback and peer interaction, and group settings present various distractions. Furthermore, some speech/language disorders (i.e. Childhood Apraxia of Speech) require consistent repetitions of targeted productions for optimal progress to be made. These patients would therefore benefit from one-on-one intervention.

J While clinical judgment is an important factor to determine the direction of care, it is essential to continue the assessment process as treatment advances to track the patient's progress and ensure that goals remain appropriate. If treatment goals have been achieved, discharge may be warranted. If no progress has been made, treatment frequency may increase or re-evaluation by a physician may be recommended. Occasionally, referrals for additional evaluations may be appropriate (i.e. behavioral and developmental). If a patient is discharged, follow-up testing at a 3 or 6-month interval is recommended, particularly for patients who are diagnosed with progressive diseases.

SUGGESTED READING

Heilmann J, Ellis Weismer S, Evans J, et al. Utility of the MacArthur–Bates communicative development inventory in identifying language abilities of late-talking and typically developing toddlers. Am J Speech Lang Pathol. 2005;14(1):40-51.

Kaufman NR. Kaufman Speech Praxis Test for Children. Detroit, MI: Wayne State University Press; 1995.

Rice ML, Smolik F, Perpich D, et al. Mean length of utterance levels in 6-month intervals for children 3 to 9 years with and without language impairments. J Speech Lang Hear Res. 2010; 53(2):333-349.

Scarborough HS, Fletcher-Campbell F, Soler J, et al. Connecting early language and literacy to later reading (dis)abilities: Evidence, theory, and practice. In: Approaching Difficulties in Literacy Development: Assessment, Pedagogy, and Programmes, 2009. pp. 23-39.

Strand E, Stoeckel R, Baas B. Treatment of severe childhood apraxia of speech: a treatment efficacy study. J Med Speech Lang Pathol. 2006;14:297-307.

Williams AL, McLeod S, McCauley RJ. Direct speech production interventions. In: Williams AL, McLeod S, McCauley RJ (Eds). Interventions for Speech Sound Disorders in Children. Baltimore, MA: Paul H. Brookes Publishing; 2010. pp. 27-39.

CHAPTER 118
Management of Disorders of the Professional Voice

Lyndsay L Madden, Libby J Smith

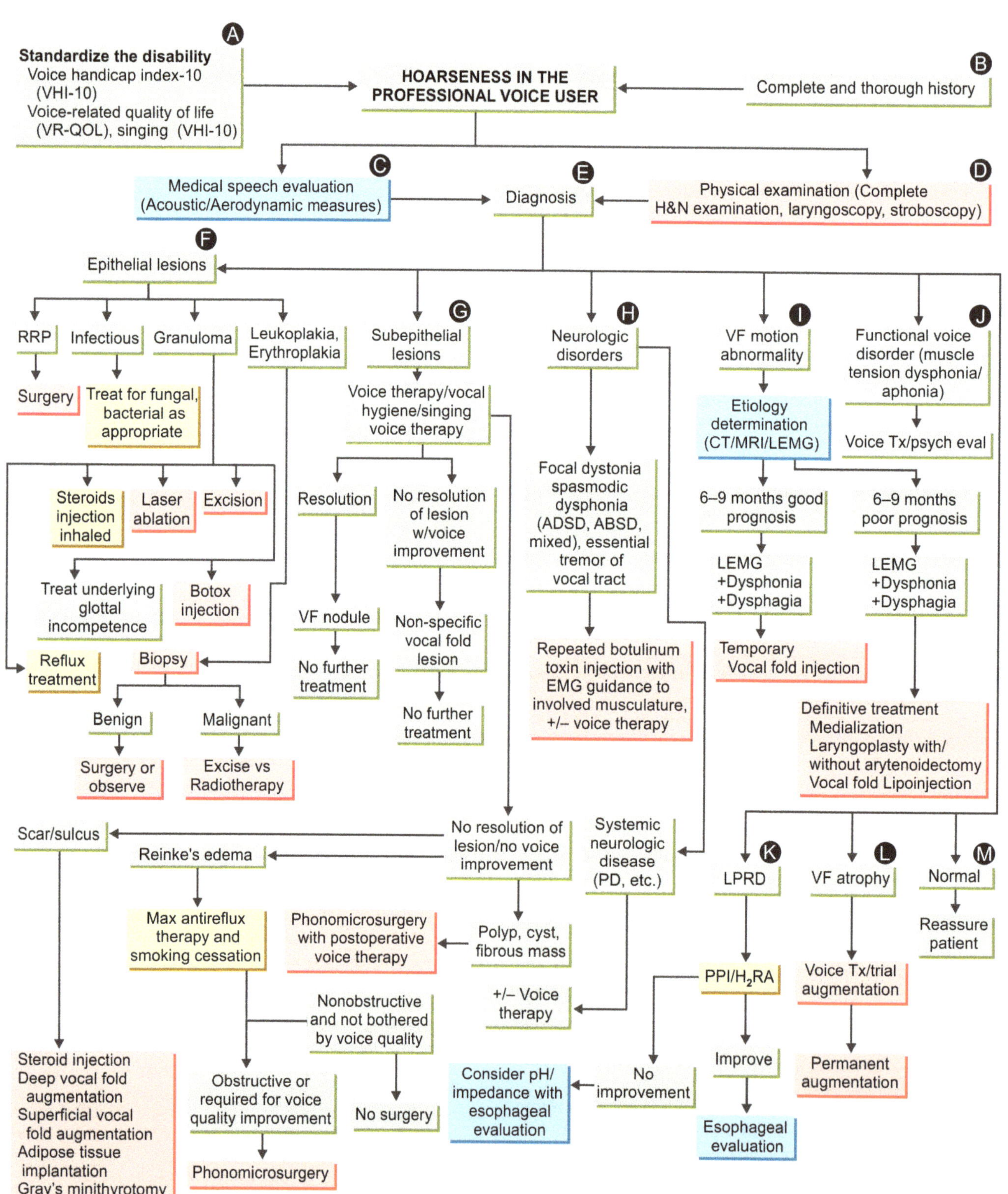

Abbreviations: (Botox: Botulinum toxin; CA: Cancer; CIS: Carcinoma-in-situ; CT: Computed tomography; H&N: Head and neck; H2RA: Histamine type 2 receptor antagonist; LEMG: Laryngeal electromyography; LPRD: Laryngopharyngeal reflux disease; MRI: Magnetic resonance imaging; PD: Parkinson's disease; PPI: Proton pump inhibitor; Tx: Treatment; VF: Vocal fold; XRT: External beam radiation therapy)

When a professional voice user presents with a complaint of "hoarseness," it is important to first determine what aspects of impaired voice production for which the patient seeks help. Patient perceptions of voice problems are individualized and directly related to voice use demands. Hoarseness broadly describes decreased quality of the voice such as raspiness, vocal fatigue, decreased projection, change in pitch, difficulty singing, and increased effort to vocalize. The patient's perception of their voice disorder and its effect on their quality of life, both personally and professionally, is important. This is often the driving force for proceeding with voice care treatment.

A To better characterize the patient's voice complaint and to distinguish the degree of disability, validated voice quality of life questionnaires such as the voice handicap index-10 (VHI-10), voice-related quality of life (VR-QOL), and singing VHI-10 (SVHI-10) were created. These surveys are useful to better understand the patient complaint; however, they do not diagnose the etiology of hoarseness. They can also be used pre- and post-treatment as a means of assessing outcomes.

B In addition to obtaining pertinent medical, surgical, and social histories, key elements of the voice-specific case history include patterns of voice use, upcoming voice needs or performances, diagnoses and treatment of previous voice disorders, previous laryngeal surgery, hearing level, smoking status, symptoms of reflux disease, and medications. Independent of the aforementioned aspects of history, the patient should be questioned on their vocal demands, amount and intensity of their voice use, as well as excessive voicing, talkativeness, and extroverted personality. Making the distinction between demand and personal proclivity toward talkativeness is important in medical decision-making. Although the patient often needs to take responsibility for their voice problem, simply blaming the patient for their vocal dilemma is neither productive nor helpful in the treatment plan. Patient education on prevention and causes of dysphonia is more important.

C A speech-language pathologist (SLP) adds significant input to the evaluation of professional voice users with the complaint of "hoarseness." The medical speech evaluation, including perceptual analysis, acoustic and aerodynamic measures, as well as the assessment of stimulability for improvement with voice therapy are important. The perceptual voice evaluation includes evaluating behavioral issues affecting voice. The SLP characterizes voice quality by using the Grade, Roughness, Breathiness, Asthenia, and Strain (GRBAS) scale and the Consensus Auditory-Perceptual Evaluation of Voice while the speaker uses his or her voice in normal speech conditions. A baseline assessment of the acoustic parameters of the voice to determine differences from normal and to establish specific abnormal acoustic parameters is also necessary to document change. These aerodynamic findings provide an indication of patient effort level, glottal flow, and thus glottic closure.

D The first element of a good voice evaluation is using the ear as a diagnostic instrument. Gross vocal aberrations will be easily identifiable, while other, more subtle anomalies require specific phonatory tasks to identify the abnormality. The laryngeal examination is paramount in determining the cause of hoarseness, accomplished by using flexible or rigid endoscopy. Flexible endoscopic examinations are well tolerated and allow laryngeal visualization during connected speech, making it the instrument of choice if one suspects neurologic disorders of the larynx, vocal fold motion abnormalities, or functional voice disorders. Whereas, the rigid 70° endoscope offers a superior means of evaluating lesions or other anatomic abnormalities of the vocal folds. Stroboscopic light examination uses a pulsed light source to create the illusion of continuous, slow motion mucosal wave movement. Stroboscopy is indispensable in evaluation of the vocal fold mucosal wave, and thus the impact of the vocal fold pathology on that mucosal wave.

E The diagnosis is based on the history, medical speech evaluation, physical examination, and laryngeal imaging. This multidisciplinary approach to diagnosis of voice problems in professional voice users is ideal. The diagnostic categories include benign vocal fold lesions, malignant vocal fold lesions, vocal fold motion abnormalities, neurologic voice disorders, functional voice disorders, and normal examination. In each of these cases, a treatment program is outlined. In addition to the pertinent laryngeal pathology, behavioral modifications are addressed such as smoking cessation, avoiding dry environments, eliminating extraneous and loud voice use, avoiding eating prior to lying down, avoiding high fat foods, avoiding foods containing natural diuretics, and increasing free water intake. These in themselves have been shown to provide relief and provide, in some cases, elimination of the problem altogether.

F Benign epithelial vocal fold lesions (leukoplakia/erythroplakia) often require treatment for possible underlying causes such as reflux, smoking, or suspected fungal, viral, or bacterial infections. If these do not resolve with conservative management or if suspicion for dysplastic or malignant vocal fold lesions exists, the patient's risk factors should be assessed and a biopsy should be taken. Dysplastic conditions can then be monitored. In the presence of higher grade dysplastic lesions (severe dysplasia and carcinoma-in-situ [CIS]) and carcinoma (CA), definitive treatment includes surgical excision, potassium-titanyl-phosphate laser ablation, or external beam radiation therapy. Appropriate post-treatment surveillance is scheduled.

G Benign vocal fold lesions can carry with them a complex diagnosis algorithm. As with any voice disorder, improving the functional status of the voice is imperative through treatment of associated medical conditions, voice therapy, and phonomicrosurgery. Benign vocal fold lesions usually arise from the superficial layer of the lamina propria due to presumed greater sensitivity to phonotrauma associated with voice misuse, coughing and inflammation. Mid-membranous vocal fold lesions treatment often involves voice therapy, either with curative intent or in the perioperative period. Vocal fold nodules, by definition, resolve with voice therapy. Some patients with vocal pathology requiring voice therapy improve with the therapy to a functional status with no resolution of lesions (termed nonspecific vocal fold lesions). Other vocal fold lesions such as polyps, cysts, fibrous masses, Reinke's edema, scar/sulcus vocalis, vocal process granulomas, and vascular ectasias are treated with a combination of voice therapy, surgery, and medical treatment. When voice therapy alone is insufficient for the patient to achieve their desired vocal status, phonomicrosurgery is then considered.

H Neurologic disorders of the voice may also be diagnosed including spasmodic dysphonia, essential tremor of the vocal tract. These conditions are often treated with voice therapy and electromyographical botulinum toxin injection into the implicated laryngeal muscles. Consultation with a Neurologist is recommended to evaluate for systemic causes of neurologic disorders. Deep brain stimulation is an option for some patients.

I Vocal fold (VF) motion abnormalities should always include testing to determine the etiology of the abnormality. In the case of iatrogenic vocal fold immobility, imaging is not needed. For the evaluation of idiopathic vocal fold motion, immobility and hypomobility, appropriate testing may include computed tomography scan with contrast enhancement from skull base to aortic arch to evaluate for lesions along the course of the recurrent laryngeal nerves (RLN), magnetic resonance imaging of the brain with gadolinium if superior laryngeal nerve involvement is suspected, and appropriately chosen laboratory studies based upon history (i.e. Lyme titer). Laryngeal electromyography provides both diagnostic confirmation of neuropathy and prognostic information regarding vocal fold motion recovery. Proceeding with treatment of glottic incompetence from vocal fold motion deficiencies depends upon the deleterious effect on the patient (i.e. thin liquid dysphagia, debilitating dysphonia). Within the first 6-9 months after time since onset, temporary vocal fold augmentation is performed. After 6–9 months for suspected peripheral RLN injury and after 12–18 months for suspected central vagus nerve injury, definitive vocal fold medialization with Gore-tex or Silastic implants, with or without arytenoid adduction, should be considered.

J Functional voice disorders, such as primary muscle tension dysphonia and muscle tension aphonia, are treated with voice therapy. These spectra of disorders are often maladaptive, compensatory voice disorders that affect many patients. Treatment may also include complimentary and adjunctive manual therapies such as myofascial release, massage therapy, and physical therapy. If a psychological component is suspected, then collaboration with psychological services is helpful.

K Laryngopharyngeal reflux disease (LPRD) is an extraesophageal reflux disorder. Symptoms of LPRD include dysphonia, throat clearing, post nasal drip, chronic cough, laryngospasm, paradoxical vocal fold motion, dyspnea, excessive phlegm, and globus sensation. Rarely does laryngeal visualization confirm diagnosis of LPRD, except when a granuloma is present. Rather, the presumptive diagnosis of LPRD is made by history. Treatment of LPRD includes specific dietary and lifestyle modifications including weight loss, decreasing meal size, avoiding lying down within 2 hours of eating a meal, low fat/low acid diet, avoiding carbonated beverages, avoiding spicy foods and caffeine (i.e. chocolate), smoking cessation, and reducing alcohol intake. If failure of symptomatic relief with dietary and lifestyle modifications, an empirical 3-month trial of proton pump inhibitor therapy can be initiated. Antisecretory therapy may then be titrated to patient symptomatic improvement. H_2 receptor antagonists may also be added to the treatment regimen. Diagnostic reflux testing, pH testing with or without impedance, may be used if the diagnosis of LPRD is questionable. Patients on long-term antireflux therapy should undergo esophagoscopy to rule out any esophageal or gastric pathology resulting from chronic acid exposure (i.e. Barrett's metaplasia or esophageal prior to carcinoma).

L Age-appropriate vocal fold atrophy should also be considered in patients with the complaint of vocal fatigue, decreased projection, and raspy vocal complaints. Voice therapy is often a successful first-line therapy for mild vocal fold atrophy, to teach the patient to more efficiently use their laryngeal anatomy. If voice therapy is not sufficient to achieve desired voice improvement, then trial vocal fold injection can be offered. If the patient does well with the trial augmentation, then permanent vocal fold augmentation procedures may be considered. It is important to discuss the unpredictable nature of treatment for vocal fold atrophy, as it is a problem of not only vocal fold bulk, which is addressed with augmentation, but also of muscle tone, for which there is no current treatment.

M Normal examinations do occur. In this case, the patient should be reassured and offered general vocal hygiene measures.

SUGGESTED READING

Akbulut S, Gartner-Schmidt JL, Gillespie AI, et al. Voice outcomes following treatment of benign midmembranous vocal fold lesions using a nomenclature paradigm. Laryngoscope. 2015; 126(2):415-420.

Carroll TL, Rosen CA. Trial vocal fold injection. J Voice. 2010; 24(4):494-498.

Gillespie AI, Gartner-Schmidt J. Immediate effect of stimulability assessment on acoustic, aerodynamic, and patient-perceptual measures of voice. J Voice. 2016:30(4):507.e9–507.e14.

Hirano M. Psycho-acoustic evaluation of voice. In: Arnold GE, Winckel F, Wyke BD (Eds). Disorders of Human Communication, 5 Clinical Examination of Voice. New York and Wien: Springer-Verlag; 1981. pp. 81-84.

Hogikyan ND, Sethuraman G. Validation of an Instrument to measure voice-related quality of life (V-RQOL). J Voice. 1999;13(4): 557-569.

Kepmster GB, Gerratt BR, Verdolini-Abbott K, et al. Consensus auditory-perceptual evaluation of voice: development of a standardized clinical protocol. Am J Speech Lang Pathol. 2009; 18(2):124-132.

Rosen CA, Gartner-Schmidt J, Hathaway B, et al. A nomenclature paradigm for benign midmembranous vocal fold lesions. Laryngoscope. 2012;122(6):1335-1341.

Rosen CA, Lee AS, Osborne J, et al. Development and validation of the voice handicap index-10. Laryngoscope. 2004;114(9): 1549-1556.

Roy N, Weinrich B, Gray SD, et al. Voice amplification versus vocal hygiene instruction for teachers with voice disorders: a treatment outcomes study. J Speech Lang Hear Res. 2002;45(4): 625-638.

Zeitels SM, Burns JA. Oncologic efficacy of angiolytic KTP laser treatment of early glottis cancer. Ann Otol Rhinol Laryngol. 2014; 123(12):840-846.

Velopharyngeal Dysfunction

Noel Jabbour

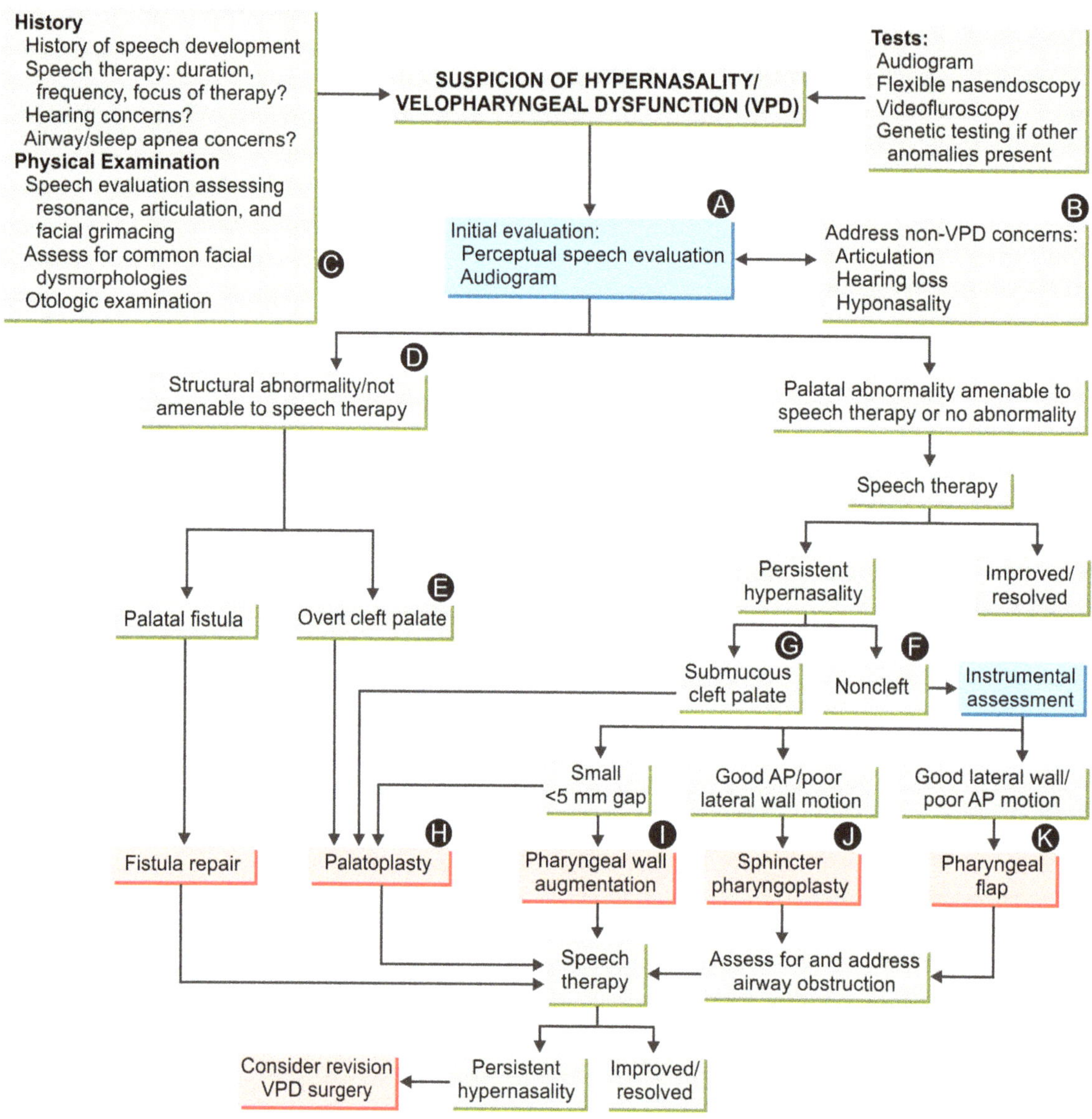

Velopharyngeal dysfunction (VPD) refers to resonance abnormalities that result from the inability to completely close the velum to the posterior pharyngeal wall or adenoid during speech, often resulting in increased nasal air escape, or hypernasality. All phonemes in the English language require velopharyngeal closure except /m/, /n/, and /ng/, which are nasal sounds. Evaluation and management of VPD is often a team approach between a surgeon and a speech language pathologist. The algorithm above highlights the importance of careful speech assessment and speech therapy in identifying and treating VPD.

A *Initial evaluation*: Patients are rarely referred with the diagnosis of VPD but rather for a variety of speech concerns or the nonspecific description of "nasal speech." A thorough history, physical examination, and perceptual speech evaluation are crucial, with careful attention to resonance, articulation, and nasal air emissions during spontaneous and provoked speech.

B Common presenting problems that are not hypernasality should be addressed, including hearing loss, airway obstruction, hyponasality, and nonresonance-related articulation errors or voice disorders.

C Palatal fistulas or unrepaired overt cleft palates may be a cause of nasal air escape or hypernasality during speech. These are not typically amenable to speech therapy and should be addressed surgically prior to continued speech therapy.

D Speech therapy is the first-line treatment for VPD in the presence of a normal palate examination or submucous cleft palate. An argument may be made to proceed directly with palatoplasty for patients with overt submucous cleft palate.

E Careful assessment of the palate may reveal signs of submucous cleft (zona pellucida, bifid uvula, and notch of the hard palate) or more subtle features of vault-shaped elevation of the palate as is common with occult submucous cleft palate, indicating anterior position of the levator veli palatini (LVP) muscles.

F For patients with persistent velopharyngeal dysfunction but no evidence of submucous cleft, instrumental assessment with videonasendoscopy or videofluoroscopy is helpful to assess velopharyngeal gap size and closure pattern.

G Videonasendoscopy or videofluoroscopy during speech assessment may be employed to assess the pattern of velopharyngeal closure and velopharyngeal gap.

H Palate lengthening and redirecting of the abnormal, anteriorly positioned LVP muscles can be accomplished with Furlow double-opposing Z-plasty. This is a common first-line surgical treatment for overt cleft palate, submucous cleft palate, and even for small velopharyngeal gaps in the setting of properly oriented LVP muscles.

I Injection pharyngeal wall augmentation has been described for closing small gaps, especially in woodwind/brass musicians with stress VPD.

J Sphincter pharyngoplasty uses the posterior tonsillar pillars or superior constrictor muscles to create a narrower velopharyngeal port; it relies on anterior-to-posterior (AP) movement of the palate and pharyngeal wall. It may be combined with Furlow palatoplasty for patients with large AP gaps.

K Pharyngeal flap involves a central, superiorly pedicled myomucosal flap of the posterior pharyngeal wall that is inset to the soft palate to create two lateral velopharyngeal ports and relies on motion of the lateral pharyngeal wall for closure. It is also useful in patients with large AP gaps.

SUGGESTED READING

Kummer AW. Perceptual assessment of resonance and velopharyngeal function. Semin Speech Lang. 2011;32(2):159-167.

Rotgers SA, Ford M, Cray J, et al. An algorithm for application of Furlow palatoplasty to the treatment of velocardiofacial syndrome-associated velopharyngeal insufficiency. Ann Plast Surg. 2011;66:479-484.

Shprintzen RJ, Marrinan E. Velopharyngeal insufficiency: diagnosis and management. Curr Opin Otolaryngol Head Neck Surg. 2009;17:302-307.

Sie KC, Chen EY. Management of velopharyngeal insufficiency: development of a protocol and modifications of sphincter pharyngoplasty. Facial Plast Surg. 2007;23(2):128-139.

Willging JP. Superiorly based pharyngeal flap and posterior pharyngeal wall augmentation. Oper Tech Otolaryngol. 2009;20(4):268-273.

CHAPTER 120

Chronic Cough

Libby J Smith

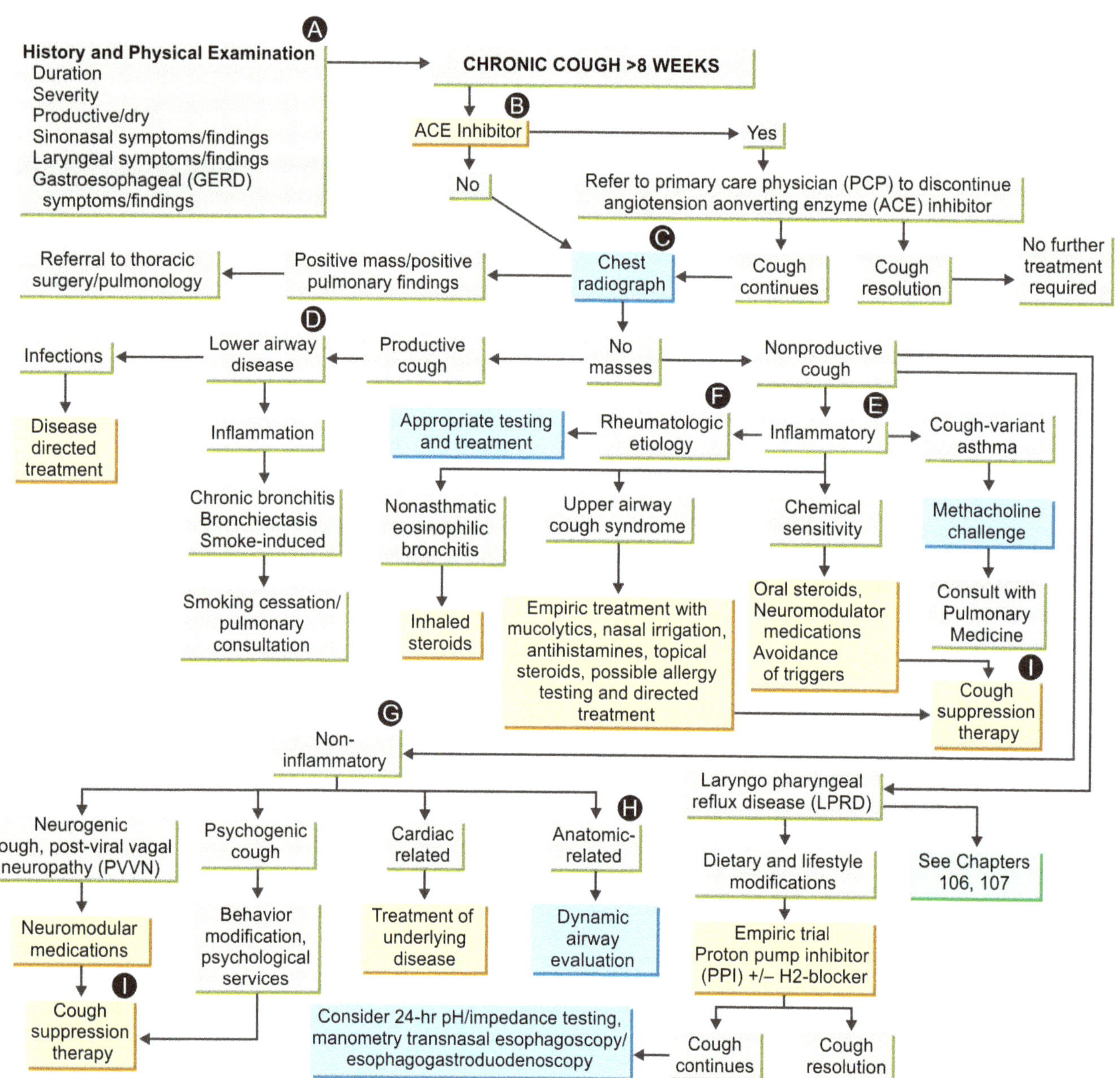

The evaluation and treatment of chronic cough can be challenging. Otolaryngologists often play a role in the multidisciplinary care of these complex patients, usually in collaboration with Pulmonary Medicine. Cough severity can range from being a nuisance to being debilitating, often adversely affecting the patients quality of life. The impact on quality of life should not be discounted. Patients may avoid social situations due to the commotion related to the cough itself and the associated urinary incontinence and vomiting. It is also important to remember that there are often multiple etiologies of cough that contribute to the patients' cough complaints, which demands a step-wise approach to determine the cause of cough, and thus the appropriate treatment.

A A thorough history is required to help determine the etiology of the cough. An acute cough lasts <3 weeks, and if often precipitated by a viral upper respiratory tract infection (URI). A subacute cough, lasting 3–8 weeks, is also often postinfectious. *Bordetella pertussis*, bacterial sinusitis, asthma, bronchiectasis, and chronic bronchitis must be considered. *Bordetella pertussis* is characterized by a biphasic course (worsens after initially improving) and has a characteristic "whooping cough." Laboratory tests for *B. pertussis* are often delayed due to its biphasic nature. Therefore, the vaccine against *B. pertussis* is recommended. The physical examination must include particular attention to the sinonasal and laryngeal regions, as these areas often provide clues to determining the etiology of cough. Evaluation for chronic cough, for >8 weeks, requires evaluation for some infectious causes, but also noninfectious etiologies.

B Medications taken by the patient must be closely evaluated. Angiotensin-converting enzyme (ACE) inhibitors are commonly used to treat hypertension. Unfortunately, it is also known to cause cough in some patients, ~2%. Cough may begin at any time while taking an ACE inhibitor medication. Any patient complaining of cough and taking an ACE inhibitor medication should work with their primary care physician to find an appropriate replacement medication from a different class of antihypertensive medication prior to further evaluation.

C Malignancy is the most feared cause of chronic cough. All patients with chronic cough should have a chest radiograph to screen for malignancy. If a mass is found, then the patient is referred to a Thoracic Surgeon for evaluation and treatment. For benign pulmonary findings, consultation with a Pulmonologist is suggested.

D A productive cough should raise the clinical suspicion of lower airway disease and possible sinonasal disease. Lower inflammatory disease, such as chronic bronchitis, and bronchiectasis are often best treated by a Pulmonologist. If the patient smokes, this must be strongly discouraged. Infectious etiologies of cough, such as tuberculosis and pertussis, are suggested by history and appropriate testing. This highlights the importance of close collaboration in a multidisciplinary model of care.

E Nonproductive chronic cough is often described as a "throat clearing" cough. Inflammatory causes of nonproductive cough include lower airway inflammation, such as nonasthmatic eosinophilic bronchitis (NAEB). These patients often respond well to corticosteroid inhalers. Upper airway cough syndrome (UACS) must also be considered. Sinonasal conditions may result in cough through tissue inflammation or direct stimulation. These patients describe having the sensation of postnasal drip. Physical examination often reveals mucoid secretions or cobblestoning of the posterior pharynx. Unfortunately, neither the complaint of postnasal drip nor physical examination findings is specific to UACS. Therefore, empiric treatment trials are needed to confirm the presence of UACS. Mucolytics are often helpful. Irritant-induced cough is often described as "chemical sensitivity" by patients, often most sensitive to strong odors such as perfume, cleaning supplies, and cigarette smoke. Patients with this self-described chemical sensitivity often report a history of URI precipitating the onset of cough. Treatment includes short-term oral steroids, neuromodulator medications (*see* step G), and avoidance of cough triggers.

Coughvariant asthma will require the aid of a pulmonologist, who will confirm the diagnosis and treatment.

F Rheumatologic causes of inflammatory chronic cough are rare and often overlooked. A detailed history of rheumatologic symptoms can help to determine if laboratory testing should be performed.

G Noninflammatory, nonproductive chronic cough incorporates several categories of cough. Chronic cough related to cardiac etiology is extremely rare, but must not be forgotten due to the morbidity and mortality associated with it, such as heart failure, edema of the extremity, cardiomyopathy, and pulmonary hypertension. Neurogenic cough is a diagnosis of exclusion, and should be made with caution. This is thought to be the result of a postviral vagal neuropathy (PVVN) after URI. Neuromodulator medications, such as pregabalin, gabapentin, and amitriptyline, are often titrated to the patient's cough complaints. Diagnosis of psychogenic cough requires ruling out all other possible etiologies. Since cough can result in increased patient anxiety and depression, the diagnosis of psychogenic cough should not be made on those findings alone. Tic disorders should be ruled out. Behavior modification and psychological care are helpful for these patients.

H Anatomic considerations are infrequently the cause of chronic cough. Tracheomalacia and bronchomalacia can be considered. Diagnosis is confirmed with dynamic airway evaluation. Treatment is directed by our thoracic surgery colleagues.

I Cough suppression therapy is an adjunctive treatment for patients with protracted nonproductive cough, especially with known cough triggers. This behavioral therapy is performed by a trained speech–language pathologist. The patient is taught to ameliorate cough severity and associated repercussions (such as urinary incontinence, postcough dyspnea, and syncope) by using specific breathing and swallowing techniques.

SUGGESTED READING

Altman KW, Irwin RS. Cough specialists collaborate for an interdisciplinary problem. Otolaryngol Clin North Am. 2010;43(1):xv-xix.

Altman KW, Noordzij JP, Rosen CA, et al. Neurogenic cough. Laryngoscope. 2015;125:1675-1681.

Canning BJ, Mori N, Mazzone SB. Vagal afferent nerves regulating the cough reflux. Respir Physiolo Neurobiol. 2006;152(3): 223-242.

Gibson P, Wang G, McGarvey L, et al. Treatment of unexplained chronic cough: CHEST Guideline and Expert Panel Report. Chest. 2016;149(1):27-44.

Ling B, Novakovic D, Sulica L. Cough after laryngeal herpes zoster: a new aspect of post-herpetic sensory disturbance. J Laryngol Otol. 2014;128:209-211.

Morrison RJ, Schindler JS. Evaluation and treatment of the patient with chronic cough referred to the otolaryngologist. Laryngoscope. 2011;121(Suppl 5):S256.

Pratter MR. Unexplained (idiopathic) cough: ACCP evidence-based clinical practice guidelines. Chest. 2006;129(1):220S-221S.

Tarlo SM, Altman KW, French CT, et al. Evaluation of occupational and environmental factors in the assessment of chronic cough in adults: a systematic review. Chest. 2016;149(1):143-160.

Cough in the Pediatric Age Group

Swathi Appachi, Samantha Anne

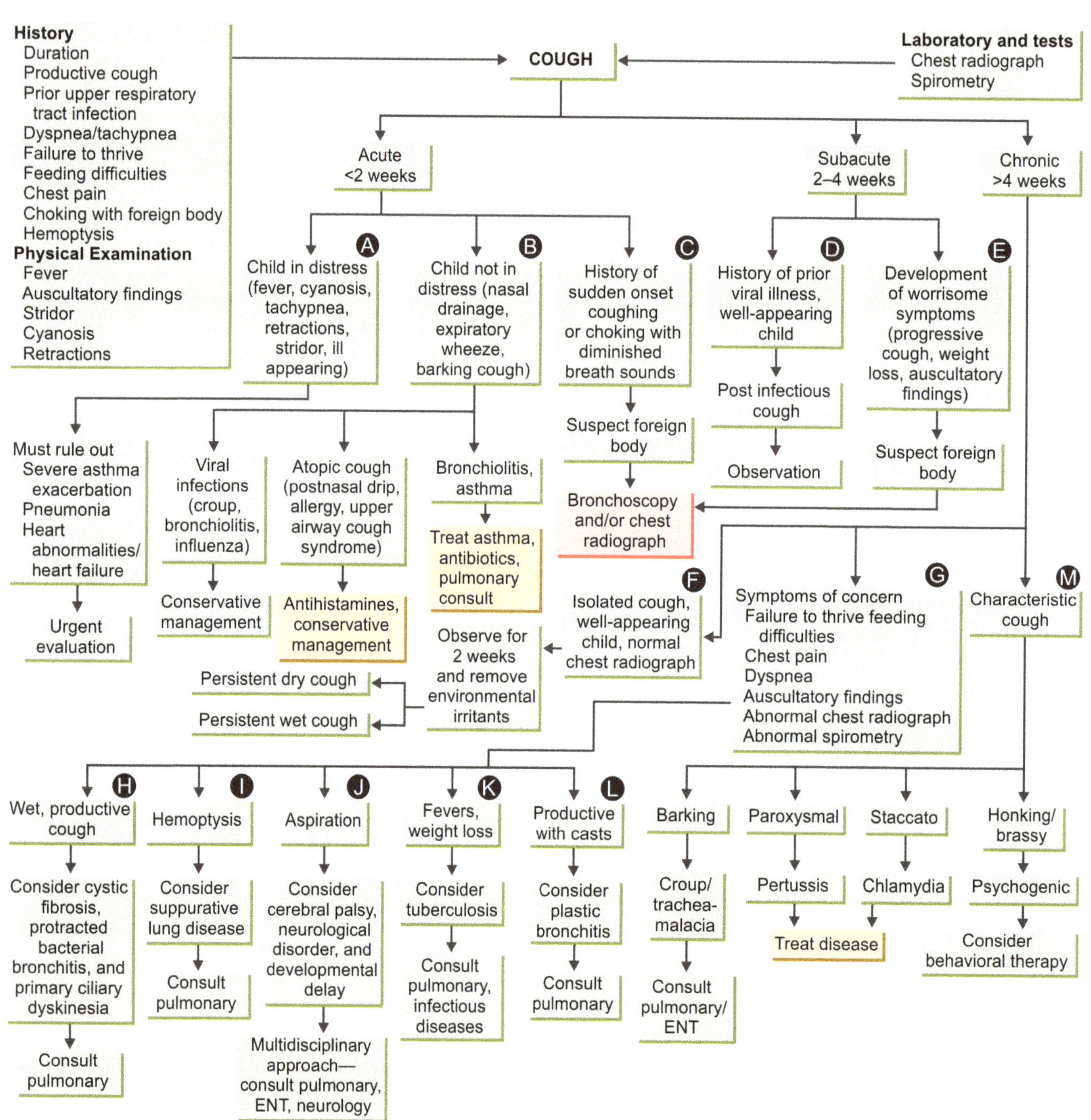

Cough in children can be a normal physiologic reflex to an airway irritant but, when persistent or severe, can be a sign of an underlying disease process. Diagnosis and management of cough in children (<18 years of age) is largely different than in adults and it is important to be cognizant of the unique differential diagnosis of cough in a child. Cough can be characterized by duration, with acute cough lasting <2 weeks, subacute cough being present for 2–4 weeks, and chronic cough as lasting over 4 weeks. When a child presents to the office with a cough, it is imperative to attain a complete history and perform a physical examination, including chest auscultation. In-office endoscopy, chest radiograph, and spirometry are adjuncts to the physical examination that can be performed at the discretion of the practitioner, depending on length of symptoms or level of concern.

A If a child presents in visible distress and is febrile, tachypneic, ill-appearing, or having visible retractions, serious and severe illnesses must be considered; this includes acute asthma exacerbation, pneumonia, heart abnormalities, or heart failure. Urgent evaluation and treatment must be instituted including chest radiograph, admission to the hospital, inhaled β-agonists, and/or intravenous antibiotics.

B If the child is not in distress upon presentation and presents with nasal drainage, expiratory wheeze, or barking cough, likely causes include viral infections, atopic cough, bronchiolitis, or asthma. These children may also present with mild stridor or retractions. Viral infections are the most common cause for acute cough and can be treated with conservative management. Atopic cough could be due to allergies, postnasal drip, or upper airway cough syndrome. A trial of antihistamines, nasal steroids, and conservative management are appropriate treatment. If asthma or bronchiolitis is suspected, inhaled corticosteroids should be administered and a consult to Pulmonology is warranted.

C If history and physical examination reveal sudden onset cough, witnessed choking, or diminished breath sounds, aspiration of foreign body should be suspected. Chest radiograph and/or bronchoscopy should be performed.

D A well-appearing child with a history of recent upper respiratory illness or viral infection presenting with subacute cough is most likely experiencing postinfectious cough. Observation is recommended.

E If a child presents with a subacute cough that was initially treated conservatively, but is starting to develop worrisome signs or symptoms, such as progressively worsening cough, weight loss, or abnormal auscultatory findings, further investigation is warranted. This includes a chest radiograph, possible spirometry, and a consult to Pulmonology (*see* G, H).

F A well-appearing child presenting with an isolated cough lasting >4 weeks, no concerning history or physical examination findings, and normal chest radiograph can be observed for resolution of symptoms for 2 weeks. In this time period, any environmental irritants (such as tobacco, allergens) should be removed. After 2 weeks, a persistent dry cough suggests asthma and a trial of inhaled corticosteroids is suggested. A persistent wet cough is likely protracted bronchitis and should be treated with antibiotics.

G If history and physical examination reveal worrisome signs and symptoms (such as history of heart or neurologic abnormalities, failure to thrive, feeding difficulties, auscultatory findings of diminished breath sounds or wheezing, chest pain, and dyspnea), and chest radiograph and spirometry are abnormal, further categorizing of the cough and accompanying symptoms should be done in order to consult the appropriate specialty services. Pulmonary consultation may be indicated from onset for these more serious conditions.

H If the cough is characterized as wet or productive, one should consider cystic fibrosis, protracted bacterial bronchitis, or primary ciliary dyskinesia. Pulmonology should be consulted.

I If the patient presents with hemoptysis, suppurative lung disease should be high on the differential list and a pulmonology consult is recommended.

J Chronic aspiration may be indicative of a neurologic disorder such as cerebral palsy, or a developmental delay. For these children, a multidisciplinary team approach, including Otolaryngology, Pulmonology, and Neurology, is warranted.

K Accompanying symptoms of fevers, weight loss, or history of recent overseas travel, should increase suspicion for tuberculosis, and pulmonology and infectious diseases should be consulted.

L If the cough is productive with casts especially in the setting of recent cardiac surgery, plastic bronchitis should be considered and the child should be seen by pulmonology. In addition, bronchoscopy with removal of casts may be necessary.

M Lastly, a characteristic cough, such as one that could be classified as barky, paroxysmal, staccato, or honking, may help provide diagnostic clues. For example, a barking cough is associated with laryngotracheomalacia. Paroxysmal or staccato coughs can be caused by pertussis or chlamydia, respectively, and the underlying disease should be treated appropriately. A honking or brassy cough is usually psychogenic or habitual, and behavioral therapy may help.

SUGGESTED READING

Chang AB, Glomb WB. Guidelines for evaluation chronic cough in pediatrics: ACCP evidence-based clinical practical guidelines. Chest. 2006;129(Supp):260S-283S.

Kelly LK, Allen PJ. Managing acute cough in children: evidence-based guidelines. Pediatr Nurs. 2007;33(6):515-524.

Shields MD, Bush A, Everard ML, et al. Recommendations for the assessment and management of cough in children. Thorax. 2008;63(Supp III):iii1-iii15.

Worrall G. Acute cough in children. Can Fam Phys. 2011;57:315-318.

Aspiration

Mark A Dettelbach

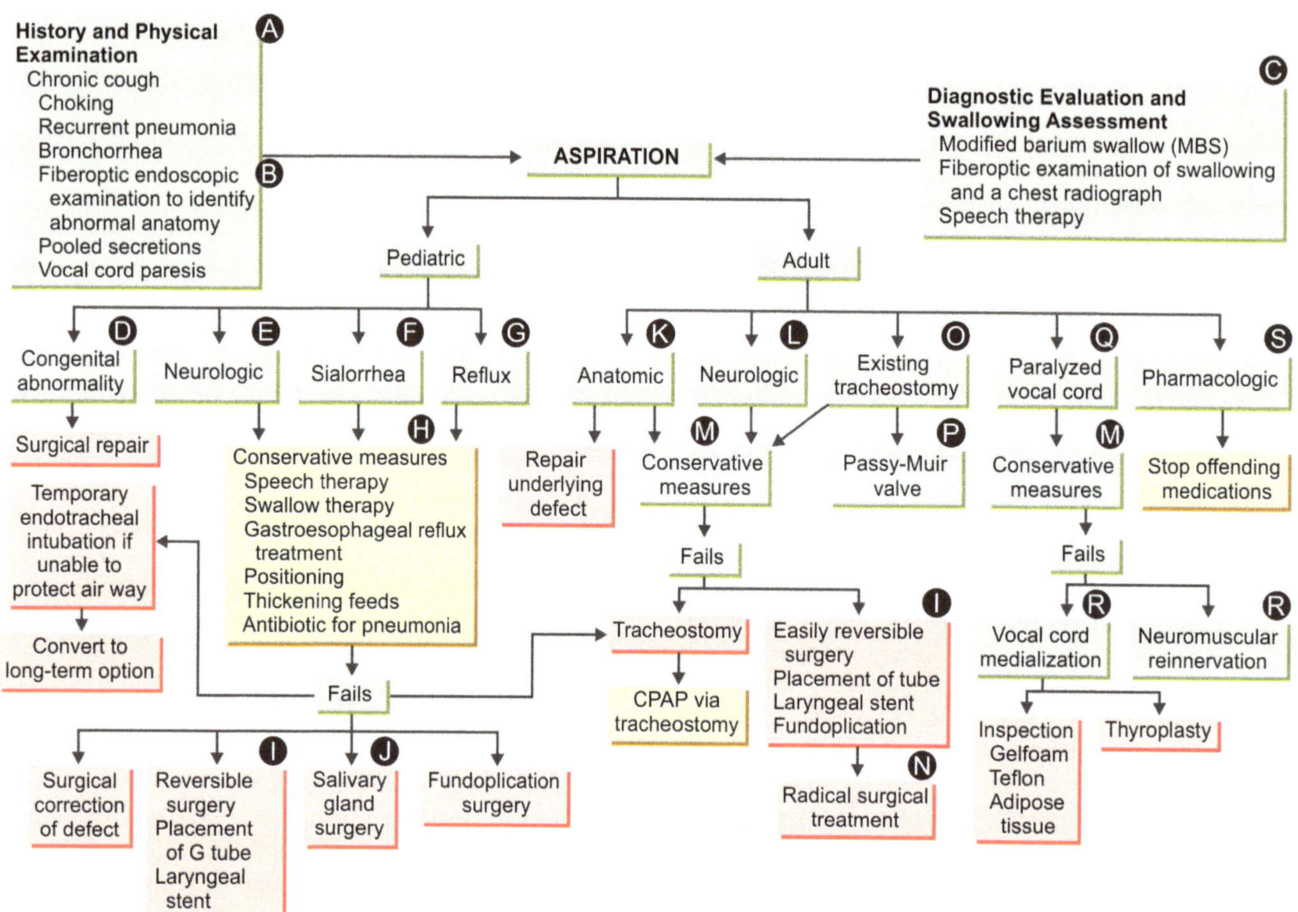

The primary goal is to stop aspiration and allow safe respiration and swallowing. A secondary goal is to permit ongoing phonation, but not at the expense of adequate pulmonary toilet and nutrition. Minimally invasive and reversible treatments are given priority. It is incumbent upon the treating practitioner to refer to an appropriate specialist when a required treatment is outside his or her expertise.

A Not all symptoms may be present. It is important to determine how and when the aspiration originated (e.g. at birth, postsurgical, etc.) and what is being aspirated (e.g. oral intake, oral secretions, refluxed material). Premature birth and a history of poor sucking and frequent gagging make aspiration more likely in children. Timing relative to feeding is also critical.

B Examination should include assessment of cranial nerves and observation for abnormal laryngeal elevation or coughing with swallowing, which suggests aspiration. It is crucial to determine whether the patient is aspirating swallowed or refluxed material.

C Initial evaluation before studies is indicated. Barium is preferred to gastrografin in radiologic studies, because

gastrografin is pneumotoxic. Functional endoscopic examination of swallowing is reliable and can replace modified barium swallow. A normal videofluoroscopic study does not rule out episodic aspiration. Computed tomography or magnetic resonance imaging from the thoracic inlet to the skull base can rule out recurrent laryngeal nerve lesions or anatomic defects such as Arnold–Chiari malformation, causing vocal cord paralysis. Salivary scintigraphy can assess salivary aspiration.

D Congenital abnormalities, including tracheoesophageal fistula, esophageal atresia, bifid larynx, and laryngotracheoesophageal cleft require surgical repair to prevent aspiration. Craniofacial abnormalities such as micrognathia or cleft palate may also predispose to aspiration.

E Neurologic impairment in children includes vocal cord paresis (congenital or acquired) and various neuromuscular disorders such as cerebral palsy. Aspiration is likely in patients with a decreased level of consciousness even with G tube feeding (see Step G).

F Drooling or sialorrhea is seen in children with neuromuscular dysfunction affecting the oral or pharyngeal phase of swallowing. Anticholinergics or similar medications (e.g. glycopyrrolate, topical scopolamine) to reduce secretions is a first step, but not very effective.

G See Chapters 106 and 107 on reflux evaluation and treatment. Rarely is fundoplication required for reflux alone.

H It is crucial to first rule out chemical pneumonitis and aspiration pneumonia or else stabilize these patients. Once stable, conservative measures for children include speech and swallow therapy and reflux medications (H2 blockers or proton pump inhibitors). Decreased meal size may also prevent reflux and aspiration. Children who drool and are cognitively intact can be cued to swallow frequently. Vertical positioning will help in the management of infants who aspirate during meals. Reflux must be confirmed before surgical management of reflux because surgery can worsen aspiration.

I In addition to the listed standard procedures, supraglottic closure with epiglottic sew-down have been reported in adults.

J Surgical management of sialorrhea is reserved for patients with severe aspiration and for those with socially embarrassing drooling. Bilateral excision of the submandibular gland and diversion of the parotid ducts help manage this condition. An alternative is the salivary glands Botox injections into that show more promise than oral and topical medications.

K Esophageal stricture or web may present in adults with dysphagia or food impaction. Even temporary esophageal obstruction can cause aspiration. A Zenker's diverticulum presents with coughing shortly after eating. Management of esophageal obstructions by dilation, cricopharyngeal myotomy, or Zenker's resection is usually curative. In less significantly affected patients, conservative measures (Step M) suffice.

Aspiration can be lethal in patients with surgically altered anatomy (e.g. total glossectomy). These patients are treated aggressively with conservative measures (Step M) and, if unsuccessful, surgery to prevent further disability.

L Neurologic and neuromuscular diseases in adults are frequently progressive and terminal. Parkinson's disease, multiple sclerosis, and amyotrophic lateral sclerosis are examples of diseases that can progress to crippling aspiration. Although each can affect a different phase of swallowing, all may require surgical intervention (Step I or Step N).

M It is imperative to determine if a chemical pneumonitis or an infectious pneumonia has occurred and to treat appropriately. Once stable, a patient can undertake conservative measures such as swallowing therapy, lifestyle changes (diet change, head elevation, decreased meal size), and medications (proton pump inhibitors, H2 blockers). These techniques are first-line treatments of adult aspiration and are used with more invasive therapy when required.

N Laryngotracheal diversion or separation (LTS) is standard treatment for intractable aspiration unresponsive to conservative measures. LTS leaves patients with a permanent stoma and unable to speak and is reserved for those with life-threatening aspiration. Total laryngectomy is an alternative last resort.

O The presence of a tracheostomy will contribute to aspiration. Retrieval of dyed secretions from a tracheostomy after oral administration of dyed food is confirmatory. Recurrent bronchorrhea may also indicate aspiration.

P An expiratory speaking valve facilitates speech in the patient with a tracheostomy and may enable swallowing without aspiration. By restoring a more physiologic pressure gradient in the larynx and upper airway, an expiratory valve seems to reduce aspiration. A patient with a valved tracheostomy can often cough more forcefully to clear secretions.

Q Vocal cord paralysis often results in glottic incompetence with aspiration as well as hoarseness. For aspiration pneumonia prevention or voice improvement, surgical intervention is warranted. Otherwise, conservative measures (Step M) suffice.

R Vocal cord augmentation or medialization corrects glottic incompetence from vocal cord paralysis. Injection of Gelfoam deep to the vocalis muscle provides ~6 weeks of augmentation for new-onset paralysis when recovery remains uncertain. Other temporary injectables include hyaluronic acid and glycerin gel. Long-term vocal cord augmentation is achieved with the injection of calcium hydroxylapatite or autologous adipose tissue. Teflon, another permanent injectable, has fallen out of favor due to side effects. An Isshiki type I thyroplasty (with or without arytenoid adduction) provides reversible medialization of the vocal cord and is standard treatment for unilateral vocal cord paralysis in many centers. Neuromuscular reinnervation of the larynx has been reported with varying success.

S Any medication that depresses consciousness or contributes to neuromuscular dysfunction can lead to aspiration. Discontinuation of the offending medication and substituting is appropriate.

SUGGESTED READING

Dettelbach MA, Gross RD, Mahlmann J, et al. Effect of the Passy-Muir valve on aspiration in patients with tracheostomy. Head Neck. 1995;17:297-302.

Eibling DE. Management of intractable aspiration. In: Bailey B (Ed). Head and Neck Surgery-Otolaryngology, 2nd edition. Philadelphia: Lippincott-Raven; 1998. p. 1773.

Eliachar I, Miller FR. Aspiration. In: Gates G (Ed). Current Therapy in Otolaryngology Head and Neck Surgery. St Louis: CV Mosby; 1994.

Langmore SE, Schatz K, Olson N. Endoscopic and videofluoroscopic evaluation of swallowing and aspiration. Ann Otol Rhinol Laryngol. 1991;100:678-681.

Logemann J. Evaluation and Treatment of Swallowing Disorders. San Diego: College-Hill Press; 1983.

Mallur PS, Rosen CA. Vocal fold injection: review of indications, techniques, and materials for augmentation. Clin Exp Otorhinolaryngol. 2010;3(4):177-182.

Mark PE. Aspiration pneumonitis and aspiration pneumonia. NEJM. 2001;344(9):665-671.

Naumann M, Dressler D, Hallett M, et al. Evidence-based review and assessment of botulinum neurotoxin for the treatment of secretory disorders. Toxicon. 2012;67:141-152.

Smith Hammond CA, Goldstein LB. Cough and aspiration of food and liquid due to oropharyngeal dysphagia: ACCP evidence based clinical practice guidelines. Chest. 2006;129(1 suppl):154S-168S.

Strahan RC, Meyers AD. Aspiration. In: Bluestone CD, Stool SE (Eds). Pediatric Otolaryngology, 3rd edition. Philadelphia: WB Saunders; 1996. p. 1245.

Aspiration in Children

Deepak Mehta, Elton Ashe-Lambert

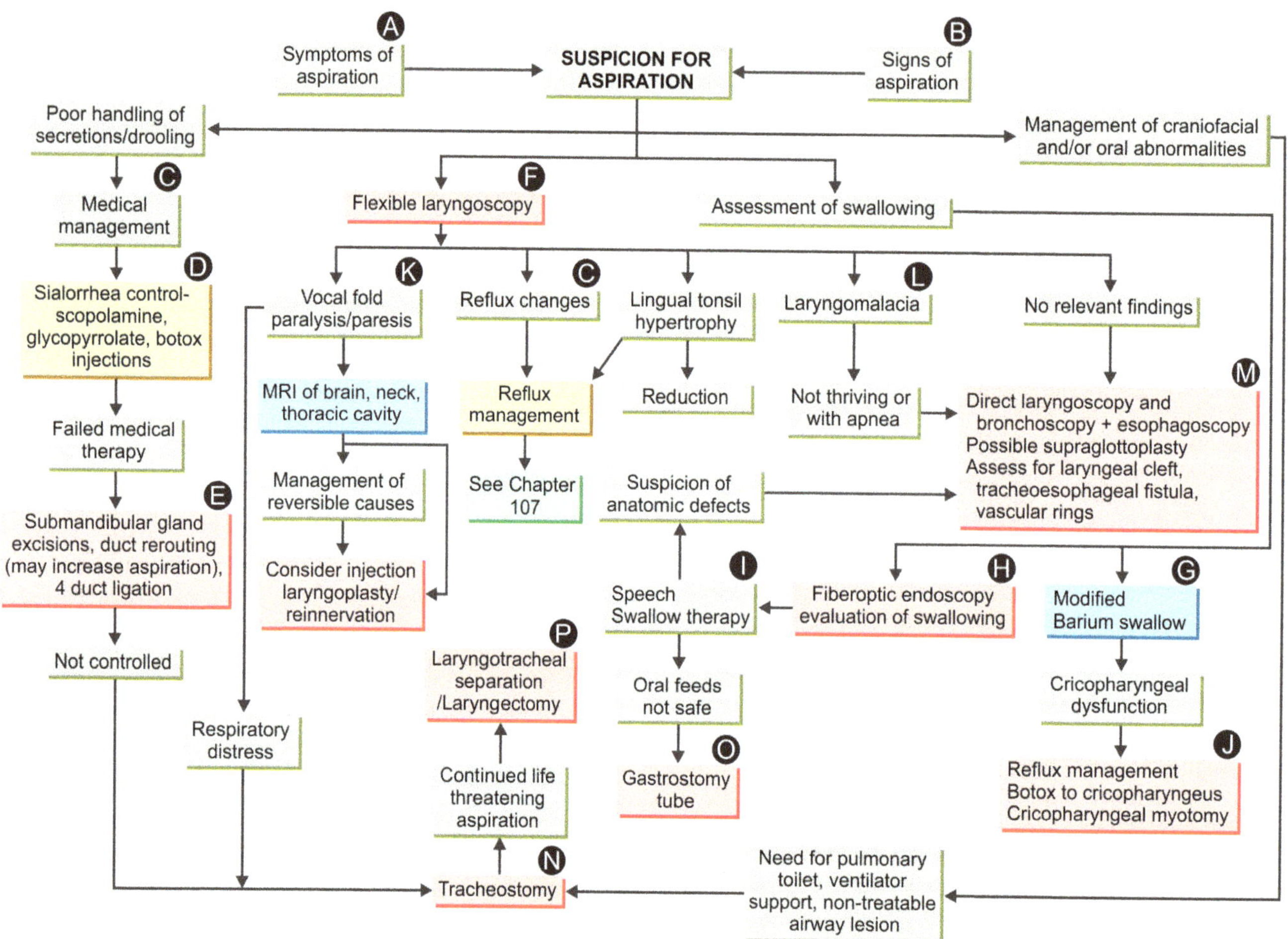

A variety of etiologies can lead to failure of the glottic protective function and resultant aspiration; however neurologic disability is the most common cause in children. Aspiration can vary in severity, from minor coughing with feedings to recurrent episodes of pneumonia.

A Symptoms of aspiration may include, choking, gagging, stridor, increased work of breathing, and coughing in the context of feeding. Drooling may indicate an inability to handle saliva and other secretions, and can be associated with aspiration in neurologically handicapped children, e.g. cerebral palsy. There must be a high index of suspicion for aspiration in any child who has recurrent pneumonias.

B The child should be observed for signs of aspiration. Asking the parent or guardian to feed the child may provide useful information. Craniofacial abnormalities such as cleft lip/palate, micrognathia, and Pierre-Robin can contribute to swallowing difficulties and aspiration. Neurologic devastation and hypotonia can also contribute to swallowing difficulty. Up to 48% of patients with cerebral palsy will have swallowing difficulty and recurrent aspiration pneumonia. Patients with oral abnormalities such as ankyloglossia or craniofacial abnormalities such as micrognathia should be managed to aid in swallow rehabilitation.

C A child who has difficulty in handling their secretions may have poor salivary control, gastroesophageal reflux, or both. Gastroesophageal reflux can be aspirated into the airway. Thus, control of reflux must be considered in any patient with concerns for aspiration.

D Sialorrhea can be managed by a number of anticholinergic agents which can have neurologic and urinary side effects associated with them. Botulinum toxin injection of the submandibular and parotid glands is effective in managing sialorrhea. Botox may reduce the episodes of aspiration pneumonia, especially in neurologically handicapped children (see Chapter 75 on drooling).

E In cases of parental preference or failed medical therapy including Botox injections, salivary gland surgery can be performed to help manage sialorrhea. Duct ligation, rerouting or bilateral submandibular gland excision can be performed. Success rates for bilateral submandibular gland excision with parotid duct ligation can be as high as 87.8%.

F Awake flexible laryngoscopy should be performed in cases where laryngeal penetration or aspiration is suspected to assess vocal fold mobility, the presence of laryngomalacia, lingual tonsillar hypertrophy, and reflux changes. Sensation of the larynx can also be assessed.

G Modified barium swallow should also be performed in the presence of a speech pathologist for patients in whom aspiration is suspected. This can detect the presence of laryngeal penetration or aspiration, anatomic aberrations such as cricopharyngeal hypertonicity, or detect problems with the coordination of swallow. Laryngeal penetration occurs when food, liquid, saliva, or refluxed stomach contents enter the laryngeal introitus, but do not pass the vocal folds into the airway. Aspiration occurs when food, liquid, saliva, or refluxed stomach contents pass the vocal folds into the airway. The study can also be therapeutic as the consistency of food and liquid that will allow for safe swallow can be assessed.

H Flexible endoscopic evaluation of swallowing, performed with the help of a speech pathologist, allows for direct visualization of the larynx during swallow. Laryngeal penetration or aspiration can be diagnosed using this modality as well.

I Speech and swallow therapy can be effective in cases where there is an issue with coordination of swallowing. Diet modification may be necessary to prevent aspiration of thin liquids.

J Cricopharyngeal hypertonicity or achalasia can cause dysphagia and resulting aspiration. It can be diagnosed by barium swallow, modified barium swallow, or esophageal manometry. Management includes Botox injections, endoscopic and open cricopharyngeal myotomy, and cervical plexus neurectomy.

K Ineffective cough, aspiration, recurrent pneumonia, and feeding difficulties can be associated with unilateral or bilateral vocal fold paresis or paralysis. Patients with vocal fold weakness should have an evaluation for intrathoracic, cervical, or intracranial etiologies. Dysphonia and aspiration caused by unilateral vocal fold paralysis can be treated with injection laryngoplasty, reinnervation procedures, or thyroplasty.

L Up to 20% of patients with laryngomalacia can have aspiration. Conservative therapy can be used in patients with laryngomalacia who are thriving and do not have life-threatening events. Supraglottoplasty should be performed in patients who are not thriving, have apneas or life-threatening events. Aspiration associated with laryngomalacia can resolve after supraglottoplasty, but there are patients who will have persistent aspiration or will have transient or permanent aspiration after supraglottoplasty.

M Direct laryngoscopy, bronchoscopy with or without esophagoscopy should be performed in any patient in whom there is a high level of suspicion for an anatomic lesion as the etiology for aspiration. A supraglottoplasty can be performed for laryngomalacia. The presence of laryngeal clefts, tracheoesophageal fistulas, and vascular rings should be evaluated. Repair of the defects would be performed as indicated.

N A tracheostomy may be necessary in the chronically aspirating patient who requires frequent suctioning for pulmonary toilet, suffers from chronic hypoxic or hypercarbic respiratory failure, is ventilator-dependent, or has an airway lesion that is nontreatable.

O Children who aspirate—in whom no nutrition is safe orally—should have enteral nutrition. This can be delivered via orogastric or nasogastric tubes temporarily to allow for reversal or treatment of anatomic lesions, or while undergoing speech therapy. Prolonged need for enteral nutrition requires a gastrostomy tube.

P In patients with continued life-threatening aspiration, laryngotracheal separation is a reversible procedure where a tracheostoma is created with closure of the subglottis. Laryngotracheal diversion is also a reversible procedure where a tracheostoma is created, but the proximal trachea is anastomosed to the esophagus. Laryngectomy is an irrevesible procedure that can be considered.

SUGGESTED READING

Butskiy O, Mistry B, Chadha NK. Surgical interventions for pediatric unilateral vocal cord paralysis: a systematic review. JAMA Otolaryngol Head Neck Surg. 2015;141:654-660.

de Jong AL, Kuppersmith RB, Sulek M, et al. Vocal cord paralysis in infants and children. Otolaryngol Clin North Am. 2000;33: 131-149.

Erasmus CE, van Hulst K, Rotteveel JJ, et al. Clinical practice: swallowing problems in cerebral palsy. Eur J Pediatr. 2012;171: 409-414.

Faria J, Harb J, Hilton A, et al. Salivary botulinum toxin injection may reduce aspiration pneumonia in neurologically impaired children. Int J Pediatr Otorhinolaryngol. 2015;79(12):2124-2128.

Gurberg J, Birnbaum R, Daniel SJ. Laryngeal penetration on videofluoroscopic swallowing study is associated with increased pneumonia in children. Int J Pediatr Otorhinolaryngol. 2015;79: 1827-1830.

Reed J, Mans CK, Brietzke SE. Surgical management of drooling: a meta-analysis. Arch Otolaryngol Head Neck Surg. 2009;135: 924-931.

Rastatter JC, Schroeder JW, Hoff SR, et al. Aspiration before and after supraglottoplasty regardless of technique. Int J Otolaryngol. 2010;2010.

Unilateral Vocal Fold Paralysis

Hailun Wang, Clark A Rosen

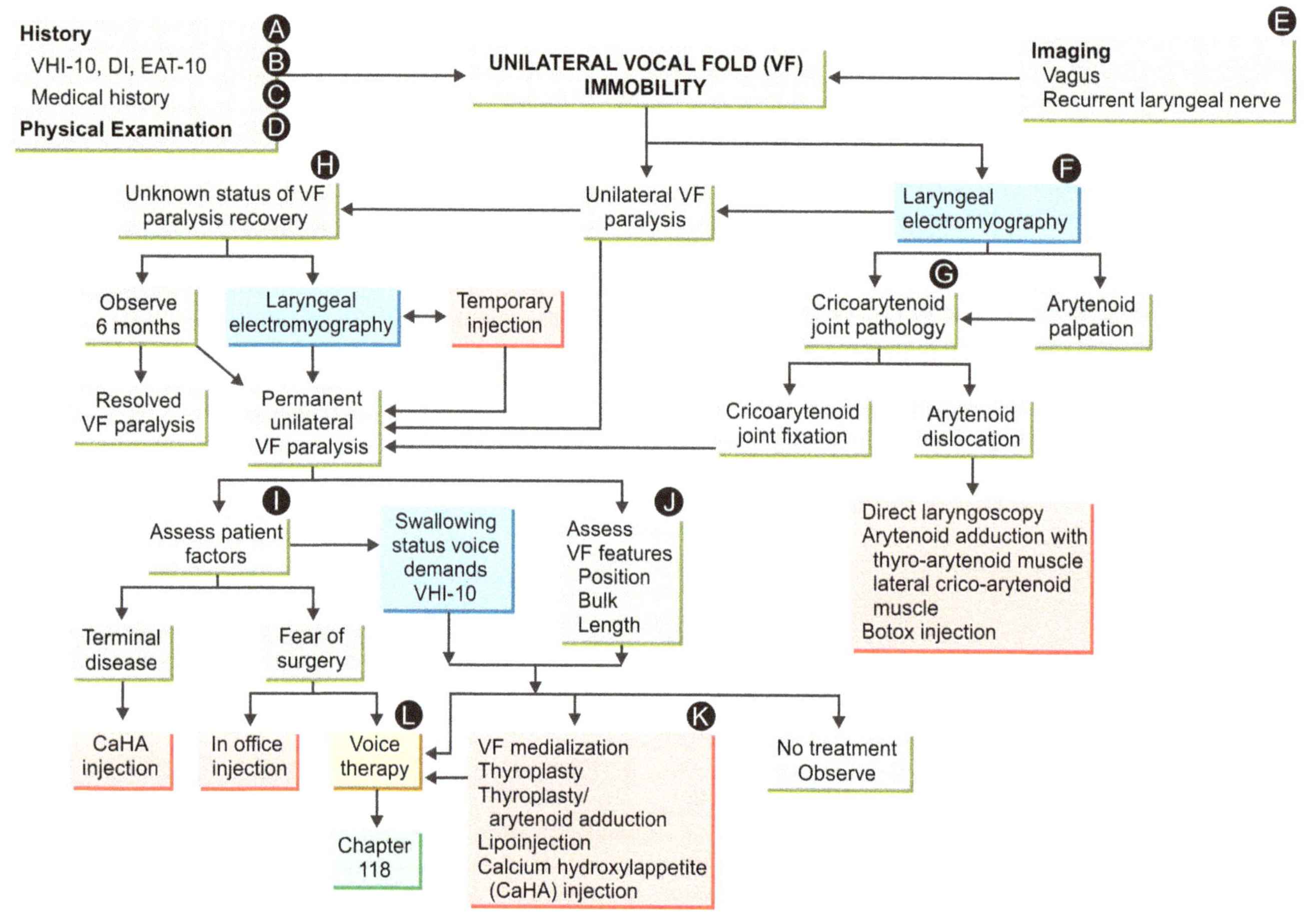

Unilateral vocal cord paralysis is usually apparent from the characteristic breathy voice. The symptom mandates laryngoscopy, and once confirmed, a search for the etiology. Laryngeal electromyography (LEMG) is valuable in diagnosis and prognostication. A wide range of interventions are feasible.

A Dysphonia associated with a unilateral vocal fold paralysis (UVFP) is usually a breathy, rough, raspy voice. Patients may notice that they are short of breath, "run out of air" when talking or experience vocal fatigue. Symptom onset may correlate with surgeries or respiratory infections. Other common complaints include weak cough, increased mucous, and/or choking while drinking liquids.

B The Voice Handicap Index-10 (VHI-10) is a standardized outcome measure that quantifies the patient's perception of vocal handicap. This is a useful, simple 10-question survey that quantifies the impact of the voice problem according to the patient's perception. The Eating Assessment Tool-10 (EAT-10) and Dyspnea Index (DI) are also validated questionnaires, which can help quantify the level of dysphagia and shortness of breath experienced by these patients.

C Over 50% of cases of UVFP are iatrogenic in nature. Therefore, a detailed surgical history involving the head, neck, chest, and any intubations, should be obtained. Medical history should include smoking and alcohol as risk factors for head and neck, esophageal, and lung cancer that can present with UVFP. In addition, it is important to note medications, history of reflux laryngitis, anticoagulation status, and overall health, with respect to tolerating surgical interventions as part of the treatment for UVFP.

D Physical evaluation of a person with UVFP should include a complete examination of the head and neck, including the otologic inspection and cranial nerve examination to rule out a glomus or skull base tumor. A thorough examination of the aerodigestive tract should be performed to rule out a mucosal cancer. Laryngeal examination can be done in a variety of ways (Step J).

E Imaging is indicated if the etiology of UVFP is not obvious—patients with new onset UVFP following surgery near the recurrent laryngeal or vagus nerve do not need imaging. Computed tomography (CT) of the neck with contrast is the most cost-effective initial imaging for workup of UVFP with similar efficacy to magnetic resonance imaging. The entire course of the vagus and recurrent laryngeal nerves should be included. This extends from the skull base through the arch of the aorta for left-sided UVFP and to the apex of the lung on for right-sided UVFP. Signs of UVFP on CT include ipsilateral piriform sinus dilatation, medial rotation of the aryepiglottic fold, ipsilateral laryngeal ventricle dilatation, and anteromedial displacement of the arytenoid cartilage.

F Laryngeal electromyography is the most accurate method of differentiating between a unilateral vocal fold paralysis and cricoarytenoid joint disease. This technique is done percutaneously and studies the thyroarytenoid-lateral cricoarytenoid muscle complex during phonation and Valsalva maneuvers. Prognostic information can also be obtained, which can help to determine the timing and method of intervention (see Step H). For instance, in the presence of neural degeneration, definitive surgery can be confidently undertaken at an earlier stage (4–6 months since onset), thereby shortening the voice rehabilitation process. There is rarely an indication for LEMG after 6 months of UVFP and the optimal time for determining UVFP prognosis from LEMG is most likely between 1.5 and 5 months since the onset of the UVFP.

G The differential diagnosis of vocal fold immobility that is caused by cricoarytenoid joint pathology is either an arytenoid dislocation or cricoarytenoid joint fixation. A cricoarytenoid joint dislocation typically is associated with either orotracheal intubation or laryngoscopy trauma or blunt trauma to the neck. Cricoarytenoid joint fixation is rare; however, it usually occurs from a severe arthritic process, especially rheumatoid arthritis.

H Decision-making regarding the treatment of a person with a UVFP with an unknown status for spontaneous recovery is based on the results of the laryngeal examination, LEMG, and the patient's needs and desires. In cases of unclear prognosis, observation only or temporary augmentation (collagen, hyaluronic acid gel, or carboxymethylcellulose) is the treatment of choice. While these are believed to last between months 2 and 3, depending on the substance used, clinical effects may last longer. Earlier timing of injection is shown to improve patient voice outcome in many and, in some cases of permanent paralysis, eliminating the need for laryngeal framework surgery.

I Patient factors play a significant role in deciding the treatment options for permanent UVFP. This involves the determination of patients' current quality of life with their present dysphonia, voice demands, and expectations. While treatment based on voice handicap is elective, more urgent intervention is needed in the presence of dysphagia leading to aspiration. With the advent of distal chip scopes allowing for high-resolution imaging, in-office vocal fold injections under local anesthetic is an attractive alternative to direct laryngoscopy, especially for patients medically unstable for general anesthesia or those with iatrogenic UVFP weary of repeat surgery.

J Vocal fold features that should be included in the decision-making process for the different treatment options of permanent UVFP include the vocal fold position, length, and bulk. These can be addressed by different treatment modalities (see Step K).

K Multiple methods can be used to successfully medialize a unilateral paralyzed vocal fold. Medialization laryngoplasty is a common method of medialization. However, this technique only corrects the vocal fold position and the bulk deficit associated with UVFP. It does not address the shortened aspect of the paralyzed vocal fold, if present. For this reason, many surgeons combine medialization laryngoplasty and an operation on the arytenoid, usually arytenoid adduction, to position the paralyzed vocal fold optimally. At present, combined medialization laryngoplasty and arytenoid adduction is the surgical treatment of choice for UVFP. Lipoinjection of the vocal fold is an excellent choice for patients who have a paralyzed vocal fold in the median and paramedian position and have good length. This procedure has the advantage of being completely autologous as well as not requiring an external neck incision. It can also be used in conjunction with framework surgery. In those patients wishing to avoid open surgery, in-office injections with a durable substance (i.e. calcium hydroxylapatite) that can last up to 1–2 years can help.

L Voice therapy can be used as primary treatment when the paralyzed VF is relatively close to midline or postoperatively to maximize the patient's vocal recovery. Voice therapy for vocal fold paralysis is typically of limited duration (four to six sessions). Voice therapy will address reducing maladaptive compensatory behavior (secondary muscle tension dysphonia), improved use of respiration for phonation, and optimizing the vocal environment to adapt to the softer, weaker voice associated with vocal fold paralysis.

SUGGESTED READING

Carroll TL, Rosen CA. Long-term results of calcium hydroxylapatite for vocal fold augmentation. Laryngoscope. 2011;121(2):313-319.

Gartner-Schmidt JL, Shembel AC, Zullo TG, et al. Development and validation of the dyspnea index (di): a severity-index for upper airway-related dyspnea. J Voice. 2014;28(6):775-782.

Ingle JW, Young VN, Smith LJ, et al. Prospective evaluation of the clinical utility of laryngeal electromyography. Laryngoscope. 2014;124(12):2745-2749.

Mallur PS, Rosen CA. Vocal fold injection: review of indications, techniques, and materials for augmentation. Clin Exp Otorhinolaryngol. 2010;3(4):177-182.

Prendes BL, Yung KC, Likhterov I, et al. Long-term effects of injection laryngoplasty with a temporary agent on voice quality and vocal fold position. Laryngoscope. 2012;122(10):2227-2233.

Rosen CA, Mau T, Remacle M, et al. Nomenclature proposal to describe vocal fold motion impairment. Eur Arch Otorhinolaryngol. 2016;273(8):1995-1999.

Bilateral Vocal Fold Immobility

VyVy N Young, Clark A Rosen

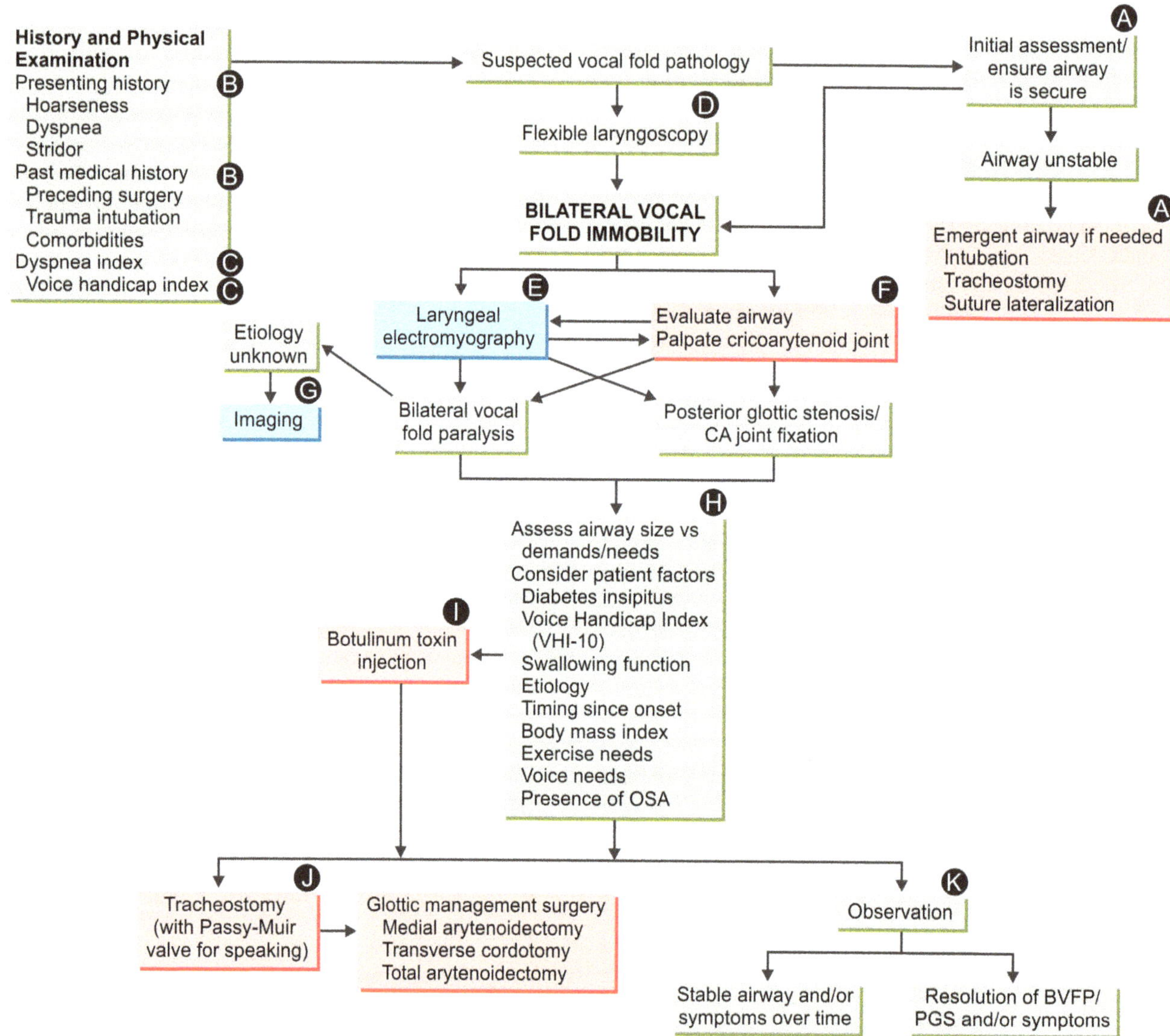

Bilateral vocal fold immobility (BVFI) has an underlying neurologic or mechanical etiology. Differentiating bilateral vocal fold paralysis from posterior glottic stenosis (PGS) or cricoarytenoid (CA) joint dysfunction has important implications in the treatment algorithm, especially related to timing of intervention(s). Patients with BVFI have varying degrees of symptoms and need for treatment and should be assessed on an individualized basis. However, securing the airway remains the highest treatment priority.

A Patients with BVFI may present with acute or chronic symptoms, including hoarseness/aphonia, aspiration, dyspnea, or stridor. It is essential to evaluate immediately if the airway is at risk. Urgent intervention to temporarily secure the airway (e.g. endotracheal intubation,

cricothyrotomy, or tracheostomy) may be required. If bilateral vocal fold paralysis is known (e.g. known referral, pre-existing condition), suture lateralization may be used as a temporizing measure. This procedure is generally contraindicated in cases of mechanical fixation and/ or mucosal erosion in the posterior commissure (e.g. following recent intubation).

B Presenting history will provide important information about the underlying etiology and will influence both the timing and nature of surgical intervention. The circumstances surrounding symptom onset (e.g. preceding surgery, trauma, intubation, or illness) as well as duration and severity of symptoms should be noted. Comorbidities such as anticoagulation status, baseline cardiopulmonary status, obstructive sleep apnea (OSA), body mass index (BMI), and history of tobacco use may impact patient's candidacy for surgical intervention.

C The Voice Handicap Index-10 (VHI-10) and Dyspnea Index (DI) are validated 10-item questionnaires assessing patient's perception of voice handicap and symptoms of upper airway related dyspnea, respectively.

D Complete head and neck examination should identify signs of recent surgery (e.g. incisions, scars) or malignancy (e.g. lymphadenopathy). Note signs of patient distress including stridor, positioning (i.e. sniffing), drooling, accessory muscle use, and/or decreased oxygen saturations. Laryngeal examination via flexible laryngoscopy [particularly with alternating sniff and phonation (i.e. sustained /i/) maneuvers] is critical to verify BVFI diagnosis. Transnasal flexible laryngoscopy is superior to peroral mirror exam or Hopkin's rod rigid laryngoscopy to assess vocal fold motion status.

E Laryngeal electromyography (LEMG) (*see also* Chapter 124) can differentiate between a neurologic (e.g. paralysis) or mechanical (e.g. PGS, CA joint dysfunction) cause of BVFI. LEMG may provide useful information regarding prognosis for spontaneous recovery of vocal fold motion, guiding decisions about appropriate timing and side (i.e. lesser degree of appropriate re-innervation) for destructive glottic enlargement surgery (GES).

F Endoscopic airway evaluation allows direct visualization of anatomic abnormalities and may be performed under local or general anesthesia. For otolaryngologists who are experienced in performing laryngeal intervention under local anesthesia, the ability to evaluate the airway in the office in this way allows immediate examination, can be efficient and cost-effective, and may facilitate decision-making regarding next step in treatment. The CA joints can be palpated, and the posterior glottis can be more thoroughly examined for PGS. In addition, evaluation of the lower airway to rule out concurrent anatomic abnormalities (e.g. subglottic or tracheal stenosis, or laryngotracheomalacia) may also be performed. However, it is important to beware the possibility of laryngospasm (with risk of airway compromise) resulting from airway manipulation in this situation.

G If the history does not provide adequate explanation for BVFI, then imaging such as CT or MRI may be useful. Similar to unilateral vocal fold immobility, as discussed in Chapter 124, imaging should encompass the entire course of the vagus and recurrent laryngeal nerves on either side. In most cases, neurogenic etiology is clear from the history, and for mechanical etiology, imaging is rarely indicated or helpful.

H Decision about next step in treatment varies based on patient's symptoms and exam findings. Factors to consider include airway size and associated symptoms, timing since symptom onset, etiology, voice and exercise needs, dysphagia, BMI, and underlying pulmonary disease. Patients with OSA are more likely to require additional intervention, including supplemental oxygen, continuous positive airway pressure (CPAP), or surgery; however, CPAP may be less effective in the presence of a fixed obstruction at the level of the glottis.

I Injection of botulinum toxin into one or both vocal fold(s) may provide some degree of temporary symptom relief. This may be helpful in patients who refuse tracheostomy. Botulinum toxin injection may be useful in the short-term, but is not a good option for long-term management of BVFI.

J If there is concern for airway compromise (e.g. symptomatic stridor, significant oxygen desaturations, or cyanosis) and the airway cannot be easily secured with endotracheal intubation, then a surgical airway such as tracheostomy should be considered. Some patients may choose permanent tracheostomy (with or without Passy Muir valve) for management of their airway. This strategy is often preferred in patients who wish to avoid change to their voice, as would occur from GES, or for those who are unlikely to be decannulated following GES due to significant OSA or underlying pulmonary disease.

K Observation with serial airway examinations may be appropriate in carefully selected patients. Factors to consider include patient symptomatology, airway size, patient and otolaryngologist comfort level, patient reliability and/or proximity to the hospital, and availability of emergency/difficult airway equipment and personnel. Timing of onset of symptoms is also an important consideration as patients with acute onset of symptoms will likely require higher degree of scrutiny than those with longstanding, potentially stable symptoms. Appropriate monitoring (e.g. pulse oximetry, monitored or ICU setting) should be utilized whenever available, especially in the acute setting. Over time, patients may develop stable symptoms and/or airway size or experience resolution of BVFI (and thus, no intervention may be required) or their symptoms may progress (necessitating temporary or permanent surgical intervention).

SUGGESTED READING

Ingle JW, Young VN, Smith LJ, et al. Prospective evaluation of the clinical utility of laryngeal electromyography. Laryngoscope. 2014;124(12):2745-2749.

Krishna P, Rosen CA. Office-based arytenoid palpation for diagnosis of disorders of bilateral vocal fold immobility. Ear Nose Throat J. 2006;85(8):520-522.

Lichtenberger G, Toohill RJ. Technique of endo-extralaryngeal suture lateralization for bilateral abductor vocal cord paralysis. Laryngoscope. 1997;107(9):1281-1283.

Rosen CA, Simpson CB. Bilateral vocal fold paralysis. In: Operative Techniques in Laryngology. 1st ed. New York, NY: Springer; 2008. pp. 168-173.

Young VN, Rosen CA. Arytenoid and posterior vocal fold surgery for bilateral vocal fold immobility. Curr Opin Otolaryngol Head Neck Surg. 2011;19(6):422-427.

Neonatal Vocal Fold Paralysis

Adrienne L Childers, Jay Werkhaven

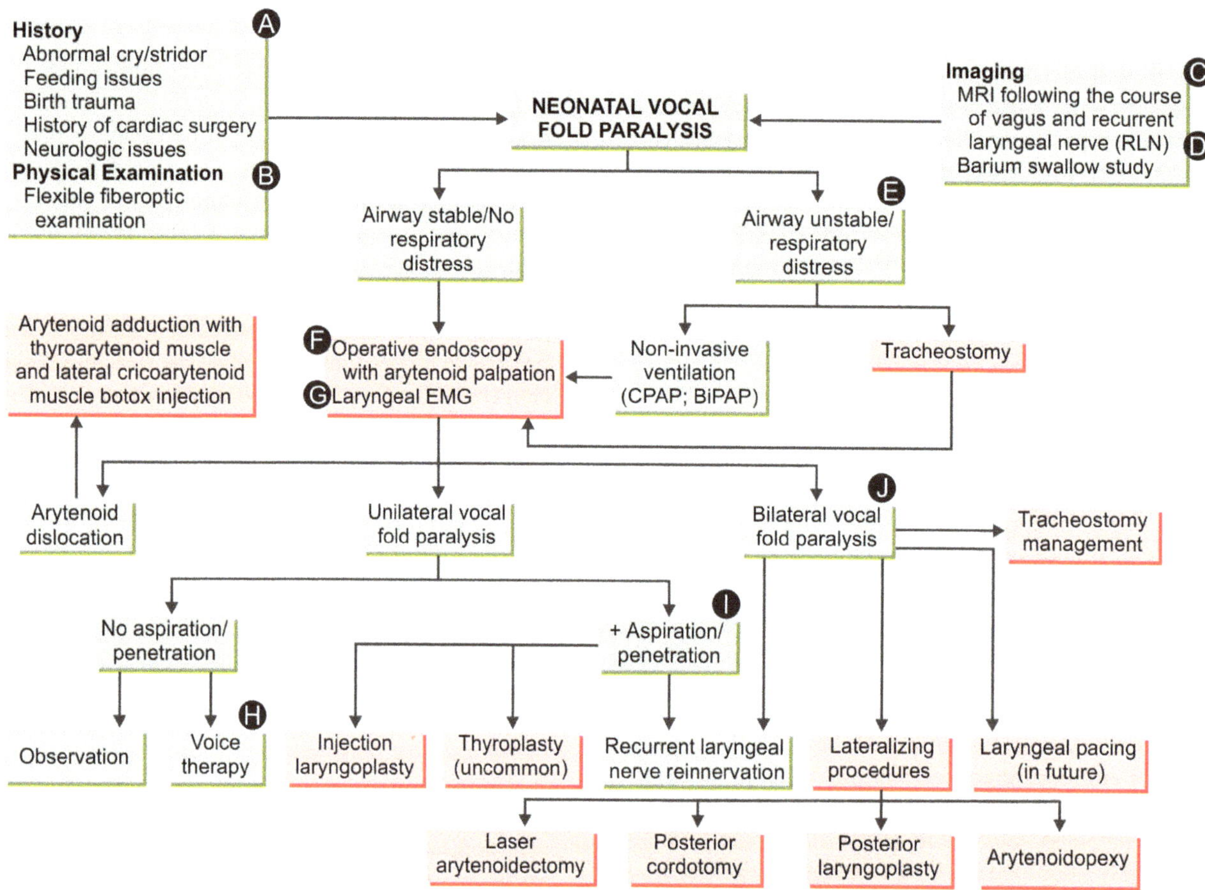

Vocal fold paralysis in the neonate is a unique entity as the etiology is varied and often idiopathic. The diagnostic pathway is focused on management of airway and feeding issues. Surgical interventions are tailored to the patient but are often not indicated with unilateral involvement. Bilateral vocal fold paralysis requires immediate airway evaluation, and it has been reported that >65% require tracheostomy during the course of treatment.

A Medical history of neonates with vocal fold paralysis (unilateral or bilateral) can be highly variable with the most common symptoms being respiratory distress, stridor, abnormal cry, and feeding difficulties. Etiologies include idiopathic, previous cardiac surgery, birth trauma, and neurologic conditions (Chiari malformation, hydrocephalus).

B Physical examination and evaluation should include a complete examination of the head and neck, including a flexible fiberoptic evaluation of the larynx in order to determine whether one or both vocal folds are involved.

C Imaging of the path of the vagus and recurrent laryngeal nerve (RLN) is important when the cause for the vocal fold paralysis is unknown. When the paralysis is on the left side, the imaging should be done from the exit of the vagus nerve from the brainstem (skull base) through the midchest to evaluate the RLN as it wraps around the arch of the aorta and returns cephalad in the tracheoesophageal groove. For a right vocal fold paralysis, the imaging should extend from the base of the skull to the upper lobe of the right lung.

D In the neonate presenting with dysphagia, it is also important to evaluate swallowing function with a modified barium swallow study once the airway has been deemed stable. If a child has evidence of aspiration and/or penetration this will direct future management (discussed in steps G and I).

E Airway stability will be evident on initial clinical evaluation and may require surgical intervention in the form of tracheostomy tube placement. This is typically reserved for patients with bilateral vocal fold paralysis who have failed conservative medical management.

F Operative endoscopy with palpation of the arytenoid complex is generally indicated to further delineate possible anatomic etiology and for thorough laryngeal evaluation. This is performed under mask ventilation with spontaneous respiration to allow for unimpeded view of the larynx, subglottis, and lower airway structures.

G Laryngeal electromyography (LEMG) is the most accurate method of differentiating between a vocal fold paralysis and cricoarytenoid joint disease. A neuropathy associated with paralysis can be identified, and then definitive diagnosis of the vocal fold paralysis is made. An important consideration in the neonatal population is that this must be obtained under general anesthesia when the patient is unable to cooperate with cued phonation.

H In most causes of neonatal unilateral vocal fold paralysis, observation is the mainstay of treatment as spontaneous resolution can be seen up to 4 years of age. In asymptomatic children, no surgical intervention is recommended. In older children who are able to participate, voice therapy can be a useful adjunctive tool for rehabilitation.

I Neonates who have evidence of aspiration/penetration on swallow evaluation and failure to thrive can be offered several treatment modalities. The most common is injection laryngoplasty using various materials including Gelfoam, collagen, and calcium hydroxylapatite. The option of surgical treatment in the pediatric population is RLN reinnervation with ansa-RLN anastomosis. This procedure has had good results in early reports but may be reserved for older children as it removes opportunity for possible spontaneous recovery. Thyroplasty is an uncommon procedure in neonates. During any vocal fold augmentation in pediatrics, the size of the airway must be considered as small changes in the glottic aperture can have significant ramifications on the respiratory stability of the child postoperatively.

J In neonates with bilateral vocal fold paralysis, the number one goal of therapy is to stabilize/secure the airway. Spontaneous resolution of paralysis has been noted to occur within weeks to up to 11 years of age, more commonly associated with an idiopathic rather than a neurologic etiology. In select patients, the use of noninvasive positive pressure airway support may alleviate the need for surgical intervention. Endoscopic techniques that may improve the quality of laryngeal patency include lateralizing procedures (see list on algorithm for more specific details), RLN reinnervation and possibly in the future, laryngeal pacing. Lateralizing procedures should not be performed in cases with overt aspiration on swallow evaluation as these will likely exacerbate the issue. Also note that voice quality is typically worsened subsequent to tissue resection. Placement of a tracheostomy tube generally occurs at around 3 months of age in those requiring this intervention. Many patients with bilateral involvement will also have airway comorbidities necessitating more aggressive surgical therapy with more protracted course toward decannulation. In children requiring tracheostomy tube placement initially, continued management with routine care and surveillance endoscopy should be performed with the ultimate goal of decannulation once the laryngeal issues are managed effectively.

SUGGESTED READING

Butskiy O, Mistry B, Chadha NK. Surgical interventions for pediatric unilateral vocal cord paralysis: a systematic review. JAMA Otolaryngol Head Neck Surg. 2015;141(7):654-660.

Daya H, Hosni A, Bejar-Solar I, et al. Pediatric vocal fold paralysis: a long-term retrospective study. Arch Otolaryngol Head Neck Surg. 2000;126(1):21-25.

Funk RT, Jabbour J, Robey T. Factors associated with tracheostomy and decannulation in pediatric bilateral vocal fold immobility. Int J Pediatr Otorhinolaryngol. 2015;79:895-899.

Jabbour J, Martin T, Beste D, et al. Pediatric vocal fold immobility: natural history and the need for long-term follow-up. JAMA Otolaryngol Head Neck Surg. 2014;140(5):429-433.

Sipp JA, Kerschner JE, Braune N, et al. Vocal fold medialization in children: injection laryngoplasty, thyroplasty or nerve reinnervation? Arch Otolaryngol Head Neck Surg. 2007;133(8):767-771.

Vocal Cord Dysfunction

Raymond Maguire

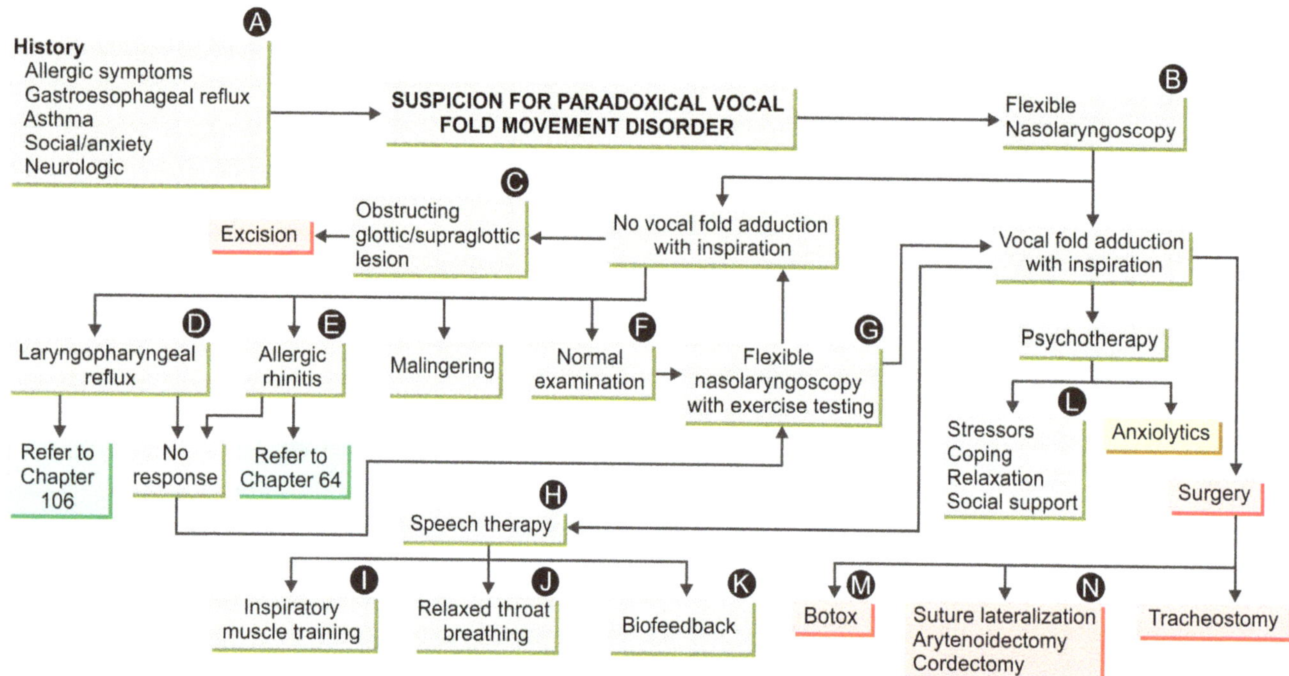

Paradoxical vocal fold movement disorder is a voice disorder in which there is adduction of the vocal folds during inspiration. These episodes occur with differing frequencies and are often seen in the setting of intense physical exertion. The onset is sudden and heralded by inspiratory stridor that usually rapidly subsides with rest or separation from the stimulus.

A The diagnosis of paradoxical vocal fold movement disorder is primarily reached with a thorough history. In the patient interview it is important to review symptoms relating to potential causes of laryngeal irritation such as environmental allergies, gastroesophageal/laryngopharyngeal reflux, underlying asthma, neurological disease, as well as any psychosocial stressors.

B Visualization of the larynx is essential in the diagnosis of paradoxical vocal fold movement disorder and endoscopic evidence of vocal fold adduction during inspiration is the gold standard for the diagnosis of paradoxical vocal fold movement disorder.

C Endoscopic examination of the supraglottic airway may reveal obstructing lesions or dynamic collapse of the pharyngeal/hypopharyngeal tissue that may be corrected with surgery.

D Laryngopharyngeal reflux may be revealed during laryngoscopy as sulcus vocalis and laryngeal edema. Appropriate treatment of laryngopharyngeal reflux is necessary in successful management of paradoxical vocal fold movement disorder.

E Nasal congestion and mucopurulent exudate secondary to allergic rhinitis can be evident upon nasolaryngoscopy. The subsequent mouth breathing and failure of inspired air to be properly filtered, humidified and warmed through the nasal cavity precipitate episodes of paradoxical vocal fold movement disorder.

F When the flexible nasolaryngoscopic examination is negative and the history is suggestive of paradoxical vocal fold movement disorder then performing an endoscopic examination in conjunction with exercise testing (if exercise is the trigger) should be considered.

G Flexible nasolaryngoscopy with exercise-induced asthma testing is a method of confirming the diagnosis of paradoxical vocal fold movement disorder as well as identifying any co-existing exercise-induced bronchospasm. During this study, the patient will undergo a known stimulus to an episode, usually intense physical exertion simulated by running as per modified Bruce protocol on the treadmill. While running they are connected to a mouthpiece measuring flow/volume loops. Attenuation or "flattening" of the inspiratory phase of respiration is suggestive of paradoxical vocal fold movement disorder. During or immediately following the test (when their symptoms develop) flexible nasolaryngoscopy is performed to visualize the larynx and confirm the diagnosis.

H Speech therapy is the basis for the treatment of paradoxical vocal fold movement disorder and is aimed at analyzing the situations in which episodes occur and modifying behaviors that encourage normal laryngeal function.

I Inspiratory muscle training is a method of treatment for paradoxical vocal fold movement disorder in which the patient performs exercises inspiring through a mouth piece that adds resistance to airflow. The muscles of respiration (diaphragm and accessory muscles) are thereby strengthened, reducing the patient's discomfort during episodes.

J Relaxed throat breathing consists of many techniques aimed at restoring normal vocal fold function by encouraging relaxation of the intrinsic and extrinsic laryngeal muscles.

K Biofeedback empowers patients to learn about their disorder with visual reinforcement (via the endoscope monitor) so that they may make appropriate interventions and gain immediate visual feedback to the result of therapy and reassurance of airway patency.

L Many patients have psychosocial stressors that precipitate episodes. Development of open communication and initiation of therapy aimed at coping with these stressors is essential. Paradoxical vocal fold movement disorder is also anxiety provoking and recognition of this is crucial in the successful treatment of these individuals.

M Recalcitrant cases may be treated in a variety of minimally invasive ways. Botox may be used to temporarily weaken the thyroarytenoid muscles especially in patients with severe symptoms who are unable to participate in therapy. The temporary effect of the botulinum toxin can allow time for other therapies to become effective.

N In situations where more permanent adduction of the vocal folds is desired endoscopic procedures may be considered although are less desirable due to the destructive nature of the surgeries.

SUGGESTED READING

Brøndbo K. Paradoxical vocal cord movement in newborn and congenital idiopathic vocal cord paralysis: two of a kind? Eur Arch Otorhinolaryngol. 2008;265:803-807.

Franca MC. Differential diagnosis in paradoxical vocal fold movement (PVFM): an interdisciplinary task. Int J Pediatr Otorhinolaryngol. 2014;78:2169-2173.

Ibrahim WH, Gheriani HA, Almohamed AA, et al. Paradoxical vocal cord motion disorder: past, present and future. Postgrad Med J. 2007;83(977):164-172.

Maturo S, Hill C, Bunting G, et al. Pediatric paradoxical vocal-fold motion: presentation and natural history. Pediatrics. 2011; 128(6):e1443-1449.

Morrison M, Rammage L, Emami AJ. The irritable larynx syndrome. J Voice. 1999;13(3):447-455.

Powell DM, Karanfilov BI, Beechler KB, et al. Paradoxical vocal cord dysfunction in juveniles. Arch Otolaryngol Head Neck Surg. 2000;126:29-34.

Sandage MJ, Zelazny SK. Paradoxical vocal fold motion in children and adolescents. Lang Speech Hear Serv Sch. 2004;35:353-362.

Vasudev M. Evaluation of paradoxical vocal fold motion. Ann Allergy Asthma Immunol. 2012;109:233-236.

Laryngeal Trauma

Ricardo L Carrau

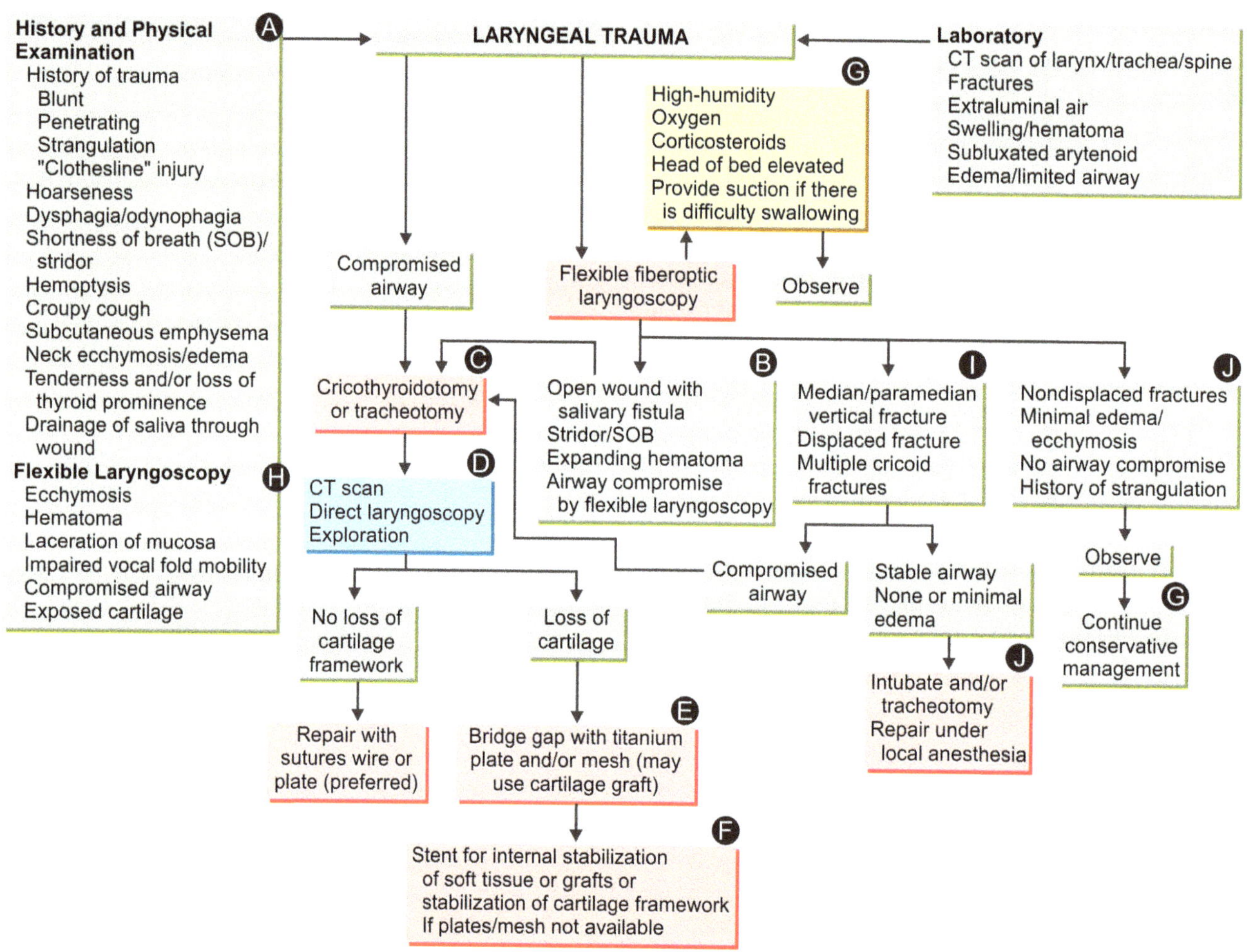

Laryngeal fractures are rare occurring in 1/30,000–1/5,000 emergency room visits and accounting for <1% of all blunt trauma and <5% of penetrating trauma. In developed countries, where the use of seat belts and airbags is mandatory, the most common mechanisms for the trauma are sports and acts of violence. It is important to note that a significant number of these injuries will be associated with trauma to the surrounding structures (i.e. esophagus, c-spine, and great vessels of the neck).

Laryngeal fractures inherently pose a major risk to the affected patient due to their propensity to lead to sudden, or progressive airway obstruction. Failure to recognize and manage these fractures can lead to the death of the patient, or at the very least, long-term tracheostomy dependence and/or severe voice disorders.

Ⓐ Patients with a history of trauma to the neck and those presenting with any of the listed signs or symptoms should be suspected to have suffered significant trauma to the larynx.

Ⓑ An emergency tracheostomy or cricothyroidotomy is indicated in patients presenting with clinical evidence of severe trauma to the neck, such as that associated with damage to neurovascular structures, and those presenting with airway compromise.

Ⓒ A cricothyroidotomy is safer and faster than a tracheostomy in an emergency situation, especially when performed by less experienced surgeons; however, patients with a history of a "clothesline" injury should be suspected to have suffered a laryngotracheal separation, for which a tracheostomy is a preferable option.

Ⓓ After the airway is secured, the patient can be evaluated with direct laryngoscopy and exploration. Patients with a C-spine injury or patients in whom a spine injury cannot be ruled out should not have their neck extended; thus, a direct laryngoscopy is contraindicated. A flexible laryngoscopy and videolaryngoscopy are reasonable alternatives in this clinical situation.

E In patients with severe disruption, comminution or loss of cartilage, titanium plates or mesh provide the best means to stabilize and reconstruct the laryngeal cartilaginous framework. Fractures that are not associated with loss of cartilage can be reduced and fixated with a variety of techniques using wires, sutures, a combination of these (with or without battens), or using adaptation plates. Adaptation plating is advantageous as it provides immediate stabilization of the framework and avoids the use of an internal stent.

F An internal stent is recommended to stabilize and bolster avulsed or severely lacerated soft tissue, or mucosal grafts. Stenting may also provide additional stability for cartilage to heal in proper position if adaptation plates or titanium mesh are not available.

G Patients without significant airway compromise should be provided with high-humidity air via facial mask. The head of the bed is elevated to reduce edema and help with the control of oral secretions. Patients with difficulty swallowing are provided with an oropharyngeal suction tip to better dispose of oral and pharyngeal secretions. Systemic corticosteroids can be used to further prevent ensuing edema of the laryngeal airway.

H A flexible laryngoscopy should be performed urgently to identify signs of endolaryngeal trauma or impending airway compromise that may not be detectable clinically. If deemed to have a stable and adequate airway, the patient can be transferred to the radiology suite for a high-resolution computed tomography of the larynx, trachea, and c-spine. If deemed to have significant fractures or if airway compromise develops, the patient is managed as described in steps C through F.

I Those patients who require surgical repair of laryngotracheal fractures but present minimal or no edema of the airway, can be safely intubated. This should only be performed in the presence of an experienced team with the ability and resources to either intubate or obtain a surgical airway, and when adequate monitoring facilities are available. A tracheostomy, however, is a safer option for most patients, especially if adequate monitoring facilities are not available. Select patients with median or paramedian thyroid cartilage fractures and minimal endolaryngeal edema may undergo repair using a wide-field block and sedation, with a surgical exposure similar to that described for a thyroplasty. The repair follows the concepts described in steps B through F.

J Patients with nondisplaced fractures that do not involve the median, upper, or paramedian area and who have no airway compromise are admitted to a monitored unit and observed for 24–48 hours. Treatment as described in step G is continued during observation.

SUGGESTED READING

Becker M, Leuchter I, Platon A, et al. Imaging of laryngeal trauma. Eur J Radiol. 2014;83(1):142-154.

Bent JP III, Porubsky ES. The management of blunt fractures of the thyroid cartilage. Otolaryngol Head Neck Surg. 1994;110:195-202.

de Mello-Filho FV, Carrau RL. The management of laryngeal fractures using internal fixation. Laryngoscope. 2000;110(12): 2143-2146.

Jewett BS, Shockley WW, Rutledge R. External laryngeal trauma analysis of 392 patients. Arch Otolaryngol Head Neck Surg. 1999;125:877-890.

Juutilainen M, Vintturi J, Robinson S, et al. Laryngeal fractures: clinical findings and considerations on suboptimal outcome. Acta Otolaryngol. 2008;128(2):213-218.

Kim JP, Cho SJ, Son HY, et al. Analysis of clinical feature and management of laryngeal fracture: recent 22 case review. Yonsei Med J. 2012;53(5):992-998.

Lykins CL, Pinczower EF. The comparative strength of laryngeal fracture fixation. Am J Otolaryngol. 1998;19:158-162.

Schaefer SD. Management of acute blunt and penetrating external laryngeal trauma. Laryngoscope. 2014;124(1):233-244.

Stanley RB, Cooper DS, Florman SH. Phonatory effects of thyroid cartilage fractures. Ann Otol Rhinol Laryngol. 1987;96:493-496.

Laryngotracheal Stenosis

Deepak Mehta

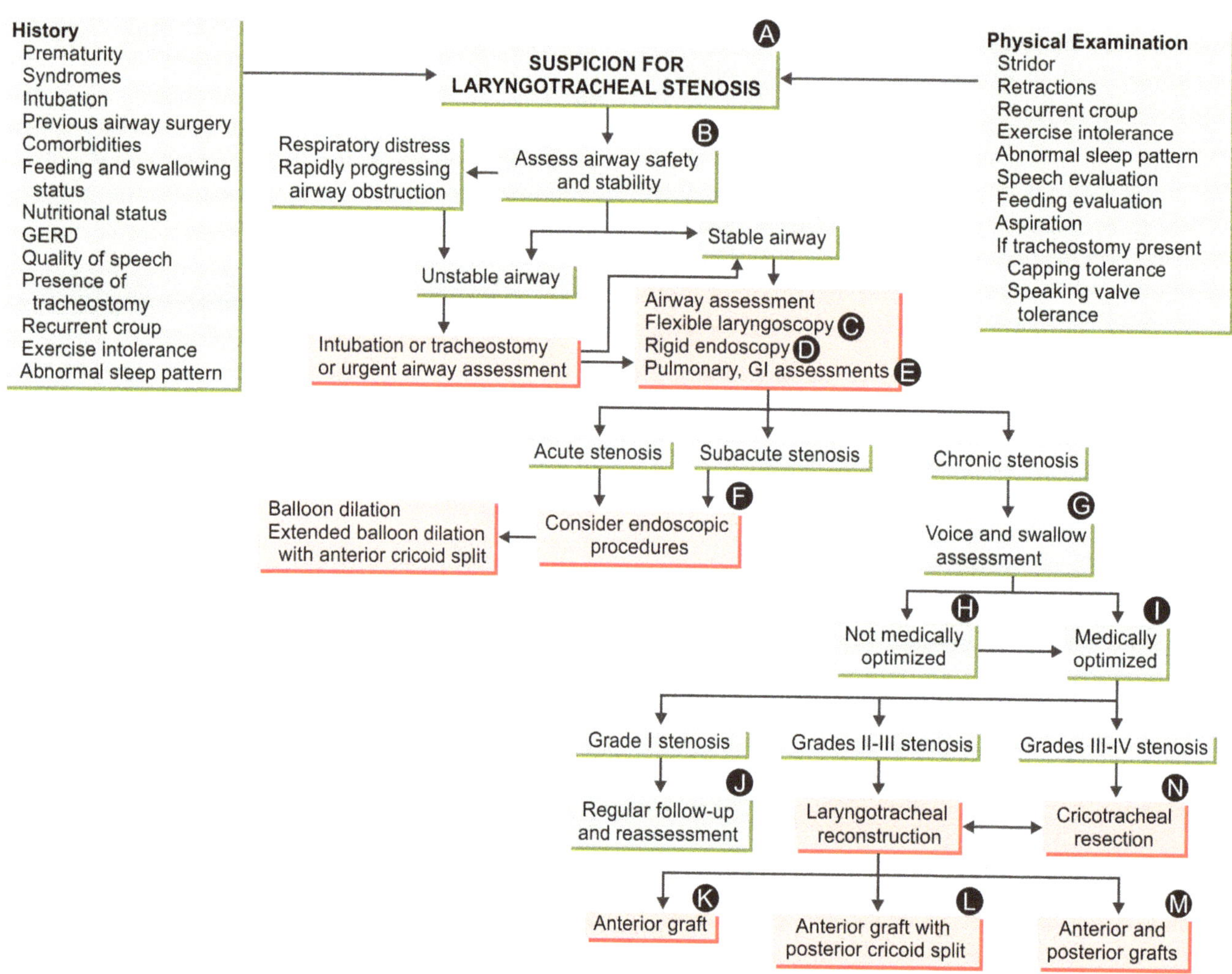

Pediatric patient laryngotracheal stenosis in the can be broadly classified as congenital or acquired, with severity ranging from asymptomatic to complete airway obstruction and tracheostomy dependent. Appropriate patient selection is critical when planning laryngotracheal surgery and treatment should be individualized.

A A complete history and physical examination will guide the diagnosis and management of the patient with laryngotracheal stenosis.

B Assessing the safety and stability of the airway is the first step in managing the patient with suspected laryngotracheal stenosis. A child in respiratory distress or one with rapidly progressing airway obstruction requires immediate intervention; intubation or tracheostomy may be necessary.

C Endoscopic airway evaluation confirms the diagnosis of laryngotracheal stenosis and provides objective information needed for further management. Flexible laryngoscopy can demonstrate glossoptosis, vocal cord dysmotility, as well as dynamic conditions such as upper airway collapse and laryngomalacia.

D Rigid endoscopy allows for direct visualization of the stenotic segment. Special attention should be paid to the level(s), length, and quality of the stenosis. Airway sizing can be performed using the Myer-Cotton staging system. The surgeon should look for secondary lesions such as tracheobronchomalacia, as well as any signs of ongoing inflammation that could impact a surgical repair.

E Evaluating for concurrent pulmonary and gastrointestinal disease is an important part of the initial assessment. In some cases, it may be appropriate to perform the airway endoscopy in coordination with the pulmonary and gastrointestinal services. A key aspect in managing patients with airway stenosis is identifying and managing medical comorbidities.

F Acute and soft subacute stenoses may be amenable to early intervention, particularly endoscopic procedures. An acute stenosis typically consists of soft granulation tissue or immature scar. Early intervention with balloon dilation or extended balloon dilation with anterior cricoid split may be options. Endoscopic procedures have the advantage of being minimally invasive and do not preclude future open procedures. Less symptomatic patients may respond to medical management with control of inflammatory diseases. Early intervention may prevent progression to firm and fixed scar tissue.

G Patients with chronic stenosis should be assessed for voice, swallowing, and sleep patterns. These can be the indicators of the patient's candidacy for surgery/decannulation.

H In patients with higher-grade stenoses, intervention depends on the patient's medical status. It is important to control ongoing inflammation prior to considering definitive surgery, particularly open or graft procedures, to maximize success and prevent restenosis. Consider conditions such as aspiration, laryngopharyngeal reflux, eosinophilic esophagitis, and bacterial colonization. Screening for methicillin-resistant *Staphylococcus aureus* can be done with a triple swab (nose, tracheostoma, and anus) at the time of rigid endoscopy. Staph carriers can be treated with perioperative antibiotics to prevent graft infection and failure. Medical comorbidities, particularly cardiopulmonary status, should be optimized before considering reconstructive procedures. The goals of treatment should be clearly defined. Is decannulation an achievable endpoint? Having realistic goals and choosing the appropriate patient is invaluable in successful management of the patient with laryngotracheal stenosis.

I Once a patient is medically optimized, the family and physician can start to work toward decannulation or surgical planning. Any patient with multilevel airway obstruction should be staged to optimize success. Supraglottoplasty or adenotonsillectomy should be done before definitive repair of stenosis if obstruction is significant. Patients should be considered individually to determine if single-stage reconstruction or double-stage reconstruction is indicated.

J Patients with grade I stenosis and mild symptoms can be observed or undergo capping trials for decannulation.

Regular reassessment allows the treating physician to intervene early if the patient becomes more symptomatic. Symptoms may improve with the growth of the child.

K Patients with grade II–III stenosis are often good candidates for expansion procedures. Patients with stenosis on the lower end of this spectrum may be amenable to anterior graft alone.

L Splitting the posterior cricoid in addition to an anterior graft will add a few more millimeters to the airway reconstruction. This is more often used in children of <3 years of age.

M Patients with more severe stenosis are more likely to require both an anterior and a posterior graft to create an acceptable airway lumen. The surgeon should be prepared to change the surgical plan intraoperatively based on airway findings and needs.

N Patients with high-grade stenosis, particularly high grade III or grade IV subglottic stenosis, may have more successful airway results from a cricotracheal resection. Cricotracheal resection is contraindicated for long stenoses or those that are too close to the vocal folds.

SUGGESTED READING

Boardman SJ, Albert DM. Single-stage and multistage pediatric laryngotracheal reconstruction. Otolaryngol Clin North Am. 2008;41:947-958.

De Alarcon A, Rutter MJ. Revision pediatric laryngotracheal reconstruction. Otolaryngol Clin North Am. 2008;41(5):959-980.

Greifer M, Santiago MT, Tsirilakis K, et al. Pediatric patients with chronic cough and recurrent croup: the case for a multidisciplinary approach. Int J Pediatr Otolaryngol. 2015;79(5):749-752.

Gustafson LM, Hartley BE, Liu JH, et al. Single-stage laryngotracheal reconstruction in children: a review of 200 cases. Otolaryngol Head Neck Surg. 2000;123:430-434.

Horn DL, Maguire RC, Simons JP, et al. Endoscopic anterior cricoid split with balloon dilation in infants with failed extubation. Laryngoscope. 2012;122(1):216-219.

McGuirt WF Jr. Gastroesophageal reflux and the upper airway. Pediatr Clin North Am. 2003;50:487-502.

Mirable L, Serio PP, Baggi RR, et al. Endoscopic anterior cricoid split and balloon dilation in pediatric subglottic stenosis. Int J Pediatr Otolaryngol. 2010;74(12):1409-1414.

Yamamoto K, Jaquet Y, Ikonomidis C, et al. Partial cricotracheal resection for paediatric subglottic stenosis: update of the Lausanne experience with 129 cases. Eur J Cardiothorac Surg. 2015;47(5):876-882.

Laryngocele

Cristine Klatt-Cromwell, Trevor Hackman

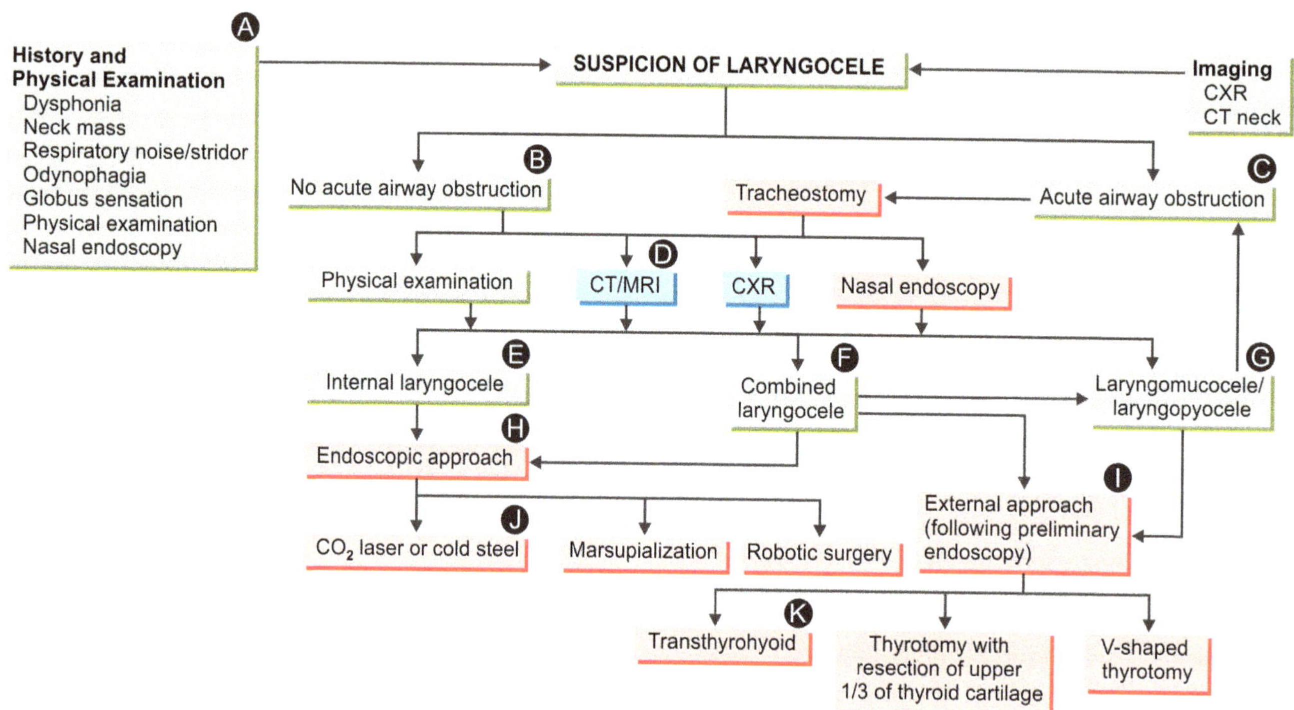

A laryngocele is an abnormal dilation of the laryngeal saccule, the anterior end of the laryngeal ventricle. The dilation extends into the false vocal fold, and is filled with air due to its communication with the laryngeal lumen. Theoretically caused by congenital factors, increased laryngeal pressure, or mechanical obstruction. Occasionally, this occurs due to obstruction of the laryngeal ventricle by malignancy. It is more common in men in the sixth decade of life.

A Physical examination can reveal dysphonia (most common symptom), neck mass or odynophagia, in addition to airway symptoms.

B Patient presents with no evidence of airway obstruction. Patient able to converse in full sentences, maintain oxygen saturations, and lie supine without difficulty.

C In comparison, patients can present with evidence of acute airway, obstruction. Such patients may present with dyspnea inability to lie supine or handle secretions, or stridor. Should complete evaluation of physical examination and if imaging findings demonstrate concern for the patient's airway, an emergency awake tracheostomy may be performed. In addition to acute airway obstruction, patients can present with signs and symptoms of sepsis.

D Fiberoptic transnasal endoscopy is used to carefully evaluate the airway. The laryngocele will not be visible before phonation. With phonation or Valsalva, the saccule inflates and at the peak, the laryngocele can obstruct

the laryngeal airway. When phonation ends, the laryngocele is deflated and hidden from view. Endoscopy is vital as it is used to assess for causes of obstruction such as carcinoma, chondroma, or amyloidosis. Computed tomography (CT) is the imaging modality of choice, and will demonstrate the relationship of the laryngocele to the thyrohyoid membrane. Chest radiograph (CXR) can demonstrate the air-filled laryngocele on inspiration.

E Internal laryngoceles are confined within the false vocal fold, medial to the thyrohyoid membrane. This can be visualized clearly on CT and will dictate the surgical treatment.

F Combined laryngoceles are formed due to extension of the laryngocele through the thyrohyoid membrane into the soft tissues of the neck, and are the more frequent type of laryngocele seen clinically. These patients may present with more acuity, as the narrow neck of the laryngocele within the thyrohyoid membrane can become obstructed with continued distal expansion of the external component of the laryngocele.

G Should this happen, a laryngomucocele, or mucous-filled laryngocele, may form. Should this become infected, a laryngopyocele may occur. Patients with this finding, typically, are quite ill and require an emergency awake tracheostomy for stabilization of their airway.

H An endoscopic approach is most commonly used for internal laryngoceles. This approach allows for direct visualization of the surgical field and airway. Disadvantages may include difficult surgical exposure, possible scarring, and need for special equipment. Incomplete surgical resection may occur. Benefits include no external incisions, faster recovery, and less morbidity. Some smaller combined laryngoceles may also be approached in this fashion.

I External approaches are the most common method for managing laryngoceles, especially combined laryngoceles. Advantages to these methods include wider field exposure and more precision for surgical resection. Because of the improved exposure through the neck, recurrence is typically low. Disadvantages include a visible scar, higher morbidity, longer duration of surgery, and hospitalization. These techniques are the method of choice for complicated laryngoceles such as laryngomucoceles and laryngopyoceles. Endoscopic examination of the laryngeal ventricle is important in both external and endoscopic approaches to rule out an obstructing lesion such as transglottic cancer.

J Endoscopic approaches include the use of the CO_2 laser and laryngeal cold knife instrumentation. With this approach, marsupialization is typically performed to eliminate the bulk of the laryngocele. Often, ipsilateral false vocal fold resection is performed to fully expose the ventricle and ensure lack of obstructing tumor at the sacculus. With the introduction of the robot into laryngeal procedures, its use for management of laryngoceles has also been proposed.

K The most commonly used external approach is the transthyrohyoid membrane approach. With this approach, no resection of the thyroid cartilage is performed. Used most commonly for combined laryngoceles, visualization is ideal with this method. The limitation of this method is visualization into the paraglottic space. The thyrotomy with resection of the thyroid cartilage and V-shaped thyrotomy approaches are less commonly used, but both provide better exposure to the paraglottic space. Any of these procedures may require the use of a temporary tracheostomy in order to secure the airway.

SUGGESTED READING

De Santo LW. Laryngocele, laryngeal mucocele, large saccules and laryngeal saccular cyst: a developmental spectrum. Laryngoscope. 1974;84(8):1291-1296.

Devesa PM, Ghufoor K, Lloyd S, et al. Endoscopic CO_2 laser management of laryngocele. Laryngoscope. 2002;112:1426-1430.

Dursun G, Ozgursoy OB, Beton S, et al. Current diagnosis and treatment of laryngocele in adults. Otolaryngol Head Neck Surg. 2007;136:211-215.

Zelenik K, Stanikova L, Smatanova K, et al. Treatment of laryngoceles: what is the progress over the last two decades? BioMed Research International. 2014;2014: Article ID 819453. doi:10.1155/2014/819453.

Recurrent Respiratory Papillomatosis

Farrel J Buchinsky, Joseph E Dohar

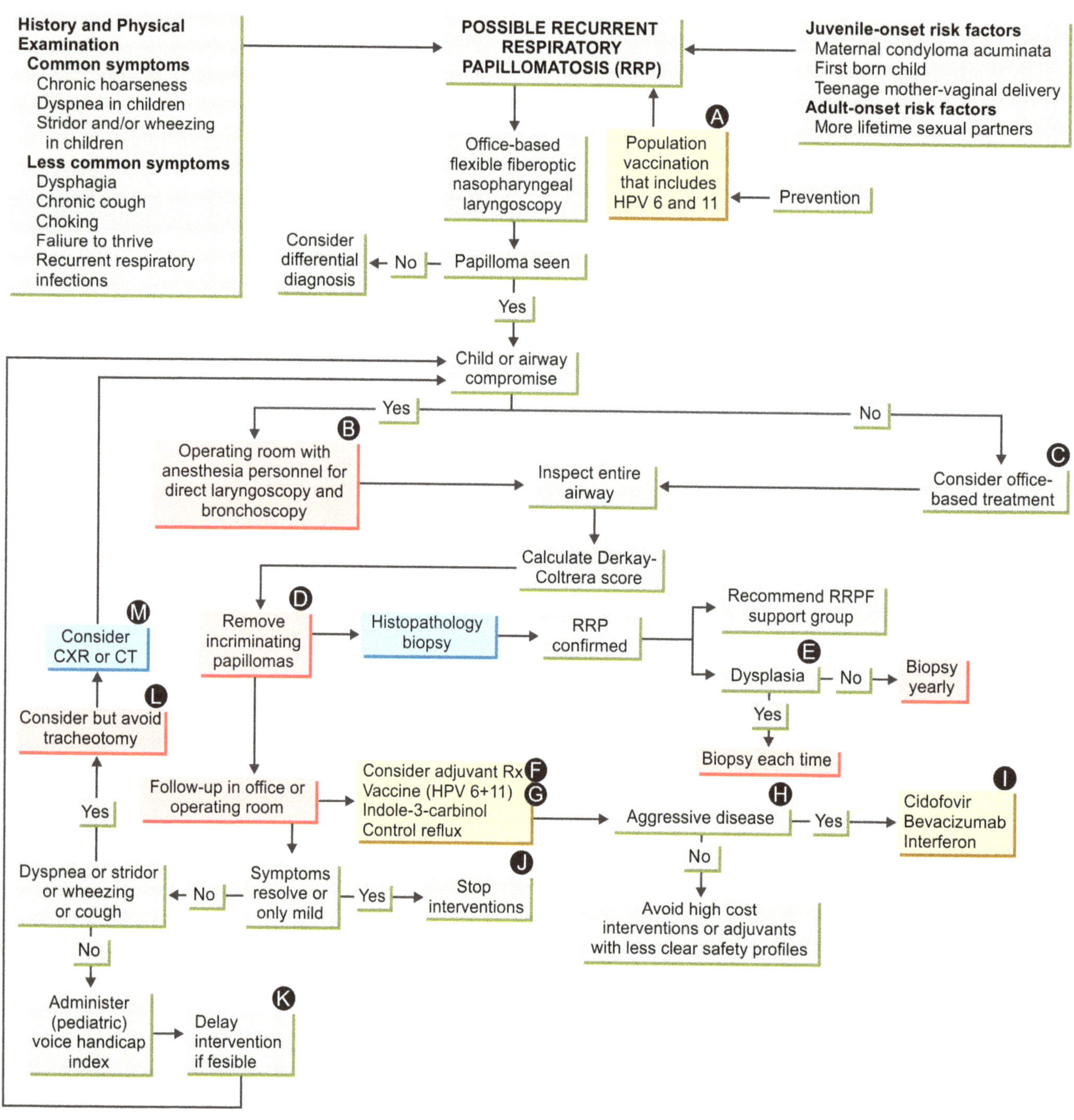

Recurrent respiratory papillomatosis (RRP) is a rare disease (about 1 per 100,000 children or adults per year) most commonly causing chronic hoarseness. Diagnosis is often delayed until an Otolaryngologist inspects the larynx. These benign epithelial lesions [caused by human papillomavirus (HPV) 6 and 11] can occur anywhere in the airway, most commonly the larynx. The clinical course is variable. With no cure, management focuses on debulking grossly visible papillomatous lesions as needed. Most spontaneously remit (after ~ 4 years); some suffer aggressive disease, requiring hundreds of surgeries, experience distal spread, pulmonary involvement, malignant transformation and mortality. Despite remission, many remain permanently dysphonic.

(A) The vaccine's efficacy relies upon administration before sexual debut and widespread adoption for herd immunity.

(B) Airway management is preoperatively planned with the anesthesiologist. Appropriate size rigid ventilating bronchoscopes are selected.

(C) Some adults are treated in the office. A fiber passed through the working channel of a flexible scope delivers laser energy to the papillomas. Recently, enthusiasm for addressing both sides of the anterior commissure with the KTP laser has increased (vs. staged procedures to avoid a web).

(D) Spontaneous ventilation is safest in children while optimizing exposure and access to papillomas. Endotracheal intubation, most common in adults, may be necessary in children to secure a precarious airway. Suspension laryngoscopy with a telescope or microscope facilitates papilloma removal with a microdebrider (commonest method) or a laser (CO_2 or KTP).

(E) Malignant transformation occurs in < 5% of papilloma cases and is less likely in children and with serotype HPV 6 (vs. 11). HPV typing is not compelling clinically since it does not change management.

(F) Rigorous prospective randomized and blinded studies of new agents often fail to confirm initial optimistic anecdotal reports and small case series. Rarely, where the disease is aggressive and possibly devastating, adjuvants for which the level of supporting evidence is poor are nonetheless appropriate, based on compassionate use. Our philosophy is to sequentially use adjuvants, prioritizing safety. Each agent's particular administration protocol is beyond the scope of this text. Efficacy is assessed by comparing pre-intervention inter-surgical intervals and Derkay-Coltrera scores to that of the post-intervention period. Less papilloma burden and persistent aggressive course warrants continued adjuvant therapy or initiation of a new agent.

(G) Vaccination against HPV 6 and 11 may conceivably reduce the incidence of distal spread. Early non-controlled studies suggest diminished disease burden following vaccination. Vaccine licensing studies limited to the genitourinary tract revealed no efficacy for treating existing disease.

(H) Aggressive disease has no absolute definition but many use the following somewhat arbitrary criteria: ≥ 10 RRP procedures OR ≥ 4 RRP procedures in the previous 12 months OR involvement distal to the subglottis OR tracheostomy required.

(I) Interferon alpha is the only adjuvant intervention that has been demonstrated by a randomized controlled trial to be efficacious but its use has been limited by multiple adverse effects and a failure to sustain remission.

(J) In the absence of symptoms, ongoing endoscopy, surgery and adjuvant therapy can be stopped. It is thought that repeated surgeries may be a cause of hoarseness persisting despite durable remission (18 months without recurrence). While relapse has been noted there is no evidence or consensus that interventions or adjuvants change the relapse rate.

(K) When hoarseness is the only symptom, and quality of life only mildly affected we reduce the frequency of interventions to diminish the economic and emotional burden and the potential for permanent scarring. Objective measures of quality of life related to voice include the pediatric voice handicap index (see Zur 2007) and the voice handicap index-10 (see Arffa 2012).

(L) When airway issues drive frequent surgical interventions, consider tracheostomy. The severity of airway obstruction does not follow a linear path and the threat of sudden exacerbation can be reduced by the presence of a tracheostomy. On the other hand, the target tissue for the papillomavirus is the juxtaposition of squamous and ciliated epithelial surfaces, including tracheostomy sites. For this reason, many have suggested avoiding tracheostomy to prevent spread to the lower airway.

(M) Pulmonary involvement is rare but life-threatening. Parenchymal papilloma can coalesce into cavitating lesions. Malignant transformation is common in pulmonary RRP. Bronchial papilloma can cause distal post-obstructive pneumonia. Pulmonary involvement is first suspected or diagnosed by chest radiograph and confirmed by CT chest and CT-guided biopsy. Care is coordinated with Pulmonologists and Oncologists. There is no guideline, evidence or consensus concerning initial or interval imaging to screen for pulmonary involvement. The incidence is low and radiography and CT may increase the risk of malignancy. Imaging is prompted by symptoms such as hemoptysis, dyspnea and exercise-intolerance more severe than would be expected given the visualized papilloma burden, or copious tracheal or bronchial papillomas.

SUGGESTED READING

Arffa RE, Krishna P, Gartner-Schmidt J, et al. Normative values for the voice handicap index-10. J Voice. 2012;26:462-465.

Buchinsky FJ. et al. Age of child, more than HPV type, is associated with clinical course in recurrent respiratory papillomatosis. PLoS One 3, e2263 (2008).

Derkay CS, Wiatrak B. Recurrent respiratory papillomatosis: a review. Laryngoscope 2008;118:1236-1247.

Derkay CS. et al. A staging system for assessing severity of disease and response to therapy in recurrent respiratory papillomatosis. Laryngoscope 1998;108:935-937.

Derkay CS. et al. Current use of intralesional cidofovir for recurrent respiratory papillomatosis. Laryngoscope 2013;123:705-712.

Gallagher TQ, Derkay CS. Pharmacotherapy of recurrent respiratory papillomatosis: an expert opinion. Expert Opin. Pharmacother. 2009;10:645-655.

RRPF. org. Available at: http://www.rrpf.org/index.shtml. (Accessed: 1st November 2015)

Taliercio S. et al. Adult-onset recurrent respiratory papillomatosis: a review of disease pathogenesis and implications for patient counseling. JAMA Otolaryngol. Head Neck Surg. 2015;141:78-83.

Zur KB. et al. Pediatric Voice Handicap Index (pVHI): a new tool for evaluating pediatric dysphonia. Int. J Pediatr. Otorhinolaryngol. 2007;71:77-82.

Leukoplakia

Karen T Pitman

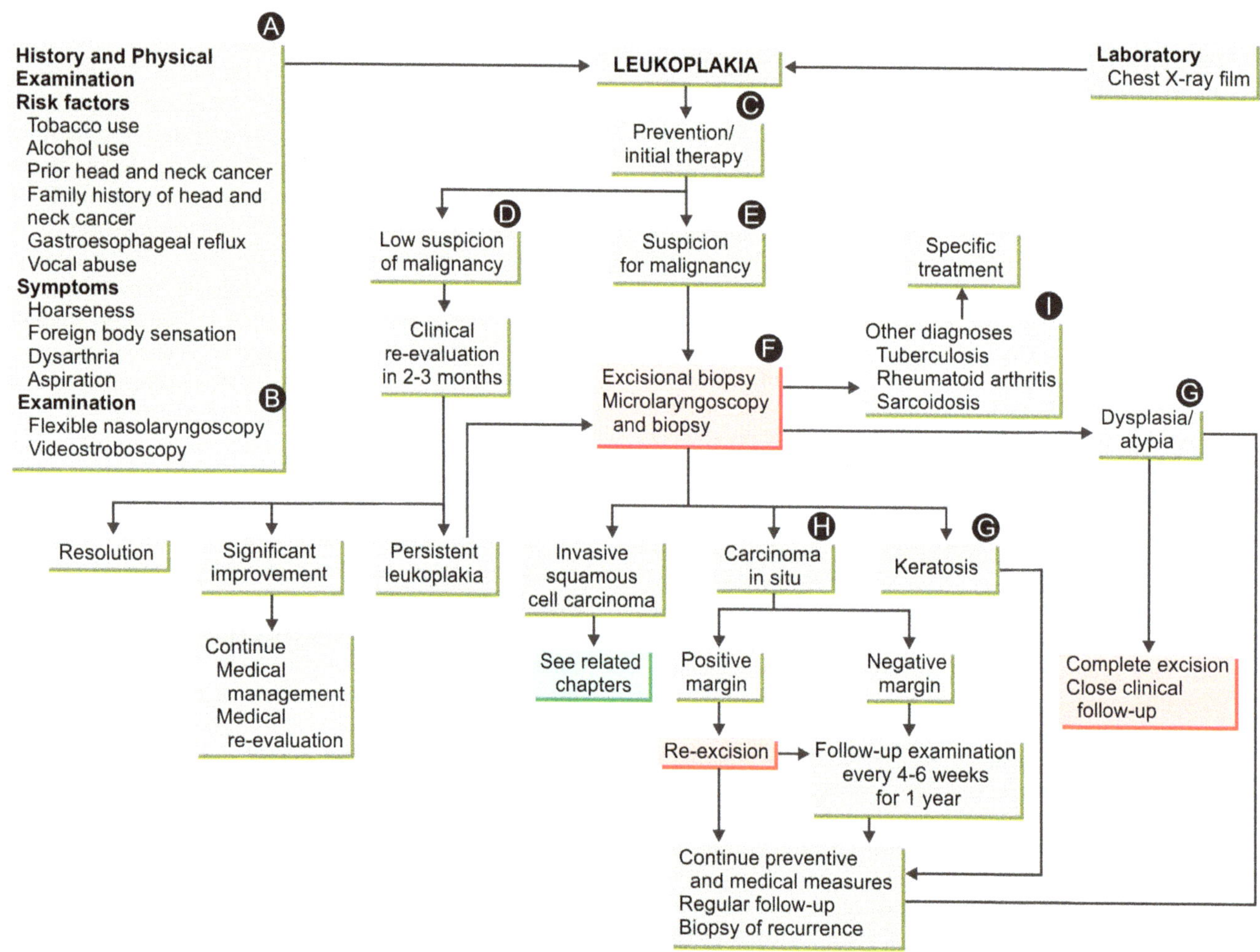

Leukoplakia is a clinical description of a white lesion that occurs most commonly on the glottis but can occur on any mucosal surface of the upper aerodigestive tract (UADT). It is not a pathologic diagnosis and, therefore, requires further evaluation. A significant percentage of lesions described as leukoplakia are premalignant or contain carcinoma. Although tailored to management of oral cavity and laryngeal lesions, the principles outlined for leukoplakia of these sites can be applied to any white lesion of the UADT. Histologic evaluation will usually demonstrate retained keratin adherent to the surface and other mucosal changes, which may or may not represent malignancy or premalignancy.

A The history assesses the patient's risk for malignancy of the UADT. Risk factors for cancer include alcohol and tobacco abuse, prior head and neck squamous cell carcinoma (HNSCC), and a family history of HNSCC. Although not a risk factor for malignancy, symptoms indicative of vocal abuse, gastroesophageal reflux (GER), or extraesophageal acid reflux are also sought because they are suspect in the etiology of leukoplakia.

B The head and neck examination documents the location of the lesion and presence of synchronous lesions, the appearance of the surrounding mucosa, and vocal fold function. Fiberoptic examination of the laryngopharynx is required to rule out additional sites of leukoplakia not visible with oral examination.

C Initial therapy is directed at eliminating inciting factors. Patients who use tobacco are advised to discontinue its use. Patients with acid reflux are treated with H_2 blockers or proton pump inhibitors and counseled about lifestyle modifications. Patients with a history of vocal abuse or overuse are referred for speech therapy and professional voice coaching. Vocal hygiene also includes hydration and humidification of inspired air.

D There is a low suspicion of malignancy among nonsmoking patients with a history of vocal abuse or GERD. Assessment of the tobacco history is important because patients who have stopped smoking are considered to be at risk for tobacco-related illness for at least 10 years.

E One should be suspicious for malignancy in those patients with a history of alcohol and tobacco abuse, previous HNSCC, head and neck radiation, or a family history of HNSCC. Lesions located on the superior/ventricular surface of the glottis with or without extension onto the medial edge are highly suspect of tobacco-induced disease.

F Panendoscopy is performed to rule out synchronous UADT lesions. Excisional biopsy is recommended because leukoplakia contains significant intralesional variability, and excision is a potentially therapeutic intervention that does not jeopardize additional therapies. Submucosal injection of dilute epinephrine aids dissection in the plane between the basement membrane and superficial lamina propria and preserves three-dimensional vocal fold structure. The specimen is carefully oriented and submitted for pathologic examination. Acid reflux therapy is continued perioperatively.

G Excise to negative margin, continue tobacco cessation, vocal hygiene, and treatment of GERD. Schedule a program of regular clinical follow-up, including biopsy of recurrent leukoplakia. Consider entry into a clinical trial to evaluate chemopreventive agents.

H For carcinoma in situ, one must ensure that the margins of excision are negative. If positive, one should consider re-excision. If the margin is negative, one should continue treatment as outlined in Step H. Follow-up examinations are scheduled at 4- to 6-week intervals for the first year after treatment.

I Tuberculosis, rheumatoid arthritis, and sarcoidosis of the larynx can present as "white lesions." If biopsy results show "other" lesions, appropriate consultation is obtained and treatment is initiated accordingly.

SUGGESTED READING

Gillis TM, Incze J, Strong MS, et al. Natural history and management of keratosis atypia, carcinoma in situ, and microinvasive cancer of the larynx. Am J Surg. 1983;146:512-516.

Jones KB, Jordan R. White lesions in the oral cavity: clinical presentation, diagnosis, and treatment. Semin Cutan Med Surg. 2015;34(4):161-170.

Lodi G, Sardella A, Bez C, et al. Interventions for treating oral leukoplakia. Cochrane Database Syst Rev. 2006;(4):CD001829.

Papadimitrakapoulou VA, Clayman GL, Shin DM, et al. Biochemoprevention for dysplastic lesions of the upper aerodigestive tract. Arch Otolaryngol Head Neck Surg. 1999;125:1083-1089.

Zeitels SM. Premalignant epithelium and microinvasive cancer of the vocal fold: the evolution of phonomicrosurgical management. Laryngoscope. 1995;105:1-51.

Cancer of the Supraglottis

John I Song

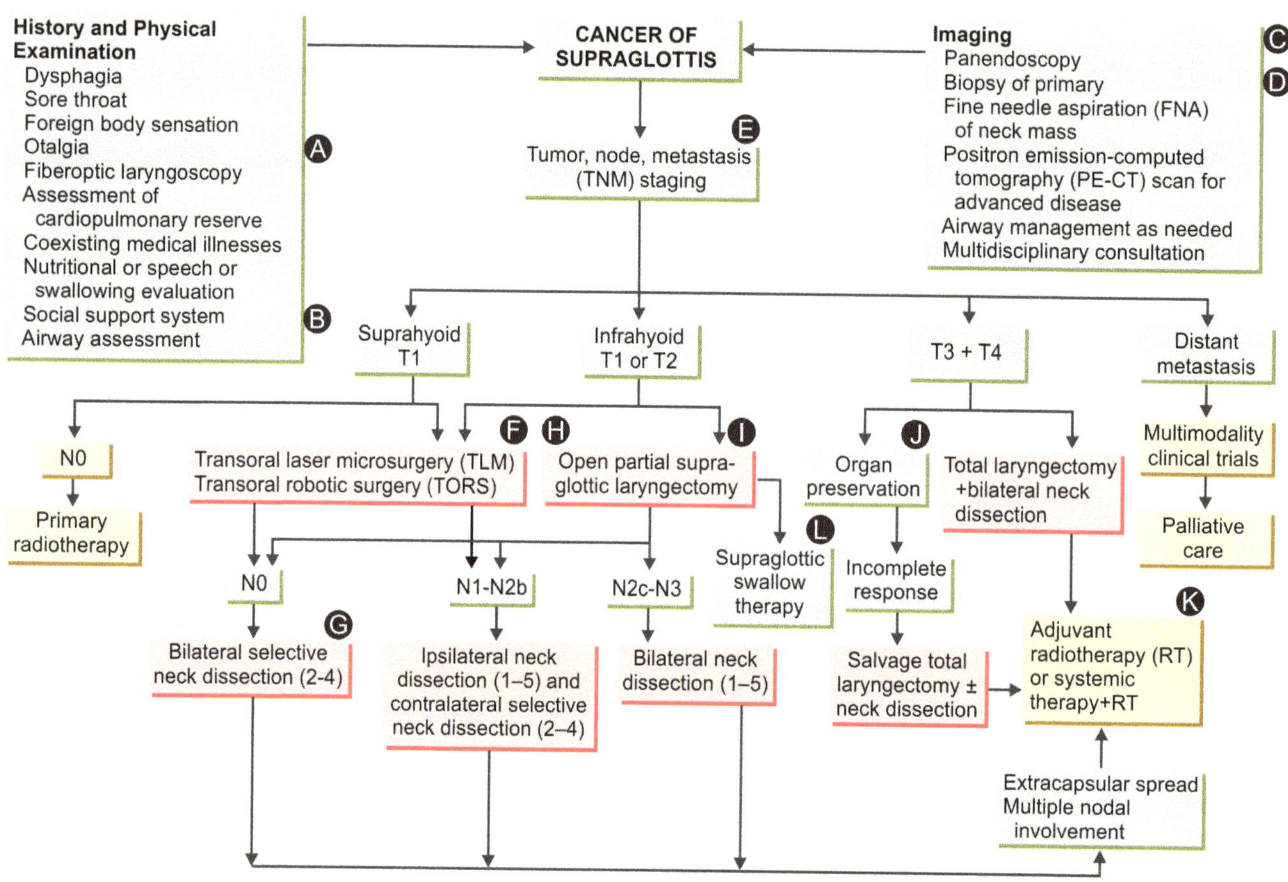

Cancers arising on the supraglottic structures of the larynx often present later and exhibit different growth patterns than do glottic cancers. Selection of treatment and optimization of outcomes requires careful assessment of the extent of the primary tumor, and the physiologic status of the patient. Treatment of the neck is required in nearly all patients due to the rich-lymphatic drainage of the supraglottis.

A Patients being considered for conservation surgery should have pulmonary assessment. They must be able to tolerate some degree of aspiration in the early postoperative period. Methods to estimate cardiopulmonary reserve include arterial blood gas measurement, pulmonary function testing, and assessment of exercise tolerance. Poor candidates for conservation surgery include those with previous pulmonary resection and nonambulatory patients.

B Nutrition, speech and swallow evaluation should be obtained as needed. Preoperative therapy is often helpful to prepare the patient for postoperative rehabilitation. Family and social support involvement can also be assessed during this period.

C Computed tomography (CT) with contrast and magnetic resonance imaging (MRI) with and without gadolinium can be used to assess the larynx with special attention to paraglottic space invasion and lymph node metastasis (nodes >1 cm or with central necrosis). CT is better in assessing thyroid cartilage invasion; MRI is better in assessing submucosal extension and invasion of the pre-epiglottic space. Fluorodeoxyglucose-positron emission tomography (FDG-PET) or CT should be obtained in advanced-stage disease to search for distant metastasis.

D Intraoperative endoscopy should assess the mobility of the vocal cords as well as a close examination of (1) the ventricles; (2) piriform sinus apex and medial wall involvement; (3) arytenoids; (4) anterior commissure; (5) base of tongue and (6) valleculae. If a tracheostomy is needed, it should be placed inferior enough so as not to compromise definitive surgery.

E Multidisciplinary consultation with Radiation Oncology and Medical Oncology should be obtained. Definitive treatment planning should occur through a multidisciplinary tumor board.

F Endoscopic surgery for supraglottic tumors includes transoral laser microsurgery (TLM) resection and transoral robotic surgery (TORS). These approaches are most successful in limited suprahyoid or aryepiglottic fold lesions without invasion of the pre-epiglottic space. Some have advocated TLM or TORS resection in more advanced-infrahyoid lesions, including those that involve the pre-epiglottic space. Because advanced-stage tumors have significant risk of pre-epiglottic space invasion, this approach may result in difficulty obtaining inferior margins endoscopically.

G Bilateral neck dissection is recommended in almost all stages of supraglottic cancer with the exception of small T1 lesions, even in the clinically negative neck. Selective neck dissection (zones II–IV) is used in N0 and some N1 and N2a necks; modified-radical neck dissection (zones I–V) is used in greater than N2a necks. This rationale is based on the following observations:

– Cervical metastasis for supraglottic cancer ranges from 25% to 50%.

– The contralateral side of the neck is the most common site of failure, with recurrence rates as high as 26%; a significant portion of these recurrences cannot be salvaged.

– In our experience, no recurrence in the neck was noted after bilateral selective neck dissection.

– Forty percent of patients with ipsilateral nodal disease have contralateral disease; 10% of patients without ipsilateral nodal disease have contralateral disease.

– Radiation alone is ineffective in controlling all nodal disease.

H Contraindications to supraglottic laryngectomy:

– Bilateral arytenoid involvement.

– Involvement of the apex of the piriform sinus.

– Extension of tumor beyond the circumvallate papillae.

– Involvement of the paraglottic space.

– Invasion of thyroid cartilage or involvement of anterior commissure.

– Invasion of cricoid cartilage.

I Supraglottic laryngectomy can be extended for involvement of (1) the superior and lateral piriform sinuses (partial laryngopharyngectomy), (2) one arytenoid (arytenoidectomy), and (3) tongue base up to the circumvallate papillae (resection of tongue base). Extending the supraglottic laryngectomy will increase complications with dysphagia and aspiration and increase the chance of local recurrence.

J Patients with T3 or T4 tumors may be considered for organ-sparing protocols using induction chemotherapy (platinum-based therapy) followed by radiotherapy with salvage surgery reserved for partial responders and nonresponders. Overall cure rates are no better than standard therapy; although up to 50% organ preservation has been reported.

K Adjuvant therapy may be indicated if there is (1) extracapsular spread and/or positive margins, (2) perineural or angiolymphatic invasion, (3) pT4 primary tumor, (4) N2 or N3 nodal disease, (5) vascular embolism. Radiation therapy (RT) alone or systemic therapy and RT should be considered in these cases.

L Patients are taught the supraglottic swallow (inspiration—Valsalva maneuver to close glottis—swallow—cough) once they have undergone decannulation. Removal of the nasogastric tube and a nonpourable pureed diet facilitates supraglottic swallowing.

SUGGESTED READING

Benito J, Holsinger FC, Pérez–Martín A, et al. Aspiration after supracricoid partial laryngectomy: incidence, risk factors, management, and outcomes. Head Neck. 2011;33:679-685.

Dhiwakar M, Robbins KT, Vieira F, et al. Selective neck dissection as an early salvage intervention for clinically persistent nodal disease following chemoradiation. Head Neck. 2012;34:188-193.

Forastiere AA, Goepfert H, Maor M, et al. Concurrent chemotherapy and radiotherapy for organ preservation in advanced laryngeal cancer. N Engl J Med. 2003;349:2091-2098.

Hinni ML, Salassa JR, Grant DG, et al. Transoral laser microsurgery for advanced laryngeal cancer. Arch Otolaryngol Head Neck Surg. 2007;133:1198-1204.

Johnson JT. Surgery for supraglottic cancer. In: Myers EN (Ed). Operative Otolaryngology: Head and Neck Surgery. Philadelphia, WB Saunders; 1997. p. 403.

Lutz CK, Johnson JT, Wagner AL, et al. Supraglottic laryngectomy: Patterns of recurrence. Ann Otol Rhinol Laryngol. 1990;99(1):12-17.

Peretti G, Piazza C, Cattaneo A, et al. Comparison of functional outcomes after endoscopic versus open-neck supraglottic laryngectomies. Ann Otol Rhinol Laryngol. 2006;115:827-832.

Weinstein GS, O'Malley Jr BW, Snyder W, et al. Transoral robotic surgery: supraglottic partial laryngectomy. Ann Otol Rhinol Laryngol. 2007;116(1):19-23.

Weinstein GS, Laccourreye O, Brasnu D, et al. Organ Preservation Surgery for Laryngeal Cancer. San Diego, CA, USA: Singular Publishing Group; 2000.

Cancer of the Glottis and Subglottis

Guy J Petruzzelli, Chelsea R Metzger

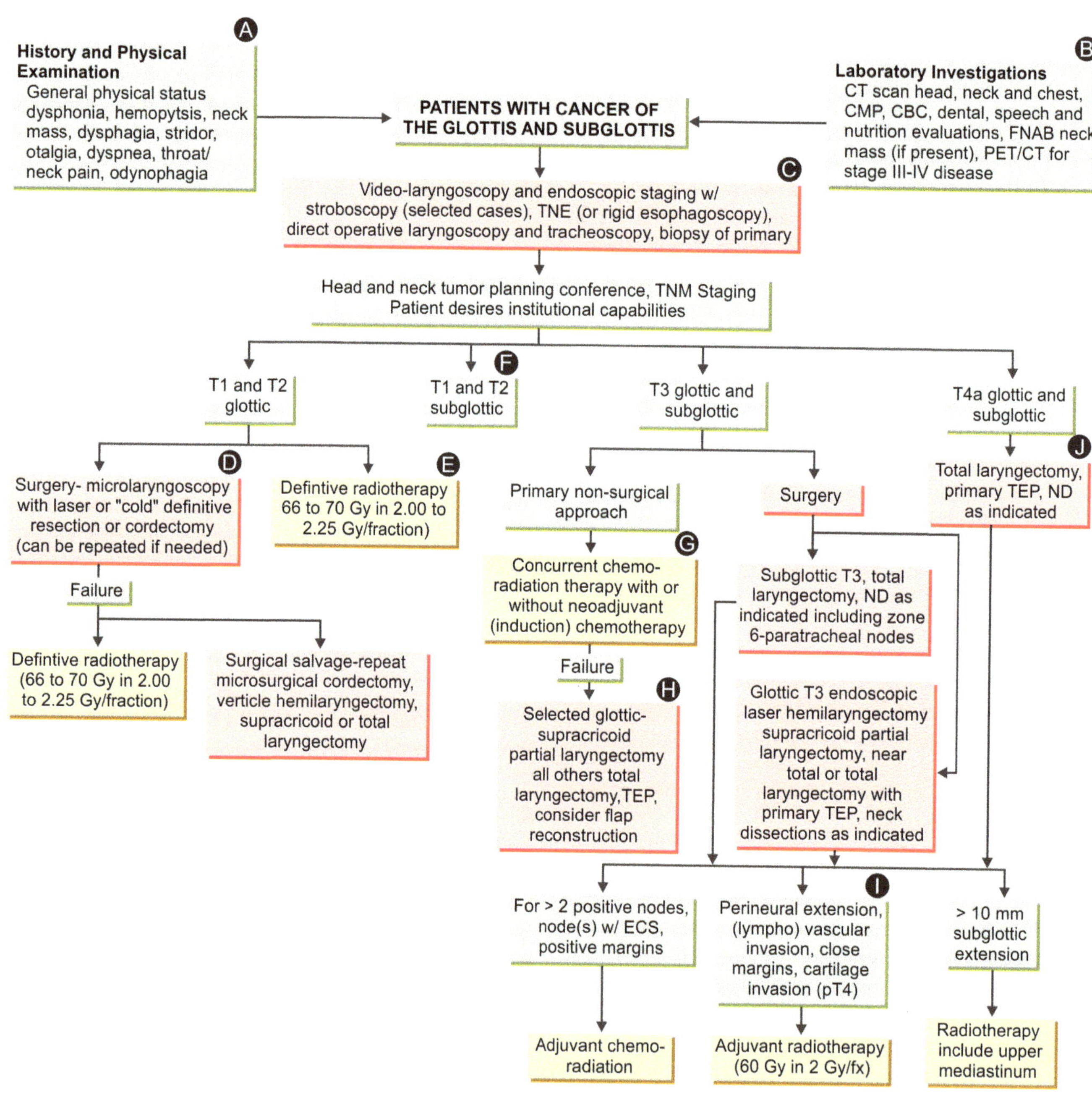

In 2017, there will be an estimated 13,560 new cases of laryngeal cancer diagnosed in the United States resulting in ~3,640 cancer deaths. The overall incidence of laryngeal cancer is decreasing by 2–3% per year consistent with reductions in per capita tobacco consumption; however, the incidence of advanced stage disease remains stable. Early stage disease is curable with either external beam radiation (EBRT) or transoral microlaryngeal surgery with differences in outcome and cost. Advanced stage cancers require combined modality treatment with concurrent chemoradiation therapy. While these studies report improvements in larynx preservation rates, significant local toxicities, reduced opportunities for effective surgical salvage, and a failure to improve survival are also observed.

A The gradual development of hoarseness is the most common chief complain in patients with cancer of the glottis. Otalgia and odynophagia indicate spread to the hypopharynx or tongue base. Stridor is associated with airway compromise due to either a transglottic tumor, usually with vocal cord fixation, or a subglottic tumor with airway obstruction. A neck mass is indicative of metastatic lymphadenopathy or extralaryngeal extension through the cricothyroid or thyrohyoid membranes.

B There is increasing use of positron emission tomography/CT during pretreatment in advanced stage cancer to guide biopsy and procedure planning. Its utility is greatest in detecting recurrent cancer. Chemistry panels, nutrition and dental consultation, as well as consideration of vocal demand, are important components of the pretreatment evaluation.

C The assessment of vocal cord mobility is critical to the accurate TMN staging of laryngeal carcinoma. In-office video-laryngoscopy should be used to evaluate the larynx and may be used in conjunction with stroboscopy to observe finer detail in mucosal wave pliability. Determination of subglottic extension may be difficult. Transnasal esophagoscopy provides the option for in-office biopsy of most laryngeal lesions; otherwise traditional direct operative laryngoscopy and tracheoscopy should be performed.

D Advances in microinstrumentation and laser technology have expanded the capabilities of surgeons to successfully treat in-situ and invasive carcinomas of the glottis. Economic analyses have demonstrated significant savings by reducing the fixed and variable treatment-related costs. Both surgery and EBRT are available for salvage of recurrences following transoral microsurgical resection. Tumors recurring or persisting bilaterally on the vocal cords can be treated with the supracricoid laryngectomy and cricohyoid-epiglottopexy. A history of prior radiation therapy has been associated with delays in decannulation and resumption of oral intake.

E Historically, EBRT was the preferred treatment for early glottic cancer. Intensity-modulated radiation therapy (IMRT) employing carefully designed highly conformal CT-based treatment plans allows for precise dose delivery and limits toxicity to surrounding tissues. Partial laryngectomy remains an option for surgical salvage in highly selected and very carefully restaged patients.

F Primary cancer of the subglottis constitutes between 1% and 8% of all laryngeal carcinomas. Early tumors are extremely rare. The location of these tumors is the cricoid prohibits larynx sparing surgery. These patients should be treated with IMRT 2–2.5 Gy per fraction including the paratracheal nodes.

G Multiple clinical trials have demonstrated the efficacy of concurrent platinum-based chemoradiotherapy as primary "organ sparing" treatment for patients with T2, T3, and some T4 glottic carcinomas. First reported in 2003, data from Radiation Oncology (RTOG) 91-11 demonstrated up to 84% larynx preservation with concurrent cisplatin and EBRT compared to EBRT alone or induction cisplatin/5-fluorouracil followed by radiation with no differences in overall survival. Improvements in overall survival were demonstrated in the TAX trials that examined neoadjuvant chemotherapy (cisplatin, fluorouracil, docetaxel vs cisplatin, fluorouracil alone) followed by definitive EBRT with carboplatin.

H Patients with local failure require thorough restaging including re-evaluation of medical comorbidities, pulmonary reserves, functional and anatomical assessment (including repeat imaging) of the larynx, and careful repeat biopsy of suspicious lesions. Total laryngectomy remains the safest and most reliable salvage alternative in this setting for glottic and subglottic primaries. Increased incidence of wound complications, pharyngocutaneous fistulae, length of stay, and delayed recovery are reported in these patients. The use of vascularized flaps to reinforce or augment the pharyngoesophageal reconstruction is associated with reduced complications. Salvage laryngectomy based on frozen section is ill-advised.

I The laryngeal ventricle defines the pattern of lymphatic drainage from the larynx such that the glottis and subglottis drain inferiorly to the inferior jugular (Zone 4) and prelaryngeal, pretracheal, and paratracheal (Zone 6) regions. Glottic cancer with <10 mm of subglottic extension and primary subglottic cancers have a higher propensity for paratracheal node metastasis, therefore a formal paratracheal node dissection should be considered in these patients. Although associated with greater toxicity, treatment volumes of adjuvant EBRT should be designed to include the stomal and peristomal regions to reduce the risk of recurrence.

J The use of primary chemoradiation for advanced cancer is frequently associated with long-term laryngeal dysfunction and gastrostomy tube dependence. Salvage total laryngectomy in this setting is often made more difficult by extensive local tissue toxicity, malnutrition, the need for flap reconstruction, and exacerbation of underlying comorbidities. All of these could be avoided by an expedient well-performed expedient total laryngectomy. Primary tracheoesophageal puncture, aggressive speech therapy, and enhanced psychosocial support systems can successfully mitigate the difficult sequelae of total laryngectomy and help provide these patients an improved quality of life.

SUGGESTED READING

Chu EA, Kim YJ. Laryngeal cancer: diagnosis and preoperative work-up. Otolaryngol Clin North Am. 2008;41:673-695.

Gourin CG, Conger BT, Sheils WC, et al. The effect of treatment on survival in patients with advanced laryngeal carcinoma. Laryngoscope. 2009;119:1312-1317.

Higgins KM. What treatment for early-stage glottic carcinoma among adult patients: CO_2 endolaryngeal excision versus standard fractionated external beam radiation is superior in terms of cost utility. Laryngoscope. 2011;121:116-134.

Pfister DG, Laurie SA, Weinstein GS, et al. American Society of Clinical Oncology Clinical Practice Guideline for the use of larynx-preservation strategies in the treatment of laryngeal cancer. J Clin Oncol. 2006;24:3693-3704.

Yoo J, Henderson S, Walker-Dilks C. Evidence-based guideline recommendations on the use of positron emission tomography imaging in head and neck cancer. Clin Oncol. 2013;25:e33-e66.

Pharyngocutaneous Fistula

Jason I Kass

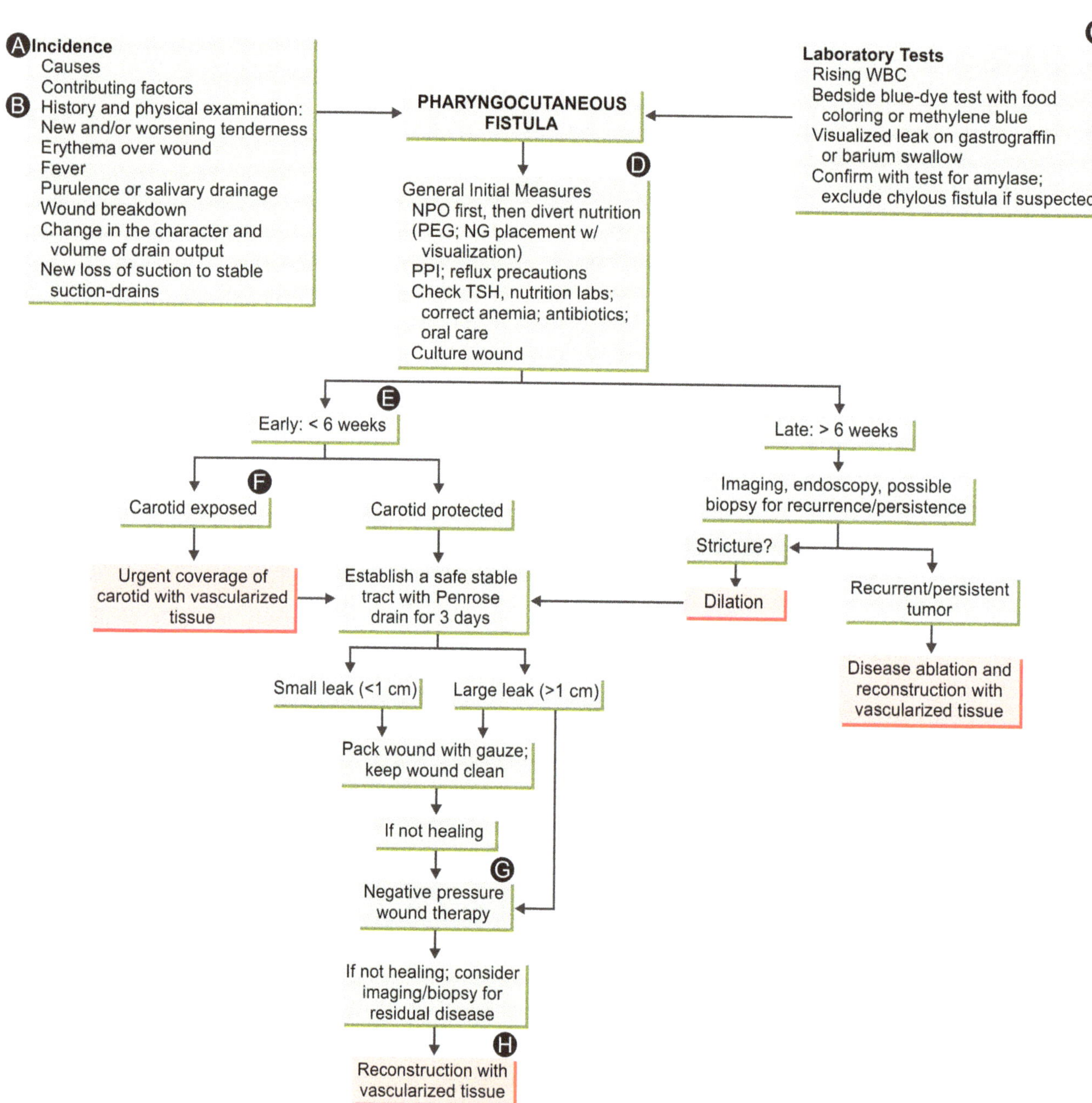

(*Abbreviations*: NPO: Nothing by mouth; PPI: Proton pump inhibitor; PEG: Percutaneous gastrostomy; NG: Nasogastric; WBC: White blood cell count; TSH: Thyroid-stimulating hormone).

A salivary leak, as a result of a pharyngocutaneous fistula, is a major complication of ablative surgery of the upper aerodigestive tract. It often leads to significant morbidity through prolonged hospitalization, protracted dysphagia, and delays in adjuvant chemoradiotherapy. In cases of carotid exposure, a salivary leak can also cause a life-threatening carotid blowout.

A This complication is typically caused by a breakdown in the pharyngeal suture line. The incidence of pharyngocutaneous fistula after total laryngectomy varies widely but has been reported as 15–65%. It is highest in the setting of prior chemoradiation without the use of vascularized tissue outside the radiation field for reconstruction. The usual causes include errors in surgical technique, hormone imbalances (particularly, hypothyroidism), malnutrition, anemia, hyperglycemia, infection, and tumor persistence/recurrence. Too much tension on the suture line from inadequate mucosa is the usual cause. Ideally, one should be able to pass a 36-French dilator through the lumen after closure.

B Early identification of a fistula is essential to minimize neck contamination and avoid major complications. New point tenderness in the neck around the pharyngeal closure is a herald sign of leak. As the saliva accumulates, there will be overlying erythema of the skin, fever, leukocytosis painful swelling, and finally skin breakdown.

C A barium or Gastrografin esophagram looks for extravasation of contrast through the suture line. Methylene blue or food coloring swallow test will give visual evidence of a fistula.

D Certain general measures should be taken when a pharyngocutaneous fistula is diagnosed. Diversion of food may be accomplished with a nasogastric tube (placed under direct visualization), endoscopic or open gastrostomy tube. Contributing factors should be addressed using antireflux medication, correcting of hypothyroidism, anemia, maintaining adequate nutrition, and using broad-spectrum antibiotics.

E If a fistula is suspected in the very early postoperative period (POD 0-2), it is reasonable to consider reoperation with a washout of the wound and revision of the suture line.

F An exposed carotid artery represents the risk of carotid artery blowout. Urgent coverage with locoregional or free tissue is necessary for prevention.

G Negative pressure wound therapy is very effective in accelerating the closure of large pharyngocutaneous fistula and should be considered before attempting a secondary reconstruction.

H Pharyngocutaneous fistula may be reconstructed with various techniques. Locoregional musculocutaneous flaps (pectoralis major, deltopectoral, and supraclavicular) or musculocutaneous/fasciocutaneous free flaps (anterolateral thigh and radial forearm) are most common. Rarely, a jejunal free flap, gastro-omental free flap, or gastric pull-up may be necessary in the persistent fistula despite other treatment modalities.

SUGGESTED READING

Asher SA, White HN, Golden JB, et al. Negative pressure wound therapy in head and neck surgery. JAMA Facial Plast Surg. 2013;35233:1-7.

Bohannon IA, Carroll WR, Magnuson JS, et al. Closure of post-laryngectomy pharyngocutaneous fistulae. Head Neck Oncol. 2011;3:29.

Mäkitie AA, Irish J, Gullane PJ. Pharyngocutaneous fistula. Curr Opin Otolaryngol Head Neck Surg. 2003;11(2):78-84.

Myers EN. The management of pharyngocutaneous fistula. Arch Otolaryngol. 1972;95(1):10-17.

Paleri V, Drinnan M, van den Brekel MWM, et al. Vascularized tissue to reduce fistula following salvage total laryngectomy: a systematic review. Laryngoscope. 2014;124(8):1848-1853.

Qureshi SS, Chaturvedi P, Pai PS, et al. A prospective study of pharyngocutaneous fistulas following total laryngectomy. J Cancer Res Ther. 2005;1(1):51-56.

Stephenson KA, Fagan JJ. Effect of perioperative proton pump inhibitors on the incidence of pharyngocutaneous fistula after total laryngectomy: a prospective randomized controlled trial. Head Neck. 2015;37(2):255-259.

Postlaryngectomy Voice Restoration

Anna M Pou

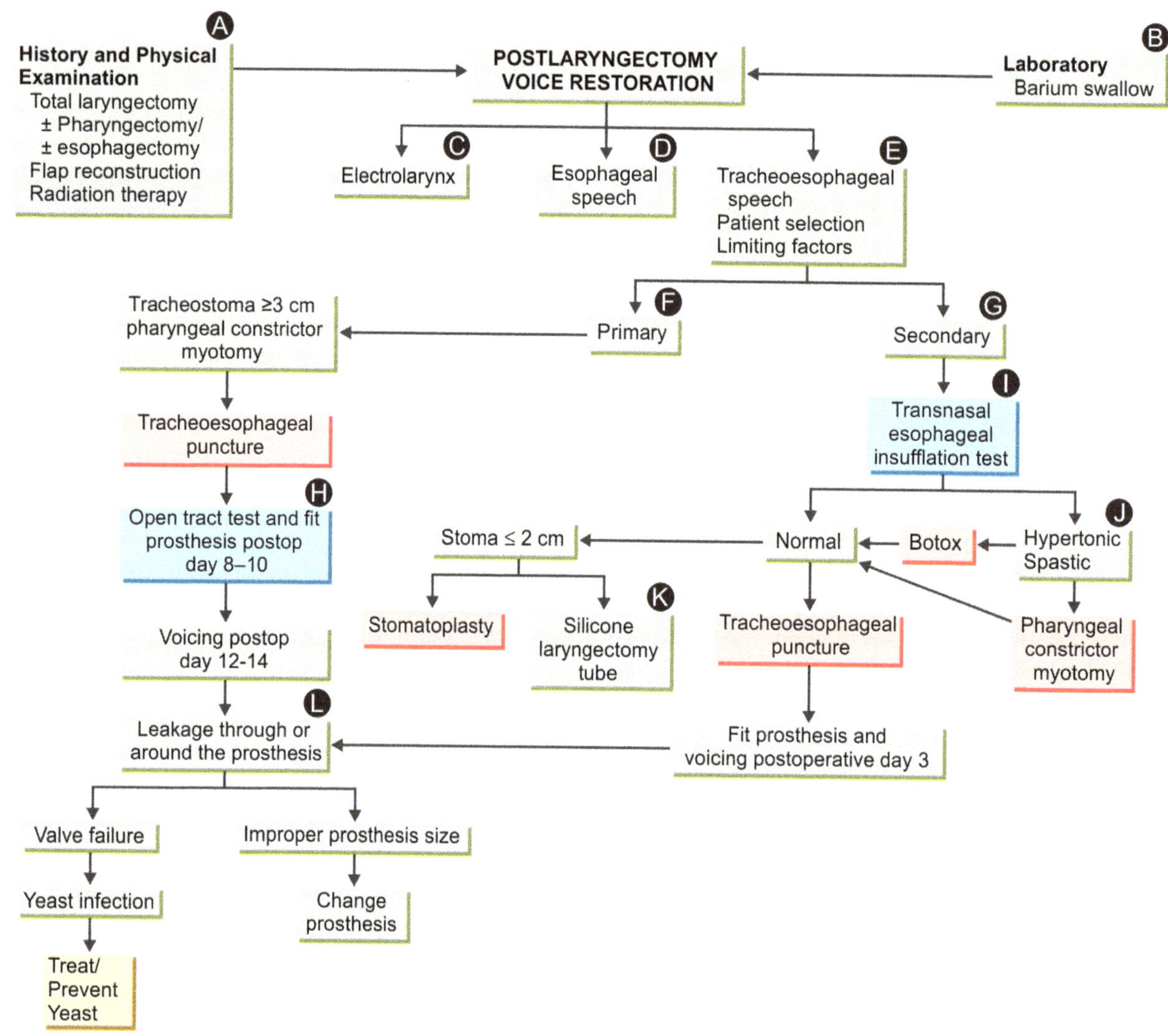

Total laryngectomy changes respiration, swallowing, and the way in which one communicates. It is the loss of voice that has the greatest effect on quality of life. There are three methods of alaryngeal speech: electrolarynx, esophageal speech, and tracheoesophageal (TE) speech, which is the preferred method today. In 1979, Singer and Blom introduced this method using a TE puncture (TEP) and a one way silicone valve, which, when placed through the fistula forces, inspired air up through the pharyngoesophageal (PE) segment causing mucosal vibrations while preventing food and saliva from spilling into the stoma.

A The extent of the resection, flap reconstruction, and the effects of radiation therapy may affect the timing and quality of postlaryngectomy speech.

B Modified barium swallow with esophageal follow through is used to evaluate the function of the pharynx, PE segment, and esophagus in patients undergoing secondary TEP *who complain of dysphagia.*

C All patients are referred to the speech and language pathologist for preoperative counseling and education regarding types of alaryngeal speech. The electrolarynx is the easiest method to learn but requires the use of batteries. Esophageal speech is difficult to learn but there are no additional costs/materials. Tracheoesophageal speech is the most natural form of alaryngeal speech but it requires maintenance of the prosthesis.

D Patients must be motivated to learn TE speech. Relative contraindications include poor pulmonary reserve, moderate-to-severe sensorineural hearing loss, impaired mental status, poor manual dexterity, and the inability to afford the costs of the prostheses.

E The only absolute contraindication to primary TEP is separation of the TE party wall at the level of the puncture site. Successful primary voice restoration requires construction of tracheostoma, TEP, unilateral pharyngeal constrictor myotomy (PCM), and buttressing of the TE party wall. A 16–20-French catheter is placed into the esophagus through the puncture site through which these patients can be fed until the pharyngeal suture line is healed. Alternatively, the prosthesis can be placed primarily (Provox) through a retrograde approach and the patient fed via a nasogastric tube.

F In primary TEP, the prosthesis is fitted between postoperative days 7 and 10 if there is no fistula and the patient is taking adequate oral intake. Before fitting the prosthesis, an open tract test is performed to assess airflow across the constrictor muscles. If the open-tract test is poor, the prosthesis is placed nevertheless. Voicing is not initiated until postoperative days 12–14 to allow the pharyngeal suture line to heal. If hypertonicity or spasticity is present after speech therapy, botulinum toxin A (Botox) injection is performed.

G Secondary TEP can be performed as early as 1–2 weeks postlaryngectomy and/or pharyngectomy; it is typically delayed for 6 weeks postadjuvant radiation therapy, 6–12 weeks poststomal radiation boost, and 3 months postgastric pull up. If a stomatoplasty is required, it is performed at the same time as the secondary TEP. However, secondary TEP and/or stomatoplasty should not be performed until the stoma is healed of radiation toxicity.

H A transnasal esophageal insufflation test is performed on all patients before undergoing secondary TEP. This test assesses pharyngeal constrictor response to esophageal distention. Four responses are possible: fluent, hypotonic, hypertonic, and spastic speech. Many speech therapists forgo this test nowadays due to popular and ease use of Botox injections for spasm.

I Hypertonicity and spasm are characterized by extremely effortful or no speech and dysphagia resulting from dysfunction of the pharyngeal muscles. This can be treated with Botox (a total of 100 units), which is injected into the pharyngeal bar under fluoroscopy or electromyography guidance. Secondary PCM is rarely, if ever, performed any longer.

J A silicone laryngectomy tube can be used to dilate the stoma if the stenosis is not severe. In patients who are at risk for stenosis, a laryngectomy tube can be worn continuously or at nighttime only. The posterior wall of the tube can be fenestrated so that TE speech can continue.

K Tracheoesophageal puncture is no longer a relative contraindication in patients with poor dexterity or mental status changes due to the advent of the indwelling prosthesis that allows the prosthesis to be cared for by a second party.

L Leakage through and around the prosthesis is among the most common problems with TE prostheses due to failure of the valve or to improper size. Yeast is a very common cause of valve failure; the life of the prosthesis can be extended by using antifungals swish and swallow or by using a valve imbedded with Candida-resistant fluoroplastic (Teflon-like) material.

SUGGESTED READING

Hilgers FJ, Ackerstaff AH, Balm AJ, et al. A new problem-solving indwelling prosthesis, eliminating the need for frequent Candida- and "underpressure" –related replacements: ProvoxActiValve. Acta Otolaryngol. 2003;123(8):972-979.

Lewin JS, Bishop-Leone JK, Forma AD, et al. Further experience with Botox injection for tracheoesophageal speech failure. Head Neck. 2001;23:456-460.

Pou AM. Voice rehabilitation following laryngectomy. In: Johnson JT, Rosen CA (Eds). Head and Neck Surgery—Otolaryngology, 5th edition. Philadelphia, PA: Wolters/Lippincott Williams and Wilkins; 2014. p. 1978.

Foreign Body of the Airway

Brian K Reilly, James S Reilly

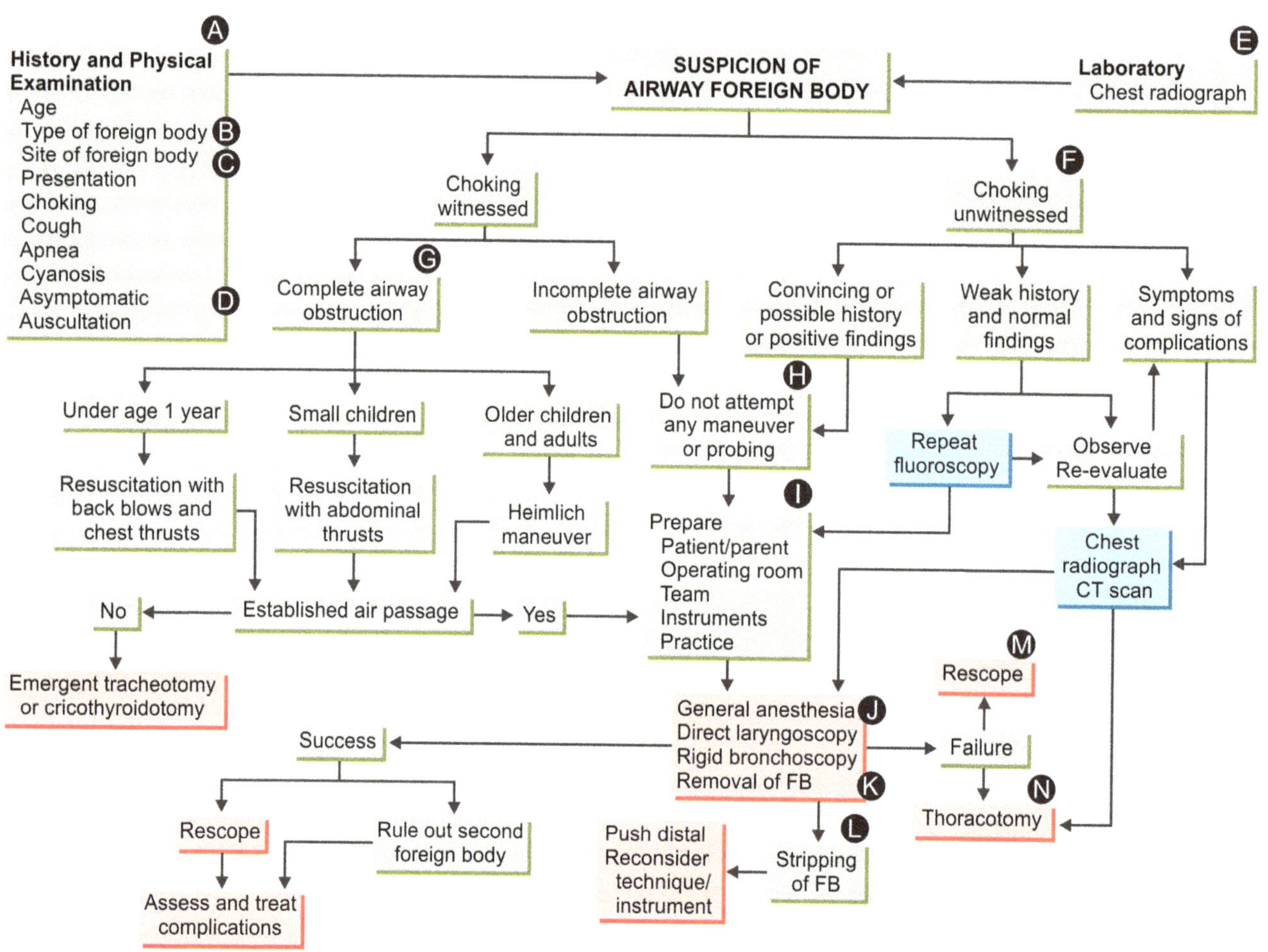

Most foreign bodies (FBs) are coughed out or swallowed. An FB in the larynx or trachea that causes complete obstruction prevents the ability to speak, cough, or in older children, gestures or signals of choking and will cause respiratory collapse and result in death if not expelled promptly.

Ⓐ Foreign bodies of the airway occur frequently in children of <5 years (84%) and boys (2:1). These are vegetables (95%) and metal or plastic objects (5%).

Ⓑ Foreign bodies that pass the larynx and trachea will become lodged more peripherally; right bronchus more so than in left bronchus. Laryngeal FBs present with stridor, hoarseness, or croupy cough. Decreased lung sounds are the most common sign on auscultation. The new Lithium batteries cause erosive injuries within 2 hours and can cause injuries that are fatal, even after emergency removal.

Ⓒ Eighty percent of patients are diagnosed in the first 7 days (first phase). Remaining 20% of individuals with FBs are evaluated after the first week (second phase). The third phase includes complications when infection develops.

Ⓓ Specificity of a history of choking is 91% and of coughing is 80%. Sensitivity is <40%. One third of patients have minimal symptoms.

Ⓔ A "normal chest radiograph" is not sufficient (sensitivity, 68%).

Ⓕ If there is a suspicious history, symptoms, a bronchoscopy is required.

Ⓖ Infants of <1 year should be positioned face down. If this fails, the earlier steps should be repeated. Young children (2-6 years) should be placed in a supine position; and perform 10 abdominal thrusts, tongue–jaw lift, mouth examination, and finger sweep, and mouth-to-mouth ventilation. Older children (≥7 years) should be treated similar to adults, with abdominal thrusts (Heimlich maneuver) in a standing, sitting, or supine position.

Ⓗ Foreign bodies of the airway require prompt endoscopic removal under the conditions of maximum safety and minimum trauma. Most patients with an airway FB presenting to the Otolaryngologist have passed the first phase. The primary exemption is that lithium disc batteries may severely damage the larynx or trachea.

I Proper training, experienced personnel, and planning are critical. A full range of laryngoscopes, open-tube bronchoscopes, suction catheters and FB forceps, and/or balloon catheters is needed.

J Preoperative sedation is avoided. General anesthesia is required. The anesthesia staff should gently, but purposefully, take over ventilation by mask and control the induction of deep anesthesia. After induction, the larynx is sprayed with topical lidocaine to reduce the risk of laryngospasm. During the actual attempted removal, 100% oxygen is administered. Positive pressure is avoided to prevent distal displacement of the FB. If complete airway obstruction occurs, the FB is removed with a direct laryngoscope and forceps without anesthesia.

K Granulation tissue may be vasoconstricted with a saline/epinephrine 1:10,000 lavage. Peanuts should be grasped lightly to avoid fragmentation. Fluoroscopic guidance of flexible bronchoscopy may be useful. The bronchoscope is reinserted immediately after removal to check for a second FB.

L If the FB strips off the instrument in the larynx, remove rapidly with Magill forceps or push back to one (preferably previous) bronchus, and the removal technique is reassessed.

M When an initial attempt is not successful, antibiotics, steroids, and pulmonary percussion therapy for 3–7 days are recommended.

N Thoracotomy with bronchotomy may be necessary for distal or large FB cases (<1%).

SUGGESTED READING

Darrow DH, Holinger LD. Foreign bodies of the larynx, trachea, and bronchi. In: Bluestone CD, Stool SE, Kenna MA (Eds). Pediatric Otolaryngology, 4th edition. Philadelphia: WB Saunders; 2003. pp. 1543-1557.

deCaen AR, Maconochie IK, Aickin R, et al. Part 6: Basic Life Support and Advanced Life Support; 2015 International Consensus on Cardiopulmonary Resuscitation and Emergency Cardiovascular Care Science with Treatment Recommendations. Circulation. 2015;132: S177-203.

Kleinman MD, Brennan ED, Goldberger ZD, et al. Part 5: Adult Basic Life Support and Cardiopulmonay Resuscitation Quality; 2015 American Heart Association Guidelines Update for Cardiopulmonary Resuscitation and Emergency Cardiovascular Care. Circulation. 2015;132;S4141-4435.

Postoperative Tracheostomy Care

Karen M Kost

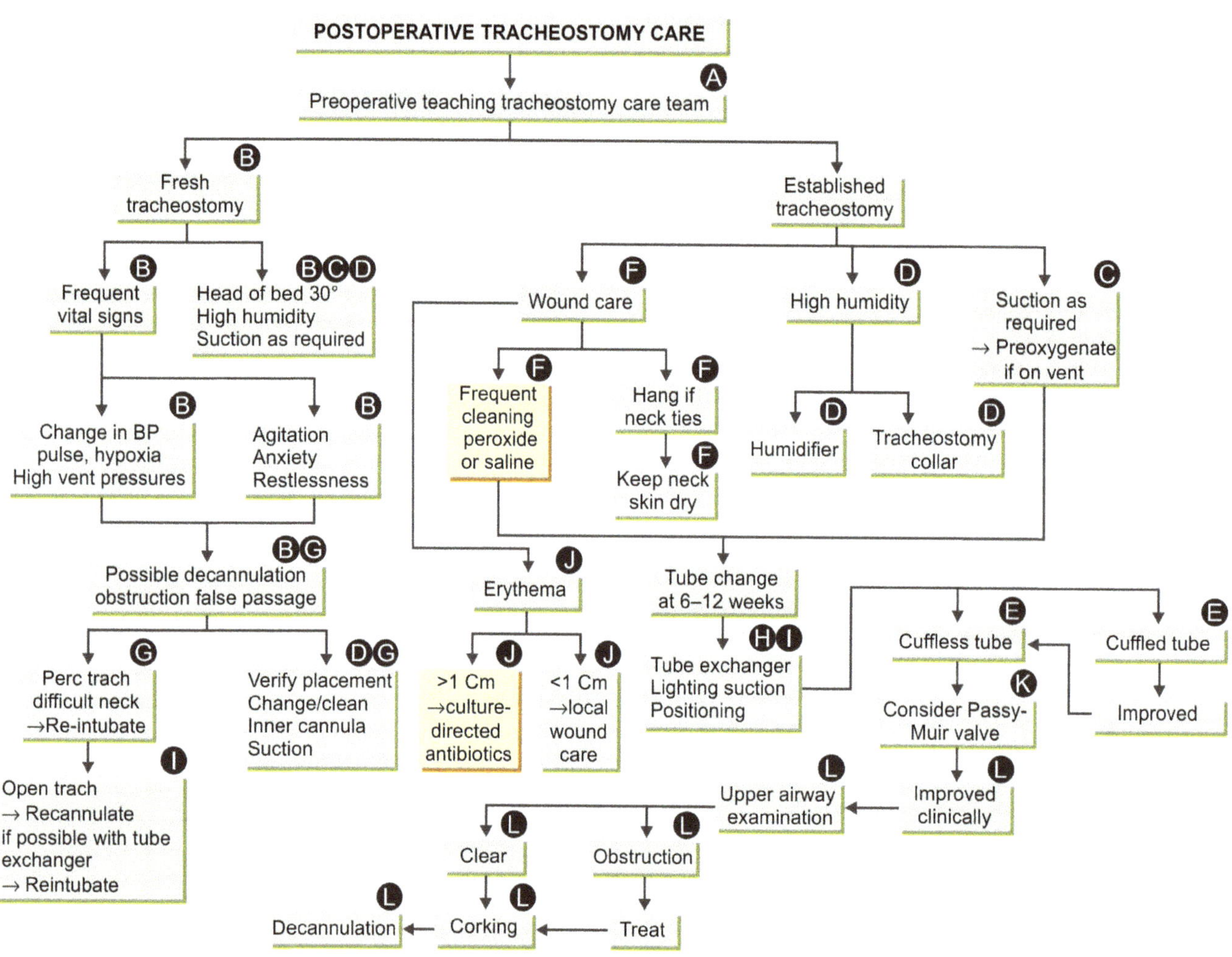

Careful management of the post-tracheostomy patient is critical in assuring an optimal outcome. Adverse events following tracheostomy are common, and can occasionally be fatal. This algorithm separates patients with fresh and established tracheostomies, recognizing that adverse events may occur in both groups.

A Preoperative teaching greatly facilitates postoperative tracheostomy care. Evidence indicates that patients undergoing tracheostomy experience a reduced quality of life. Teaching with visual aids, family counseling, and highly skilled nursing care are all key factors in reducing anxiety and ensuring a smooth postoperative course. A multidisciplinary tracheostomy team consisting of a physician, nurse, respiratory therapist and speech-language pathologist has been shown, with measurable results, to play a critical role in coordinating and delivering the complex care tracheostomy patients' require. The team assists with wound care, tracheostomy tube changes, deglutition, communication, decannulation, and teaching of the patient and caregivers.

B In the initial postoperative period, patients should be positioned with the head of the bed elevated 30–45° to maximize comfort, and facilitate coughing, deep breathing, and suctioning. Patients should be closely watched, in a special care unit for at least 24 hours. Vital signs, including continuous pulse oximetry, require frequent monitoring. Changes in blood pressure, respiratory rate, or pulse rate may indicate a new or ongoing respiratory problem. Tube obstruction due to plugging or displacement out of the trachea is a serious, life-threatening event that must be recognized rapidly. Agitation, anxiety and restlessness may indicate hypoxia and should never be dismissed or treated with anxiolytics.

C Tracheal suctioning is performed to maintain pulmonary toilet and patency of the tracheostomy tube. Initially, this should be done frequently, and as aseptically as possible. Suctioning should be tailored to the patient's needs and may be necessary four or more times daily. Patients on mechanical ventilation are at risk for hypoxia and cardiac arrhythmias during suctioning because oxygen-rich air is suctioned and catheters may be too large. This problem can be prevented by ventilating the patient on 100% O_2 for at least five breaths before and after suctioning, and limiting suctioning to less than or equal to 12 seconds with a small catheter. As an alternative to this open technique, a closed, multiple-use suction catheter contained within a sheath may be used.

D Humidity facilitates mucociliary transport of secretions and prevents serious complications such as crusting, accumulation of secretions, mucus plugging, and eventual obstruction of the airway. Tracheostomies with disposable or reusable inner cannulas are available. When present, the inner cannula should be frequently cleaned or changed, if encrusted. The use of a T tube should be avoided because the torque exerted on the tube, traumatizes the tissue every time the patient moves.

E Decisions regarding tracheostomy tube cuff presence or inflation are patient-dependent. Cuffed tracheostomy tubes are often used initially to reduce the risk of aspiration of blood and/or saliva. Typically, the cuff can be deflated after the immediate postoperative period.

F Meticulous local wound care is an essential component of post-tracheostomy care. The tracheostomy site should be cleaned as often as necessary with normal saline or hydrogen peroxide to prevent breakdown of the skin and the progression from wound colonization to infection. Initially, this is likely to be at least three or four times daily. The tapes holding the tracheostomy tube in place should be changed as necessary when soiled. The skin under the tracheostomy neck plate should be kept dry with a thin nonadherent dressing such as Telfa to prevent skin maceration.

G Early tracheostomy tube changes should be avoided until adhesions form between the overlying soft tissues and the trachea. Accidental decannulation in the early postoperative period can be very dangerous because the tissues collapse, sealing off the airway, and increasing the possibility of tube misplacement in a false passage when reinsertion is attempted. Patients should not be ventilated through an urgently replaced tracheostomy tube unless the tip of the tube is verifiably within the trachea. Forcefully bagging when a tube is displaced can lead to pneumothorax and death. Accidental decannulation in a patient with difficult anatomy, or following percutaneous tracheostomy in the early postoperative period should be managed with reintubation.

H Changing the tracheostomy tube requires skill and preparation. Early tube changes are not necessary unless the tube is to be changed from a cuffed to an uncuffed tube or if the cuff fails. Safe tube replacement in the first 48 hours requires the following—optimal patient positioning, assistance, adequate light, a tracheal hook, suction, an ideally sized and smaller tracheostomy tube, and a tracheostomy tube exchanger.

I A tracheostomy tube exchanger is very helpful for early tube changes and adds an important measure of safety. The exchanger is a long semiflexible tube with a central lumen through which ventilation is possible. The exchanger is inserted into the tracheostomy tube, which is then removed. The new tube is then "guided" into the trachea over the exchanger. If the new tracheostomy tube proves difficult to replace, ventilation may be temporarily continued through the exchanger.

J Postoperative antibiotics are not indicated and serve only to select out resistant organisms. Within 24–48 hours, the tracheostomy site is colonized by a variety of organisms, including *Pseudomonas*, *Klebsiella*, *Candida*, and *Proteus*. Fastidious wound care is the most important element in preventing infection. Culture-directed antibiotics should only be used when cellulitis extends one centimeter or more beyond the wound edges.

K Patients who do not require a cuffed tube should be considered for a Passy-Muir or speaking valve in the postoperative period. This one-way valve allows inspiration through the tracheostomy tube and closes on expiration, deflecting air through the vocal folds and permitting phonation. Additional benefits include improved cough and management of secretions. Swallowing also improves through restoration of subglottic pressure. Contraindications for use of a speaking valve include a cuffed tracheostomy tube, upper airway obstruction, bilateral vocal fold paralysis, severe tracheal stenosis, copious inspissated secretions, and cognitive dysfunction. The patient must understand the mechanics of the valve and be able to easily and rapidly remove the valve in the event of tube obstruction or respiratory distress.

L Decannulation should be considered as the patient's clinical condition improves. This is facilitated in cognitively intact patients who understand the process and the steps that will be followed. The first step involves examining the upper airway to make sure there is no obstruction. Patients with a cuffed tracheostomy tube should be fitted with a cuffless tube with an internal diameter of 6 mm or less to allow airflow around the tube up through the vocal folds and upper airway. Prior to "corking" the tracheostomy tube, the patient should be able to independently position and remove the cork. Once "corked", the patient should be observed closely for a few minutes to ensure that the occluded tube is well tolerated. Patients who are cognitively or otherwise impaired must be carefully observed throughout this process. Once the patient is comfortable carrying out all daily activities with the tracheostomy tube occluded, generally over a 24-hour period, the tracheostomy tube may then be safely removed, and the site occluded with an airtight dressing. Complete closure usually occurs in 7–10 days.

SUGGESTED READING

Bryant LR, Trinkle JK, Mobin-Uddin K, et al. Bacterial colonization profile with tracheal intubation and mechanical ventilation. Arch Surg. 1972;104(5):647-651.

de Mestral C, Iqbal S, Fong N, et al. Impact of a specialized multidisciplinary tracheostomy team on tracheostomy care in critically ill patients. Can J Surg. 2011;54(3):167-172.

Deppe SA, Kelly JW, Thoi LL, et al. Incidence of colonization, nosocomial pneumonia, and mortality in critically ill patients using a Trach Care closed-suction system versus an open-suction system: prospective, randomized study. Crit Care Med. 1990;18(12):1389-1393.

Hashmi NK, Ransom E, Nardone H, et al. Quality of life and self-image in patients undergoing tracheostomy. Laryngoscope. 2010;120 Suppl 4:S196.

Kost KM. Tracheostomy in the intensive care unit setting. In: Myers EN, Johnson JT (Eds). Tracheotomy: Airway Management, Communication, and Swallowing. San Diego: Plural Publishing; 2008. pp. 83-116.

Hemoptysis

Jeffrey M Bumpous

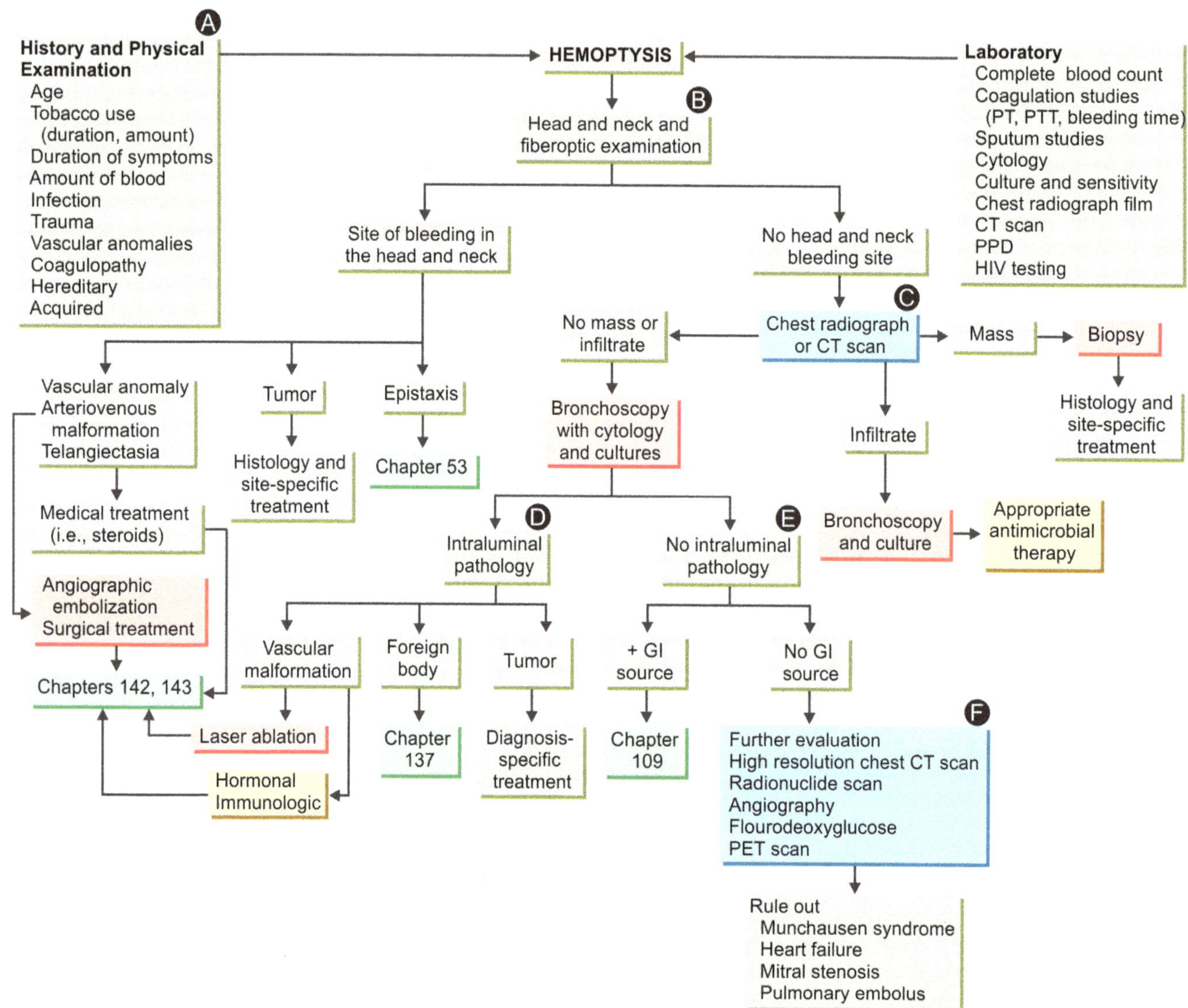

Hemoptysis is defined as the expectoration of blood, and can be classified as massive or nonmassive in volume. In general, hemoptysis can be classified as pulmonary or extrapulmonary in origin.

A The history and physical examination are critical in securing a diagnosis. The most common general causes include malignancy, inflammatory and infectious processes, blood dyscrasias, and trauma.

Common pulmonary causes include bronchitis and bronchiectasis, pulmonary neoplasms, vascular malformations, tuberculosis and histoplasmosis, and foreign bodies. One must also consider coagulopathies as well as iatrogenic causes after invasive interventions. Extrapulmonary causes include epistaxis, laryngeal malignancies, and esophageal lesions. The history will dictate appropriate laboratory tests such as coagulation profile. A complete blood count, sputum studies, human immunodeficiency virus and purified protein derivative testing.

B A thorough examination of the head and neck is critical including fiberoptic flexible nasopharyngoscopy with examination of both nasal passages, nasopharynx, larynx, and hypopharynx. This examination will often allow the examiner to distinguish between pulmonary and extrapulmonary sources of bleeding. If the practitioner discovers a laryngeal or hypopharyngeal tumor in the evaluation of a patient with hemoptysis, one must still consider a synchronous second primary malignancy in the lung as a cause of the hemoptysis.

C After potential causes of hemoptysis from the upper aerodigestive tract are ruled out, imaging of the chest is required. The initial examination is a chest radiograph. A large portion of patients with hemoptysis will have an abnormal chest radiograph. This may be suggestive of specific causes, but is rarely diagnostic. More importantly, a normal chest radiograph does not entirely exclude a malignancy or other cause of bleeding. In patients with severe chronic obstructive pulmonary disease or bullous disease, a computed tomography (CT) scan of the chest may be required. If performed in the past, it is critical that a previous chest radiograph is available for comparison. Discovery of a new mass in a smoker is nearly diagnostic of nonsmall cell carcinoma. The CT of the chest should be performed with contrast in order to better identify enhancement within lesions and to note vascularity.

Risk factors for pulmonary malignancy include age of >40, smoking history, and chronic hemoptysis. If a mass is identified, a biopsy should be obtained. There are many methods for obtaining tissue, depending on the location of the mass. These include cytology from sputum, bronchoalveolar lavage, CT-guided biopsy, biopsy via open and video-assisted thoracoscopic surgery, and endobronchial ultrasound-guided biopsy.

D Bronchoscopy is the diagnostic procedure of choice, particularly in cases of normal chest imaging. This intervention may reveal vascular malformations, a foreign body, or a mucosal-based malignancy.

E If all pulmonary and upper aerodigestive tract causes have been excluded, one must consider an upper gastrointestinal cause. This could include esophageal varices, esophagitis, gastritis, malignancy, or peptic ulcer disease. This workup will include endoscopy by a gastrointestinal specialist.

F In patients with a normal chest CT, normal bronchoscopy, and not on anticoagulation, a diagnosis of "cryptogenic" hemoptysis is made. Further investigations may include a high-resolution CT scan, radionuclide scan, pulmonary angiography, and (fluorodeoxyglucose) positron emission topography scan. Furthermore, rare causes may also include factitious hemoptysis (Munchausen's syndrome), congestive heart failure, mitral stenosis, and pulmonary embolus. In spite of an exhaustive search for the cause of hemoptysis, the cause may remain unknown in up to 19% of patients.

SUGGESTED READING

Bidwell JL, Pachner RW. Hemoptysis: diagnosis and management. Am Fam Phys. 2005;72(7):1253-1260.

Herth F, Ernst A, Becker HD. Long-term outcome and lung cancer incidence in patients with hemoptysis of unknown origin. Chest J. 2001;120(5):1592-1594.

Jeudy J, Khan AR, Mohammed TL, et al. ACR appropriateness criteria® hemoptysis. J Thorac Imaging. 2010;25(3):W67-69.

Knott-Craig CJ, Oostuizen JG, Rossouw G, et al. Management and prognosis of massive hemoptysis. Recent experience with 120 patients. J Thorac Cardiovasc Surg. 1993;105(3):394-397.

Mason RJ, Broaddus VC, Martin T, et al. Murray and Nadel's Textbook of Respiratory Medicine: 2-Volume Set. Elsevier Health Sciences; California, 2010.

Myers EN, Suen JY, Myers JN, et al. Cancer of the Head and Neck. Philadelphia, WB Saunders; 2013.

Townsend CM Jr, Beauchamp D, Evers M, et al. Sabiston Textbook of Surgery: The Biological Basis of Modern Surgical Practice. Philadelphia, PA: Saunders; 2008.

Neck

CHAPTER 140

The Mass in the Neck in the Pediatric Age Group

Minyoung Jang, Kenneth M Grundfast

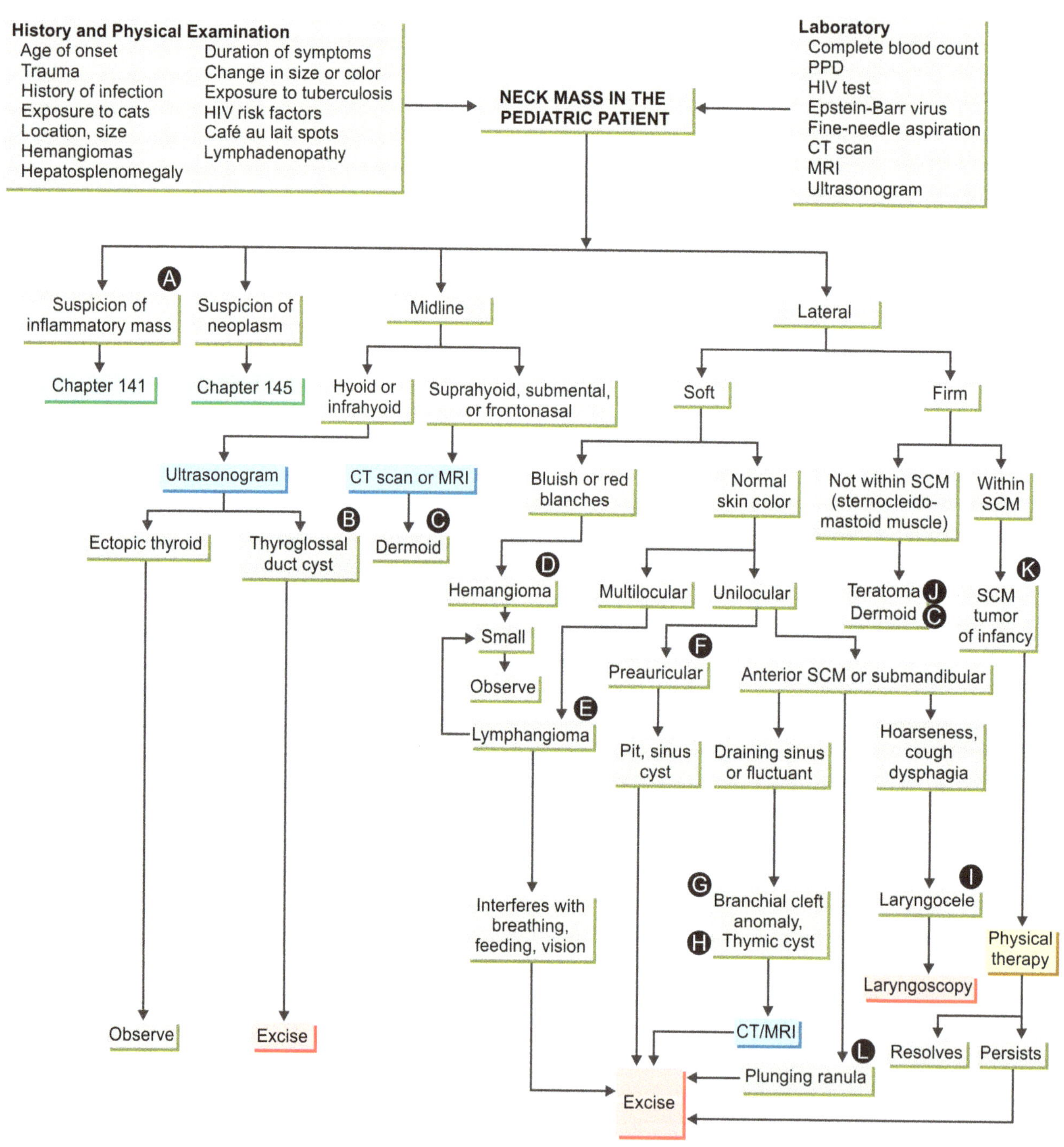

Unlike in adults, a neck mass in a child is more likely to be of inflammatory or congenital etiologies. However, malignancies, although rare, do occur.

A Inflammatory or infectious origin may be suggested by the history of recent trauma or infection; exposure to cats, ticks, or tuberculosis; recent fever, hepatospenomegaly, or weight loss; positive purified protein derivation skin test for tuberculosis; or positive tests for human immunodeficiency virus or Epstein-Barr virus. Having said this, it is important to keep in mind that nontuberculous mycobacterial infections frequently present without constitutional symptoms or history of exposures, negative laboratory testing, and with or without violaceous skin changes or draining fistula. Neoplasm should be considered when a child has a history of cervical lymphadenopathy that fails to resolve after 6–8 weeks with appropriate treatment, or is associated with systemic manifestations of neoplasm (i.e., café au lait spots) or constitutional symptoms (fever, weight loss, decrease in appetite).

B Thyroglossal duct cysts (TDCs) are the most common congenital midline mass in the neck. Most TDCs appear in children between 2 and 10 years of age, are found at or below the level of the hyoid bone, and elevate with swallowing or protrusion of the tongue. Rarely, the TDC may contain the patient's only functioning thyroid gland, and preoperative ultrasonography should be used to establish the presence of a normal thyroid gland. The treatment of choice is a Sistrunk operation, with excision of the cyst as well as any remnant duct by excising the center of the hyoid bone and a cuff of tissue at the base of tongue. Infected cysts should be treated with warm soaks and antibiotics: excision should be delayed until the infection has resolved.

C Dermoid cysts occur along embryonic lines of fusion, most commonly in the midline above the hyoid or along the bridge of the nose, but, uncommonly they can also occur lateral to the midline. Midline dermoid cysts may be difficult to distinguish from TDCs. Dermoid cysts are more superficial, do not elevate with swallowing or tongue protrusion, and are filled with sebaceous material. However, if uncertainty remains, it is advisable to proceed with a Sistrunk operation in order to avoid incomplete excision, as there will be a high chance of recurrence with a superficial excision as for a dermoid if histopathology reveals that the mass is a actually a partially excised TDC.

D Hemangiomas are the most common benign neoplasm of the head and neck in infants. Classified as a vascular tumor, they undergo a period of active growth usually during the first year of life, usually followed by spontaneous involution. About 30% are present during the first week of life, but most appear after the first month. They are red-to-blue-colored soft lesions that blanch with pressure and may increase in size with crying. A bruit

may be heard, and other cutaneous hemangiomas elsewhere on the body may be seen. Maximum involution occurs in 50% by age 5 and in 90% by age 9. Given spontaneous regression, treatment should consist of observation unless lesions become problematic. About 3–5% of hemangiomas will grow large enough to interfere with breathing, feeding, or eyesight; cause thrombocytopenia; or cause cardiac failure. In these cases, aggressive management should be instituted. Propranolol has recently become the recommended first-line therapy for complicated infantile hemangioma. Although it is associated with a low risk of adverse events such as bradycardia, hypotension, bronchospasm, and hypoglycemia, it is widely considered to be less morbid than procedures such as tracheotomy or emergent excision, and more effective than laser ablation or corticosteroids. In a recent large randomized controlled trial, the rate of adverse events appeared higher in the propranolol group compared to placebo, but it is unclear whether this reached statistical significance. Ulceration with secondary infection may also occur, in which case systemic antibiotics and local wound care should be administered. A hemangioma that continues to have incomplete involution may be excised for cosmetic considerations.

E Lymphatic malformations (cystic hygromas or lymphangiomas) are vascular malformations derived from lymphatic vessels, and unlike vascular tumors such as hemangiomas, grow proportionately with the child. They are usually noted at birth (50–65%) but may appear or enlarge after an injury or upper respiratory infection. They are classified as microcystic, macrocystic, or combined based on imaging studies. Microcystic lesions commonly present as firm brawny edema in the oral cavity and pharynx. Macrocystic lesions are often soft, fluctuant lesions in the anterior or posterior cervical triangles that transilluminate. Small, stable, asymptomatic lesions may be observed; however, these lesions are known for their persistent growth, and larger symptomatic lesions may be treated with complete surgical excision. Sclerotherapy, while not curative, is a useful alternative for reducing symptoms for macrocystic types. No prospective studies comparing the various sclerotherapy agents exist, but OK-432 and doxycycline have been used with similar success in retrospective studies. Ethanol, bleomycin, and sodium tetradecyl sulfate are other commonly used sclerosing agents. Location may affect prognosis after surgical intervention, i.e., laterality and inferior and/or superior relationship to hyoid (the de Serres classification).

F Preauricular pits, sinuses, and cysts are due to aberrant development of the auricular tubercles. The pits are located anterior to the tragus, tend to be familial, and are often bilateral. They may drain sebaceous material or undergo recurrent infection, and excision is recommended if these symptoms are bothersome. If they are acutely infected, warm compresses and antibiotics should be used and excision delayed. Although preauricular lesions may be associated with renal anomalies in syndromes such as branchio-oto-renal, CHARGE (coloboma of the eye, heart defects, atresia of the nasal choanae, retardation of growth and/or development, genital and/or urinary abnormalities, and ear/hearing abnormalities), and Townes-Brocks, renal ultrasound is not indicated if they are not accompanied by other dysmorphic features or risk factors. Risk factors for associated renal anomalies include family history of deafness, auricular and/or renal malformations, or history of gestational diabetes. Similarly, if newborn hearing screening is normal and there is no concern for hearing loss, additional screening audiograms are not indicated. There is no evidence that bilateral lesions increase the likelihood of renal or hearing abnormalities, if there are no other risk factors, and existing studies have not risk stratified by laterality.

G Branchial cleft anomalies (BCAs) can usually be found along the anterior border of the sternocleidomastoid muscle. They result from errors of embryogenesis and include cysts, sinuses, and cartilaginous remnants. Second BCAs are the most common. They typically present as a fluctuant, mobile, and nontender mass located at the anterior border of the sternocleidomastoid muscle or with drainage from a sinus, and may get infected. Approximately 10% are bilateral. First BCAs usually present as masses or sinus tracts anterior and inferior to the ear and parotid, may end in a sinus in the external auditory canal, and may be medial or lateral to the facial nerve when located in the submandibular neck. Third and fourth branchial cleft cysts can often be misdiagnosed initially as thyroid masses. Complete surgical excision is the preferred treatment. For third and fourth BCAs, cauterization of the sinus tract through an opening in the piriform sinus has also been reported as an effective treatment method.

H Thymic cysts occur due to ectopic tissue along the tract of the thymopharyngeal duct as it descends into the mediastinum, or due to persistence of the duct itself. The duct travels with the carotid sheath, and therefore cysts present as a lateral neck mass and may appear similar to third and fourth BCAs. Because of the course of the duct, cysts may be adherent to the vagus or recurrent laryngeal nerve and cause vocal cord weakness, and may have substernal extension. Complete surgical excision is curative, and final diagnosis is determined by histopathology.

I A laryngocele is an abnormal dilation of the laryngeal ventricle and saccule. An external laryngocele extends through the thyrohyoid membrane and may present as a mass in the neck. Increased intralaryngeal pressure may increase the size. The laryngocele may become infected and form a laryngopyocele. Laryngoscopy should be performed to rule out an internal component before surgical excision, which is the treatment of choice.

J A teratoma is a germ cell tumor and may present as a bulky tumor of the head and neck in the newborn. Nearly all are benign, and complete surgical resection is the treatment of choice. If malignant elements are identified by the pathologist, chemotherapy should be added.

K Sternocleidomastoid muscle (SCM) tumors of infancy (pseudotumor of infancy, fibromatosis colli) present within the first 3 weeks of infancy. These lesions of unknown cause are fibrous tumors that are inseparable from the lower to middle third of the sternocleidomastoid muscle. The lesion causes progressive torticollis, causing the infant's face and chin to tilt away from the affected side and the head to tilt toward the ipsilateral shoulder. Most cases respond to physical therapy, which is the treatment of choice. Surgical division of the SCM and its investing fascia may be warranted in severe cases.

L Plunging ranulas: Ranulas are mucoceles that arise from sublingual salivary glands, and therefore are typically located in the oral cavity lateral to the lingual frenulum. However, large ranulas may extend across the midline or below the mylohyoid muscle and present as a neck mass (plunging ranula). They commonly result from salivary duct obstruction. Surgical excision of the ranula with the associated sublingual gland is associated with the best outcomes and lowest recurrence rates. Most plunging ranulas may be excised transorally, but occasionally a transcervical excision may be required for additional exposure.

ACKNOWLEDGMENT

The authors wish to acknowledge the contributions to the writing of this provided by Dr Jessica Levi, Pediatric Otolaryngologist at the Boston Medical Center.

SUGGESTED READING

Brown RL, Azizkhan RG. Pediatric head and neck lesions. Pediatr Clin North Am. 1998;45:889-905.

Chinnadurai S, Fonnesbeck C, Snyder KM, et al. Pharmacologic interventions for infantile hemangioma: a meta-analysis. Pediatrics. 2016;137(2):1-10.

Connolly AAP, MacKenzie K. Paediatric neck masses: a diagnostic dilemma. J Laryngol Otol. 1997;111:541-545.

Elluru RG, Friess MR, Richter GT, et al. Multicenter evaluation of the effectiveness of systemic propranolol in the treatment of airway hemangiomas. Otolaryngol Head Neck Surg. 2015;153(3):452-460.

François M, Wiener-Vacher SR, Falala M, et al. Audiological assessment of infants and children with preauricular tags. Audiology. 1995;34(1):1-5.

Léauté-Labrèze C, Hoeger P, Mazereeuw-Hautier J, et al. A randomized, controlled trial of oral propranolol in infantile hemangioma. N Engl J Med. 2015;372(8):735-746.

Mobley DL, Wakely PE, Frable MA. Fine-needle aspiration biopsy: application to pediatric head and neck masses. Laryngoscope. 1991;101:469-472.

Motz KM, Nickley KB, Bedwell JR, et al. OK432 versus doxycycline for treatment of macrocystic lymphatic malformations. Ann Otol Rhinol Laryngol. 2014;123(2):81-88.

Torsiglieri AJ Jr, Tom LW, Ross AJ, et al. Pediatric neck masses: guidelines for evaluation. Int J Pediatr Otorhinolaryngol. 1988;16:199-210.

Wang RY, Earl DL, Ruder RO, et al. Syndromic ear anomalies and renal ultrasounds. Pediatrics. 2001;108(2):E32.

CHAPTER 141

Inflammatory Neck Masses in Children

Allison Tobey, Joseph E Dohar

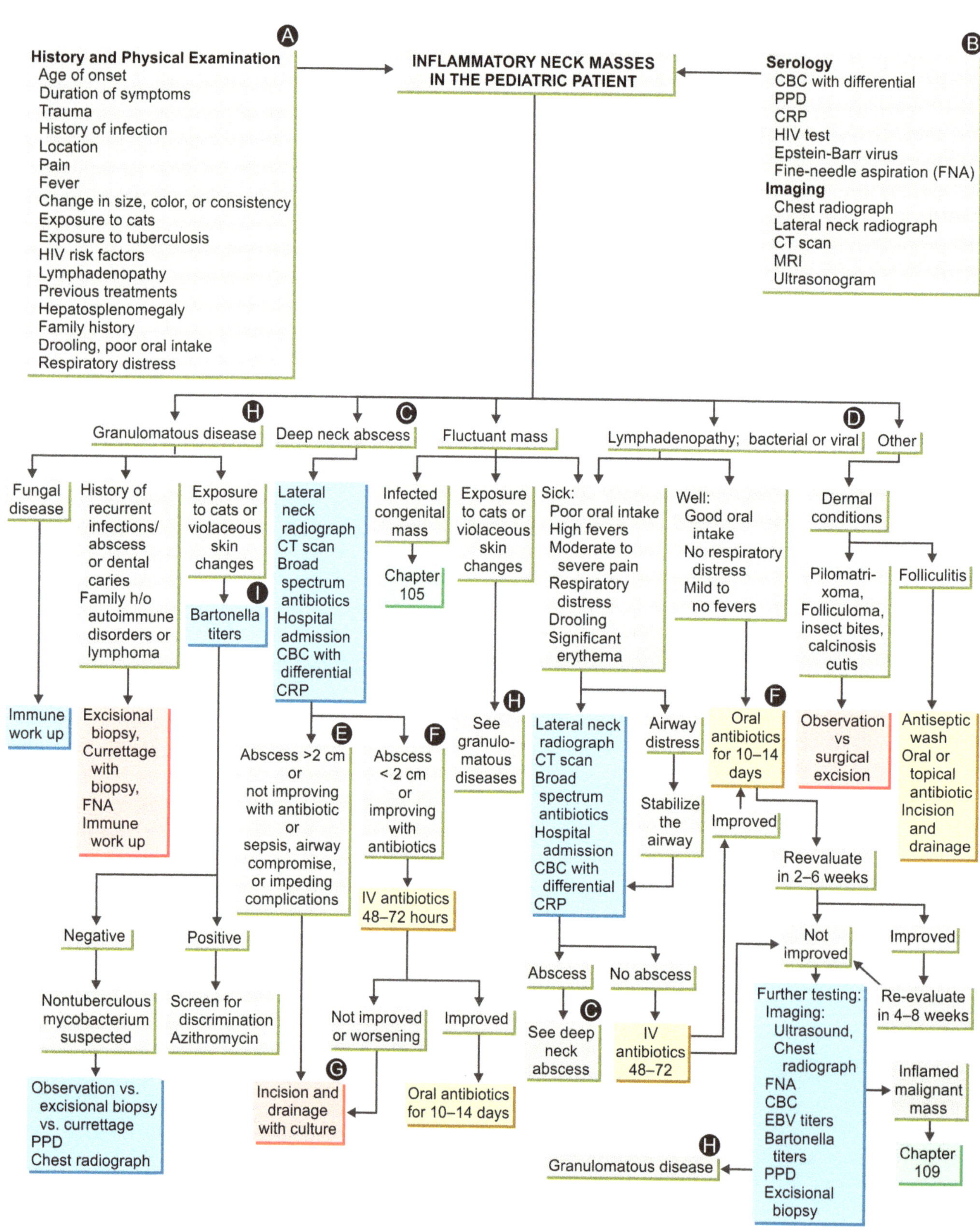

Masses in the neck are commonly inflammatory in nature, particularly in children and young adults. The differential diagnosis is very broad, consisting of localized infections or local manifestation of systemic illness. Regardless of cause, a search for the etiology is required to assure optimal outcome. Malignant neck masses can mimic inflammatory masses, so the physician must maintain a healthy skepticism that the hypothesized diagnosis is correct until confirmed.

A History of trauma, malignancy, autoimmune or immunologic disorders, known congenital masses, exposure to animals, dental issues and immunization status are important. Lethargy, decreased oral intake, fever, pain, erythema, tenderness and swelling suggest infection. Respiratory distress, limited neck extension or drooling are concerning signs of deep neck abscesses (C).

B *Serology*: Leukocytosis, neutrophilic shift, bandemia and elevated C-reactive protein (CRP) or erythrocyte sedimentation rate (ESR) suggest inflammation and can be used to follow response to therapy. Patients with leukocytosis >11 and CRP >100 are less likely to respond to medical therapy alone and have longer hospital stays and neutropenia, anemia and thrombocytopenia may suggest leukemia. Epstein-Barr virus, HIV, toxoplasmosis and Bartonella titers may be helpful.

Imaging: Lateral neck radiographs should be performed with neck extension and on inspiration. Retropharyngeal soft tissue thickening >7 mm or retrotracheal thickening >13 mm are concerning for infection. Air/fluid level diagnostic for abscess. CT scans greatly improves characteristic neck masses. Inflammatory neck masses will have fat stranding of surrounding tissue. Irregular borders with ring enhancement and central hypodensity is suggestive of abscess however, accuracy of CT for predicting abscess is at best 75%. Ultrasound does not involve risk of radiation exposure, is quick, inexpensive and can be performed without sedation. Changes in lymph node architecture, blood flow patterns, fluid density and presence calcification can aid in diagnosis. If airway compromise, patient needs to be accompanied by medical staff to radiology and closely monitored.

C Deep neck abscesses can be life-threatening secondary to airway compromise and should be treated aggressively and with urgency. Overall, most common locations are: Peritonsillar (49%), retropharyngeal (22%) and submandibular (14%). Children <1 year are more likely to present with submandibular, submental or cervical infections as opposed to pharyngeal or retropharyngeal.

D Most lymphadenopathy in pediatrics is reactive to presumed infections of the oropharynx, oral cavity or skin. Complete blood count (CBC) with differential can be used to follow medical therapy when viral or bacterial infections present. It is also helpful for detecting leukemia and some lymphomas.

E Antibiotic use alone for deep space neck abscess is ~50–75% successful. Larger abscesses (>2 cm^2), older patient and those with of recurrent infections are more likely to require surgical intervention.

F Polymicrobial growth occurs in >70% of cases. Group A beta-hemolytic *Streptococcus*, other streptococcal species and *Staphylococcus aureus* are the most common however, gram negative and anaerobic species are also present in 10–50% of specimens. Ampicillin with a beta-lactamase inhibitor or a 2nd or 3rd generation cephalosporin are recommended. Methicillin resistant *S. aureus* occurs in 22–29% of cases. Additional of clindamycin, trimethoprim-sulfamethoxazole and/or vancomycin should be considered when response is poor.

G Gram stain and bacterial cultures helpful in narrowing antibiotic usage. If findings of granulomatous disease, chest radiography and tuberculin skin test (PPD) should be performed. See H.

H Granulamatous disorders are the second most common with Bartonella and nontuberculosis mycobacterium being the most common in Northern America. *Mycobacterium tuberculosis*, fungal infections and Langerhans cell histocytosis X should also be considered.

I Cat Scratch disease (CSD) is caused by inoculation of *Bartonella henselae* species typically through exposure to cat saliva (bites, claws or licking of open wounds) but can be transmitted by fleas and dogs. CSD is typically a benign, self-limited disease and resolved without treatment in 2–3 months, but 5–14% of cases will disseminate and can be life-threatening. More than 50% of patient will have noticeable response with 5 days of azithromycin.

SUGGESTED READING

Bass JW, Freitas BC, Freitas AD, et al. Prospective randomized double blind placebo-controlled evaluation of azithromycin for treatment of cat-scratch disease. Pediatr Infect Dis J. 1998;17(6): 447-452.

Carbone PN, Capra GG, Brigger MT. Antibiotic therapy for pediatric deep neck abscesses: a systematic review. Int J Pediatr Otorhinolaryngol. 2012;76:1647-1653.

Coticchia JM, Getnick GS, Yun RD, et al. Age-, site-, and time-specific differences in pediatric deep neck abscesses. Arch Otolaryngol Head Neck Surg. 2011;130:201-207.

Gori-Ari E, Hopewell BL. Correlation between pre-operative diagnosis and post-operative pathology reading in pediatric neck masses—a review of 281 cases. Int J Pediatr Otorhinolaryngol. 2015;79:2-7.

Iversen RH, Illum P. Cervical nontuberculous mycobacterial lymphadenitis in children. Dan Med J. 2012;59(1):A43-49.

Penn EB, Goudy SL. Pediatric inflammatory adenopathy. Otolaryngol Clin North Am. 2015;48:137-151.

CHAPTER 142

Vascular Malformations of the Head and Neck

Larry D Hartzell, Gresham T Richter

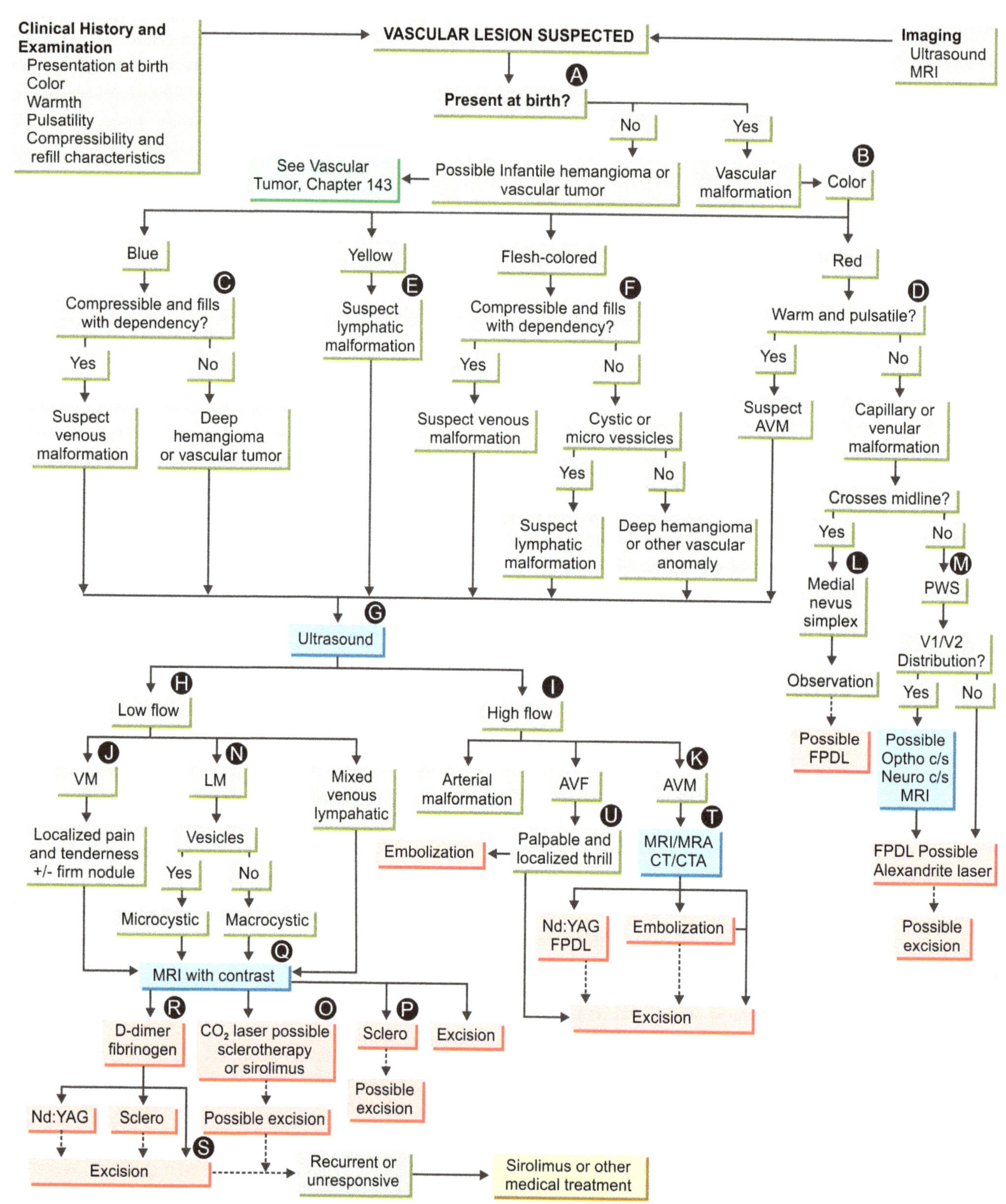

Vascular malformations (VaM) are distinguished from vascular tumors by their clinical and histological characteristics as demonstrated by the 2014 classification scheme outlined by the International Society for the Study of Vascular Anomalies.

A Vascular malformations are present at birth although their presence may not become recognized until later in life. Slow, proportionate growth is typical of VaM, although accelerated growth can be found associated with trauma, infection, and hormonal changes (i.e. pre-pubescence, pregnancy, and menopause). Although considered benign lesions, VaM can be locally aggressive and destructive creating significant disfigurement and functional problems.

B When a patient with a vascular anomaly presents to clinic, the history will provide the diagnosis in the majority of cases. The next step in the diagnostic search that often proves very revelatory is the examination of the lesion. Specific analysis of the color of the lesion subcategorizes these anomalies effectively. The major colors encountered are: blue, red, yellow, and flesh-colored.

C For "blue" lesions, the ability to engorge or fill with dependent positioning (i.e. head down) will help separate venous malformations (VMs) from vascular tumors or other possible lesions.

D "Red" lesions are most commonly infantile hemangiomas or other capillary malformations such as a Port Wine Stain (PWS). However, if it is found to be pulsatile and warmer than surrounding tissues, ateriovenous malformation (AVM) should be suspected.

E "Yellow" vascular lesions are likely lymphatic malformations (LMs) and are frequently cystic in nature.

F "Flesh-colored" lesions can be vascular in nature. Many times this occurs early in presentation while still fairly small in size or before associated findings like telangiectasias are recognized. If a vascular lesion is suspected, the compressibility and filling with dependency should be explored. If negative, then the cystic nature should be questioned. Lymphatic malformations will frequently be flesh-colored especially if located deep to the skin. If not cystic, a deep vascular tumor or malformation should be suspected and ultrasonography performed.

G Vascular malformations are best sub-divided into slow-flow or fast-flow lesions based on ultrasonography findings. These ultrasound flow characteristics help to accurately define the different classes of VaM. The addition of vessel type as discovered by physical examination, radiographic imaging, and pathologic evaluation helps to confirm the diagnosis. Capillary or venular malformations (including medial nevus simplex and PWS) that are not vascular tumors do not need ultrasound testing and are diagnosed predominantly with history and physical examination findings based mostly on color and location.

This modality alone will to help distinguish slow versus fast flow lesions, and can even help differentiate vascular tumors (hemangiomas) from compressible vascular malformations (venous and lymphatic).

Venous malformations are compressible, have low vascular flow, and demonstrate areas of echogenicity with a monophasic duplex waveform.

Lymphatic malformations are also compressible but without flow. These must be distinguished from one another as macrocystic, microcystic, or mixed lesions. They may also occur along with venous malformations.

Arteriovenous malformations are defined by duplex ultrasound as high flow lesions with distinct arterial waveforms with vascular clusters and poorly demarcated borders.

H Vascular malformations can be mixed lesions composed of multiple vascular sub-types, however, most VaM are of a single type.

Low flow is the most common class of VaM. Their predominant vessel allows for subcategorization of these lesions. Therefore they are separated into VM, LM, and mixed venous lymphatic malformations. Mixed venous lymphatic may have characteristics of either or both components.

I High-flow vascular malformations are less frequently encountered and are divided into arterial malformations, arteriovenous fistulas (AVF), and AVMs. Arteriovenous malformations are the most complex and difficult to treat high flow extracranial vascular malformations. Arterial malformations and AVF are uncommon and will not be discussed further within this algorithm. Their clinical findings and treatment are often similar to that of AVMs.

J A few specific history and physical examination findings may help to confirm or in some cases further clarify the diagnosis after obtaining the ultrasound findings. Periodic pain indicates the likely presence of a VM as most VaM are painless. Pain related to VM is thought to be secondary to local intravascular coagulation (LIC), swelling, or phleboliths. These are spherical and well-organized, calcified clots found in the ectatic veins of venous malformations. Despite the cause, pain in these lesions responds well to anti-inflammatory treatment. Because of discomfort and LIC, prophylactic aspirin therapy and subcutaneous lovenox can be used to manage pain in these lesions. Compression garments (although these may prove difficult if not impossible within the head and neck area) and head elevation are also employed to reduce venous stasis. A firm nodule is palpable when a phlebolith is present and may be associated with localized tenderness.

As mentioned previously, VMs are compressible with a slow refilling time. This helps distinguish them from AVMs, which are limited in their compressibility and rapidly rebound upon release in addition to having increased warmth to touch.

Engorgement with dependent positioning or a Valsalva maneuver is a hallmark sign of VM. Bleeding episodes are also occasionally reported in VMs, especially when the mucosa is involved. However, massive spontaneous bleeding is rare and is more often associated with AVMs. Bleeding with dental extractions may be encountered with VMs, AVMs, or mixed lesions.

K Arteriovenous malformations are warm to palpitation relative to the adjoining skin or soft tissue in comparison to VM and LM, which are isothermal. This relative warmth is due to the high arterial flow. These lesions are also frequently pulsatile with a palpable thrill.

L Medial nevus simplex (also known as midline venular malformation, nevus flammeus, or salmon patch but is more commonly known as a "stork bite" or "angel's kiss") is an erythematous stain of the skin that is present at birth and found in the midline of the body. It may be found on the forehead, glabella, eyelids, nape of neck, lower back. It typically crosses the midline and is fairly symmetric as opposed to the typical unilateral and asymmetric nature of the PWS. During the first few years of life the skin color tends to fade with the majority resolving completely. Observation is recommended with the rare consideration for laser therapy if fading does not occur to an acceptable degree. The flash pulse dye laser (FPDL; 585 nm wavelength) would be the laser most commonly used in this circumstance. Imaging and laboratory testing are not indicated and excision is unnecessary.

M Port-wine stains (defined as capillary or venular malformations) occur in 1:10,000 to 1:40,000 newborns. They may occur anywhere on the body as a well-defined vascular stain. These lesions slowly darken with time to a more purple discoloration. They may occur in isolation or part of more complex congenital vascular disorders. The involved skin will thicken at times with age in untreated lesions to become excess, disrupted, and sessile lesions.

Early intervention with laser therapy is advocated for most superficial vascular lesions. Port-wine stains are commonly encountered in a dermatomal distribution. The location of the lesion can also have a significant impact on patient prognosis. Lesions found in the V1 or V2 distribution can be associated with Sturge-Weber syndrome, which includes the risk of meningeal involvement, glaucoma and seizure activity. A referral to Ophthalmology and/or Neurology should be considered in these circumstances. Magnetic resonance imaging (MRI) is recommended in these cases. Treatment typically consists of periodic laser treatments (typically FPDL although Alexandrite has also been successfully employed). Port-wine stains associated with soft tissue hypertrophy may also occur which in some cases may require surgical excision.

N Lymphatic malformations are subdivided into microcystic and macrocystic based on ultrasound findings although most patients have at least a small component of each type. Magnetic Resonance Imaging typically allows for further categorization and delineation of the extent of disease although computed tomography (CT) can also provide sufficient information for treatment. Typical MRI findings are: T1 isointense, T2 hyperintense, no contrast enhancement and fluid–fluid levels.

O Patients with microcystic LMs typically develop microvesicles on the skin or mucosa. These can be treated with CO_2 laser or another form of thermal destruction. Adjunctive sclerotherapy or interstitial laser treatments can help to manage the microcystic disease although surgical excision is often required.

P Macrocystic LMs are frequently very apparent at birth. These are very unlikely to spontaneously regress although some case reports of this do exist particularly in those found in the posterior triangle of the neck. Nearly all will require intervention. There are two major options for treatment with fairly equivalent results depending on the literature that is being reviewed. Injection with a sclerosing material, such as OK-432, which can be very effective especially in the setting of a single macrocyst. Alternatively, surgical excision provides an opportunity for complete disease removal with a low rate of recurrence. Surgery also allows for adjustment of tissues that may have stretched and expanded with the growth of the malformation. If surgery does not provide complete disease resolution, the use of sirolimus can be explored to slow the growth of the disease as well as possibly eradicate the lesion.

Q Magnetic Resonance Imaging with gadolinium contrast is very helpful in the delineation of the different vascular anomalies. Magnetic Resonance Imaging findings for VM are: T1 isointense, T2 hyperintense, contrast enhancement, and venous flow voids where phleboliths are present. Magnetic Resonance Imaging findings that distinguish arteriovenous malformations from other vascular anomalies are the presence of tortuous arterial feeding vessels and flow voids indicating a fast flowing lesion.

R Laboratory testing does not currently assist in the diagnosis of vascular anomalies. However, VM or mixed venous LMs may display elevated D-dimer and low fibrinogen levels due to constant local intravascular coagulation in the lesions. Histologic tissue staining, however, is frequently used to help distinguish different VaM from one another; Glut-1, GNAQ, TIE2, D2-40, and CD105 help distinguish hemangiomas, PWS, VM, LMs, and AVMs respectively.

S Venous malformations will continue to expand and grow throughout life and will require intervention for control and resolution of the disease process.

Unlike hemangiomas that stop growing and slowly involute, VaM will persist and grow slowly throughout life. Minimally invasive laser treatment of skin and mucosal involvement therefore becomes important in their control and resolution. Red or pink lesions will respond well to FPDL. Blue mucosal and skin staining indicate venous malformation which will improve with Nd:YAG laser therapy. Early treatment of all these lesions has been shown to provide better long-term results. The degree of tissue penetration will vary with each laser. For deeper lesions to benefit from laser treatment, an interstitial approach may be necessary. Caution must be taken, however, to avoid neuromuscular injury.

Laser treatment using Nd:YAG laser superficially or interstitially can prove very effective in VM. Sclerotherapy can also prove very effective as a primary treatment or as a preoperative measure to lessen blood loss as well as better define the extent of resection during surgical excision. Operative excision remains, however, as a reliable method for primary and salvage disease removal in VM although repeat procedures are common. If surgical management fails, the use of sirolimus can be considered as has been more recently described.

Mixed venous lymphatic malformations as identified by ultrasound, MRI and at times only by histological examination after excision can be managed very similar to either VM or LM. Multi-modality therapy is frequently required and found to be effective.

T Arteriovenous malformations tend to be the most difficult and challenging VaM to treat. Magnetic resonance imaging (MRI and MRA), CT, CT angiography and in some cases angiography are used to determine the diagnosis as well as extent of disease. Efforts are made to identify the nidus or center of the AVM as most feel this area is the critical growth and angiogenic center that must be removed or destroyed in order to eradicate the disease. This malformation has the greater risk of leading to progressive tissue necrosis and deformity requiring multiple procedures throughout a patient's lifespan. Massive bleeding and loss of vital organ may transpire.

Excision is almost always required in AVMs although some reports of control with embolization have been described. Prior to excision, embolization of the feeding vessels is frequently performed. For the cutaneous or mucosal staining, laser treatment can be performed as well.

U Arteriovenous fistulas are sometimes encountered although much less frequently than AVMs but more commonly than arterial malformations which are very rare and will not be discussed further. Most AVFs of any notable size will have a classic palpable thrill when touched and this will be fairly localized. Ultrasound is used to confirm the diagnosis much like the other vascular malformations. After being identified, the decision to proceed to possible embolization versus excision should be made.

Large vascular malformations are rarely fully cured as they frequently infiltrate normal tissue. The first dictum of surgery is that the treatment shall be no worse than the disease. Surgical excision can be the "gold standard" in attempting cure of vascular malformations although alternative therapies are gaining greater success and surgery is progressively becoming a salvage effort. Careful surgical planning is required to maximize disease control, minimize morbidity and limit bleeding. Referrals to centers accustomed to treating such malformations should be considered. Advanced reconstruction techniques (such as free tissue transfer) may even be required and appropriate preparation for this component of the treatment should be performed.

SUGGESTED READING

Dasgupta R, Fishman SJ. ISSVA classification. Semin Pediatr Surg. 2014;23(4):158-161.

Horbach SE, Lokhorst MM, Saeed P, et al. Sclerotherapy for low-flow vascular malformations of the head and neck: a systematic review of sclerosing agents. J Plast Reconstr Aesthet Surg. 2016;69(3):295-304.

Kransdorf MJ, Murphey MD, Fanburg-Smith JC. Classification of benign vascular lesions: history, current nomenclature, and suggestions for imagers. Am J Roentgenol. 2011;197:8-11.

Richter GT, Braswell L. Management of venous malformations. Facial Plast Surg. 2012;28(6):603-610.

Richter GT, Freidman AB. Hemangiomas and vascular malformations: current theory and management. Int J Pediatr. 2012; 2012:645-678.

Richter GT, Suen JY. Head and Neck Vascular Anomalies: A Practical Case-Based Approach. San Diego, CA, USA: Plural Publishing, Inc; 2015.

Wassef M, Blei F, Adams D, et al. Vascular anomalies classification: recommendation from the International Society for the Study of Vascular Anomalies. Pediatrics. 2015;136(1):e203-e214.

Vascular Tumors of the Head and Neck

Andrew A McCormick, Lorelei J Grunwaldt

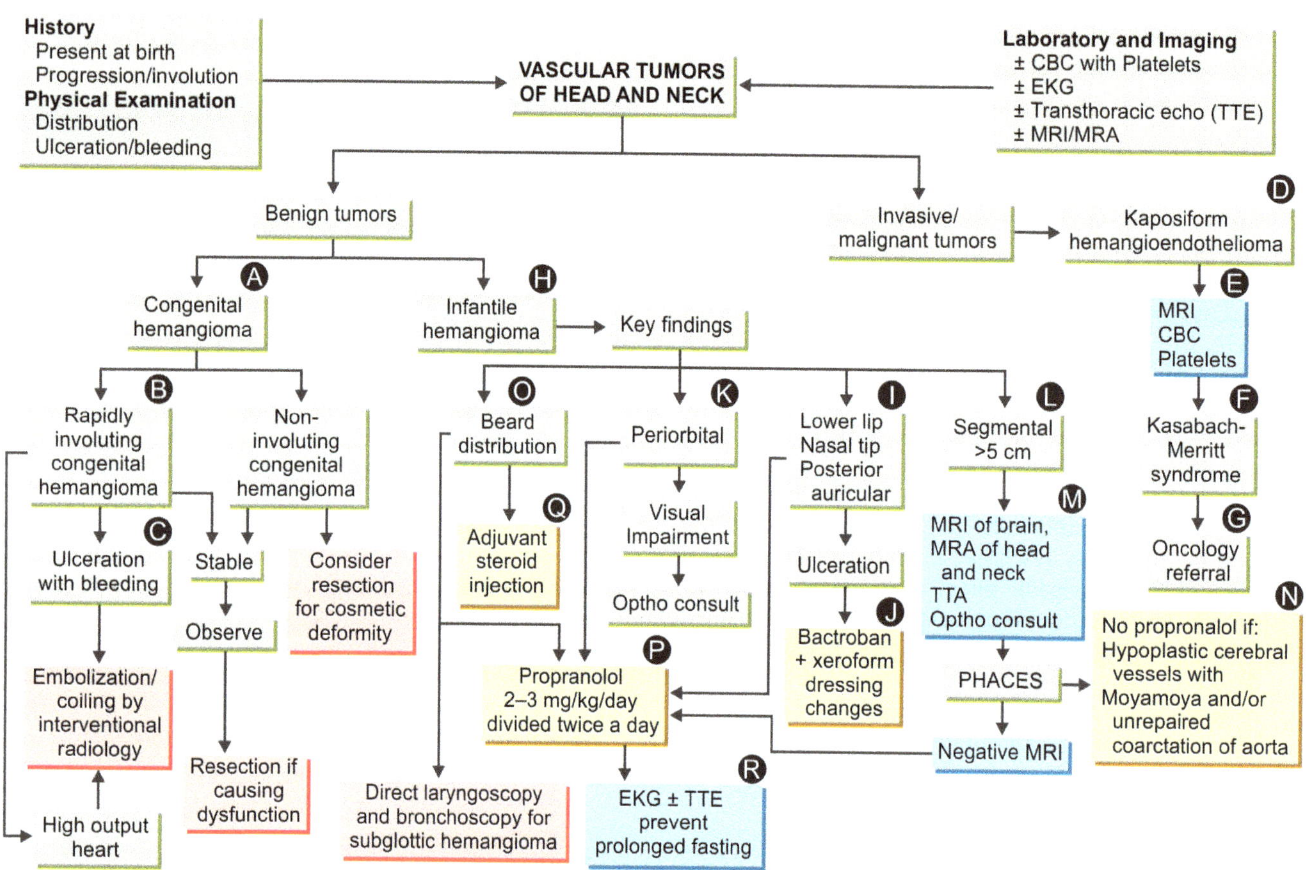

Vascular tumors of the head and neck are a rapidly evolving area of medicine. The advent of innovative medical interventions has led to shifts in treatment of these lesions. This chapter focuses on bedside evaluation of these lesions and then directs diagnostic and treatment interventions.

A The congenital hemangioma can be distinguished from the infantile hemangioma in that they are fully formed at birth and appear as ≥5 cm violaceous plaques with coarse telangiectasia and surrounding hypopigmented halo.

B There are two types of congenital hemangiomas: the rapidly involuting congenital hemangioma (RICH) that self-involutes by 1 year of life and the noninvoluting congenital hemangioma that never resolves.

C Large congenital hemangiomas can contribute to shunt physiology producing high-output heart failure. Specifically, RICH can lead to ulceration with risk of significant bleeding. When this occurs, these lesions may require coiling/embolization by interventional radiology or surgical resection.

D The Kaposiform hemangioendothelioma (KHE) is an invasive vascular tumor that has an appearance of expansive nonhealing bruise. It has a very low potential for malignancy.

E Kaposiform hemangioendothelioma is diagnostically evaluated with magnetic resonance imaging (MRI), which demonstrates an invasive vascular tumor that crosses tissue planes and complete blood count (CBC) with platelets to screen for consumptive thrombocytopenia.

F Kaposiform hemangioendothelioma is commonly complicated by Kasabach-Merritt syndrome, characterized by profound thrombocytopenia due to platelet trapping within the tumor, sometimes accompanying microangiopathic hemolytic anemia and secondary consumptive coagulopathy.

G Because of the aggressive nature of KHE, they should be managed in conjunction with an oncologist.

H The typical life cycle of an infantile hemangioma has appearance in the first month of life with rapid proliferation lasting for the first 5–9 months followed by slow involution by 10% every year (30% resolution by 3 years, 50% by 5 years, and 100% by 10 years).

I Infantile hemangiomas of the lower lip, nasal tip, and posterior auricular surface are at increased risk of ulceration; therefore, they should be treated aggressively (barrier cream + initiation of propranolol).

J Ulceration should be treated with good wound care including bactroban + xeroform dressing changes twice a day until healing occurs; then continue use of barrier cream to prevent further ulceration.

K Infantile hemangiomas in the periorbital region, which are >1 cm, have a deep component, on the eyelid, medial in orientation, associated ptosis, or proptosis, are at high risk of permanent visual impairment and therefore should be treated aggressively.

L Segmental infantile hemangiomas >5 cm that are located on the head and neck are associated with PHACES (posterior fossa anomaly, hemangioma, arterial anomalies of head and neck, cardiac defects, eye anomalies, and sternal malformations) syndrome.

M The PHACES evaluation includes an MRI of the brain to evaluate posterior fossa anomalies, magnetic resonance angiogram (MRA) head and neck to evaluate for arterial anomalies of the carotid and derivative branches, transthoracic echo (TTE) to evaluate for cardiac anomalies with coarctation of aorta most common and ophthalmology evaluation to rule out eye anomalies.

N Children with PHACES complicated by hypoplasia of the carotid and associated branches complicated by Moyamoya disease or coarctation of aorta are at increased risk of stroke when treated with propranolol and therefore should be done in conjunction with Neurosurgery and Cardiology.

O Segmental infantile hemangiomas of the beard distribution had an association with airway hemangiomas and therefore warrant direct laryngoscopy and bronchoscopy.

P The treatment of infantile hemangiomas has shifted to medical management with propranolol 2–3 mg/kg per day divided twice a day until the first birthday.

Q Subglottic hemangiomas are typically more recalcitrant to treatment with propranolol alone and require higher dosing (3 mg/kg per day) and consideration for adjuvant steroid injections.

R The most concerning complications related to propranolol use are hypoglycemia and bradyarrhythmias. Hypoglycemia can be prevented with the use of propranolol by assuring oral feeding immediately before or after every dose of the medication and holding the medication when the child is sick. Cardiac complications can by minimized by confirming a normal cardiac examination (if murmur present, then obtains transthoracic cardiac echo) and normal baseline electrocardiogram.

SUGGESTED READING

Chang LC, Haggstrom AN, Drolet BA, et al. Hemangioma Investigator Group. Growth characteristics of infantile hemangiomas: implications for management. Pediatrics. 2008;122(2):360-367.

Colmenero I, Heoger PH. Vascular tumours in infants. Part II: vascular tumours of intermediate malignancy and malignant tumours. Br J Dermatol. 2014;171:474-484.

Kim HJ, Colombo M, Frieden IJ. Ulcerated hemangiomas: clinical characteristics and response to therapy. J Am Acad Dermtol. 2001;44:962-972.

Liang MG, Frieden IJ. Infantile and congenital hemangiomas. Semin Pediatr Surg. 2014;23:162-167.

Metry D, Heyer G, Hess C, et al. Consensus statement on diagnostic criteria for PHACE syndrome. Pediatrics. 2009;124:1447-1456.

Spence-Shishido AA, Good WV, Baselga E, et al. Hemangiomas and the eye. Clin Dermatol. 2015;33:170-182.

Neck Pain

Larry A Zieske

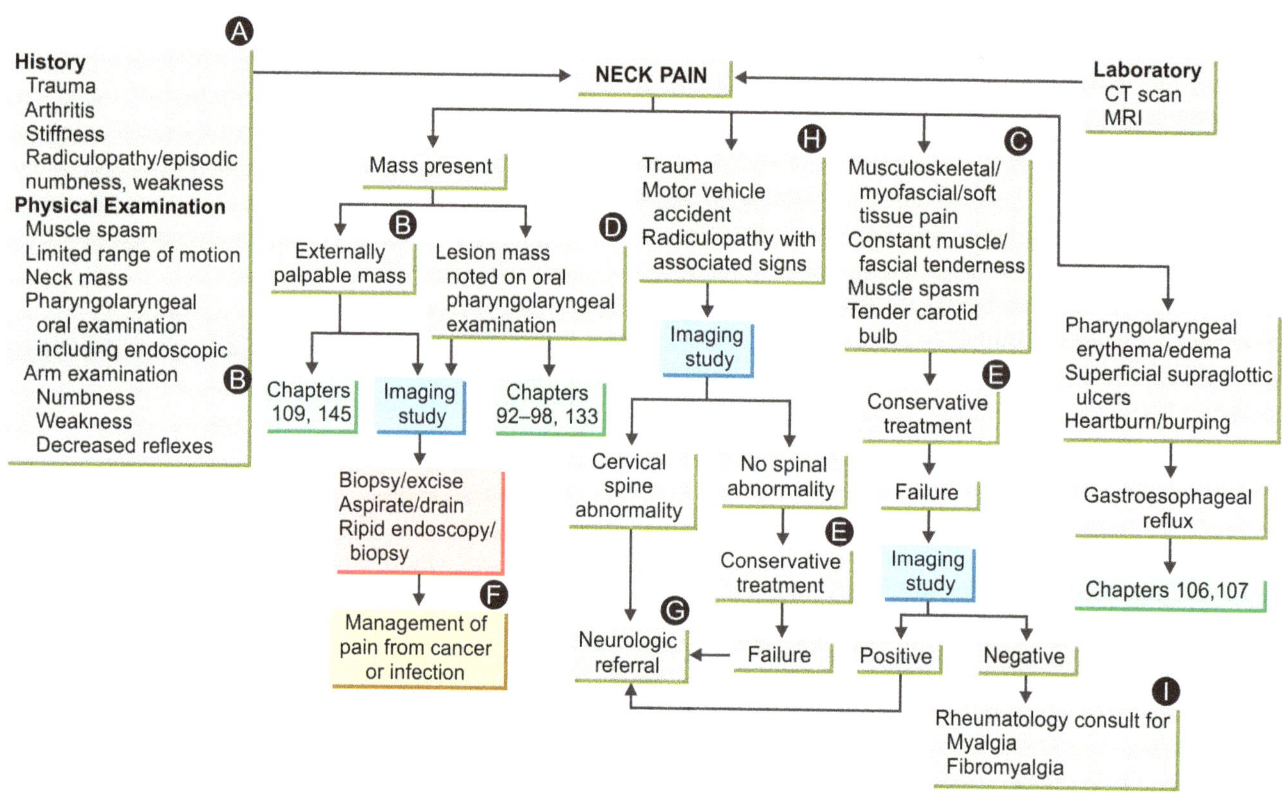

Neck pain is a common complaint. Differentiating pain originating in the cervical spine and musculotendinous tissue from other causes can be challenging and critical. Historical association with trauma, degenerative inflammatory diseases or recent infectious, dental issues, or reflux symptoms assists in guiding initial choices. Physical examination findings also assist such as masses or neurological deficits. Temporal factors, such as acute versus chronic and rapidity of evolution, are also beneficial considerations in establishing a diagnosis.

A The causes of neck pain are multiple and differ significantly with age and history. As age increases, degenerative conditions predominate, such as osteoarthritis of the cervical spine. Radiculopathy may produce pain associated with motion. Children and adolescents often have a shorter history and symptoms associated with inflammation (cough, sore throat, fever). A history of trauma is usually easily elicited but in situations of child abuse can be hidden. Establishing the diagnosis must be the primary goal to develop a rational program of pain relief.

B The presence of a palpable mass in the neck will narrow the differential diagnoses and direct examination based on location and characteristics. Imaging and biopsy usually are keys (*see* Step D and other chapters of this book, such as Chapters 145 and 146).

C Muscular-fascial tenderness with or without a history of trauma (motor vehicle accident) and no radiculopathy suggests soft tissue injury. The most frequent causes are overuse or direct injury. Pain is typically constant, although with variations in intensity. Pain activated by motion or muscle tenderness on palpation often with trigger points is typical. Trigger point-sensitive pain often increases with age or inactivity.

D The finding of a pharyngeal/laryngeal lesion or mass will focus the differential diagnosis. A complete examination of the mucosal surfaces of the upper aerodigestive tract will identify whether the lesion is single or multiple. Typically flexible endoscopic examination would be done in the office. Imaging studies will assist in determining the extent of the lesion(s). Biopsy will then direct appropriate therapies. Lesions that appear to be highly vascular should potentially be studied angiographically with potential embolization (angiofibromas and paragangliomas) (*see* Chapters 141 and 142).

E Conservative therapy generally falls into three areas: physical therapy, pharmacotherapy, and behavioral therapy.

Physical therapy includes soft tissue mobilization, body mechanics, postural exercises, cervical traction, development and management of home exercise programs with muscle balancing and strengthening exercises, heat and cold therapy, spray and stretch, ultrasonography, electrogalvanic stimulation, phonophoresis, transcutaneous electrical nerve stimulation, and acupuncture. The goal of pharmacotherapy is to relieve pain on a short-term basis, while other therapies are being instituted for more long-lasting benefit. Oral medications such as nonsteroidal anti-inflammatory drugs (NSAIDs), acetaminophen, muscle relaxants, and myoneural injections with anesthetics and steroids may be quite effective. Injection can be both diagnostic and therapeutic. Behavioral medicine includes relaxation therapy, biofeedback, behavior modification, operant conditioning, and hypnosis. Psychiatric consultation may be helpful in achieving behavioral goals as well as assisting in prescribing pharmacotherapies such as antidepressants in chronic pain situations. The use of narcotics and psychosedatives is to be avoided in patients with chronic pain. Physical medicine practitioners can design and supervise a comprehensive program of physical therapy, which may include biofeedback.

F Cancer pain resulting from infiltration of soft or bony structures and inflammation of nearby tissues often decreases with the use of cancer therapy. The use of ancillary measures is appropriate in this instance, especially in a patient who is terminally ill (Chapter 180). Narcotics administered concurrently with other medications such as NSAIDs, antipsychotics, antidepressants, steroids, and amphetamines can minimize sedation.

G Referral could be to a Neurologist, Neurosurgeon, or Orthopedic surgeon experienced in cervical spine abnormalities. The selection depends on the local clinical circumstances and preferences. Although nonsurgical treatments can be instituted by the Otolaryngologist, early consultation generally is believed to be wise for optimal patient care and litigation protection/avoidance.

H Although an examination is not the usual area of Otolaryngologists, knowledge of abnormalities is helpful in the evaluation of neck pain in patients. Pain radiating into the arm and associated paresthesias, numbness, and weakness indicate radiculopathy and the need for neurologic referral (disk degeneration and neural foramina narrowing). Decreased deep tendon reflexes can also be noted in these circumstances.

I An interesting variant of rheumatologic pain is calcifying myositis of paraspinal muscles including longus colli. It can include fluid collection in the prevertebral space to be differentiated from infectious etiology and abscess. Other inflammatory signs would be lacking, such as fever and elevated WBC count.

SUGGESTED READING

Barnsley L. Neck Pain. In: Rheumatology, vol 1, 4th edition. Spain: Mosby Elsevier; 2008. pp. 579-592.

Boyd R. Evaluation of neck pain. In: Goroll AH (Ed). Primary Care Medicine: Office Evaluation and Management of the Adult Patient, 3rd edition. Philadelphia, PA: JB Lippincott; 1994. p. 752.

Chung T, Rebello R, Booden EA. Retropharyngeal calcific tendonitis: case report and review of the literature. Emerg Radiol. 2005:11;375-380.

Clauw DJ. Fibromyalgia. In: Rheumatology, vol 1, 4th edition. Spain: Mosby Elsevier; 2008. pp. 701-711.

MacNab I, McCulloch J. Neck and Shoulder Pain. Baltimore, MD: Williams & Wilkins; 1994.

Phew Le, Katz lA, Raj PP. Evaluation and management of patients with chronic head and neck pain. In: Paparella MM, Shumrick DA, Gluckman JL, Meyerhoff WL (Eds). Otolaryngology, vol I, 3rd edition. Philadelphia, PA: WB Saunders; 1991. pp. 817-839.

Neck Mass in Adults

Johannes J Fagan

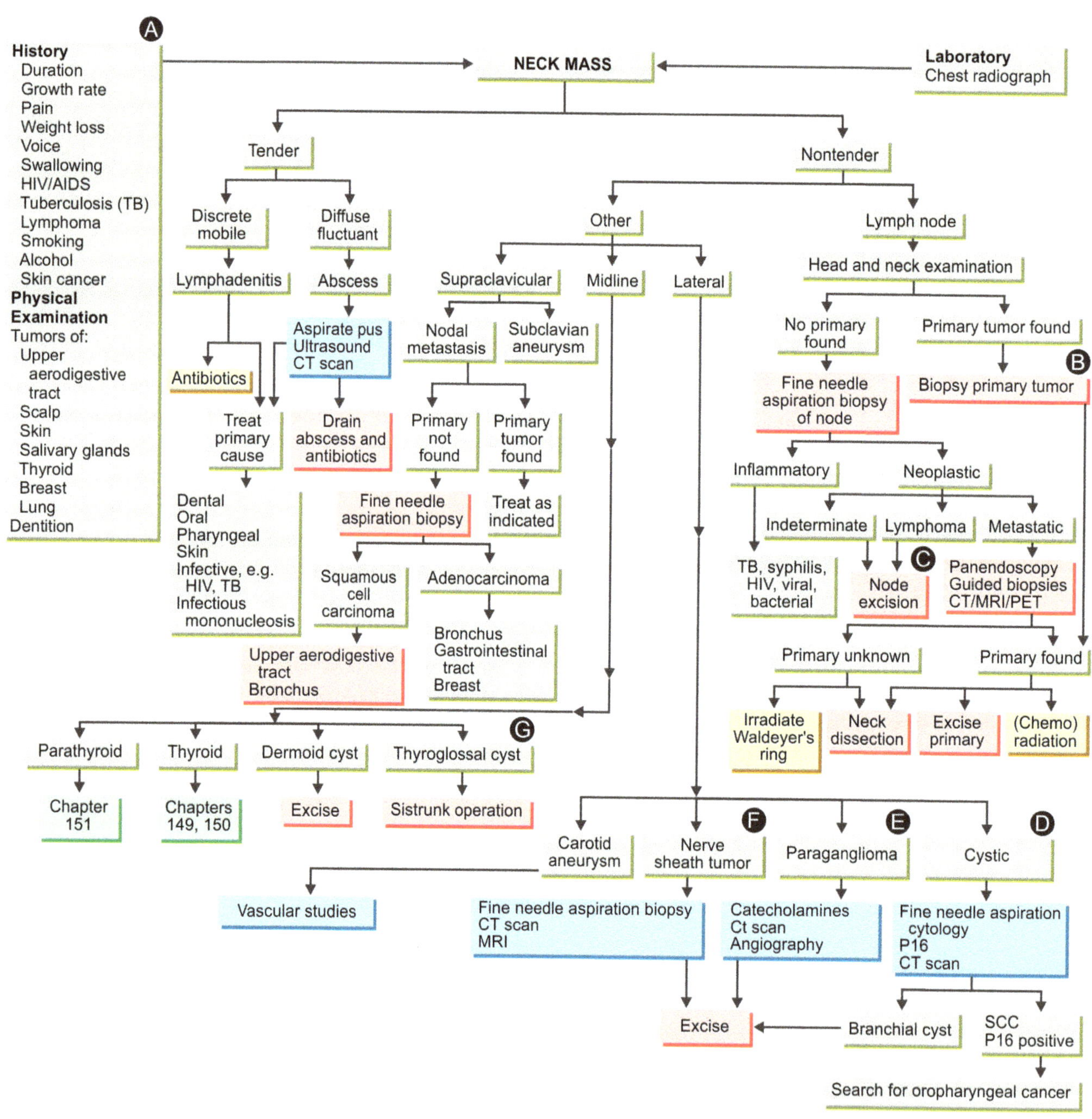

The etiology of the majority of neck masses in adults can be determined following a detailed history, examination, and if still in doubt, fine-needle aspiration. A stepwise diagnostic approach avoids unnecessary and expensive investigations such as computed tomography (CT), magnetic resonance imaging (MRI), and positron emission tomography (PET) scans being done in many cases.

A The etiology of neck masses is generally apparent following a careful history and physical examination. Primary pathology of the upper aerodigestive tract should be excluded, especially in patients presenting with pain, dysphagia, odynophagia, dysphonia, or cervical adenopathy. Tuberculosis (TB) can present with lymphadenopathy, abscesses, and, if they break through skin, as sinuses (scrofula). Tuberculosis can also mimic carcinoma of the pharynx and larynx. Diagnosis is made by microscopy, culture, and histology. Acquired immunodeficiency syndrome (AIDS) is associated with cervical adenopathy, Kaposi's sarcoma, lymphoma, and TB.

B If a primary tumor is found, confirmation that enlarged cervical nodes contain tumor is unnecessary, except when nodes are outside the expected lymphatic drainage area of the tumor. In such cases, fine-needle aspiration biopsy (FNAB) of the nodes is appropriate.

C Open biopsy is rarely required if a systematic diagnostic approach is followed. Not only may it be unnecessary, but it may compromise the design of skin incisions, preclude pedicled flaps, and necessitate the use of adjuvant irradiation. With a lymph node or a mass of uncertain nature, one should therefore avoid the temptation to perform open biopsy. Although a suspicion of lymphoma can be raised on FNAB, conclusive diagnosis and classification require histologic examination of an excised node (*see* Chapter 152, Lymphomas of the Head and Neck).

D A cystic mass should always raise the suspicion of a cystic metastasis from an oropharyngeal carcinoma, or from squamous cell carcinoma or melanoma of the skin. If the FNAB tests are positive for P16 (HPV+), then the search for the primary cancer should be directed at the oropharynx.

E Paragangliomas arise from neuroectodermal tissue but, unlike pheochromocytomas, rarely secrete catecholamines. Evaluation for catecholamine secretion is indicated in the presence of palpitations, flushing, or hypertension, and in patients with a positive family history of paraganglioma. A positive family history is associated with multiple paragangliomas. Multiple tumors can be detected by CT, MRI, or angiography.

F Nerve sheath tumors include schwannomas, neurofibromas and their malignant counterparts, malignant schwannoma, and neurofibrosarcomas. They arise from the nerve sheaths of any of the cranial, autonomic, and peripheral nerves in the head and neck. Schwannomas are slow-growing tumors, and nerve function is initially preserved. Neurofibroma may be solitary or more commonly multiple as part of neurofibromatosis (von Recklinghausen's disease). About >50% of patients with neurofibromatosis have a positive family history. Treatment is by surgical excision.

G Thyroglossal duct cysts occur anywhere between the base of the tongue and the mediastinum. They may present as a cystic mass, an abscess, a draining sinus, or a tumor, most commonly papillary carcinoma. If they occur in the region of the hyoid bone, they typically move upward on protrusion of the tongue or swallowing. Treatment is by surgical excision. The Sistrunk operation involves resection of the cyst, the infrahyoid tract, the body of the hyoid bone, and a core of muscle up to foramen cecum.

SUGGESTED READING

Fagan JJ, Taylor K, Bolding E. Head and neck lymph node and tumour biopsy techniques. In: Open Access Atlas of Otolaryngology Head and Neck Operative Surgery. [online] Available from: https://vula.uct.ac.za/access/content/group/ba5fb1bd-be95-48e5-81be-586fbaeba29d/Head%20and%20neck%20lymph%20node%20and%20tumour%20biopsy%20techniques.pdf. 2017, Open Education Consortium, Creative Commons, Mountain View, CA, Pages 1-12, Last accessed: 5.19.2018

Strojan P, Ferlito A, Langendijk JA, et al. Contemporary management of lymph node metastases from an unknown primary to the neck: II. A review of therapeutic options. Head Neck. 2013;35(2):286-293.

Strojan P, Ferlito A, Medina JE, et al. Contemporary management of lymph node metastases from an unknown primary to the neck: I. A review of diagnostic approaches. Head Neck. 2013;35(1):123-132.

Management of the Neck in Head and Neck Cancer

David E Eibling

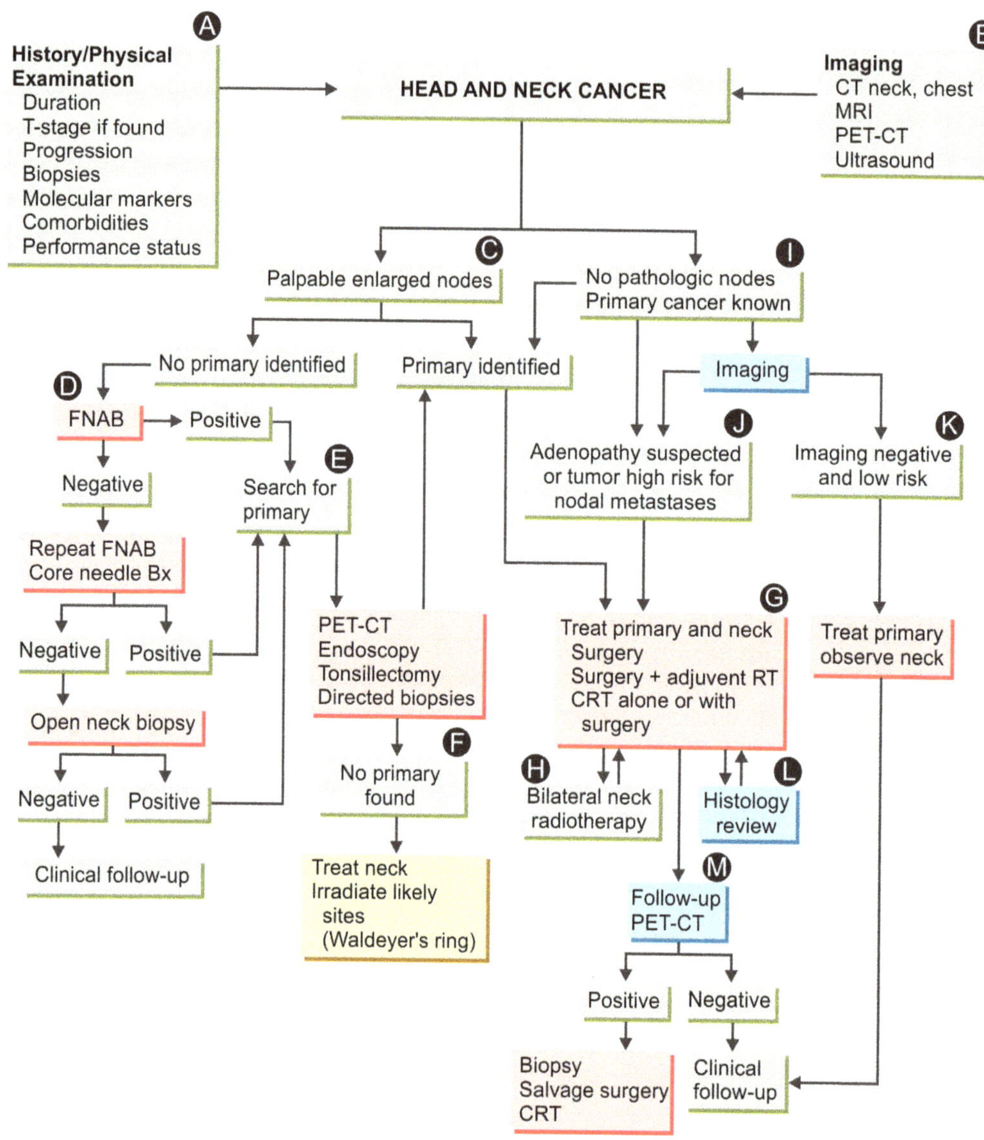

Many cancers of the head and neck metastasize to the regional lymph nodes early in the course of the disease. The impact on prognosis is dependent on primary site and stage, tumor growth characteristics, presence of distant metastases, and extent of regional adenopathy. Some sites (oropharynx and nasopharynx) and some tumor variants such as Epstein-Barr virus (EBV) and human papilloma virus (HPV)-related cancers demonstrate an early propensity to metastasize, whereas others (i.e. glottic cancers) rarely metastasize until late in the disease course. With the exception of thyroid and EBV-related nasopharyngeal cancers, the presence of cervical adenopathy reduces the likelihood of cure, and the staging system reflects this negative impact. As a result, treatment strategies for head and neck cancer must consider management of the neck, whether or not palpable adenopathy is present. Recent studies have demonstrated significant differences in the clinical behavior of HPV-related oropharyngeal (OP) cancer, with improved survival even in the presence of adenopathy, hence dramatic changes in treatment algorithms for HPV-related OP cancer may be promulgated in the near future. This algorithm will address cancers of the upper aerodigestive track and nonmelanoma skin cancer, but not thyroid, salivary gland, or melanoma.

A The history, physical examination, and imaging will determine the clinical stage of the cancer. The presence of palpable adenopathy indicates, for most head and neck cancers, stage III disease. The probability of occult adenopathy in a clinically negative neck is dependent on the site and extent of the primary tumor, as well as cell type. The presence of specific molecular markers, as currently employed in thyroid and melanoma, may be incorporated into future treatment algorithms.

B Imaging is typically obtained at the time the head and neck cancer is identified or suspected. The standard in many centers is computerized tomography (CT), although ultrasound is commonly used by those experienced with its performance. Positron-emission tomography (PET) imaging, especially combined with CT (PET-CT) is useful in demonstrating extent of disease as well as regional and distant metastases, but will fail to detect small (<1 cm) tumor deposits. Imaging of the chest is required for all patients with head and neck cancer, and is usually obtained at the same time the neck and primary tumor is imaged. Malignant neck nodes with central necrosis often resemble benign cystic masses on imaging, which can lead to delayed diagnosis. The absence of radiographic evidence of metastatic disease does not rule out the presence of histologically positive regional nodes.

C The presence of a neck mass in an adult suggests the presence of metastatic cancer until proven otherwise. Concurrent with the increasing prevalence of HPV-related cancer in nonsmokers, the probability that a neck mass in any adult represents metastatic cancer has increased. Even in the absence of a visible or palpable primary tumor, the physician must assume that a neck mass is cancer until proven otherwise.

D The initial step in the evaluation of a neck mass without an identifiable primary cancer should be a fine-needle aspiration biopsy (FNAB). Unfortunately, the false-negative FNAB rate of a cystic neck mass is ~30%. Therefore, a negative FNAB mandates a repeat FNAB, core-needle biopsy, or even eventual open biopsy to rule out malignancy. Molecular markers for HPV should be obtained in addition to histologic examination and may impact therapeutic decisions.

E Biopsy-proven metastatic cancer in the absence of primary cancer mandates a search for the primary. The search is directed by the location and histology of the positive node. If not previously performed, imaging, to include PET-CT if available, should be obtained. Laryngopharyngoscopy under general anesthesia with focused biopsies of likely sites is the next step. Most surgeons perform routine tonsillectomy as well as directed biopsies of the base of tongue. More recently, many head and neck surgeons routinely perform robotic excision of the tongue base due to the occult nature of many primary cancers. Careful histologic examination is required since large palpable nodes are often associated with very small (2–3 mm) primary cancers.

F If no primary tumor is found, most centers radiate the usual locations of occult primaries within Waldeyer's ring, including the neck nodes.

G Definitive therapy of primary and neck nodes depends on a variety of factors, including local therapeutic algorithms. Palpable adenopathy in association with a known primary tumor requires treatment (therapeutic neck dissection). If the primary and metastases are resectable with curative intent, the preferred modality is therapeutic neck dissection. If unresectable, then nonoperative treatment is selected. If primary radiation therapy is selected as the treatment modality for the primary tumor, typically the neck nodes are incorporated into the treatment plan. Larger nodes and advanced primary cancers are managed with radiotherapy with radiosensitizing doses of chemotherapy (CRT).

H Decisions regarding contralateral neck dissection (and type of dissection) are site specific. Bilateral therapeutic neck dissection is the standard therapy for patients with bilateral palpable nodes, or for specific tumor sites such as midline tongue/floor of mouth cancers, medial wall of pyriform sinus, and supraglottis.

I The presence of occult adenopathy varies widely with tumor site and histology. Imaging may identify suspicious adenopathy but has a wide margin of error. Malignant neck nodes often appear as cystic masses on imaging. Positron-emission tomography imaging, especially when combined with CT may be beneficial, but will fail to detect small (<1 cm) tumor deposits. The absence of radiographic findings to suggest metastatic disease does not rule out the presence of histologically positive regional nodes.

J In the absence of palpable or radiographic evidence of cervical metastases, decisions regarding the treatment of the neck are based on the knowledge of the biologic behavior of the specific cancer, with specific attention to the incidence of occult adenopathy. Although not included in the staging system, depth of invasion has been shown to impact the likelihood of metastasis in cancers of the oral tongue. The incidence of bilateral adenopathy is very high in supraglottic and hypopharyngeal cancers; hence, bilateral neck dissections are standard part of treatment, even in the absence of palpable nodes. Most authorities perform sentinel node biopsies (SNBs) for intermediate-thickness melanoma since the presence of positive nodes has a large impact on therapeutic decisions, whereas SNB has not yet supplanted elective neck dissection in upper aerodigestive tract squamous cell cancer.

K Treatment of the neck is not required for low-risk cancers—such as superficial (<4 mm depth) tongue cancers or superficial small (<2 cm) skin cancers—when there is no objective evidence of adenopathy.

L Histologic examination of the resected primary and neck specimens provides rich information regarding the biologic behavior of the malignancy. Histologic characteristics such as extracapsular spread of cancer, or perineural or intravascular invasion suggest a biologically aggressive tumor, information that helps drive treatment decisions.

M Most centers use post-treatment PET-CT scanning to drive decision making following completion of therapy, particularly CRT in which clinical follow-up is often difficult. The sensitivity of PET-CT for persistent cancer is high; however, specificity is not. Local inflammation following therapy persists for several months, hence early post-treatment imaging (<3 months) should be avoided. A negative PET-CT implies cure, whereas a positive scan is of less value (specificity of 50%) in driving decision making regarding biopsy and salvage therapy.

SUGGESTED READING

Byers RM, Wolf PF, Ballantyne AJ. Rationale for elective modified neck dissection. Head Neck Surg. 1998;10:160-167.

Lutz C, Johnson JT, Myers EN, et al. Supraglottic carcinoma: patterns of recurrence. Ann Otol Rhinol Laryngol. 1990;99:12-17.

Myers E (Ed). Operative Otolaryngology: Head and Neck Surgery, 2nd edition. Philadelphia, PA: WB Saunders; 2004.

Neck Trauma

Meghan T Turner, Seungwon Kim

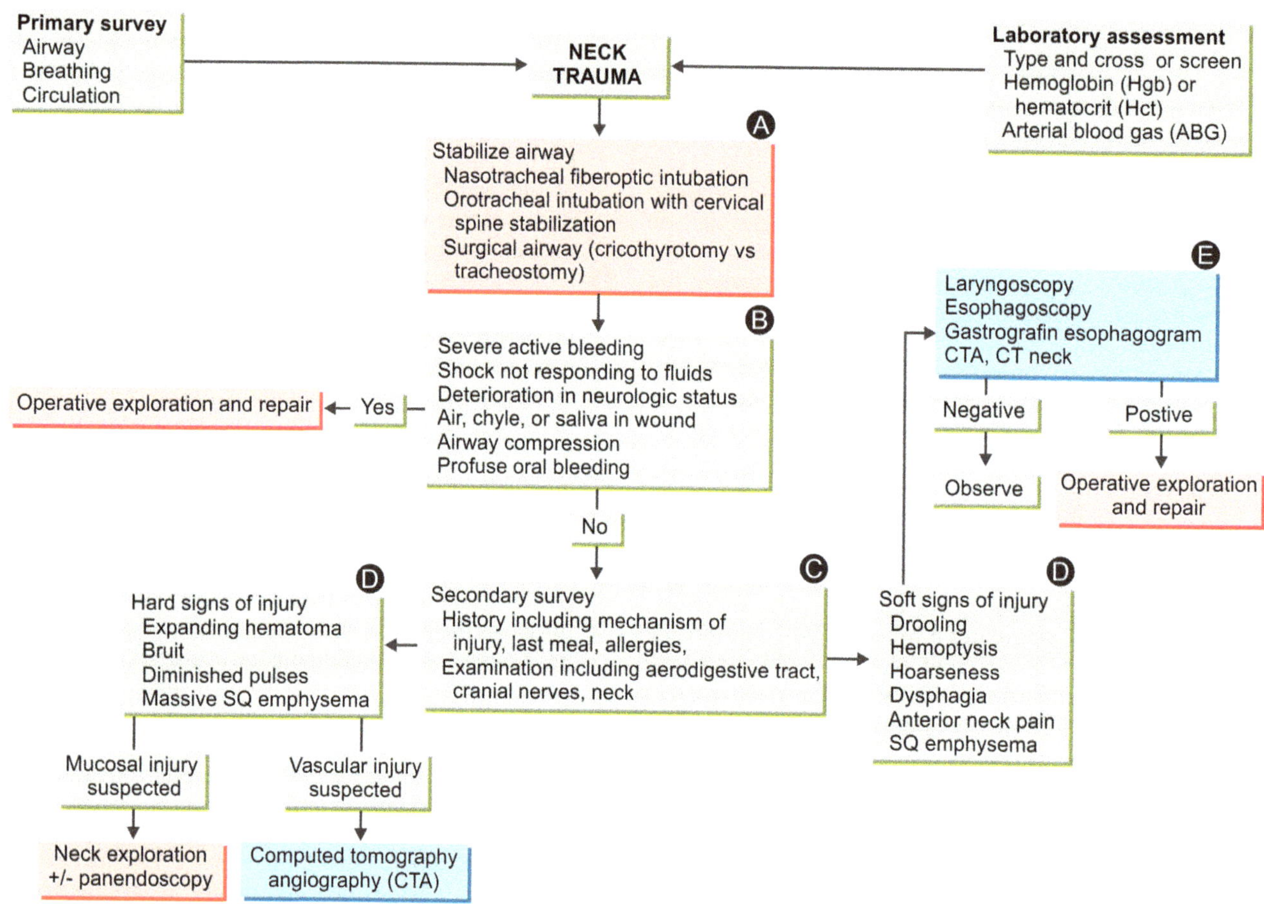

The American College of Surgeons Advanced Trauma-Life Support protocols must guide decision making in evaluation and resuscitation of patients with trauma to the neck and is ideally coordinated by trauma surgeons in a level I trauma center. Initial management begins with the primary survey. In the modern era, the mortality from penetrating neck injury of all velocities is between 3% and 10%, depending on the mechanism of injury.

(A) Approximately 10% of patients with penetrating injury of the neck will present with airway compromise. Reasons for immediate surgical intervention that are undisputed in the literature are major airway injury associated with dyspnea, stridor, hemoptysis, massive subcutaneous emphysema, or air bubbling through the wound that may be a source of immediate or impending airway compromise. Of particular importance is the mechanism and velocity of injury. High-velocity penetrating neck injury (as due to close range handgun, shotgun or rifle injury, explosives, shrapnel) has a higher likelihood of cervical (C)-spine injury, which requires immobilization of the C-spine, creates the scenario of difficult intubation, and

may result in the need for surgical airway establishment. In low-velocity injury, such as a stab-wound to the neck, C-spine injury rates are reported to be as low as 0.15%. C-spine immobilization has been associated with a significantly increased risk of death [odds ratio (OR) = 2.77, probability (p) < 0.02], perhaps due to obscuration of clinical findings and impaired intubation.

(B) After securing the airway, attention is turned to the patient's hemodynamic status. For patients with penetrating neck trauma, the cause of death is exsanguination in 50% of cases. As such, patients may arrive with active hemorrhage or expanding hematoma requiring immediate intervention in the OR. Given the high rate of mortality from exsanguination and the low-morbidity of neck explorations, neck exploration became the standard of care for all anterior neck injuries deep to the platysma after World War II. With this practice, up to 50% of neck explorations were negative for injury. The 1980s saw a paradigm-shift towards selective neck explorations in high-risk patients as determined by zone of injury and findings on computed tomography angiography (CTA).

Presently, the zone of injury is no longer useful as many studies, prospective and randomized, have demonstrated that modern imaging techniques and endoscopic evaluation serve as better screening tools than neck exploration. However, zone of injury still remains important when considering indications for immediate neurosurgical or thoracic surgery consultations.

C Modern treatment of stable patients with penetrating injury of the neck relies mostly upon the findings of the secondary survey. Assuming patients are hemodynamically stable, a pertinent history and review of symptoms with particular attention to the presence or absence of symptoms including altered mental status, dyspnea, orthopnea, dysphonia, dysphagia, hemoptysis, palpitations, weakness and numbness is required. Next, a targeted physical examination is performed, including assessment of the airway, respirations, wound (including depth, entrance wound, trajectory, and exit wound), neurovascular examination, neck and flexible evaluation of the airway. Finally, the results of preliminary imaging studies are reviewed. Altered mental status, associated-head or midface injury, acute hemorrhage, soft-tissue prolapse and/or edema may also lead to airway compromise in the setting of neck trauma and should be recognized early. Others may have evolving stroke requiring emergent repair of a major vascular injury.

D Hard and soft signs of injury should be assessed in detail. Stable patients may still display hard signs of injury requiring emergent operative management including: (1) active hemorrhage, (2) expanding hematoma, (3) bruit, (4) pulse deficit, (5) massive subcutaneous emphysema, (6) hoarseness, (7) stridor and/or respiratory distress, or (8) hemiparesis. A subset of patients who have a secure airway and stable hemodynamics may require further diagnostic work-up and CTA should be the next step. Soft signs of severe injury include nonexpanding hematoma, venous oozing, subcutaneous emphysema, dysphonia, hemoptysis, dysphagia, and proximity of injury to important structures or vessels also warrant further work-up with CTA with or without the addition of esophagography, traditional angiography, and/or endoscopy given patient factors and degree of suspicion. The current evidence supports the principle notion that conservative management is now indicated for asymptomatic patients with negative physical examinations and appropriate screening studies.

E Controversy remains in the literature about what further modalities work best in cases where injury is suspected. In the recent literature, panendoscopy has been shown to be more sensitive than esophagography with gastrografin. However, esophagography provides information on the size and extent of the leak as well as determine which cases may be managed conservatively and which may require open-repair. CTA is superior to conventional angiography in that it is noninvasive does not carry the risk of stroke, and can be performed more quickly. It does not, however, allow for simultaneous intervention and may be less desirable in the patient with hard signs of injury that may benefit from endovascular intervention at the time of angiography.

SUGGESTED READING

Brennan JA, Gibbons MD, Lopez M, et al. Traumatic airway management in operation Iraqi freedom. Otolaryngol Head and Neck Surg. 2011;144(3):376-380.

Brennan JA, Holt GR. Resident Manual of Trauma to the Face Head and Neck, 1st Edition. Alexandria, VA: American Academy of Otolaryngology—Head and Neck Surgery Foundation; 2015.

Burgess CA, Dale OT, Almeyda R, et al. An evidence based review of the assessment and management of penetrating neck trauma. Clin. Otolaryngol. 2012;37:44-52.

Inaba K, Branco BC, Menaker J, et al. Evaluation of multidetector computed tomography for penetrating neck injury: a prospective multicenter study. J Trauma Acute Care Surg. 2012;72(3):576-584.

Mazolewski PJ, Curry JD, Browder T, et al. Computer tomographic scan can be used for surgical decision making in Zone II penetrating neck injuries. J Trauma. 2001;51(2):315-319.

Schroll R, Fontenot T, Lipcsey M, et al. Role of computed tomography angiography in the management of Zone II penetrating neck trauma in patients with clinical hard signs. J. Trauma Acute Care Surg. 2015;79(6):1943-1950.

Tisherman SA, Bokhari F, Collier B, et al. Clinical practice guideline: penetrating Zone II neck trauma. J Trauma. 2008;64(2):1392-1405.

Parapharyngeal Space Lesions

Christopher H Rassekh

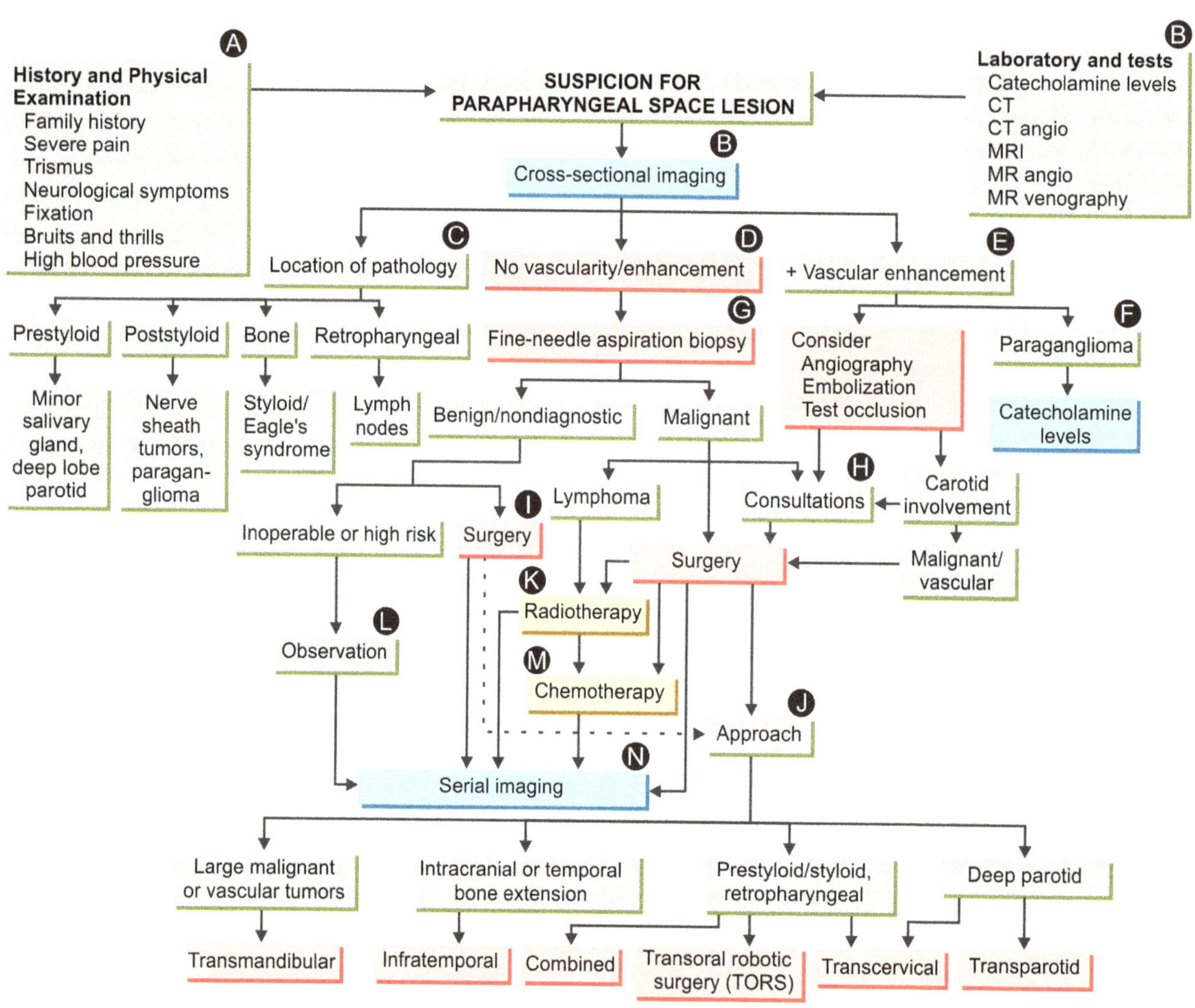

Lesions of the parapharyngeal space represent a diverse group of pathological conditions. Clinical decision making can be improved by using an algorithm that allows safe management of even the most complex lesions.

A Parapharyngeal space masses most commonly present as an asymptomatic mass in the neck, pharynx, and/or palate on routine physical examination. One should suspect malignancy if there is severe pain, trismus, or neurological symptoms. Fixation of palpable masses also suggests malignancy or vascular involvement. Vocal cord paralysis is suggestive of malignancy or paraganglioma. Bruits and thrills are also signs of vascular pathology. Family history of paraganglioma may suggest the diagnosis. Hypertension may be a manifestation of hormone secretion and catecholamine testing is warranted; *see* step (E).

B Parapharyngeal space lesions often present as incidental findings on imaging studies. Computed tomography (CT) with contrast and/or magnetic resonance imaging (MRI) with gadolinium should be performed on all patients to identify the type of lesion and the degree of vascularity.

C Classification by location is as follows: prestyloid masses are usually salivary gland tumors but nerve sheath tumors of the trigeminal nerve and lipomas and lymph nodes can present in this space also. A mass in the parotid gland will usually displace parapharyngeal adipose tissue anteromedially; a minor salivary gland mass will displace adipose tissue posteriorly; a poststyloid space mass displaces adipose tissue and carotid sheath anteriorly or anteromedially and is usually nerve sheath tumor of lower cranial nerves or paraganglioma. Retropharyngeal lesions displace the vessels anterolaterally and are most commonly lymph nodes but may be sympathetic chain lesions. Styloid process elongation is best evaluated with CT scan.

D Enhancing masses in the parapharyngeal space may be vascular, most commonly paragangliomas and angiography should be considered. Carotid body tumors splay the internal carotid artery and external carotid artery so may be both prestyloid and poststyloid. Multicentricity with paragangliomas is common: synchronous tumors are found in 10% of patients; familial tendency with multiple tumors is found in up to 25% of patients.

E Embolization and test occlusion can be considered during angiography.

F Catecholamine secretion may occur in paraganglioma patients. The most common cause is a pheochromocytoma, which can usually be identified by MRI of the abdomen. In rare cases, the paraganglioma may be the secreting tumor; *see* also step (I).

G Once vascular pathology is excluded, surgical planning is facilitated by fine-needle aspiration (FNA) biopsy. Fine-needle aspiration is usually CT-guided but may be done transorally if the lesion is easily visualized and palpable. When an FNA is nondiagnostic, it is often because the lesion is a nerve sheath tumor, a cyst, or other fibrous lesion likely to be benign. Surgery is warranted even in asymptomatic patients for definitive diagnosis and removal of the lesion.

H For malignant tumors or for lesions involving the carotid artery, consultations may be required. Consultation with a Vascular or Neurosurgeon is appropriate for patients who require cranial base surgery or carotid artery reconstruction. Consultation with Radiation Oncology and Medical Oncology may be needed for malignant tumors. Genetics consultation is appropriate for paragangliomas. Anesthesia consultation is important for patients requiring preoperative adrenergic blockade with propranolol or phenoxybenzamine for catecholamine-secreting tumors. Endocrine surgery consultation is appropriate for management of pheochromocytoma.

I The majority of patients have benign tumors, and the majority of these are benign pleomorphic adenomas of the prestyloid space. Surgery is the primary modality of treatment of these lesions.

J The transcervical approach is usually used for excision of paragangliomas and benign tumors of the prestyloid space. The transoral approach is a good option for selected prestyloid tumors but should not be used

for paragangliomas. Transoral robotic surgery (TORS) improves the visualization and facilitates manual dexterity for transoral surgery but should be done only in experienced hands. Care must be taken to close the pharynx meticulously to avoid dehiscence. Indications for TORS include prestyloid benign tumors, retropharyngeal space lesions, and Eagle's syndrome. Contraindications include malignancy by FNA, tumors extending into the stylomandibular tunnel, and poststyloid vascular lesions.

The transparotid approach is most useful for deep parotid lobe tumors. It may be used in conjunction with the transcervical approach for larger tumors.

The infratemporal fossa approach is used for tumors with intracranial or temporal bone extension (i.e. jugular or vagal paragangliomas).

The transmandibular approach is performed in conjunction with a midline mandibulotomy to give widest exposure to parapharyngeal space. It is ideal for large malignant or vascular tumors.

K Radiation is used for treatment of inoperable tumors, in poor surgical candidates, and as an adjuvant therapy for malignant tumors.

L Older patients with isolated asymptomatic neuromas, multiple tumors necessitating large functional losses, and poor surgical candidates may be observed closely.

M Chemotherapy may also be indicated as adjuvant therapy and both radiation and chemotherapy may be considered for patients with lymphoma. Major surgery should be avoided in lymphoma.

N Regardless of the treatment strategy, serial imaging is appropriate to follow patients. The interval depends on the strategy and the histology.

SUGGESTED READING

Carrau RL, Myers EN, Johnson JT. Management of tumors arising in the parapharyngeal space. Laryngoscope. 1990;100:583-589.

Garrett CR, Pillsbury HC. Parapharyngeal space masses. In: Shockley WW, Pillsbury HC (Eds). The Neck: Diagnosis and Surgery. St Louis, MO: Mosby Year Book; 1996. p. 313.

Johnson JT. Parapharyngeal space. In: Myers EN (Ed). Operative Otolaryngology: Head and Neck Surgery. Philadelphia, PA: WB Saunders; 1997. p. 656.

Olsen KD. Tumors and surgery of the parapharyngeal space. Laryngoscope. 1994;104:1-28.

Rassekh CH, Weinstein GS, Loevner LA, et al. Transoral robotic surgery for prestyloid parapharyngeal space masses. Op Tech Otolaryngol. 2013;24:99-105.

Urquhart AC, Johnson JT, Myers EN, et al. Glomus vagale: paraganglioma of the vagus nerve. Laryngoscope. 1994;104:440-445.

Thyroid Enlargement

William G Albergotti, David E Eibling

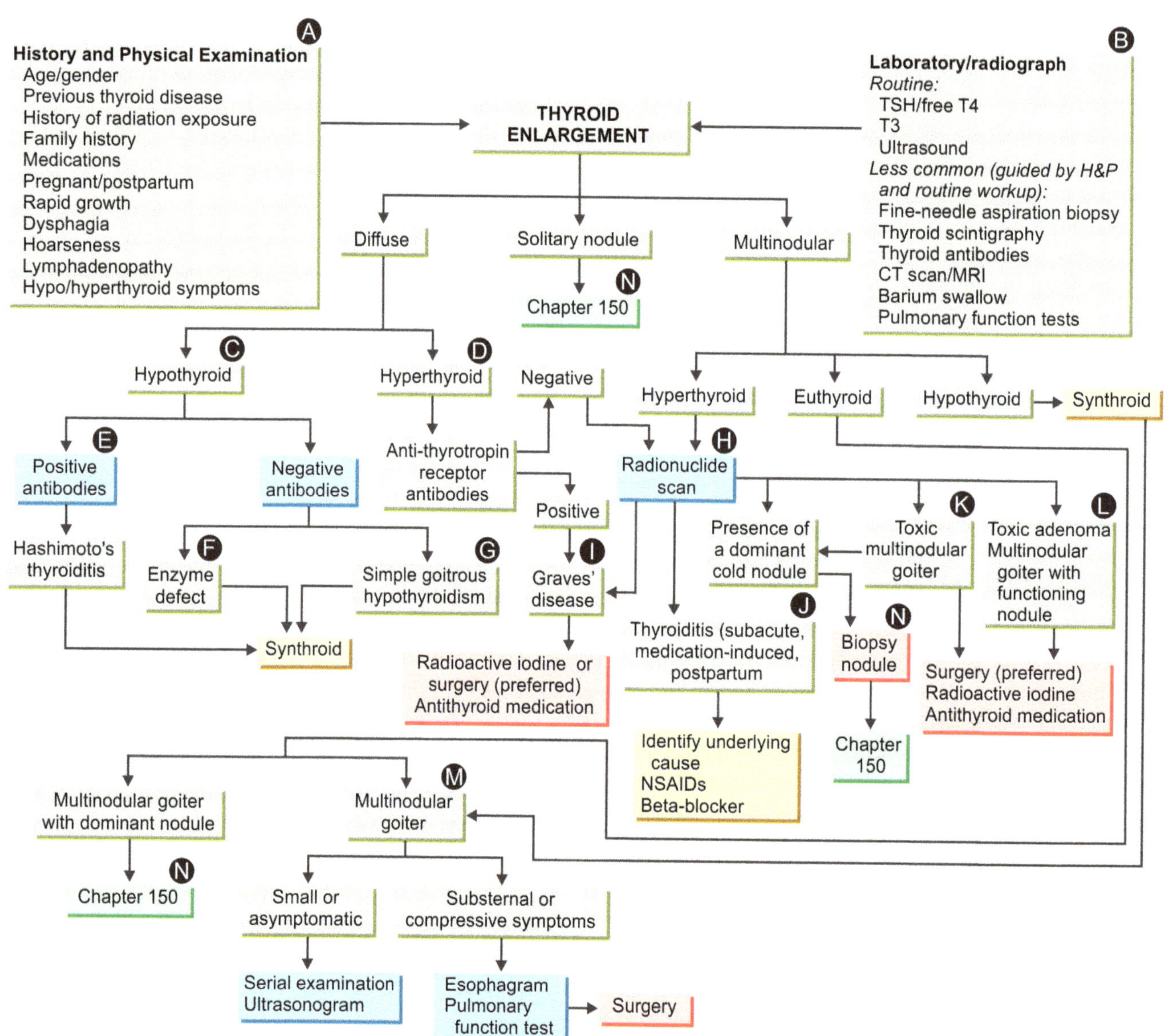

Thyroid enlargement is a common complaint encountered by Otolaryngologists and Primary Care physicians. Thyroid enlargement is an anatomic diagnosis based on physical examination of the gland itself or as an incidental finding on radiographic imaging. The majority of cases of thyroid enlargement will be found to be benign but careful evaluation must be performed to ensure both the absence of malignancy as well as correction of any hypo- or hyper-thyroid dysfunction whose symptomatology can be distressing to the patient and is correctable with appropriate evaluation and treatment. Further, benign thyroid enlargement may lead to local compressive symptoms that may be addressed surgically. The goal ultimately is to establish both anatomic and functional diagnoses.

A Patients with a family history of thyroid disease, such as multinodular goiter (MNG), Graves' disease, or thyroid carcinoma, have an increased risk of sharing that diagnosis. A history of radiation exposure and female sex increases the risk for differentiated thyroid carcinoma. Dysphagia and hoarseness may be seen in both benign and inflammatory processes as well as advanced malignancy. Flexible fiberoptic laryngoscopy is considered a routine part of the examination.

B History and physical examination guide appropriate laboratory and radiologic evaluation. For most patients, this includes a baseline laboratory evaluation of thyroid function by measurement of thyroid-stimulating hormone (TSH) and free thyroxine (T4) Occasionally triiodothyronine (T3) is obtained.

Ultrasonography (US) of the thyroid and lateral neck is also commonly used in the evaluation of thyroid enlargement. It facilitates evaluation of nodular goiter and identification of multinodularity, enables accurate fine-needle aspiration of lesions suspicious for malignancy, and may demonstrate associated lymphadenopathy. Computed tomography or magnetic resonance imaging may be helpful in evaluating substernal goiter or tracheal compression but are not routinely indicated for workup of thyroid enlargement.

Compressive symptoms may be evaluated by barium esophagram (dysphagia to solids), modified barium swallow (aspiration symptoms) or pulmonary function tests (dyspnea).

C Common symptoms of hypothyroidism include fatigue, dry skin, constipation, cold intolerance, weight gain, hair loss. TSH is elevated.

D Common symptoms of hyperthyroidism include palpitation, heat intolerance, weight loss, increased appetite, tremor, poor concentration, and irregular menses. TSH is low.

E Hashimoto's thyroiditis, the most common cause of thyroid gland failure, is a chronic autoimmune process. It is confirmed with measurement of either thyroid peroxidase or thyroglobulin antibodies. Levothyroxine is the treatment of choice.

F Genetically determined enzyme defects of hormone biosynthesis are rare causes of goitrous hypothyroidism that is not autoimmune. Treatment is levothyroxine.

G Simple goitrous hypothyroidism is the gland's compensatory response to hypersecretion of TSH secondary to impaired production of thyroid hormone. Treatment is levothyroxine.

H Thyroid scintigraphy (Technetium pertechnetate or iodine-123) is most useful in characterizing the underlying process in a hyperthyroid patient. If a patient has a diffusely enlarged gland and hyperthyroidism, the uptake pattern can reliably distinguish between Graves' disease (diffuse and homogenous) and subacute thyroiditis (low or subnormal uptake). Similarly, in a patient with nodular thyroid, scintigraphy can differentiate between toxic MNG/Plummer's disease (enlarged, heterogeneous gland with focal uptake), and single toxic nodule (localized high uptake surrounded by low uptake).

I Causes for thyroiditis include postpartum thyroiditis, subacute thyroiditis (De Quervain), medication (amiodarone, iodine). If symptomatic hyperthyroidism is present, then short-term beta-blocking medications (propranolol or atenolol) may be used. Symptoms usually resolve within several weeks.

J Graves' disease is the most common cause of thyrotoxicosis (70% of cases). It is characterized by diffuse goiter, thyrotoxicosis, and infiltrative ophthalmopathy (exophthalmos). The disorder, which has a hereditary and autoimmune component (anti-thyrotropin receptor), is more common in women. Treatment is with antithyroid medications in the short term to achieve a euthyroid state (or lifelong in those who are medically infirm) followed by iodine-131 [RAI (radioactive iodine)], or total thyroidectomy. Total thyroidectomy is preferred when there are contraindications to RAI, severe disease, progressive symptoms or suspicious nodules.

K Toxic MNG is a disorder in which hyperthyroidism arises in an MNG. It is the primary cause of hyperthyroidism in the elderly. Obstructive symptoms are more common than in Graves' disease due to the physical characteristics of the thyroid gland as well as its frequent retrosternal extension. Total thyroidectomy is the preferred treatment. RAI may be considered in patients who are poor surgical candidates.

L Toxic adenomas and functional autonomous adenomas present in an otherwise normal thyroid gland are rarely a cause of hyperthyroidism (5% of cases). Usually caused by a single adenoma, these are true follicular adenomas of the thyroid gland and are capable of functioning without stimulation by TSH. Hemithyroidectomy is the preferred treatment. RAI is reserved for those who cannot tolerate surgery.

M Simple or nontoxic goiter is any thyroid enlargement not associated with hyperthyroidism or hypothyroidism or a neoplastic process. Clinical features are due to thyroid enlargement: larger goiters cause displacement or compression of the esophagus or trachea, leading to dysphagia, a choking sensation, or inspiratory stridor. Ultrasound with fine-needle aspiration of any suspicious nodules is required before observation can be recommended. Thyroidectomy is indicated in symptomatic patients with enlarged substernal thyroid glands.

N A dominant nodule, particularly one that demonstrates suspicious features on US, requires biopsy. The use of fine-needle aspiration biopsy with a skilled cytopathologist is both sensitive and specific in differentiating malignant from benign lesions. Newer molecular tests increase the diagnostic accuracy. See Chapter 150 for a more in-depth discussion.

SUGGESTED READING

Baker JR Jr. Autoimmune endocrine disease. JAMA. 1997;278: 1931-1937.

Banks CA, Ayers CM, Hornig JD, et al. Thyroid disease and compressive symptoms. Laryngoscope. 2012;122(1):13-16.

Borman KRF, Erin A. Thyroid diseases. In: Ashley SW (Ed). Scientific American Surgery. Philadelphia: Decker Intellectual Properties; 2014. pp. 1547-1616.

Cirocchi R, Trastulli S, Randolph J, et al. Total or near-total thyroidectomy versus subtotal thyroidectomy for multinodular non-toxic goitre in adults. Cochrane Database Syst Rev. 2015;8: CD010370.

Jonklaas J, Bianco AC, Bauer AJ, et al. Guidelines for the treatment of hypothyroidism: prepared by the american thyroid association task force on thyroid hormone replacement. Thyroid. 2014;24(12):1670-1751.

Ross DS, Burch HB, Cooper DS, et al. 2016 American Thyroid Association Guidelines for diagnosis and management of hyperthyroidism and other causes of thyrotoxicosis. Thyroid. 2016;26(10):1343-1421.

Thyroid Nodule

Meghan T Turner, Robert L Ferris

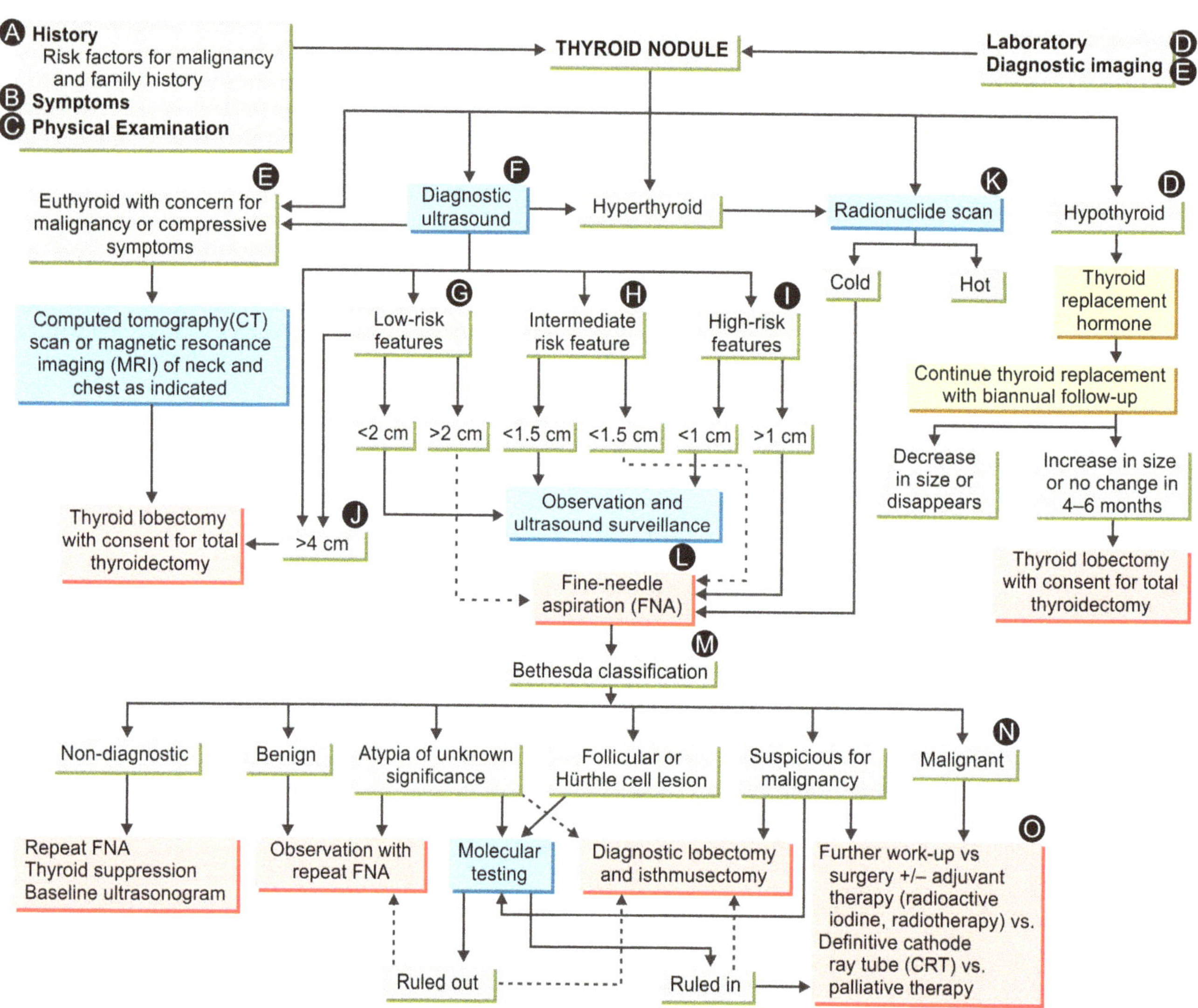

Thyroid nodules are common and found most often in women 20–40 years old. Nodules must be evaluated for malignancy. In low-risk groups, the rate of malignancy is approximately 5%, rising as high as 15% in high-risk groups. The incidence of thyroid cancer has tripled since 1975, and is attributed to increased detection on high-resolution ultrasound (US) and imaging performed during other types of medical evaluations. Well-differentiated thyroid cancer represents greater than 90% of thyroid malignancy with a 20-year survival rate greater than 80%. The National Cancer Institute's Surveillance, Epidemiology, and End Results Program (SEER) estimates that thyroid cancer accounts for 3.8% of all new cancer diagnoses, but only 0.3% of cancer deaths. In recent years, the American Thyroid Association (ATA) proposed stricter treatment guidelines to prevent overtreatment. For that reason, understanding the algorithm in the evaluation of a thyroid nodule has become important and relies on the clinician's ability to incorporate results of the history, physical examination, laboratory testing, sonographic features, cytology, and molecular testing to better treat patients.

Ⓐ The history should identify patients at high-risk of poor prognosis. Age, Metastasis, Extent of disease, Size (AMES) criteria identifies such patients, which include: females older than 51 years; males older than 41 years; children, extrathyroidal involvement metastases; size greater than 5 cm; and exposure to environmental or therapeutic irradiation. The family history also identifies at-risk patients, such as those with familial differentiated thyroid cancer or tumor syndromes [i.e. multiple endocrine neoplasia (MEN), Cowden disease, DICER-1 syndrome, familial adenomatous polyposis, Carney complex, and Werner syndrome].

B Certain symptoms raise particular concern. Pain, rapid-enlargement, hoarseness, hemoptysis and stridor are symptoms concerning for aggressive malignancy with tracheal invasion. Such cases require computed tomography (CT) of the neck with contrast and may warrant open-biopsy even with equivocal imaging or benign fine-needle aspiration (FNA) biopsy. Nodules that are distressing to patients are another indication for surgery. Compression of upper aero-digestive structures can cause dysphagia, dyspnea during exertion, or orthopnea. Cosmetic deformity of the neck may motivate patients to seek removal. Finally, patients may suffer significant anxiety about the possibility of having cancer and may choose lobectomy as an immediate diagnostic and therapeutic treatment. Surgery is indicated in these cases.

C Physical examination documents the size, mobility, and character of the nodule. It also may reveal tracheal deviation or compression, substernal extension, vocal fold paresis or paralysis, or the presence of cervical metastases. Such findings on physical examination require imaging of the thyroid, neck and/or chest. Nodules invading surrounding structures or those associated with a neck mass are suspicious for malignancy and warrant ultrasonography with FNA biopsy of the nodule and/or cervical masses to tailor the surgery.

D Patients should be evaluated for hyper- or hypothyroidism and screened appropriately with serum thyroid-stimulating hormone (TSH), Free-T4 and -T3 levels. Hypothyroid patients should undergo medical therapy. Hyperthyroid patients require imaging to rule-out hyper-functioning adenoma versus toxic multinodular goiter, which are managed medically. Surgery should be reserved for refractory enlargement or hyperthyroidism. Other tests such as serum thyroglobulin, antithyroid antibody testing, carcinoembryonic antigen (CEA), calcitonin, and catecholamine-testing may be helpful for specific pathologies and postoperative surveillance; however, these are indicated prior to FNA or diagnostic lobectomy.

E Consider preoperative contrast CT or magnetic resonance imaging (MRI) to assess tracheal deviation or compression, substernal extension, displacement of vessels, or suspected aero-digestive tract invasion, when patients have symptoms or signs concerning for invasive cancer. Diagnostic US, CT, or MRI of the neck may also help to evaluate cervical metastases. "Incidentalomas" should undergo further work-up. Fluorodeoxyglucose (FDG)-avid thyroid nodules on positron emission tomography (PET)-CT are of particular concern, and have a 40–56% chance of being malignant.

F Diagnostic US provides critical information in the evaluation. The ATA identifies size criteria and sonographic features of nodules that allow risk stratification.

G Low-risk nodules are isoechoic or hyperechoic, solid nodules, and partially cystic nodules with eccentric solid areas without suspicious features (microcalcifications, irregular margins, extrathyroidal extension, or taller than wide shape).

H Intermediate-risk nodules are hypoechoic, solid nodules with smooth margins that lack suspicious features. Intermediate-risk nodules have a 10–20% risk of malignancy.

I High-risk nodules have a hypoechoic portion with one or more of the features that include: (1) irregular margins, (2) microcalcifications, (3) taller than wide-shape, (4) rim calcifications with a small extrusive soft-tissue component, and (5) extrathyroidal extension.

J The larger the nodule, the higher the risk of malignancy. Redundant as is addressed in L.

K Radioactive-iodine scanning helps evaluate nodules in hyperthyroid patients. "Hot," or functioning, nodules on thyroid scan do not require surgical treatment unless suppressive therapy is unsuccessful. The risk of malignancy in such nodules is 4–5%. "Cold," or nonfunctioning, nodules warrant further work-up with US-guided FNA and carry a significant risk of malignancy, approximately 15%.

L FNA biopsy is the most cost-effective and sensitive test currently available in the evaluation of a thyroid nodule. Limitations include: (1) sampling error in lesions larger than 4 cm; (2) missing lesions smaller than 1 cm (difficult target); and (3) the inability to distinguish benign versus malignant follicular or Hürthle cell neoplasms.

M The Bethesda Classification system standardizes cytologic reporting and estimates the incidence of malignancy based on class. For example, Bethesda Class IV, V, and VI nodules have a 15–30%, 60–75%, and 97% chance of being malignant, respectively.

N Molecular testing for thyroid nodules has become clinically useful in ruling-in and ruling-out malignancy in Bethesda class III/IV nodules. The new ThyroSeq2.1 examines carcinogenic point mutations and gene fusions in 14 genes. It has a 90.9% sensitivity and 92.1% specificity, which make it useful to rule-in cancer. The Afirma panel detects carcinogenic mutations in 167 loci, is highly sensitive and is used to rule-out cancer. This may help clinicians decide, which patients should undergo observation, diagnostic lobectomy or total thyroidectomy for indeterminate nodules.

O Certain malignancies require further evaluation and are not necessarily treated with surgery. Suspicion of medullary thyroid carcinoma warrants further evaluation including chest radiograph, calcitonin, and MEN syndromes. Pheochromocytoma must be ruled out; if present, it is treated prior to the thyroid cancer. Family screening for the RET proto-oncogene can identify relatives, who should undergo prophylactic thyroidectomy. Surgery is based on stage and surveillance includes monitoring CEA and calcitonin levels. Lymphoma requires open-biopsy for tissue diagnosis and aids in choosing of chemotherapeutic agents. Diagnosis of anaplastic thyroid carcinoma should be confirmed, either repeat FNA or open biopsy. Airway concerns and the need for tracheostomy should be discussed. Some patients may require feeding tubes. Medical and radiation oncology services should be consulted. Most important is the establishment end-of-life care goals.

SUGGESTED READING

Cibas ES, Ali SZ. The Bethesda system for reporting thyroid cytopathology. Thyroid. 2009;19(11):1159-1165.

Davies L, Randolph G. Evidence-based evaluation of the thyroid nodule. Otolaryngol Clin North Am. 2014;47(4):461-474.

Giuffrida D, Gharib H. Controversies in the management of cold, hot, and occult thyroid nodules. Am J Med. 1995;99(6):642-650.

Haugen BR, Alexander EK, Bible KC, et al. 2015 American Thyroid Association Management Guidelines for adult patients for thyroid nodules and differentiated thyroid cancer. Thyroid. 2016; 26(1):1-133.

Nikiforov YE, Carty SE, Chiosea S, et al. Impact of the multi-gene ThyroSeq next-generation sequencing assay on cancer diagnosis in thyroid nodules. Thyroid. 2015;25(11):1217-1223.

Hyperparathyroidism

Alfred A Simental Jr

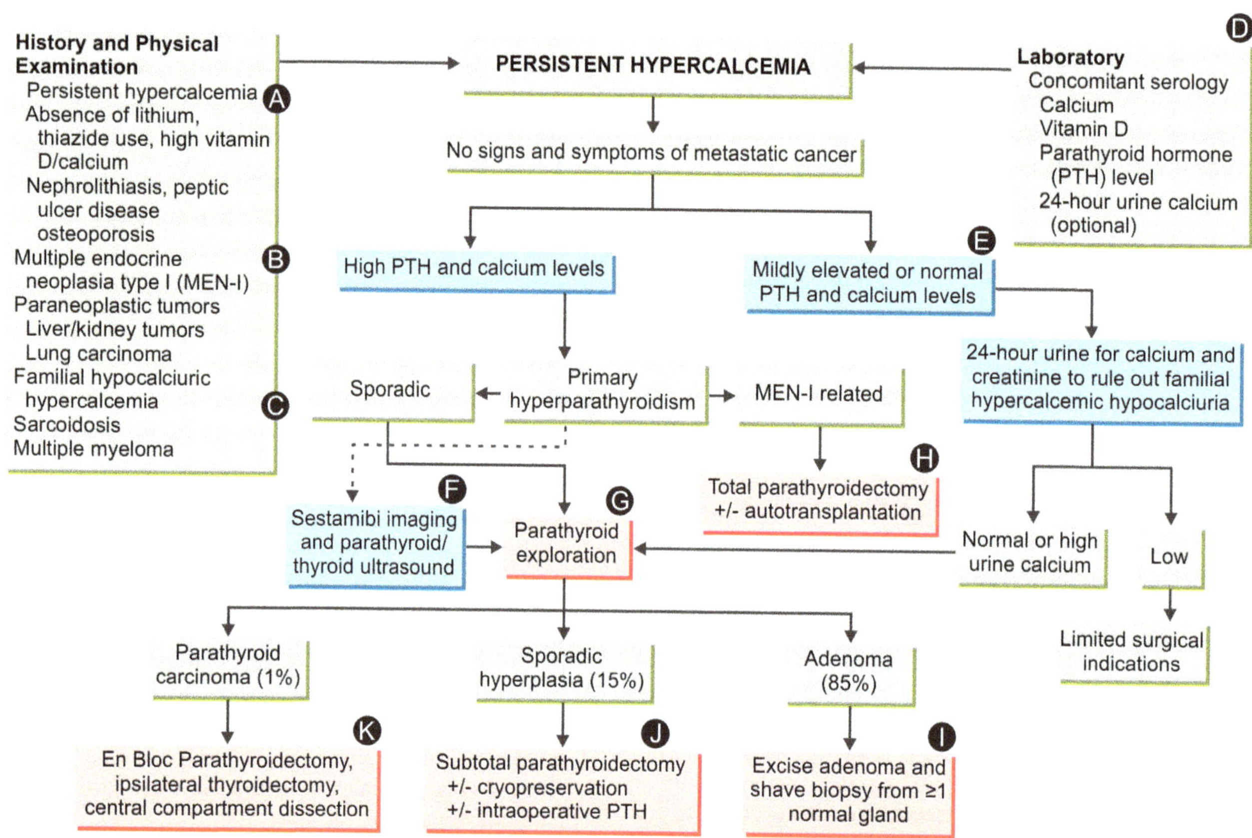

Hyperparathyroidism is hypercalcemia resulting from overproduction of parathyroid hormone (PTH) and is currently detected before traditional signs and symptoms arise, because of expanded chemical analysis. Thus, most patients today present with incidentally noted hypercalcemia on routine serology.

A History should exclude excessive calcium or vitamin D intake, uses of lithium or thiazide diuretics as these may result in nonparathyroid hypercalcemia. Some patients may experience kidney stones, stomach ulcers, fibromyalgia, and osteoporosis. More subtle signs and findings may include hypertension, history of pancreatitis, bone pain, arthritis, fatigue, depression, memory changes, polyuria–polydipsia, and constipation.

B Family history of hypercalcemia should be explored. Most cases of hyperparathyroidism are caused by a single abnormally functioning gland (adenoma) but may also be related to multiple abnormally functioning glands. Most cases are sporadic although some may be related to inherited syndromes such as the multiple endocrine neoplasia type I (MEN-I) whose features include anterior pituitary tumors, parathyroid hyperplasia, pancreatic

tumors (e.g. gastrinoma, insulinoma, and glucagonoma), carcinoid tumors, and adrenal tumors.

C Systemic disorders may result in nonparathyroid hypercalcemia, such as sarcoidosis, multiple myeloma, familial hypocalciuric hypercalcemia (FHH), and paraneoplastic tumors.

D The intact immune-fluorescent PTH assay is superior to other PTH assays and is now widely available for PTH analysis. Analysis of PTH and calcium levels is optimally measured in the fasting state. Vitamin D deficiency is also common and should be evaluated.

E In FHH, a mutated set point for renal calcium excretion produces 24-hour urine calcium levels generally well below the normal level. The disorder is autosomal dominant and should not be confused with primary hyperparathyroidism.

F Preoperative imaging should include sestamibi imaging and parathyroid ultrasound examination in an attempt to localize an enlarged parathyroid gland, rule out ectopic locations of parathyroid glands and screen for concomitant thyroid pathology. These modalities allow for more directed exploration, and when combined with intra-operative PTH monitoring, they may increase the success of unilateral exploration, avoiding routine bilateral exploration with four-gland identification. However, bilateral exploration with four-gland exploration by an experienced surgeon carries the highest cure rate. Radioguided surgery may also facilitate the intraoperative identification of abnormal parathyroid tissue, but this technique is dependent on preferential radiotracer uptake by parathyroid tissue.

G "Neck exploration with parathyroidectomy" is the most appropriate term for the operation performed, because it is impossible to accurately determine preoperatively whether a patient will have a single adenoma or multigland hyperplasia. A thorough knowledge of normal and abnormal parathyroid anatomy is essential to operative success. Enlarged parathyroid glands vary significantly in their locations throughout the neck and occasionally are located in the mediastinum. The risks of parathyroid exploration include permanent recurrent laryngeal nerve injury (1%), hypoparathyroidism (3%), bleeding, infection, and operative failure (2–30%, depending on the skill and experience of the surgeon).

H In patients with MEN-I, total thyroidectomy with autotransplantation or subtotal parathyroidectomy should be considered as residual or re-implanted parathyroid tissue will become hyperplastic and result in recurrent hyperparathyroidism, even several decades after initial parathyroidectomy. Thus, residual parathyroid tissue should be marked and left over the trachea or thyroid, away from the recurrent nerve for safe extraction at a later date. Any transplanted tissue should be placed in a region that can be removed with little morbidity such as the strap (sternothyroid/sternohyoid), sternocleidomastoid, deltoid, chest, or nondominant forearm musculature. The incidence of supranumerary parathyroid glands is increased in MEN-I, so cervical thymectomy and removal of the central compartment contents are often employed.

I Intraoperative exploration will determine the presence of a single adenoma or multigland hyperplasia after thorough exploration of all four parathyroid glands and comparison of their relative sizes, realizing that abnormal parathyroid gland is 30–60 mg in size. Frozen section pathology cannot routinely distinguish adenoma from hyperplasia.

J Subtotal parathyroidectomy involves removal of three parathyroid glands and attempting to leave a 30–50-mg remnant of one gland, preserved on its vascular pedicle.

The preserved parathyroid might not produce sufficient PTH and some patients may have >4 parathyroid glands.

K Parathyroid cancer is usually associated with a markedly elevated calcium and PTH levels. The presence of an associated ipsilateral vocal fold paralysis or palpable paratracheal mass should raise the suspicion of carcinoma but this diagnosis is considered intraoperatively by the surgeon encountering a firm gland, adherent to surrounding structures. Frozen and permanent section pathologic analysis may confirm a high mitotic rate, bizarre nuclei, fibrous bands, and possible vascular invasion. Surgery is the only cure and standardly includes en bloc parathyroid resection, ipsilateral thyroidectomy, and ipsilateral paratracheal, central compartment lymph node dissection.

SUGGESTED READING

Bilezikian JP, Brandi ML, Eastell R, et al. Guidelines for the management of asymptomatic primary hyperparathyroidism: summary statement from the Fourth International Workshop. J Clin Endocrinol Metab. 2014;99(10):3561-3569.

Bilezikian JP, Silverberg SJ. Clinical practice. Asymptomatic primary hyperparathyroidism. N Engl J Med. 2004;350(17):1746-1751.

Dy BM, Richards ML, Vazquez BJ, et al. Primary hyperparathyroidism and negative Tc99 sestamibi imaging: to operate or not? Ann Surg Oncol. 2012;19(7):2272-2278.

Eastell R, Arnold A, Brandi ML, et al. Diagnosis of asymptomatic primary hyperparathyroidism: proceedings of the Third International Workshop. J Clin Endocrinol Metab. 2009;94(2):340-350.

Marcocci C, Bollerslev J, Khan AA, et al. Medical management of primary hyperparathyroidism: proceedings of the Fourth International Workshop on the management of asymptomatic primary hyperparathyroidism. J Clin Endocrinol Metab. 2014; 99(10):3607-3618.

Marx SJ, Simonds WF, Agarwal SK, et al. Hyperparathyroidism in hereditary syndromes: special expressions and special managements. J Bone Miner Res. 2002;17(Suppl 2):N37-43.

O'Riordain DS, O'Brien T, Grant CS, et al. Surgical management of primary hyperparathyroidism in multiple endocrine neoplasia types 1 and 2. Surgery. 1993;114(6):1031-1039.

Schneider DF, Mazeh H, Sippel RS, et al. Is minimally invasive parathyroidectomy associated with greater recurrence compared to bilateral exploration? Analysis of more than 1,000 cases. Surgery. 2012;152(6):1008-1115.

Sharma J, Mazzaglia P, Milas M, et al. Radionuclide imaging for hyperparathyroidism (HPT): which is the best technetium-99m sestamibi modality? Surgery. 2006;140(6):856-865.

Steward DL, Danielson GP, Afman CE, et al. Parathyroid adenoma localization: surgeon-performed ultrasound versus sestamibi. Laryngoscope. 2006;116(8):1380-1384.

Lymphomas of the Head and Neck

Emmanuel P Prokopakis

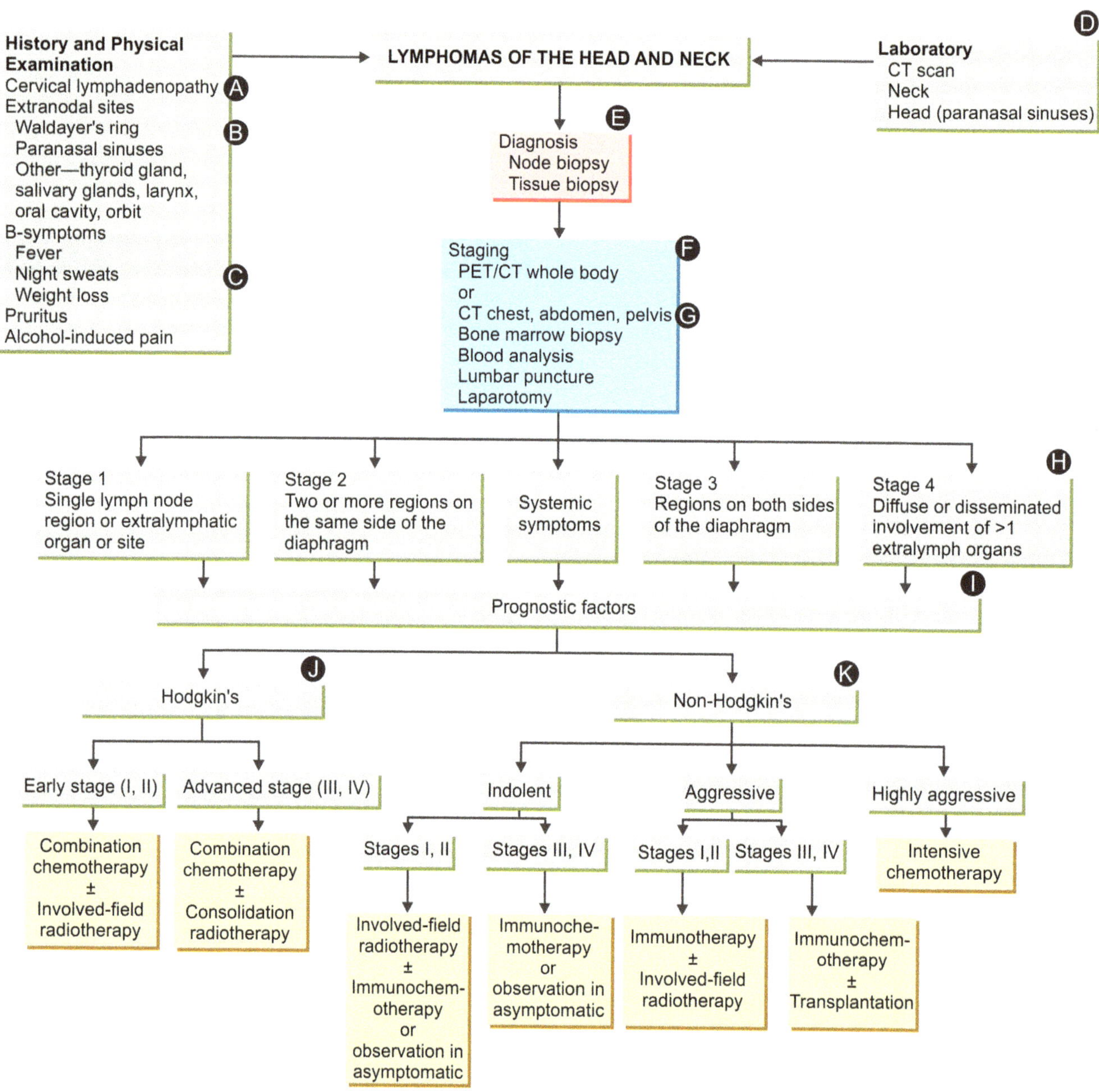

Lymphomas are malignant neoplasms of the lymphocyte cell lines. They are mainly classified as either Hodgkin's lymphoma (HL) or non-Hodgkin's lymphoma (NHL), nodal or extranodal lymphomas, and of either B-lymphocyte, T-lymphocyte, or (rarely) natural killer (NK) cell origin. Lymphoma is the second most common primary malignancy occurring in the head and neck. Hodgkin's lymphoma accounts for ~10% of all lymphomas. It has a bimodal age distribution curve—one peak in young adults (20–30 years) and one in adults of older age (>65 years). Non-Hodgkin's lymphoma is the most frequent type, usually occurs above 50 and the incidence increases with age. There are no gender differences between HL and NHL in the head and neck.

A Cervical lymphadenopathy is the most frequent head and neck presentation in both HL and NHL. The most common location of HL nodes is the lower cervical or supraclavicular region. Hodgkin's lymphoma usually arises in a single node or chain of nodes, and spreads to a contiguous node or chain. Non-Hodgkin's lymphoma spreads more commonly to noncontiguous nodes and may involve the upper, lower, and posterior cervical nodes.

B The most common extranodal site of head and neck is Waldeyer's ring (tonsil, base of the tongue, and nasopharynx), followed by nasal cavity and paranasal sinuses. Other sites include the thyroid gland, the salivary glands, larynx, oral cavity, and orbit.

C Constitutional symptoms may occur in up to one third of patients with lymphoma (more frequent in HL).

D Computed tomography (CT) scanning of the head and/or neck is mandatory in evaluating the extent of the disease.

E Diagnosis requires a lymph node biopsy. For extranodal sites, a tissue biopsy is indicated. Biopsy material should be processed fresh. Histologic, immunophenotypic, and genetic studies follow.

Fine-needle aspiration cytology is useful for the initial investigation of neck lymphadenopathy. However, the general consensus is that accurate histopathologic evaluation of lymphomas requires a tissue biopsy.

F The classification currently used is the World Health Organization system and describes >50 histological types. Non-Hodgkin's lymphoma is clinically organized in terms of aggressiveness and prognosis (indolent, aggressive, and highly aggressive).

G Computed tomography scanning of the chest, abdomen, and/or pelvis is necessary for staging. Magnetic resonance imaging (MRI) is indicated for evaluating the brain and/or spinal cord and soft tissue extension. Whole-body positron emission tomography (PET)/CT scan 2-deoxy-2-[fluorine-18]fluoro-D-glucose (18F-FDG) is recently used for the initial staging and for follow-up of many types of lymphoma-limited sensitivity for some low-grade lymphomas.

Staging evaluation also includes bone marrow biopsy and, serum chemistries. A lumbar puncture is usually performed if there is suspected central nervous system involvement. A staging laparotomy should be performed only when the results will substantially change the therapeutic plan.

H The modified Ann Arbor staging system is used to stage both HL and NHL: stage 1, involvement of a single lymph node region or a single extralymphatic organ or site; stage 2, involvement of two or more lymph node regions on the same side of the diaphragm; stage 3, involvement of lymph node regions on both sides of the diaphragm; stage 4, diffuse or disseminated involvement of one or more extralymphatic organs. Each stage is further divided into A or B (absence or presence of systemic symptoms, respectively, in HL).

I The International Prognostic Score is a predictor of treatment outcome for patients with HL calculated on the basis of the following potential unfavorable features at diagnosis: serum albumin <4 g/dL, hemoglobin <10.5 g/dL, male gender, age >45 years, stage IV disease, white blood cell count ≥15,000 per μL, absolute lymphocyte count <600 per μL, and/or <8% of the total white blood cell count. In NHL, age >60 years, serum lactate dehydrogenase (LDH) above normal, Eastern Cooperative Oncology Group (ECOG) performance status ≥2, Ann Arbor stage III or IV, number of extranodal disease sites >1.

J In HL, patients with early-stage disease (stages I–II) are usually treated with a combination of chemotherapy and radiotherapy. The doses of chemotherapy and radiation are different for patients with favorable and unfavorable prognosis disease. Combination chemotherapy is the main treatment for patients with advanced stage (stages III–IV) HL. Radiation therapy may be used for selected patients as consolidation.

For several decades, ABVD (doxorubicin, bleomycin, vinblastine, and dacarbazine) has been the standard regimen. Escalated bleomycin, etoposide, adriamycine, cyclophosphamide, vincristine, procarbazine, and prednisone (BEACOPP) and Stanford V incorporate radiation therapy and are also widely used for advanced stage HL.

K The initial treatment of NHL depends upon the histologic subtype and disease stage. Treatment options include chemotherapy, immunotherapy, radiation therapy, or a combination of these. A subset of patients is treated with high-dose chemotherapy followed by stem cell support (i.e. autologous hematopoietic cell transplantation). The general treatment principles include treatment with an anthracycline-based combination chemotherapy regimen plus the recombinant anti-CD20 antibody rituximab. In indolent NHL in asymptomatic patients observation is also an approach.

SUGGESTED READING

Barnes L, Myers EN, Prokopakis EP. Primary malignant lymphoma of the parotid gland. Arch Otolaryngol Head Neck Surg. 1998;124:573-577.

Cheson BD, Fisher RI, Barrington SF, et al. Recommendations for initial evaluation, staging, and response assessment of Hodgkin and non-Hodgkin lymphoma: the Lugano classification. J Clin Oncol. 2014;32(27):3059-3068.

National Comprehensive Cancer Network. Hodgkin Lymphoma (Version 1) 2017. [online] Available from: http://www.nccn.org/professionals/physician_gls/pdf/hodgkins.pdf.

National Comprehensive Cancer Network. Non-Hodgkin Lymphoma (Version 2). (2015). [online] Available from: http://www.nccn.org/professionals/physician_gls/pdf/nhl.pdf.

Papadakis MA, McPhee SJ, Rabow MW. Current Medical Diagnosis and Treatment, 54th edition, LANGE current series; McGraw-Hill Education/Medical; 55 edition (September 8, 2015).

Shankland KR, Armitage JO, Hancock BW. Non-Hodgkin lymphoma. Lancet. 2012;380:848-857.

Urquhart A, Berg R. Hodgkin's and non-Hodgkin's lymphoma of the head and neck. Laryngoscope. 2001;111(9):1565-1569.

CHAPTER 153

Neoplastic Involvement of the Carotid Artery

Mathew Geltzeiler, Carl H Snyderman

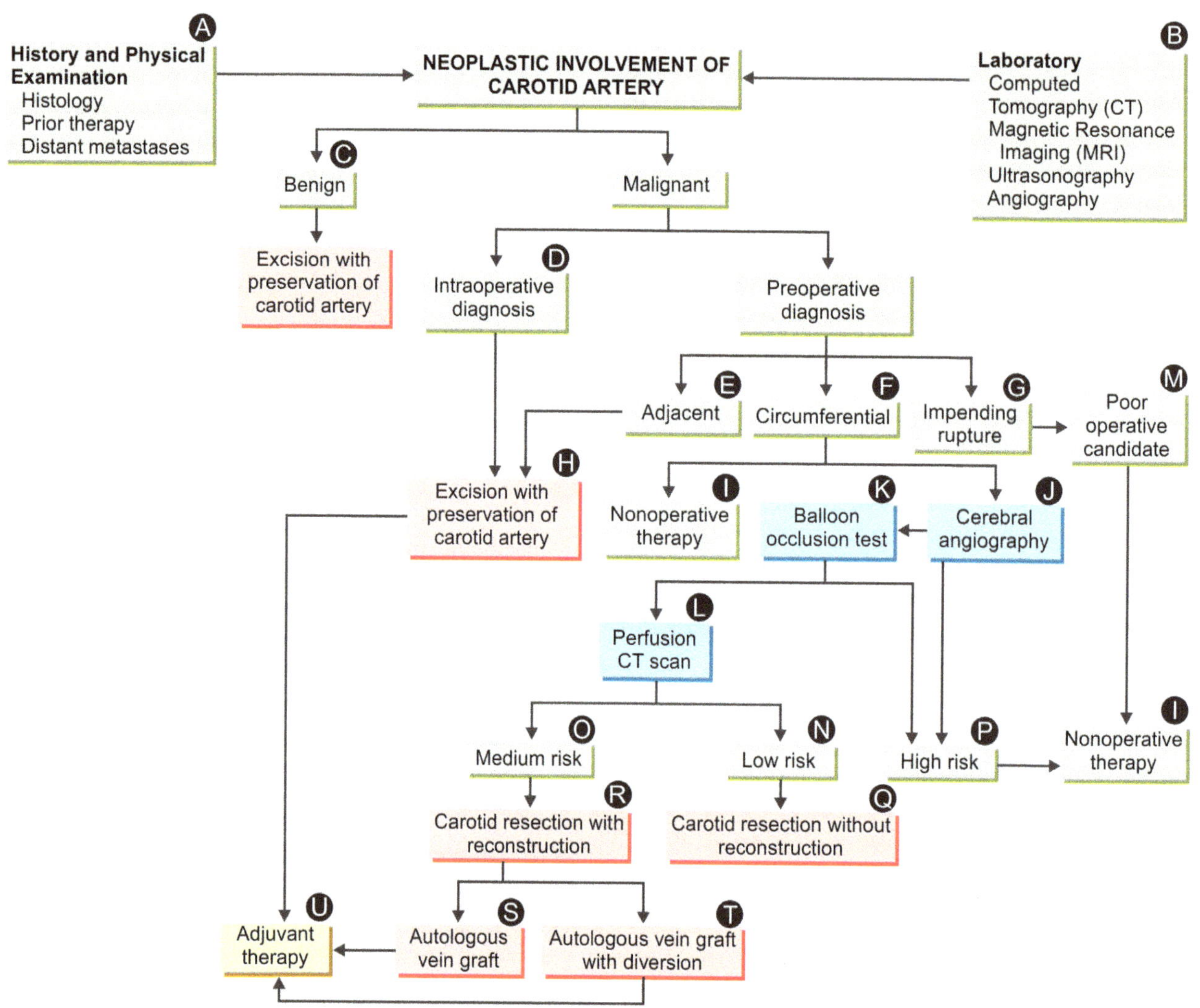

Neoplastic involvement of the carotid artery results from advanced disease (T4) or metastatic disease in the neck. Advanced cervical metastases (N3) from squamous cell carcinoma are frequently associated with extracapsular extension, which increases the likelihood of carotid artery involvement.

A Risk factors for carotid involvement include advanced-neck metastasis and recurrent cancer in the neck. Assessment of carotid involvement by physical examination is not accurate.

B Computed Tomography (CT) scan with contrast or Magnetic Resonance Imaging (MRI) with contrast, demonstrating encasement of the carotid artery or loss of usual fascial planes, best assesses involvement of the carotid artery. Angiography may also demonstrate vessel narrowing or irregularity of the vessel lumen. Ultrasonography has been used to assess "fixation" of metastatic cancer to the carotid artery.

C Benign neoplasms, which may be adherent to the carotid artery or encircle it, include paragangliomas and neurilemmomas. They can usually be separated from the carotid artery by dissection in an adventitial or subadventitial plane. Injuries to the carotid artery should be repaired primarily.

D Unanticipated detection of tumor involvement of the carotid artery intraoperatively is rare with the use of preoperative imaging. Therapeutic options are limited without knowledge of collateral cerebral blood flow. Excision of the tumor with preservation of the carotid artery should be attempted.

E Tumor in close proximity or involving less than 180° of the circumference of the carotid artery can usually be dissected from the surface of the artery. The risk of a microscopically positive margin is high, and adjuvant therapy should be considered.

F When tumor encases more than 180° of the circumference of the carotid artery, dissection from the artery is usually not possible and, even though technically feasible, is non-oncologic.

G Delaying treatment until a rupture occurs is often unsuccessful. Permanent occlusion may result in a stroke in up to 25% of unselected individuals. The adequacy of collateral cerebral circulation should be assessed preoperatively to guide further decisions. Significant palliation may be achieved even in patients with incurable cancer.

H Although dissection of cancer from the surface of the artery is non-oncologic, patients with carotid artery involvement usually have advanced neck metastasis (N3, with extracapsular extension), and the prognosis is unlikely to be altered with resection of the carotid artery.

I Treatment options in patients who are not candidates for surgery include radiotherapy with or without chemotherapy and palliative care. Radiation therapy can be delivered to the entire neck or more focally to the region adjacent to the vessel with stereotactic radiosurgery (SRS) or brachytherapy.

J Four-vessel angiography is performed to evaluate the patency of the carotid arteries and circle of Willis and to detect the presence of significant extracranial-intracranial collaterals. Significant arteriosclerosis with narrowing of the contralateral carotid artery may make the patient a poor-operative candidate. Despite complete occlusion of the ipsilateral carotid artery, the patient may be at risk for stroke during periods of hypotension or with loss of important collaterals.

K Balloon test occlusion of the internal carotid artery (ICA) is performed with clinical or electroencephalographic monitoring. If the patient becomes symptomatic, further testing is not performed. If successful, a perfusion CT scan is performed to quantitate cerebral blood flow within the distribution of the occluded vessel.

L Perfusion CT during balloon occlusion of the ICA allows calculation of cerebral blood flow and categorization of patients into stroke risk categories. Other techniques for evaluating collateral cerebral blood flow during balloon occlusion include xenon gas CT, transcranial Doppler and single-photon emission CT.

M Treatment choices depend on an assessment of the patient's prognosis for disease-free survival. The risks of carotid resection outweigh the benefits in patients with distant metastases or excessive comorbidity, unless there is evidence of imminent carotid hemorrhage.

N Patients with cerebral blood flow greater than 30 mL/100 g brain tissue per minute can usually tolerate permanent interruption of carotid blood flow with low risk of a cerebral infarction.

O Patients who pass the test clinically but have cerebral blood flow less than 30 mL/100 g brain tissue per minute may tolerate temporary interruption of carotid blood flow but are at increased risk for a delayed cerebral infarction as a result of marginal collateral cerebral circulation.

P Patients who fail the test clinically (onset of neurologic symptoms) are at high risk for cerebral ischemia after temporary or permanent interruption of carotid blood flow.

Q If the carotid artery is ligated below the carotid bifurcation, there is a theoretical risk of a "steal" phenomenon with retrograde flow from the ICA through the external carotid artery. Distal occlusion is typically performed angiographically just proximal to the ophthalmic artery in order to minimize the dead space (and risk of distal thromboembolism); proximal ligation of the vessel is performed intraoperatively.

R Autologous saphenous vein graft is preferred for reconstruction of the carotid artery.

S If there is no communication of the wound with the upper aerodigestive tract after tumor resection, the carotid artery may be reconstructed with a vein graft using end-end anastomoses.

T If the wound communicates with the upper aerodigestive tract after tumor resection, the risk of a postoperative wound infection increases the potential for blow-out of the vein graft. The graft may be protected by diversion posteriorly beneath the trapezius muscle from the subclavian artery to the ICA or middle cerebral artery. Closure of the communication should be performed primarily or with vascularized tissue (local, regional or free-flap).

U Patients with carotid artery involvement are at high risk for recurrence in the neck and distant sites. Treatment options include radiotherapy (external beam and brachytherapy), chemotherapy, and immunologic therapy. Greater tumor control and more accurate delivery of radiation may be achieved by SRS. Placement of brachytherapy catheters at the time of tumor dissection is also an option. Low-dose or high-dose interstitial radiation may be administered adjuvantly.

SUGGESTED READING

Hage ZA, Alaraj A, Arnone GD, et al. Novel imaging approaches to cerebrovascular disease. Transl Res. 2016;175:54-75.

Lim CM, Clump DA, Heron DE, et al. Stereotactic body radiotherapy (SBRT) for primary and recurrent head and neck tumors. Oral Oncol. 2013;49(5):401-406.

Sekhar LN, Linskey ME, Snyderman CH. Surgical management of neoplastic involvement of the internal carotid artery. In: Carter LP, Spetzler RF, Hamilton MG (Eds). Neurovascular Surgery. New York: McGraw-Hill; 1996. p. 1263.

Snyderman CH, Carrau RL, deVries EJ. Carotid artery resection: Update on preoperative evaluation. In: Johnson JT, Derkay CS, Mandell-Brown MK, et al. (Eds). Instructional Courses, American Academy of Otolaryngology—Head and Neck Surgery, 6th volume. St. Louis, MO: CV Mosby; 1993. pp. 341-346.

Snyderman CH, D'Amico F. Outcome of carotid artery resection for neoplastic disease. A meta-analysis. Am J Otolarynol. 1992;13:373-380.

Snyderman CH, Sekhar LN. Carotid artery problems. In: Gates GA (Ed). Current Therapy in Otolaryngology—Head and Neck Surgery, 5th edition. St. Louis, MO: Mosby-Year Book; 1994. p. 328.

Orbital Involvement by Tumor

Susan Tonya Stefko

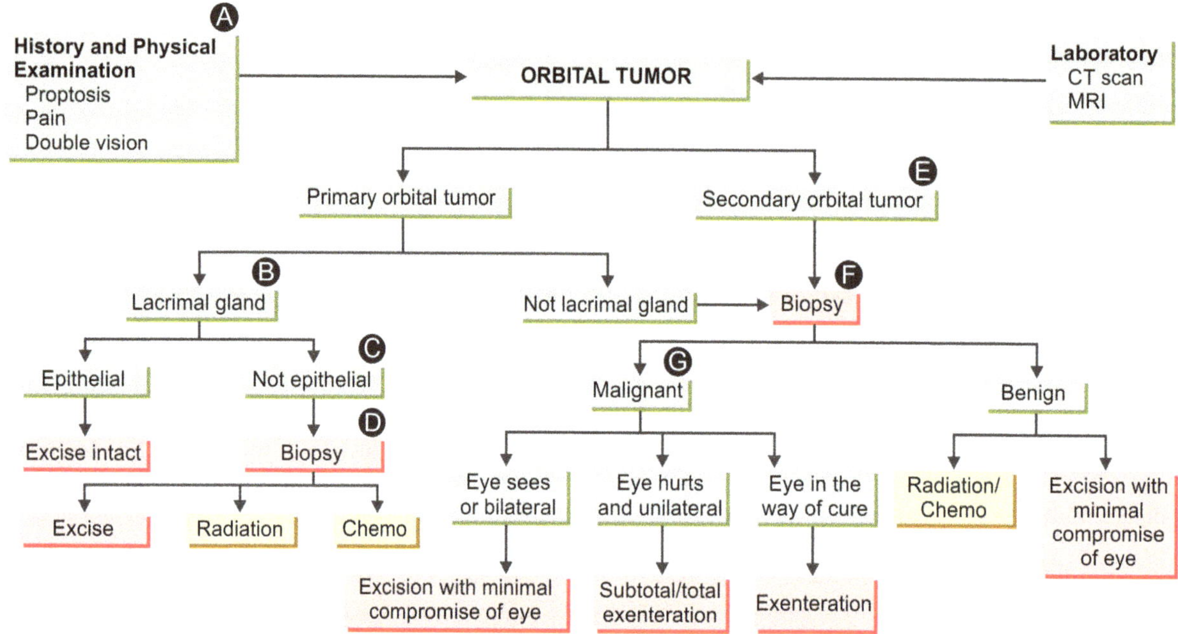

Patients may present to the Otolaryngologist with a primary tumor of the orbit and sent for treatment, or may have contiguous spread of masses from sinuses or brain. The decision to remove the eye or not must be guided by the overall health and function of the patient, with some consideration of the pathology, not by the pathology itself.

A The presence of pain, proptosis, and/or diplopia all suggest orbital involvement by tumor, but do not indicate whether the mass is likely arising from the orbit or secondarily involving it. The patient should be examined by an Ophthalmologist, preferably one experienced in the treatment of orbital tumors, in order to assess the function and health of both eyes, which is important in decision making.

B Lacrimal gland masses present with inferior and medial displacement of the eye. These will require either excision intact (in the case of a probable benign mixed tumor), or biopsy via an incision in the lid crease. Pain, <6 months' duration of symptoms, and bone destruction suggest a malignant process that should be biopsied before further decisions are made regarding management. A painless, indolent course with only bone remodeling on CT suggests a benign mixed tumor and this should be excised intact via a lateral orbitotomy to prevent future degeneration into malignancy.

C Lymphoid tumors which are small, low grade [usually Mucosa Associated Lymphoid Tissue (MALT)] anterior, and determined by complete staging workup to be isolated, may be excised entirely. Those which are larger and isolated may be treated with radiation alone. Those which are part of a systemic disorder will be treated with chemotherapy, with or without targeted radiation to the area (for symptom relief if needed).

D Some benign orbital entities will be treated with chemotherapy or radiation: lymphangioma, in particular, is often amenable to sclerotherapy by an experienced interventionalist. Radiation is occasionally used in the treatment of orbital inflammation, which may look impressive enough on imaging to warrant biopsy. Meningioma of the orbit, particularly optic nerve sheath meningiomas, is treated with radiation as soon as the vision begins to decline, either conventional or stereotactic fractionated.

E Orbital invasion by tumor may originate from three primary organs: skin, brain, and sinuses. Each of these requires a different approach to biopsy and treatment, likely involving surgeons of different specialties. Benign tumors that secondarily involve the orbit often will not violate the periorbita, or the periosteal lining on the interior of the bone, allowing for resection with less risk of harm to the eye. Malignancies that have spread to the orbit often do not respect these boundaries, and much more serious consideration of orbital exenteration must take place.

F In the case of benign or malignant tumors that spread to the orbit, three questions should be asked primarily: does the eye see, is the eye painful, and is the eye in the way of a potential cure of malignancy? If, for example, the patient is a young, healthy individual with an otherwise resectable cancer, even with a healthy eye, exenteration may be an appropriate option. If, on the other hand, the patient's other eye is not useful, or the patient is older or has other comorbidities, keeping the eye and subtotal resection with adjuvant therapy might be a better choice.

G In planning for subtotal resection, or for resection of tumor involving only the orbit, adequate plans for protection of the eye must be in place. In the situation of a malignancy invading the orbit, the eye may be the "margin" of tumor needed for a cure. In cases where the mass is benign, or the globe itself is uninvolved, but the eye is already painful, or will become painful due to lack of its natural defenses (lids, muscles, etc.), exenteration may be offered. A common example of this is orbital involvement by skin tumor, where extensive resection of the lids would quickly render the eye blind and painful.

SUGGESTED READING

Hoffman GR, Jefferson ND, Reid CB, et al. Orbital exenteration to manage infiltrative sinonasal, orbital adnexal, and cutaneous malignancies provides acceptable survival outcomes: an institutional review, literature review, and meta-analysis. J Oral Maxillofac Surg.; 2016;74(3):631-643.

Sakata K, Maeda A, Rikimaru H, et al. Advantage of extended craniofacial resection for advanced malignant tumors of the nasal cavity and paranasal sinuses: long-term outcome and surgical management. World Neurosurg. 2016;89:240-254.

Stefko S. Exenteration. In: Myers E (Ed). Operative Otolaryngology: Head and Neck Surgery, 2nd edition. Elsevier; 2008.

Wellman BJ, Traynelis VC, McCulloch TM, et al. Midline anterior craniofacial approach for malignancy: results of en bloc versus piecemeal resections. Skull Base Surg. 1999;9(1):41-46.

Plastic and Reconstructive Surgery

- Cleft Lip and Palate Deformities
- Nasal Deformity with and without Nasal Obstruction
- Deformity of the Nasal Tip
- Revision Rhinoplasty
- Soft Tissue Injuries of the Face
- Maxillofacial Trauma
- Orbital Fractures
- Fractures of the Mandible
- Craniomaxillofacial Trauma in Children
- Reconstruction of Major Head and Neck Defects
- Reconstruction of Cutaneous Defects of the Head and Neck
- Maxillofacial Prosthetic Rehabilitation
- Scar Revision
- Aging Face and Neck
- Cancer of the Skin of the Head and Neck
- Malignant Melanoma

Cleft Lip and Palate Deformities

Jesse Goldstein, Joseph E Losee

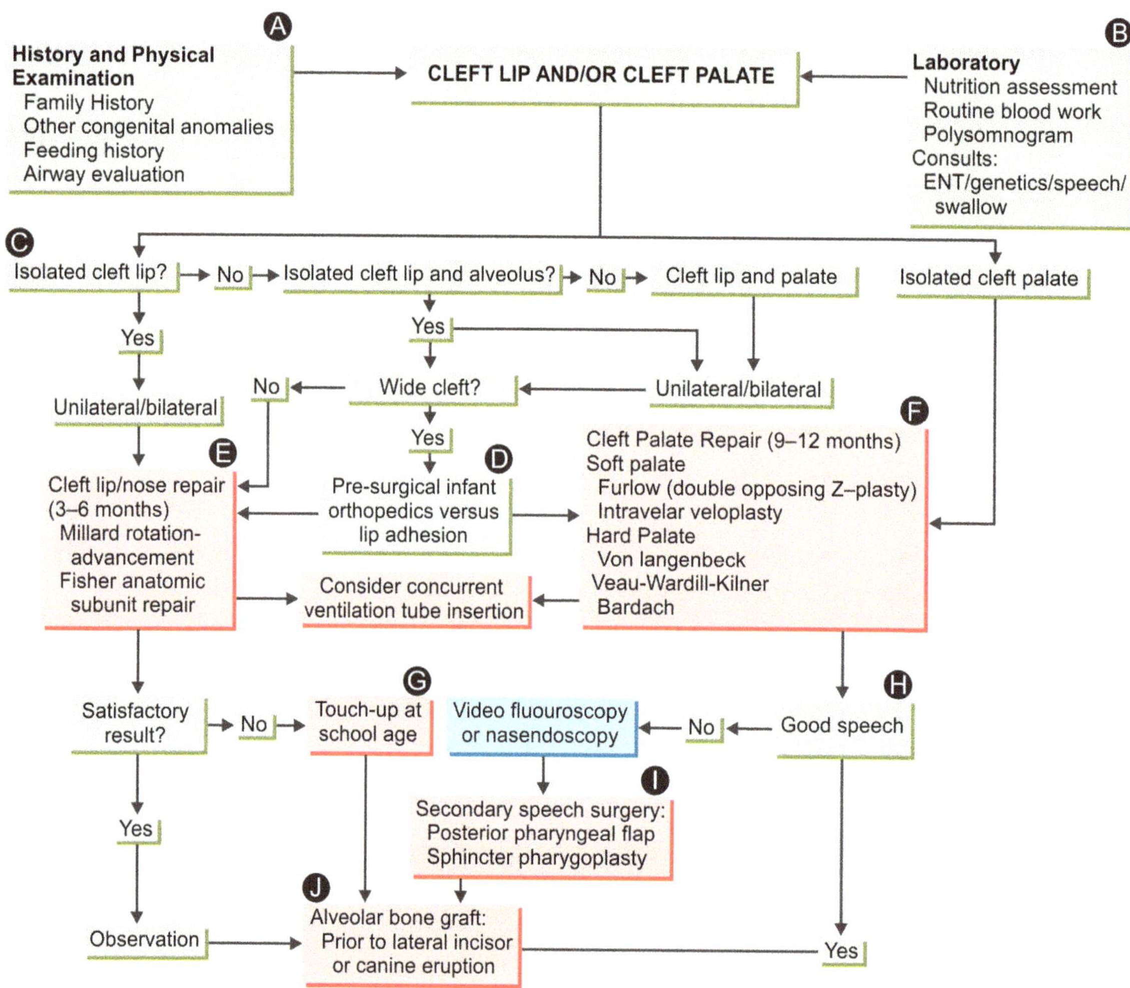

Cleft lip and/or palate (CL/P) deformities have a broad range of severity and can be associated with disorders in multiple systems. They affect 1:750 to 1:1,000 live births, with a slightly increased incidence in Asians (1:500) and a slightly reduced incidence in African Americans (1:1,500). Although there are few known genetic links, most cases of CL/P are multifactorial or sporadic. Therefore, multidisciplinary care is the mainstay of treatment. The team should include Plastic Surgeons, Otolaryngologists, Dentists, Orthodontist, Speech Pathologists, and Nutritionists.

A Evaluation of a patients with CL/P should begin with a detailed history and physical examination. In the neonatal period, particular attention should be paid to feeding and airway concerns. Patients with a cleft palate cannot form suction and therefore cannot breastfeed or use conventional nipples. Families will need specific training by Speech Language Pathologists and/or Nutrition Services. Patients with cleft palate may also have tongue-base airway collapse in association with Pierre Robin sequence (*see* Chapter 113) and a careful airway evaluation should be undertaken.

B Routine tests, including nutritional assessment and blood work, are often performed. In patients in whom Pierre Robin sequence is suspected, a polysomnogram may help to determine the severity of obstruction. In addition to these routine tests, consultation with Audiology, Otolaryngology, Genetics, and Speech/swallow is routine.

C There are many ways to characterize the extent of the CL/P deformity. Patients with no alveolar or palatal involvement are considered to have an isolated cleft lip, which can be unilateral or bilateral. The addition of an alveolar cleft may contribute to the severity of the cleft nasal deformity and can lead to more widely diastatic lip elements. In patients with bilateral cleft lips, the cleft alveolus can also be bilateral. Such clefts require a more structured treatment plan. The addition of a cleft palate to the cleft lip and alveolus further accentuates the soft tissue deformity which causes the lesser segment to be positioned inferiorly, posteriorly, and laterally to the greater segment or primary palate.

D Presurgical infant orthopedics (either nasoalveolar molding [NAM] or Latham device) or lip adhesion can significantly reduce the width of the cleft at the level of the alveolus and lip. Additionally, NAM has the added benefit of lengthening the columella, which is often foreshortened, especially in patients with wide bilateral lip/palate deformities.

E The basic principles of cleft lip repair concern restoring symmetry to the nose, philtral column, Cupid's bow, and vermilion. Many techniques exist to accomplish this, but all involve lengthening the cleft-sided philtrum by rotating it inferiorly and interposing tissue from the lateral lip element. The Millard rotation advancement, and variations thereof, is the classic and most practiced technique, but other techniques, based on similar principles can achieve similar results in skilled hands. Although there is variation regarding when to perform a cleft repair, most centers plan for repair between 3 and 6 months of age. Many authors advocate performing a primary cleft rhinoplasty at the time of lip repair. This may range from a few percutaneous (McComb) sutures to a limited open approach, which directly resuspends the hypoplastic lower lateral cartilage and lengthens the columella.

F Cleft palate repair is performed some time before speech develops but late enough so that maxillary growth is not impaired by scar. The most common age range is 9–12 months old. However, there is substantial controversy regarding the optimum age to perform the repair. Most techniques for palate repair are concerned with how the levator muscle is reoriented. Some perform an aggressive straight line repair (intravelar veloplasty) while others elect to overlap the muscle and lengthen the soft palate with a Furlow (double-opposing) Z-plasty. There are also multiple approaches to the hard palate based on how the mucoperiosteal flaps are elevated and apposed.

G The goal of a well-performed lip repair is to create symmetry in both the lip and the nasal repair. When this is not achieved, revisionary surgery may be employed. There is great variation with respect to timing of cleft lip/nasal revisions, and much depends on the degree of

deformity as well as the preferences of the patient and families preferences. The transition to school age poses thin particular challenges to patients with unfavorable results, and this is when many surgeons chose to offer limited lip revisions. Nasal revisions at this age are more controversial; however, minor nasal tip work may often be added to a lip revision.

H Cleft palate repair is a functional surgery, and the key to adequate palatal function is appropriate speech production. Specifically, production of pressure sounds such as /b/, /p/, /d/, /t/, /k/, and normal resonance are indicators that the palate is functioning appropriately. When pressure sounds are weak or absent, or when hypernasal resonance is noted, the palate may be functioning suboptimally leading to velopharyngeal dysfunction.

I Video fluoroscopy and nasendoscopy can identify areas of impaired velopharyngeal port closure as well as what secondary speech operation should be employed. Depending on what closure patterns are observed, a posterior pharyngeal flap or a sphincter pharyngoplasty can eliminate hypernasality and allow for improved speech.

J Neither CL/P repair addresses the bony cleft in the alveolus or the associated oronasal fistula. In order for healthy adult tooth eruption into the region, patients with a cleft of the alveolus will require bone grafting and closure of the oronasal fistula usually between 7 and 9 years of age. Most surgeons prefer iliac crest bone; however, some use other sources including demineralized cadaveric bone. Alveolar bone grafting should be performed sometime after orthodontic palatal expansion and prior to the eruption of the lateral incisor or canine, and should be performed with close coordination with an experienced orthodontics.

SUGGESTED READING

Fisher DM, Sommerlad BC. Cleft lip, cleft palate, and velopharyngeal insufficiency. Plast Reconstr Surg. 2011;128(4):342e-360e.

Guyuron B. MOC-PS(SM) CME article: late cleft lip nasal deformity. Plast Reconstr Surg. 2008;121(4 Suppl):1-11.

Losee JE, Kirshner RE. Comprehensive Cleft Care, 2nd edition. New York: McGraw Hill; 2015.

Millard DR. Refinements in rotation-advancement cleft lip technique. Plast Reconstr Surg. 1964;33(1):26-38.

Mulliken JB. Bilateral cleft lip. Clin Plast Surg. 2004;31(2):209-220.

Nasal Deformity with and without Nasal Obstruction

Grant S Gillman

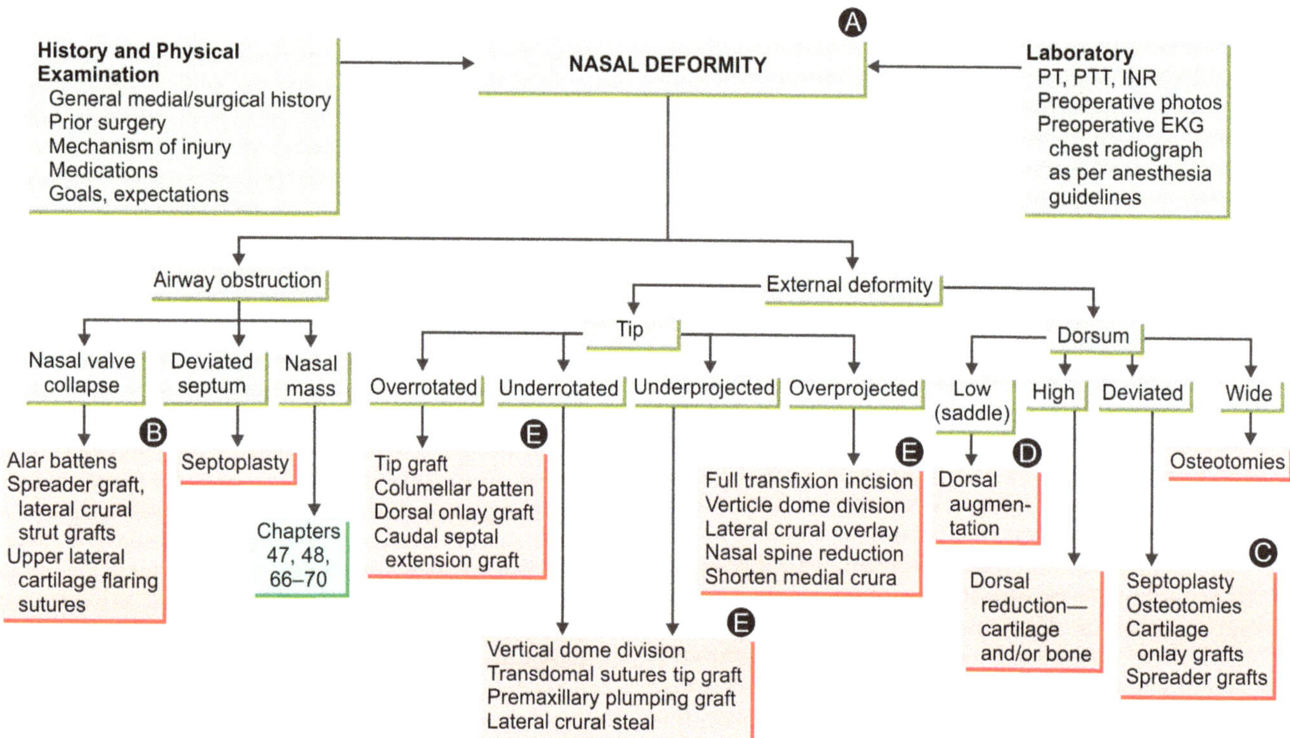

Nasal obstruction remains one of the most common patient concerns presenting to the Otolaryngologist. Structural problems manifested by nasal obstruction can be simple and the management decisions clear, or they can be subtle and deceptively complex. Once inflammatory and other nonstructural causes have been ruled out on examination, a very critical analysis of the nose—internally, externally, while at rest, and with inspiration—can define the source of obstruction and guide the necessary intervention.

A The history should inquire about previous nasal surgery or trauma and the patient's symptoms, goals, and motivation for considering surgery. The use of any medication that would contraindicate surgery such as cocaine or anticoagulants should be determined. The physical examination should evaluate septal position, stability of the nasal sidewall (internal and external valves) and external alignment. Thoughtful preoperative analysis is essential for guiding appropriate management. A realistic and thorough review of attainable objectives and potential complications will help to maximize patient's satisfaction.

There are frequently several ways to address a given problem, as indicated in this algorithm. In many instances, more than one maneuver may be required to achieve the desired result: a graduated approach is recommended. In all instances, the techniques and approach (endonasal vs external) chosen will vary with the comfort and experience of the surgeon.

With children, for traumatic deformities, any intervention must be conservative to minimize the potential for interfering with nasal and midfacial growth. The emphasis is on closed reduction techniques when possible and when open reduction is required, repositioning of tissues is favored over resection. For nontraumatic deformities in children, intervention is often best deferred until facial growth is largely complete.

If any change in external appearance is planned, preoperative photodocumentation is an essential part of the medical record.

B Spreader grafts (cartilage grafts placed between the septum and upper lateral cartilages) and upper lateral cartilage flaring sutures are used to improve on the narrowed internal nasal valve. Alar battens and lateral crural strut grafts address dynamic inspiratory collapse of the nasal sidewall (external nasal valve).

C Correction of the deviated external nasal pyramid begins with correction of the septum internally. Spreader grafts can be used to address asymmetries or narrowing in the middle nasal vault. Cartilage onlay grafts are a very efficient means of effacing or camouflaging depressions along the lateral nasal wall. To reposition the pyramid the bony vault osteotomies are required; a very wide upper third or severely deviated pyramid may require intermediate osteotomies in addition to standard lateral and medial osteotomies.

D The nasal dorsum can be augmented with autologous (septal, auricular, or costal cartilage) or alloplastic materials. The use of autologous materials is considered the gold standard although there are situations in which an alloplastic implant may be preferred (e.g. patient objection to other incisions or donor sites, limited availability of donor tissue).

E A variety of techniques are available to increase or decrease the projection or rotation of the nasal tip. Typically, these involve maneuvers that influence tip support mechanisms or alter the volume, length, or orientation of the medial and lateral crura of the lower lateral cartilages. Over-resection is to be avoided in all cases to prevent a stigmatized nasal appearance postoperatively. The use of a particular method will vary among surgeons. Ultimately, having more than one technique in one's armamentarium is optimal.

SUGGESTED READING

Ballert JA, Park SS. Functional rhinoplasty: treatment of the dysfunctional nasal sidewall. Facial Plast Surg. 2006;22:49-54.

Chand MS, Toriumi DM. Treatment of the external nasal valve. Facial Plast Surg Clin North Am. 1999;7:347-355.

Daniel RK. Mastering Rhinoplasty, 2nd edition. New York: Springer; 2010.

Dixon TK, Toriumi DM. Nasal tip surgery. In: Johnson JT, Rosen CA (Eds). Bailey's Head and Neck Surgery, 5th edition. Philadelphia, PA: Lippincott Williams & Wilkins; 2014. pp. 2964-3297.

Gunter JP, Friedman RM. Lateral crural strut graft: technique and clinical applications in rhinoplasty. Plast Reconstr Surg. 1997;99(4):943-952.

Lee J, White WM, Constantinides M. Surgical and nonsurgical treatments of the nasal valves. Otolaryngol Clin North Am. 2009;42:495-511.

Toriumi DM, Ries WR. Innovative surgical management of the crooked nose. Facial Plast Surg Clin North Am. 1993;1:63-78.

Deformity of the Nasal Tip

Rebecca E Fraioli

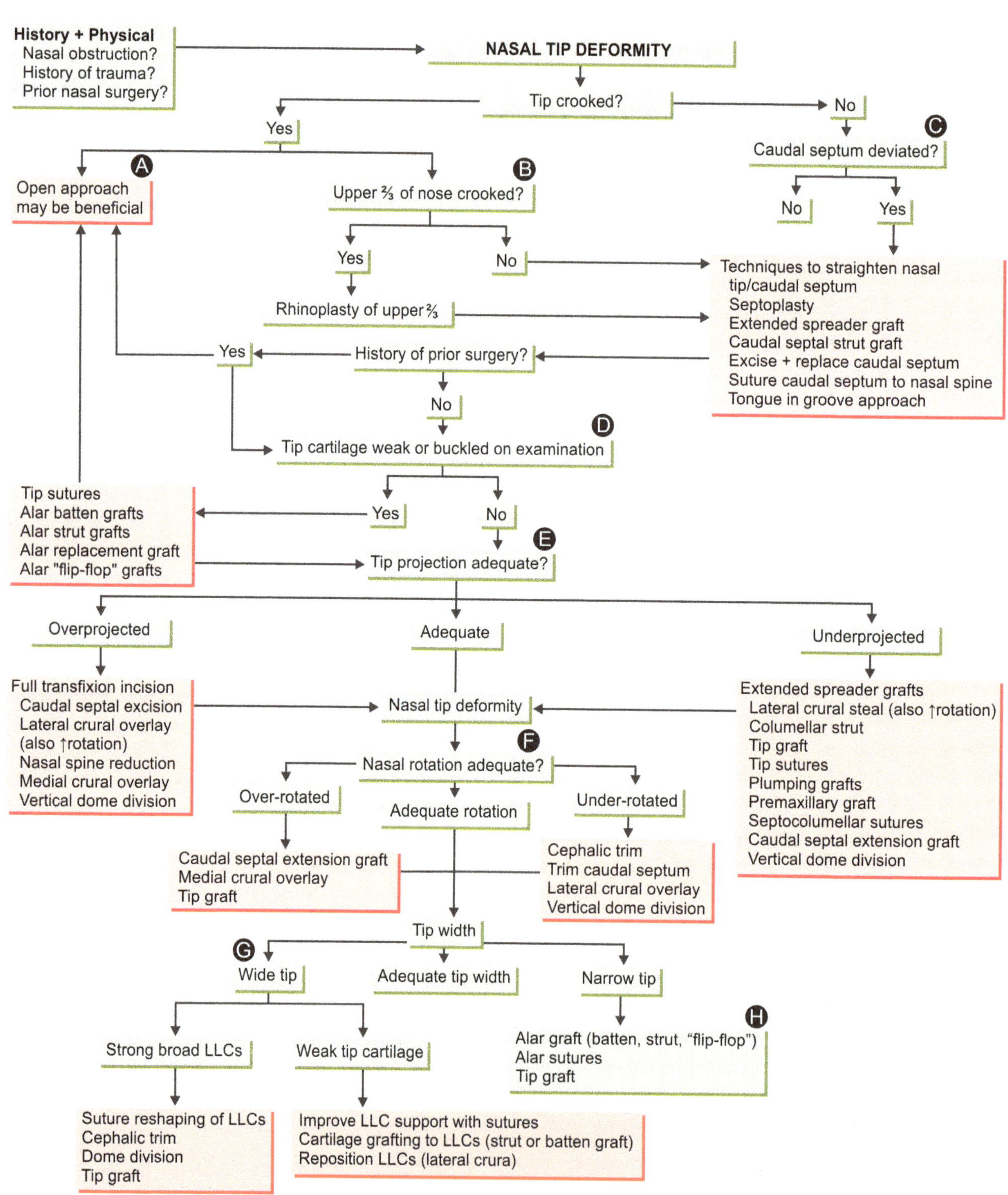

Nasal tip dynamics require that many factors are considered simultaneously in determining which interventions will achieve the desired result. Surgeon preference and experience should supplement and at times supersede this algorithm.

A The initial history and physical examination guides the choice of surgical approach to the nasal tip. If the nasal tip itself, the caudal septum, or both are deviated, then the external (open) rhinoplasty approach is preferred. Other indications for the external approach include a weak, ptotic, or buckled nasal tip, or a patient with a history of prior tip rhinoplasty. In each of these situations, there is a high likelihood that multiple grafts will be necessary to reconstruct the nasal tip, and the external approach provides excellent exposure to facilitate proper positioning of the grafts.

B If the nasal tip is crooked, a determination of the cause of this deviation can usually be obtained from a physical examination of the nose. If the upper two-thirds of the nose is also crooked, a full rhinoplasty with osteotomies will likely be necessary in order to straighten the nasal tip.

C Deviations of the caudal septum can cause tip deviation. Straightening a caudal septum can be difficult, and the choice of which method to use is beyond the scope of this chapter. Some techniques that may be useful include nasal septoplasty, separation of the upper lateral cartilages from the dorsal septum with release of scar tissue, extended spreader grafts, caudal septal strut graft, suture of caudal septum to nasal spine, tongue in groove approach, excision and replacement of the caudal septum.

D Physical examination of the nasal tip can help to determine whether the tip cartilages have adequate strength to support the nasal tip, or whether they are too weak and nonsupportive. In the event that tip cartilages are weak and causing buckling and collapse of the tip, an open rhinoplasty approach may be helpful. Depending on the severity of the deformity, options to regain tip support include tip sutures, alar batten grafts, alar strut grafts, or alar replacement grafts. In some cases, a combination of the above methods may be the most useful solution.

E Nasal projection describes the anterior-posterior distance that the nasal tip extends outward from the facial plane. An overprojected nose may result from an overdeveloped nasal septum or nasal spine, from overdeveloped lower lateral cartilages (LLCs), or from all of the above. Several potential methods exist for deprojecting the nasal tip. The choice of technique will depend on the cause of the overprojection as well as on the other desired changes to be made in the nasal tip. Deprojection options include full transfixion incision, caudal septal excision, lateral crural overlay (also increases tip rotation), nasal spine reduction, medial crural overlay, vertical dome division. As with the overprojected nose, the underprojected nose can be caused by deficient support from the caudal septum or LLCs. Options to increase nasal projection include vertical dome division, lateral crural steal (also increases

rotation), columellar strut graft, tip graft, tip sutures, plumping grafts, premaxillary graft, septocolumellar sutures, a caudal septal extension graft, or extended spreader grafts.

F Tip rotation is a term used to describe the degree to which the nasal tip is upturned or downturned; it is frequently measured by the nasolabial angle. The over-rotated nose may be corrected using a caudal septal extension graft if the over-rotation is due to a deficient caudal septum, a medial crural overlay if it is due to overly long medial crura, or a tip graft for camouflage if the patient has thick skin. Tip grafts are more likely to become visible in thin-skinned patients and should be avoided or used with caution in this situation. Vertical dome division may also decrease tip rotation; however, the amount of derotation achieved is difficult to predict. An under-rotated nose may be corrected using cephalic trim of the ULCs, trim of the caudal septum if it is overly long, or a lateral crural overlay if deprojection is also desired.

G Assessment of the width of the tip is another major decision point in tip rhinoplasty. A wide nasal tip may be due to overly strong and broad LLCs, in which case cephalic trim, tip suture techniques, or both may be useful to narrow the nasal tip. Tip grafts may also be useful to give the appearance of a more narrow nasal tip. Conversely, if the wide tip is due to a lack of tip support with collapse and splaying of the LLCs, then techniques to increase the strength and support of the nasal tip will be necessary. These techniques include replacing or reinforcing the caudal septum if it is deficient, suture techniques to reshape the domes, cartilage grafting such as lateral crural strut grafts, or repositioning of the lateral crura via either lateral crural steal or lateral crural overlay. As with other aspects of rhinoplasty, the ultimate choice of which technique to use depends on the other desired effects in a particular patient. For example, the decision to use lateral crural steal versus lateral crural overlay would depend on whether the goal is to increase or decrease nasal projection; the former technique will increase nasal projection, whereas the latter technique will decrease it.

H A narrow nasal tip is likely to be caused by weak or buckled LLCs. Accordingly, management of the narrow nasal tip is focused on strengthening or reconstructing these cartilages. Tip sutures or structural grafts (alar batten grafts, alar strut grafts, tip onlay grafts) may be used.

SUGGESTED READING

Ahmad J, Rohrich RJ. The crooked nose. Clin Plast Surg. 2016;43: 99-113.

Apaydin F. Projection and deprojection techniques in rhinoplasty. Clin Plast Surg. 2016;43:151-168.

Christophel JJ, Park SS. Structural support and dynamics at the tip. Facial Plast Surg. 2012;28:145-151.

Friedman O, Koch CA, Smith WR. Functional support of the nasal tip. Facial Plast Surg. 2012;28:225-230.

Quatela VC, Kolstad CK. Creating elegance and refinement at the nasal tip. Facial Plast Surg. 2012;28:166-170.

Revision Rhinoplasty

Paul Leong

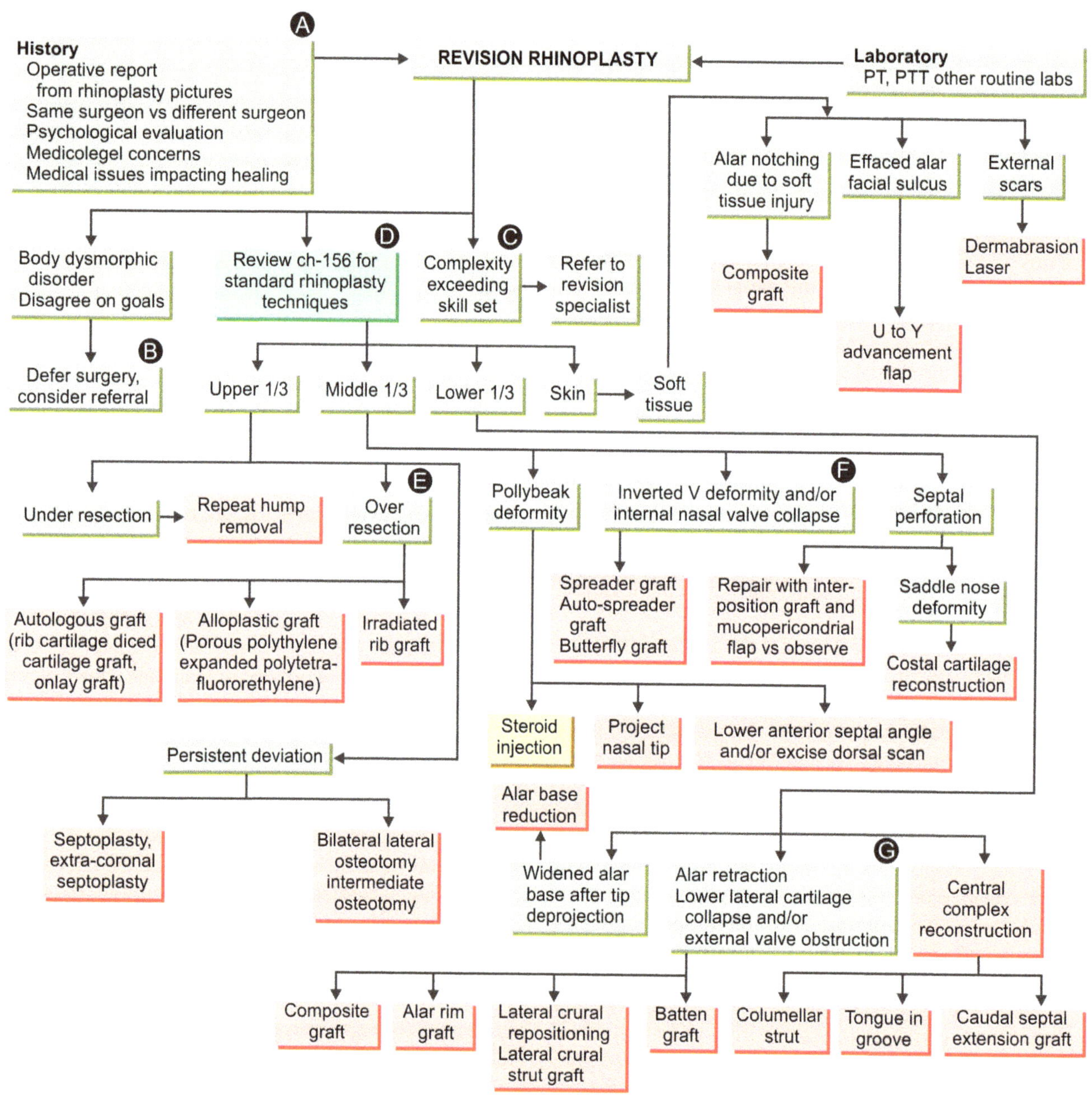

Revision rhinoplasty is arguably the most challenging commonly performed surgery by a facial plastic surgeon. The complex interaction between the soft tissue, cartilage, and bony components of the nose provides a multidimensional and unpredictable terrain even in the setting of primary rhinoplasty. Revision rhinoplasty superimposes issues of uncertain anatomy, scar contracture, structural compromise, and increased psychological burden to further elevate the intensity of the treatment encounter. Being prepared to respond effectively to difficult revision rhinoplasty cases is part of a facial plastic surgeon's practice, and comprehensive planning is a precondition to success.

A The evaluation begins with a complete history and physical examination, with emphasis on the status of the nose prior to the first procedure, the operative changes made during that procedure, and the postoperative course. An important distinction is whether the first rhinoplasty was performed by the same surgeon or a different surgeon. If a different surgeon performed the initial surgery, the operative and perioperative notes from the prior procedure should be obtained, as well as the standard rhinoplasty photographs from the first procedure. The motivation of revision rhinoplasty patients must be closely examined. Any concern about body dysmorphic disorder (BDD) or other inappropriate motivations should be evaluated closely. The surgeon should be alert to whether there are any medicolegal issues regarding the first rhinoplasty. Any medical issues that may have predisposed to a poor outcome after the first surgery (diabetes, connective tissue disorders) should be sought.

B Given the intrinsically subjective nature of all cosmetic surgery outcomes, the surgeon and patient may disagree that a revision rhinoplasty is necessary. The patient might conclude that, while there is no frank defect, the nose simply does not have the appearance he or she would like. Such a difference of opinion does not necessarily imply that the patient is unreasonable or has BDD; there is merely a difference of opinion. Conversely, the surgeon must be alert for the presence of BDD is the revision rhinoplasty population, which has an incidence of up to 13% in patients seeking cosmetic surgery. Whatever the source of the disagreement between the surgeon and patient, there are circumstances in which the surgeon must decline doing further surgery.

C Not all revision rhinoplasty procedures are within the capabilities of all facial plastic surgeons. Difficult revision rhinoplasty surgery is amongst the most daunting challenges a facial plastic surgeon can confront and there should be no false pride in admitting that some cases are beyond one's present skill set. Particularly difficult cases can only reasonably expect moderate improvement from the most experienced surgeons in the world. In such cases, referral to a more experienced revision rhinoplasty expert is warranted.

D It should be noted that the fundamental surgical maneuvers in revision rhinoplasty surgery are not markedly distinct from those used in primary rhinoplasty. Revision cases may involve greater emphasis on reestablishing structural support and more effort in dissecting within a scarred field, but the differences in surgical technique are more a matter of degree than different maneuvers. Understanding this, please refer to Chapter 156 to review standard rhinoplasty technique. The maneuvers emphasized in this chapter are not meant to be an exhaustive review; rather they are more likely to be used in revision cases.

E While aggressively reductive primary rhinoplasty is now widely discouraged, it still occurs. When the revision rhinoplasty surgeon confronts an overly reduced dorsum,

some form of augmentation is necessary. The source of ideal graft material is on an ongoing controversy. Autologous sources (rib cartilage, diced cartilage, and onlay grafts) suffer the disadvantages of increased operative time, donor site morbidity, resorption, and warping. Alloplastic implants (porous polyethylene, expanded polytetrafluoroethylene) can cause infection and extrusion. Irradiated rib cartilage has been criticized for absorption difficulties, but some surgeons have used it successfully. The choice of graft material requires weighing the advantages and disadvantages for each surgical case in the context of each surgeon's experience and preferences.

F Nasal obstruction and/or cosmetic deformities caused by asymmetries or collapse of the middle third of the nose are common finding in revision rhinoplasty. Spreader grafts can be used to treat internal nasal valve stenosis and inverted V deformities. The evidence supporting the use of spreader grafts to address nasal obstruction is conflicting and some authors prefer the use of a butterfly graft in this setting. Spreader flaps, also known as auto-spreaders, are frequently unavailable due to lack of cartilage in the revision setting, but can be useful in selected cases.

G As with all rhinoplasty procedures, addressing cosmetic and functional challenges of the nasal tip are often the most elusive elements of revision rhinoplasty surgery. Deformities of the lateral crura can result in retraction and/or collapse causing stigmata of prior surgery and external nasal valve collapse leading to airway obstruction. Alar retraction is traditionally addressed with composite grafts, but can also be treated with alar rim grafts, lateral crural struts, and lateral crural repositioning. These same grafts, as well as alar batten grafts, are used to restore the external nasal valve.

SUGGESTED READING

Calvert JW, Patel AC, Daniel RK. Reconstructive rhinoplasty: operative revision of patients with previous autologous costal cartilage grafts. Plast Reconstr Surg. 2014;133(5):1087-1096.

Chauhan N, Alexander AJ, Sepehr A, et al. Patient complaints with primary versus revision rhinoplasty: analysis and practice implications. Aesthet Surg J. 2011;31(7):775-780.

Fedok FG. Costal cartilage grafts in rhinoplasty. Clin Plast Surg. 2016;43(1):201-212.

Katira K, Guyuron B. Contemporary techniques for effective nasal lengthening. Facial Plast Surg Clin North Am. 2015;23(1):81-91.

Loyo M, Wang TD. Revision rhinoplasty. Clin Plast Surg. 2016; 43(1):177-185.

Roostaeian J, Unger JG, Lee MR, et al. Reconstitution of the nasal dorsum following component dorsal reduction in primary rhinoplasty. Plast Reconstr Surg. 2014;133(3):509-518.`

Soft Tissue Injuries of the Face

Mark Mandell-Brown

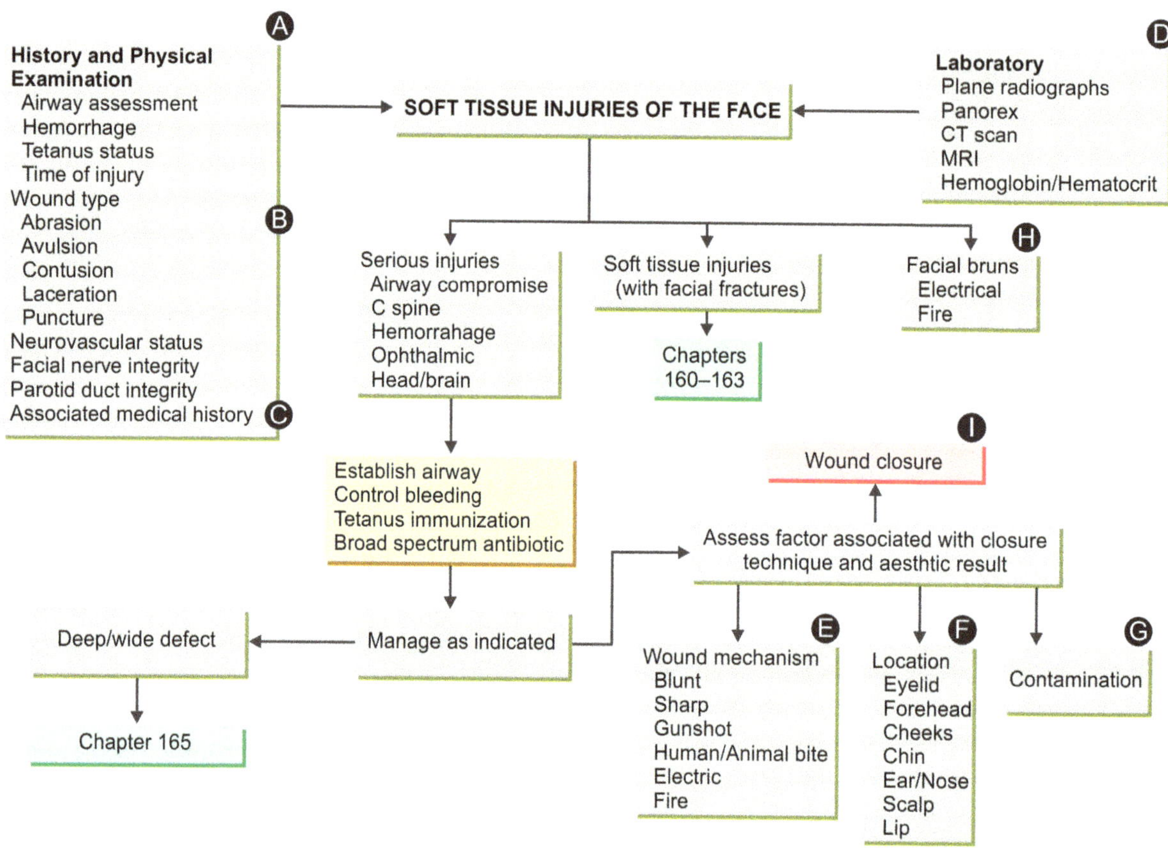

Soft tissue injuries can have a devastating effect on the individual's appearance and self-esteem. Motor vehicle injuries, violence, falls, and animal bites are among the most common causes of soft tissue facial injuries.

A With major traumatic injuries, establish an airway and control bleeding. Unless the patient was recently immunized, give 0.5 mL of tetanus toxoid. Consider broad-spectrum antibiotics. Assess facial nerve function and parotid duct integrity. Lacerated facial nerve branches can be approximated with loupes and 6-0 or 7-0 Prolene. A greater auricular nerve interposition can be used for missing facial nerve segments. The parotid duct injury can be managed conservatively, reapproximated, or the duct can be ligated. Stents can be difficult to place although reported in the literature.

B It is important to assess the type of wound that will help dictate antibiotic coverage and wound treatment. Puncture wounds and contaminated wounds will require more vigorous cleaning. Puncture wounds should be allowed to heal secondarily. Avulsed ear or nose tissue may be resutured or treated as a composite graft. Failure to heal properly will require a later flap reconstruction.

Abrasions generally heal well. Foreign bodies along with dirt must be removed to avoid skin tattooing.

C Associated disease states should be assessed including diabetes, drug history, coagulopathies, malignancy, smoking history, liver, or thyroid disease. Use of steroids, anticoagulants, and antineoplastic drugs may affect wound healing.

D Radiographic evaluation may be required depending on the history. Plain films, panorex, and computed tomography (CT) of facial bones with midsagittal views to assess the orbital floor may be helpful. For altered mental status or severe head trauma, a head CT should be added.

E Knowledge of wound mechanism is essential to obtain a good cosmetic result. Intensity of blunt trauma may determine if facial bones or mandible fractures are likely. There may be more subclinical damage with blunt trauma. Sharp trauma may leave foreign body debris and result in injury to the parotid duct and branches of the facial nerve. Bleeding typically requires ligation of the injured vessel. Gunshot wounds create severe deformities. Airway management and bleeding control are critical. Large defects may require delayed repair once devitalized tissue is ascertained. Dog, cat, or other animal bites may require animal quarantine to assess for rabies. Wild animals (skunks, raccoons, and bats) should be considered rabid unless captured and brain tests prove negative. Rabies vaccines may be initiated if the animal is not captured. Consider loose approximation, placing a drain, or packing open extensive bite injuries.

F Location will affect closure techniques. Eyelid and lip have functional and cosmetic importance. Proper alignment is essential. The vermillion border and eyebrow must be aligned properly. Deep injuries of the cheek will require assessment of the parotid duct and facial nerve. Chin injuries are prone to hypertrophic scarring. Revisions with W-plasty, Z-plasty, dermabrasion, or laser resurfacing may be required. Scalp lacerations should be thoroughly cleaned and outer table skull fractures can be assessed.

G Thorough irrigation should be performed. Antibacterial cleaning such as Betadine or Hibiclens should be used. Avoid using Hibiclens around the eyes.

H Electrical, chemical, and fire burns can be devastating. It is important to preserve and maintain tissue integrity as well as functionality. Muscle injury is more like to occur in electrical burns. Extensive delayed reconstruction may be required. Chemical and electrical burns typically occur in children through ingestion or biting on electric cords. Chemical burns respond to conservative treatment with minimal debridement. Severe lip electrical or flame burns may require prosthetic splints. Flame burns to the face are classified as superficial or deep. First-degree burns can be treated conservatively. Deep second- and third-degree burns require debridement of eschar with skin grafting or flap reconstruction. Facial masks may reduce scarring.

I Superficial wounds can be closed in one or two layers. Deep injuries require a layered closure, elimination of dead space, and avoidance of excess tension. Wide defects should be closed primarily, if possible, with minimal debridement. Advancement flaps, rotation flaps, or skin grafts may be required but generally should be performed after initial healing. Close deep layers using absorbable suture that maintains tensile strength for several weeks such as a 3-0 or 4-0 PDS or Vicryl. Skin can be closed with subcuticular 5-0 Monocryl or 5-0 and 6-0 Nylon. Particularly in children, consider fibrin glue or mild chromic fast absorbing sutures. Surgical staples may be used in the scalp.

SUGGESTED READING

Bhattacharya V. Management of soft tissue wounds of the face. Indian J Plastic Surg. 2012;45:436-443.

Futran N. Maxillofacial trauma reconstruction. Facial Plast Surg Clin North Am. 2009;17:239-251.

Kretlow J, McKnight A, Izaddoost S. Facial soft tissue trauma. Semin Plast Surg. 2010;4(24):348-355.

Kumar R, Devireddy S, Gail R, et al. A clinician's role in the management of soft tissue injuries of the face: a clinical paper. J Maxillofac Oral Surg. 2013;12(1):21-29.

Wainwright D. Burn reconstruction: the problems, the techniques, and the applications. Clin Plast Surg. 2009;36:687-700.

Maxillofacial Trauma

David M Johnson, Eric W Wang

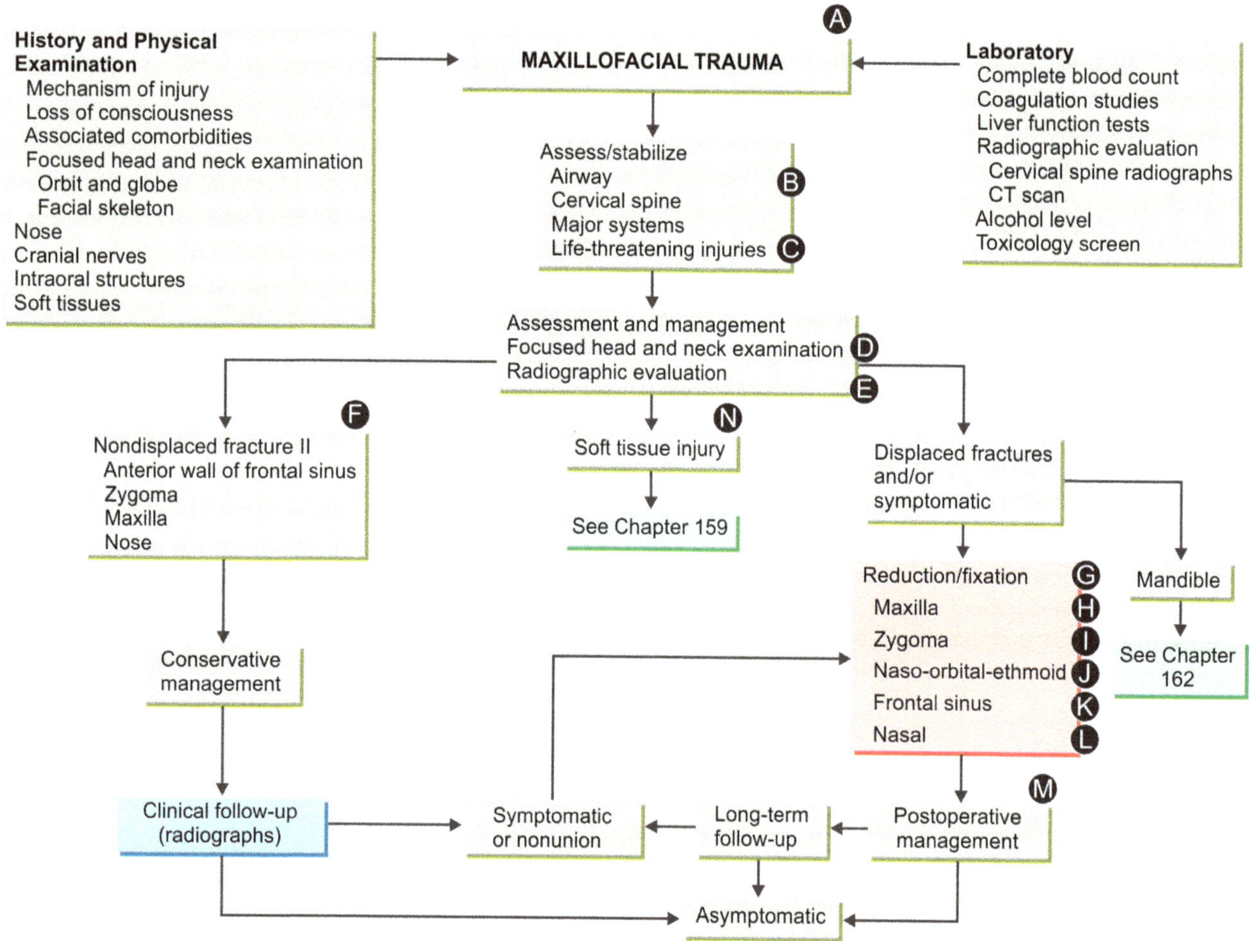

Maxillofacial trauma is usually the result of motor vehicle accidents, industrial injuries, sports injuries, or altercations. Accordingly, facial injuries may be but one component of multisystem injuries typically managed by a specialized trauma team. Superficial soft tissue injuries can be managed by team members from many disciplines (e.g. emergency medicine and general surgery), but due to the anatomic complexity of the head and neck, patients with more serious wounds may benefit from assessment by an Otolaryngologist, Plastic Surgeon, Oral-Maxillofacial Surgeon, or other individuals with advanced training.

A In the setting of trauma, an accurate and complete history may be impossible to obtain due to the patients condition (confusion, intoxication, pain). At a minimum, the presumed mechanism of injury should be obtained from first responders or family members distinguishing between low and high impact, blunt versus penetrating, and so on will guide decision-making and further testing.

B Initial evaluation requires rapid assessment of the airway and cervical spine immobilization. Facial fractures may impact the bony support of the oral cavity and pharynx; edema may impair the ability to clear secretions; a foreign body may obstruct the airway. If suctioning does not stabilize the airway, an endotracheal tube placed with inline cervical traction, cricothyrotomy, or tracheotomy is mandatory. The method used depends on the potential for continued edema of the face, oral cavity, and oropharynx as well as other injuries. The time until recovery from other injuries is also a consideration, because tracheostomy will minimize sequelae of prolonged intubation. Laryngeal crepitus, new-onset dysphonia, and other signs or history of laryngeal trauma necessitate prompt endolaryngeal examination with intervention directed by findings.

C Facial trauma is addressed once the trauma team and appropriate consultants stabilize the airway, the cervical spine, hemodynamic and neurologic status, and life-threatening injuries.

D Focused head and neck examination must include the following:

- *Orbit and globe*: Ocular mobility, visual acuity, size and position of the globe, anterior chamber, fundi, and status of the periorbital soft tissues.
- *Facial skeleton*: Orbits, maxilla, mandible, zygoma, and frontal bone are evaluated, noting the integrity of bony structures, symmetry, contour, and dental occlusion.
- *Nose*: The nasal airway is inspected for patency, blood, and cerebrospinal fluid (CSF); shape and symmetry are evaluated; septal hematoma should be drained without delay.
- *Cranial nerves*: Deficits are recorded.
- *Intraoral structures*: Dentition and soft tissues, interdental occlusion.
- *Soft tissues*: Periorbital and facial tissues and the lacrimal system are assessed, and the laryngopharynx is evaluated fiberoptically.
- Photographic documentation is recommended for postoperative counseling and for medicolegal purposes.

E Additional studies are directed by the findings on physical examination. Suspected bony injuries (aside from isolated nasal bone fractures) are best evaluated with fine-cut CT imaging with multiplanar reconstructions.

F Conservative management of the midface, zygoma, and isolated anterior wall frontal sinus fractures is recommended if the fracture is nondisplaced and there are no associated symptoms. Treatment includes pain control, measures to control edema (e.g. head of bed elevation), and soft diet.

G Fractures are repaired once soft tissue edema is resolved and before malunion of fracture and/or contracture of soft tissue occurs (within 5–10 days after injury).

H Fractures of the midface that result in malocclusion, facial asymmetry, CSF rhinorrhea, or airway compromise require reduction and fixation. Goals of reduction are to restore pretreatment occlusion and stabilize the buttresses that will restore the height, width, and projection of the maxilla. Associated mandible fractures are stabilized first; midface fracture sites are then exposed with an appropriate extended access approach as required (transcoronal, hemicoronal, transconjunctival, sublabial). Fractures are most commonly fixed with rigid internal plates and screws.

I Malar fractures that produce trismus, abnormalities of the orbit, or displacement of the lateral canthal ligament must be reduced and fixation applied.

J Naso-orbital-ethmoid fractures involve the medial orbital wall, with potential to involve the nasal bones and septum, anterior skull base, and frontal sinus; they should be suspected when telecanthus or blunting of the medial canthal angle is noted on exam. Ocular injury is common. The lacrimal system, palpebral fissures, optic nerve, nasal contour, and integrity of the nasofrontal duct and cribriform require evaluation. Ophthalmologic consultation is required, and vision must be tested early in the clinical course. Reduction is required to restore the bony anatomy of the region, integrity of the medial canthal tendon, lacrimal apparatus, and nasofrontal duct.

K Fractures of the frontal sinus are classified according to location of injury (e.g. anterior or posterior table, floor, and frontonasal duct). Associated intracranial injuries (CSF leak, subdural/epidural hematoma,

pneumocephalus) must be ruled out. Neurosurgical consultation is recommended.

Displaced fractures of the frontal sinus, especially those that involve the nasofrontal duct, have significant potential for mucocele or mucopyocele formation. Evaluation and management of the injured frontonasal duct requires either close serial radiologic observation or surgical exploration via endoscopic or open approach.

A fractured displaced anterior table is reduced to address cosmetic deformity. Displaced posterior table fractures may require exploration to assess for CSF leak and possible intracranial injuries. For through-and-through fractures and those resulting in a significant (>25%) loss of posterior table bone, the frontal sinus is cranialized via craniotomy. A pericranial flap may assist in separating the nasofrontal recess from the cranialized sinus.

L Nasal fractures can usually be treated with closed reduction. Septal fractures may require open reduction. Untreated nasal fractures account for a significant number of later corrective procedures for nasal deformity and obstruction.

M Postoperative management includes monitoring of visual acuity and neurologic status, positioning to reduce facial edema, airway management, and decannulation once airway concerns are resolved. Postoperative assessment of dental occlusion, facial symmetry, and facial nerve function ensure that the goals of surgery have been accomplished.

N Wounds are thoroughly irrigated, explored, and debrided of foreign bodies. Hemostasis can be achieved with pressure, cautery, or ligation as appropriate. Facial nerve exploration with neurorrhaphy is indicated if paralysis is present in the setting of penetrating trauma lateral to the lateral canthus.

Primary closure of lacerations is preferred and should be accomplished as soon as possible, ideally within 4–6 hours of injury. Judicious debridement of frankly devitalized tissue may be considered at this time; however, robust blood supply to the face, head, and neck often results in good outcomes even where tissue appears marginal. Lacerations should be closed in a fashion appropriate for each anatomic subunit, details of which are beyond the scope of this text. In general, multilayered, tension-free closure with good edge eversion is desired. Grossly contaminated wounds, human bites, and violation of mucosa or cartilage are indications for antibiotic prophylaxis.

SUGGESTED READING

Committee on Trauma. Resident Manual of Trauma to the Face, Head, and Neck, 1st edition. eBook published by American Academy of Otolaryngology-Head and Neck Surgery, Alexandria, Virginia, 2012.

O'Connor RC, Shakib K, Brennan PA. Recent advances in the management of oral and maxillofacial trauma. Br J Oral Maxillofac Surg. 2015;53(10):913-921.

Pawar SS, Rhee JS. Frontal sinus and naso-orbital-ethmoid fractures. JAMA Facial Plast Surg. 2014;16(4):284-289.

Shumrick KA, Kersten RC, Kulwin DR, et al. Extended access/internal approaches for the management of facial trauma. Arch Otolaryngol Head Neck Surg. 1992;118:1105-1112.

Orbital Fractures

Susan Tonya Stefko

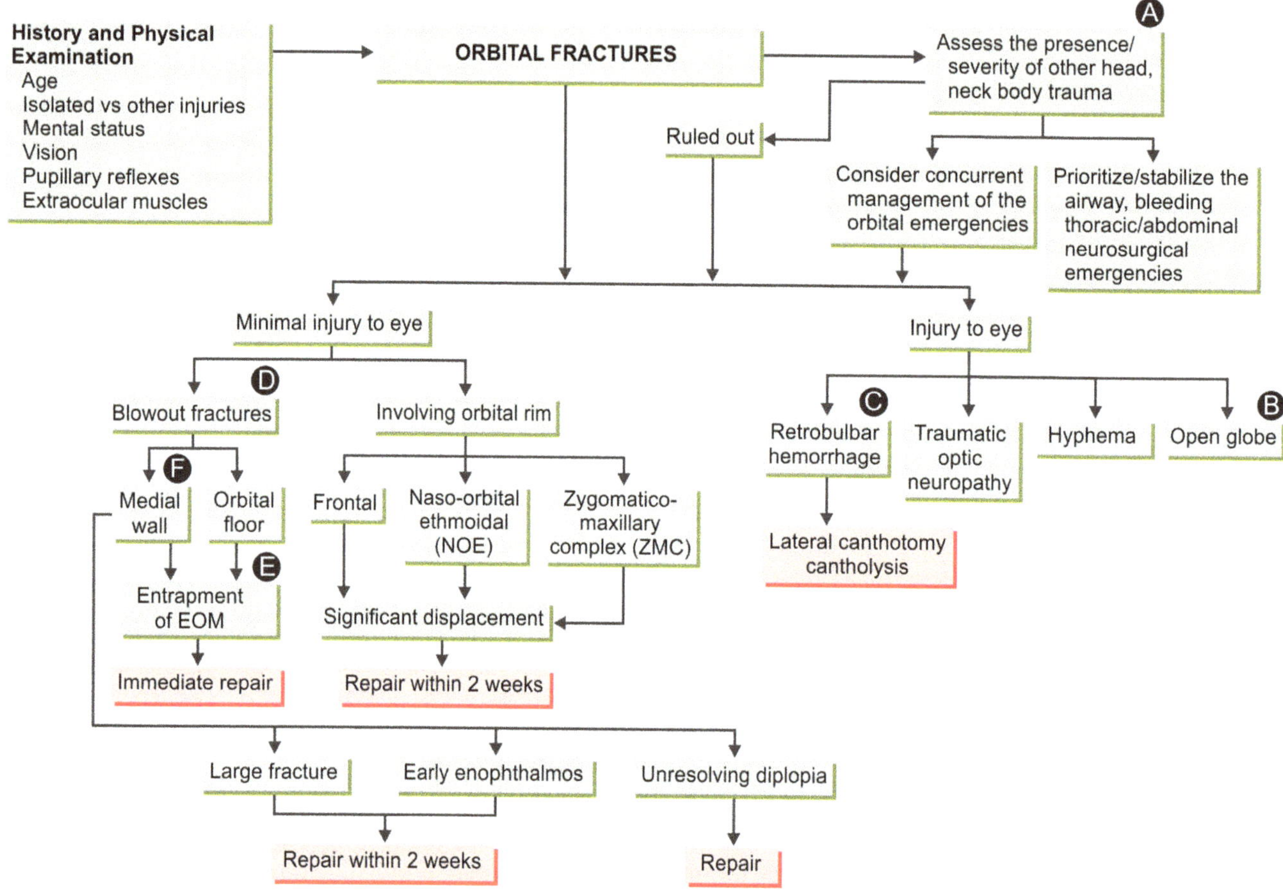

Orbital fractures occur in about one-third of patients with facial trauma in the pediatric population, and in the adult population presenting with any facial fracture. The repair of these fractures must be well thought out and meticulous, both because of structure–function relationships, as well as aesthetic concerns. Two of the horizontal beams and two of the vertical buttresses make up the rim of the orbit. Increases in the volume of the orbit (generally about 30 cc in an adult) can cause dystopia of the eye. Isolated orbital fractures are associated with an incidence of about 15% ophthalmic injury, 1/3 of which will require ophthalmic surgical intervention. In a patient with loss or alteration of consciousness, assessment of the eye and its function may be challenging and require the assistance of an Ophthalmologist.

A Orbital fractures may be part of major head and body trauma, and must always be approached with respect to the overall stability of the patient. This may require delay of evaluation until airway, thoracic/abdominal, and neurosurgical issues have been addressed.

B In the presence of open globe injury (which requires immediate microsurgical repair), hyphema (blood in the anterior chamber of the eye), or traumatic optic neuropathy (indicated by relative afferent pupillary defect), delay surgery until serial ophthalmological examinations have shown improvement. With hyphema, this will generally require at least 5 days, and with traumatic optic neuropathy, this may be 6 months.

C Retrobulbar hemorrhage, which produces severe proptosis, ophthalmoplegia, and optic neuropathy, requires immediate lateral canthotomy and cantholysis to allow reperfusion of critical ocular structures. A true emergency, this is more commonly found in patients on anticoagulants and in fractures of the lateral and medial wall.

D Blowouts are fractures of a wall of the orbit (usually medial or floor) without an associated rim fracture. Decision to repair or not is guided by the size of the fracture, its displacement, and the overall health of the patient. When the decision for surgery is made, ideally this will occur within 2 weeks of injury to minimize any development of scar, but late repair is also feasible.

E An entrapped rectus muscle is more common in younger patients, when a linear blowout fracture (greenstick) snaps closed over a herniated extraocular muscle (EOM). This is classically described as a "White-eyed blowout fracture" because the eye often appears to be unharmed. The injury usually stimulates the afferent arc of the oculocardiac reflex, producing bradycardia, nausea, and hypotension. Because of this and the potential for severe, irreversible ischemic damage to the muscle, this is a true emergency. It requires urgent surgery to release the muscle (which often requires enlarging the fracture before repairing it). Radiologic clues include a very narrow fracture and/or decreased size or disappearance of the inferior or medial rectus muscles.

F In the case of medial wall and floor fractures, most of the diplopia will resolve over the ensuing 6 months without intervention. If the patient has intractable diplopia with displacement of periorbita into the sinus, early repair is indicated.

SUGGESTED READING

Al Shetawi AH, Lim CA, Singh YK, et al. Pediatric maxillofacial trauma: a review of 156 patients. J Oral Maxillofac Surg. 2016; 74(7):1420.e1-4.

Atisha DM, Burr Tv, Allori AC, et al. Facial fractures in the aging population. Plast Reconstr Surg. 2016;137(2):587-593.

Boyette JR, Pemberton JD, Bonilla-Velez J. Management of orbital fractures: challenges and solutions. Clin Ophthalmol. 2015;9:2127-2137.

Ho TQ, Jupiter D, Tsai JH, et al. The Incidence of ocular injuries in isolated orbital fractures. Ann Plast Surg. 2016;78(1):59-61.

Stefko ST. Fractures of the orbit. In: Myers E (Ed). Operative Otolaryngology: Head and Neck Surgery, 2nd edition. Elsevier; New York, 2008.

Nandini Govil, Eric W Wang

CHAPTER 162
Fractures of the Mandible

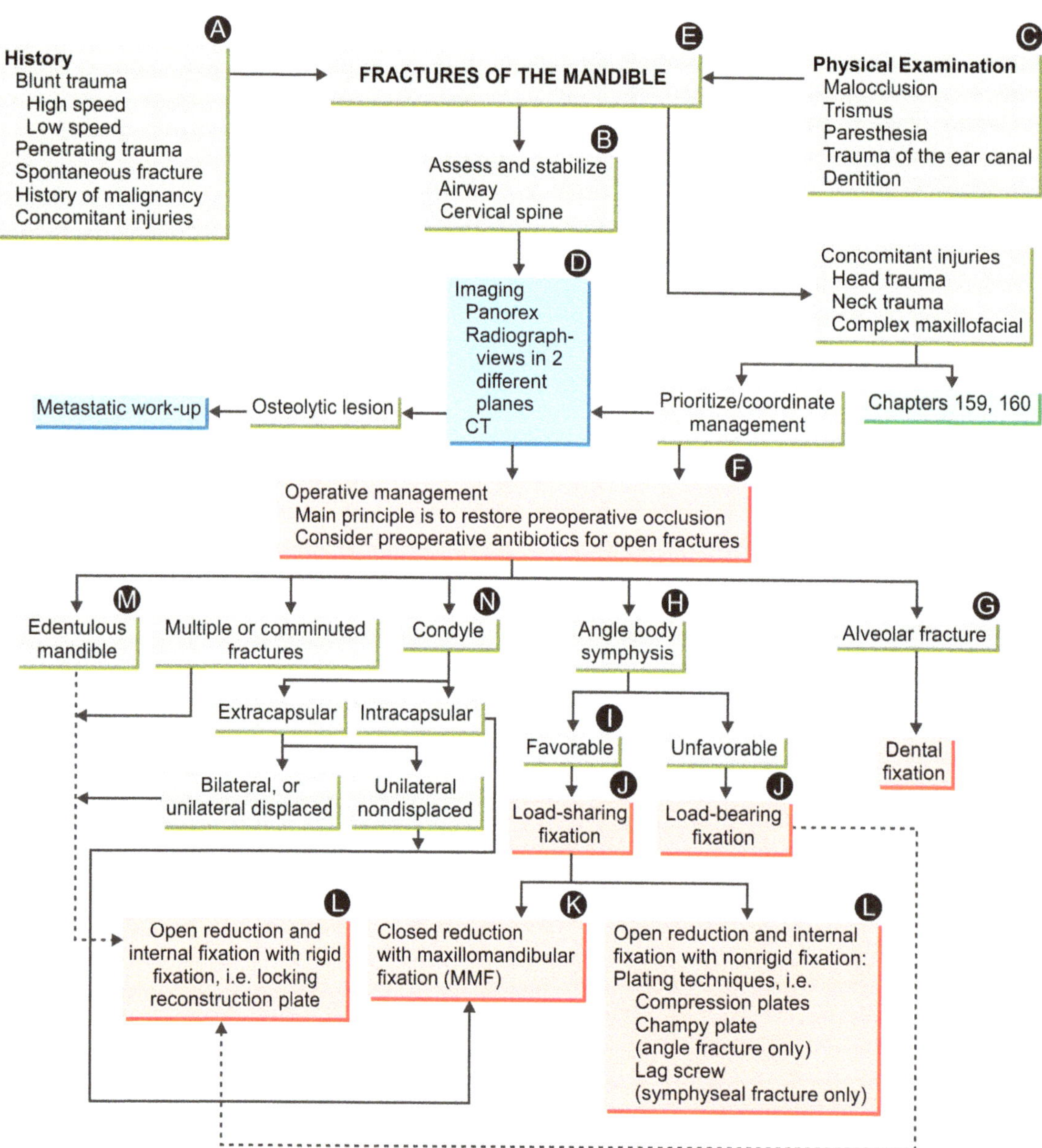

Facial trauma can be classified by the mechanism of injury. In general, the force of trauma will usually correlate with the number and severity of facial fractures.

A Mandibular injuries result as a consequence of low-speed blunt trauma such as falls and assaults, or high-speed trauma such as motor vehicle accidents; *see* Chapter 163 for pediatric mandibular fracture. Fractures of the mandible can generally be treated as separate isolated fractures.

B Examination of patients with facial trauma must begin with evaluation of the airway. Airway compromise can occur with severely displaced bilateral mandibular fractures and/or floor of mouth swelling or hematoma. Additionally, all patients should be evaluated for head injuries and assumed to have a cervical spine injury.

C Malocclusion is the hallmark for diagnosis of a mandibular fracture. This includes premature contact on mastication and failure to contact (open bite). Paresthesia of the lower lip often indicates fractures involving the inferior alveolar nerve. Point tenderness, pain on movement, and trismus are typical signs of mandible fractures. Dentition should also be assessed and the presence of missing teeth or orthodontic devices should be noted, as this can impact surgical management. Trauma to the external auditory canal may be seen with condylar fractures.

D Both plane radiographs and helical computed tomography (CT) are used to diagnose mandible fractures. Plane radiographs should include views in two different plains, such as panorex (orthopantomogram) and posteroanterior view. CT offers the advantage of evaluating concomitant facial and spinal fractures.

E The majority of mandible fractures are multiple and bilateral. The mechanism of injury often predicts the fracture pattern. An anteriorly based force results in symphyseal, parasymphyseal, and condylar fractures. A laterally based force results in angle and body fractures.

F The main principle of fracture management is to restore dental occlusion by placing the segments into anatomical alignment and limiting movement at the fracture site. Fractures of the mandible should be repaired as soon as possible for patient comfort. There is no strong evidence for preoperative antibiotics other than for patients with open or comminuted fractures. In these cases, the antibiotic of choice is penicillin since it covers oral flora; clindamycin is prescribed for patients with penicillin allergy.

G Fractures of the alveolus are fractures to the teeth and supporting bone and result in displacement of the dentition. These are best treated with closed reduction by manually replacing the dentoalveolar segment to its anatomic position. These fractures are stabilized with interdental wire or composite materials.

H The most common fractures of the mandible are fractures of the angle, body, and symphysis. These result in the classic type of malocclusion and should be initially categorized as simple versus complex and displaced versus nondisplaced. The time required for healing is usually about 6 weeks. These fractures are approached by an intraoral, or vestibular, incision. Submandibular or Risdon incisions are used for symphyseal or body fractures requiring manipulation of the lingual cortex. High-angle fractures may require submandibular, retromandibular, or rhytidectomy (facelift) incisions.

I Favorable or unfavorable is terminology referring to the angle of the fracture and its relationship to the muscles of mastication and suprahyoid muscles. The muscles of mastication tend to pull the posterior fracture segments superiorly, whereas suprahyoid muscles pull anterior fracture segments inferiorly. Favorable fractures are angled such that muscular forces reduce the fracture to an anatomical position. An unfavorable fracture is angled so that muscular forces displace the fracture. During mastication, there are also varying amounts of compressive and tensile forces acting on the mandible. Generally, the superior border of the mandible bears tensile forces, and the inferior border of the mandible bears compressive forces.

J Load bearing versus load sharing refers to the mechanics of forces at the fracture site. In load-bearing fixation, the plate bears all the forces at the fracture line. Thus, there is no motion and segments heal by primary bone healing. In contrast, in load-sharing fixation, the plate and the bone share in the forces. This results in some micromotion at the fracture site, and healing occurs by callous formation with eventual ossification. Load-bearing fixation is used in complex or unfavorable fractures of the mandible where the fractures segments require complete stabilization. Load-sharing fixation is used in simple or favorable fractures where the bone is able to bear some of the load without compromising healing.

K Closed reduction of mandible fractures involves wiring the maxillomandibular arches together with intermaxillary fixation. This fixation is maintained for 6 weeks in most patients. Maxillomandibular fixation can be used on its own if only closed reduction is needed. Alternatively, it may be used as a means to reduce the fracture intraoperatively while fixation is achieved by other techniques such as plating. The MMF may be left in place at the end of the case to act as a tensile force at the fracture site, or it may be removed if the compressive and tension forces are relieved by other fixation techniques.

L Open reduction and internal fixation (ORIF) with appropriate-sized bone plates has reduced the need for prolonged MMF. This has led to an improvement in functional outcomes by allowing movement of the mandible, and has eliminated complications associated with prolonged wire fixation such as temporomandibular joint (TMJ) dysfunction and ankylosis.

M Edentulous mandibles are vulnerable to fracture due to reduced vascularity and bone stock. Management of these patients is controversial. Most surgeons advocate that edentulous mandibular fractures should be treated by ORIF with load-bearing techniques.

N Fractures of the condyle are described as intracapsular or extracapsular. Intracapsular fractures are treated with closed reduction with 2 weeks of wire fixation. Extracapsular fractures are described as unilateral or bilateral, and displaced or nondisplaced. Displaced unilateral fractures, in which the condylar head is dislocated out of the fossa, should be treated with ORIF with rigid fixation. Patients with bilateral fractures of the condyle should have at least one side treated with ORIF to maintain the normal occlusion. If open reduction is required, fractures may be approached via submandibular, retromandibular, preauricular, or endoscope-assisted incisions.

SUGGESTED READING

Al-Moraissi EA, Ellis E 3rd. Surgical treatment of adult mandibular condylar fractures provides better outcomes than closed treatment: a systematic review and meta-analysis. J Oral Maxillofac Surg. 2015;73:482-493.

Cienfuegos R, Cornelius CP, Ellis E 3rd, Kushner G. "Mandible". AO Surgery Reference. AO Foundation [online]. 2017. Available from: https://www2aofoundation.org. Accessed July 17, 2017.

Morrow BT, Samson TD, Schubert W, et al. Evidence-based medicine: mandible fractures. Plast Reconstr Surg. 2014;134(6):1381-1390.

Mundinger GS, Borsuk DE, Okhah Z, et al. Antibiotics and facial fractures: evidence-based recommendations compared with experience-based practice. Craniomaxillofac Trauma Reconstr. 2015;8(1):64-78.

Roth FS, Kokoska MS, Awwad EE, et al. The identification of mandible fractures by helical computed tomography and panorex tomography. J Craniofac Surg. 2005;16:394-399.

CHAPTER 163

Craniomaxillofacial Trauma in Children

Bernard J Costello

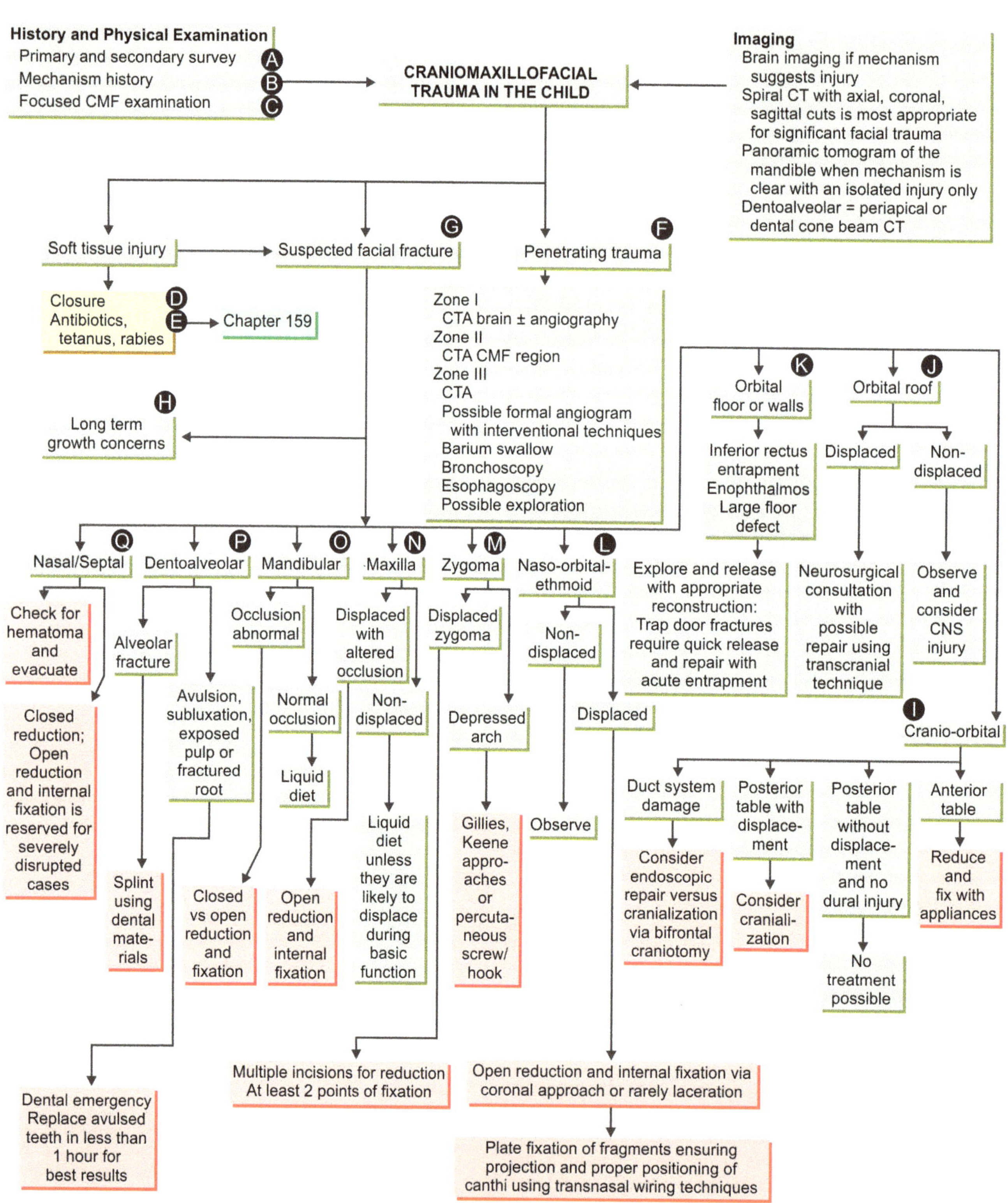

Facial trauma in children is rare, when compared with adults, and the patterns vary wildly with age. Falls and nonaccidental trauma are more common in early childhood, while sport, all-terrain vehicle, and automobile injuries tend to be more common in older children. The patterns of facial injuries are significantly different in early childhood and gradually approach the characteristics of adults by adolescence. Differences in anatomy including unerupted teeth, high cancellous-to-cortical bone ratio, limited pneumatization of the sinuses, and protected midfacial structures due to size dictate that mandible, orbital, nasal, dental, and cranial fractures occur much more commonly compared with midface and zygomatic fractures. Children also have improved healing capabilities when compared with adults and this often reduces the time required for healing. The management of these injuries is different from adults and requires an approach that respects growth. This chapter highlights some of those important differences that are important for the surgeon to consider when treating facial trauma in this population.

A A detailed history with mechanism and field information is helpful, particularly in young children who may have unwitnessed craniomaxillofacial (CMF) injuries. The epidemiologic differences in injury presentation based on age and environment are dramatic. A thorough examination coupled with imaging choices that are thoughtful are helpful. Many children with facial trauma have other injuries, usually involving the central nervous system, eye, dentition, and airway.

B Primary and secondary surveys are performed initially, but many CMF injuries are picked up on tertiary survey—including facial injuries. Airway management begins with positioning and a careful assessment of the potential for airway impingement. Intubation is preferable to tracheotomy, and most operative interventions can be done with an oral or nasal tube. Cervical spine injuries are rare when compared with those found in adults, but a careful evaluation is needed when the mechanism suggests an injury. Blood loss can be significant due to the increased vascularity in the head and neck, as well as the decreased blood volume in children.

C Often examination is difficult in young children due to cooperation issues, and imaging is relied upon for a detailed diagnosis. Increased adipose tissue of the face and the primary or mixed dentition occlusion can confound diagnosis in the younger child as well. Some soft tissue injuries can be associated with other critical structures such as the globe, lacrimal system, facial nerves, or salivary gland ducts. Many patients who present with of the condyle fractures can be difficult to diagnose on physical examination in this population.

D Local anesthetics (injected and/or topical) should be used with careful calculation of maximum dosing in small children. Primary closure can almost always be achieved due to the collateral blood supply, except in severe avulsion. The use of 5-0 or 6-0 rapidly absorbing sutures with or without tissue adhesives obviates the need for suture removal in small children. Tissue adhesives provide excellent results in small, clean wounds, or those that have been closed with deep sutures that approximate the skin very well. Scars in children can be unpredictable and should be observed for at least 12–18 months before considering revision.

E Broad-spectrum antibiotics (gram-positive, gram-negative, and anaerobic coverage) are often used prophylactically for contaminated wounds. The literature is conflicted regarding recommendations for antibiotics in typical clean-contaminated lacerations in and around the oral and nasal cavities. Consideration should be given for the use of tetanus and rabies treatment as appropriate.

F Computed tomography with angiography may be used in patients with penetrating injuries, but may volume average with smaller vessel injuries, yielding false negatives. Formal angiography with contrast may be indicated in some cases. Exploration may be indicated with some penetrating mechanisms and locations, and the approach is formalized based on the caliber or size of the penetrating element.

G While some fractures are best treated with no treatment, closed reduction or minimal intervention, the healing potential of children should not be license for inadequate reduction and fixation where needed to achieve a more symmetric and functional result. However, there is a biologic consequence and potential growth restriction associated with aggressive operative intervention in children—so a tempered approach is helpful. Restoring the functional and/or aesthetic aspects of the CMF anatomy is appropriate justification for this potential growth restriction. As such, long-term follow-up to evaluate long-term growth considerations is often necessary.

H Soft tissue elevation and periosteal stripping impair CMF bone growth. The use of conservative, minimally invasive repair techniques, when appropriate, is encouraged. Closed reduction is effective, particularly in young children. Resorbable plates or plate removal should be considered in the upper facial skeleton, but their use does not appear to alter the pattern of growth restriction. It is likely the surgery itself rather than fixation appliances has the effect of restricting growth, although there is significant controversy on this point.

I The frontal sinus does not develop in a standard pattern or time in children. It may act as a "crumple zone" and is often associated with disruption of the dura, anterior cranial fossa floor, orbital roof, and occasionally frontal lobe. Patients should be screened for concussion effects. Depressed fractures of the anterior table are reduced and repositioned with fixation via a coronal approach. Defects that are large may result in pulsatile exophthalmos, and primary reconstruction may be indicated. A team approach with a Neurosurgeon is helpful when anterior frontal craniotomy and/or cranialization of the frontal sinus is indicated. Disruption of the duct drainage system is often an indication for cranialization. I do not recommend obliterating the sinus, as an infection of the material used or the dead space left behind can occur.

This is often seen with synthetic materials. Follow-up CT scans may be helpful to identify the development of a mucocele in those patients who may be at risk for this late complication.

J and **K**
Orbital fractures of various types are common in children. The orbital floor can be reconstructed with absorbable collagen film or polymer when the defects are small. Porous polyethylene, nylon, metallic alloy floor implants, or bone grafts may be used larger defects. Orbital dimensions are different in children, and navigation can be helpful in understanding implant placement in larger floor and medial wall defects. Orbital roof fractures are often in association with cranial vault and/or fractures of the supraorbital rim.

L Naso-orbital ethmoid fractures produce substantial facial width disruption in the central third of the face. Restoration of intercanthal distance is important and can be estimated based on age-matched norms. Identifying the small fragment of bone that is typically attached to the medical canthus on one or both sides is one aspect of restoration. Placing the canthus in its appropriate posterior-superior position is another key. Transnasal wiring techniques with plating for contralateral support work best for predictable positioning.

M Fractures of the zygoma are rare in smaller children due to the high degree of force required to break this bone in childhood. The orbital floor is always involved when the zygoma is fractured. However, not all fractures of the floor of the orbit require repair. The need for orbital reconstruction should be assessed intraoperatively after the reduction of the zygoma, as the size of the defect and its effect on potential enophthalmos is not apparent until the zygoma is fully repositioned. Alternatively, the reconstruction can be staged using navigation for implant placement.

N Midface fractures are uncommon in children and present in unusual conformations. The distribution of forces is different in the growing child's facial skeleton, and this results in different fracture patterns than those seen in the adult skeleton. Consequently, LeFort midface fracture classification schemes are not particularly helpful in children. Closed reduction with maxillomandibular fixation (MMF) is not appropriate for most maxillary fractures, as this allows the mandible to distract the loose segments of the maxilla. Open reduction with internal fixation is usually indicated when the occlusion is affected significantly. It is important to avoid developing tooth structures when placing the fixation devices.

O Condyle fractures are very common in children and alter the occlusion significantly in some. Simple closed reduction for a limited time with range of motion physical therapy prevents fibrosis or ankyloses of the temporomandibular joint. Remodeling is common, despite the medial displacement of fragments due to the pterygoid muscle. However, facial asymmetry is often seen in teenagers and adults who have a history of mandibular trauma at a young age. Orthognathic surgery is often used to treat facial asymmetry. Older children typically experience fracture at the condylar neck, rather than at the condylar head itself. Some low condylar neck fractures may be treated with open reduction and internal fixation. However, closed reduction is often suitable. Maxillomandibular fixation is maintained for 10–14 days in young children. Skeletal fixation with circummandibular and piriform rim wires can be used in small children. Care is necessary to avoid the developing tooth buds when using skeletal fixation screws or arch bars using screw-based fixation. Maxillomandibular fixation techniques depend on the developmental stage of the dentition.

In other areas of the mandible, fixation appliances may be used to immobilize segments. When using fixation appliances in the small child, mandibular screws should be placed along the inferior border to avoid injury to developing teeth. Unerupted teeth within the fracture line should be maintained unless reduction is prevented. Typically, monocortical fixation is utilized in the more superior aspects of the mandible, while bicortical fixation is used whenever the neurovascular bundle and teeth can be avoided. Closed reduction techniques may be used for most fractures of any age. The techniques vary based upon the dentition present and may include:

- Primary dentition; skeletal wiring, or acrylic splints.
- Mixed dentition; ancillary methods often required, including occlusal splints and suspensory piriform and circummandibular wiring.
- Adult dentition/permanent dentition; standard arch bar or screw techniques.

Open reduction is indicated for (1) pulmonary insufficiency, seizure disorder or cognitive impairment increasing the risk of aspiration or airway compromise with MMF, (2) condyle displaced into middle cranial fossa, (3) inability to obtain occlusion using closed reduction.

P Avulsed permanent teeth should be immediately replaced or transported in isotonic solution, saline or milk to be reimplanted by a dental professional. Subluxated teeth usually require stabilization with a splinting wire or similar orthodontic device. Primary teeth are not reimplanted. Fractured teeth usually require attention from a Restorative Dentist.

Q Nasal and septal fractures are very common in children and often treated as an outpatient with closed reduction when seen as an isolated injury. "Open roof" deformities may occur more commonly in children due to the developing suture areas. Teenagers tend to have dorsal defects that may require secondary revision if adequate projection cannot be achieved primarily. Parents should be made aware of potential functional and aesthetic issues over the long term. Approximately 15% of nasal fractures may benefit from revision rhinoplasty. Secondary septorhinoplasty is typically delayed until after 5–7 years of age to allow for the majority of growth in the nasal complex to be complete. This minimizes growth restriction and optimizes the definitive result. If possible, consideration is given to waiting until the teen years unless significant psychosocial or functional issues exist.

SUGGESTED READING

American College of Surgeons. Advanced trauma life support courses. Chicago, IL: American College of Surgeons; 1997.

Amaratunga NAS. The relation of age to the immobilization period required for healing of mandibular fractures. J Oral Maxillofac Surg. 1987;45:111-113.

Costello BJ, Papadopoulos H, Ruiz R. Pediatric craniofacial trauma. Clin Pediatr Emergency Med. 2005;6:32-40.

Haug RH, Foss J. Maxillofacial injuries in the pediatric patient. Oral Surg Oral Med Oral Path Oral Radiol Endod. 2000;90:126-134.

Kaban LB, Mulliken JB, Murray JE. Facial fractures in children: an analysis of 122 fractures in 109 children. Plast Reconstr Surg. 1977;59:15-20.

Koltai PJ, Rabkin D. Management of facial trauma in children. Pediatr Clin North Am. 1996;43:1253-1275.

Posnick JC. Craniomaxillofacial fractures in children. Oral Maxillofac Clin North Am. 1994;1:169-185.

Posnick JC, Wells M, Pron GE. Pediatric facial fractures. Evolving patterns of treatment. J Oral Maxillofac Surg. 1993;51:836-844.

Scott D, Imahara MD, Hopper R, et al. Patterns and outcomes of pediatric facial fractures in the United States: a survey of the national trauma data bank. J Am. Coll Surg. 2008;207(5):710-716.

Zide MF. Open reduction of mandibular condylar fractures: indications and technique. Clin Plast Surg. 1989;16(1):69-76.

Reconstruction of Major Head and Neck Defects

Sebastian M Brooke, Mario G Solari

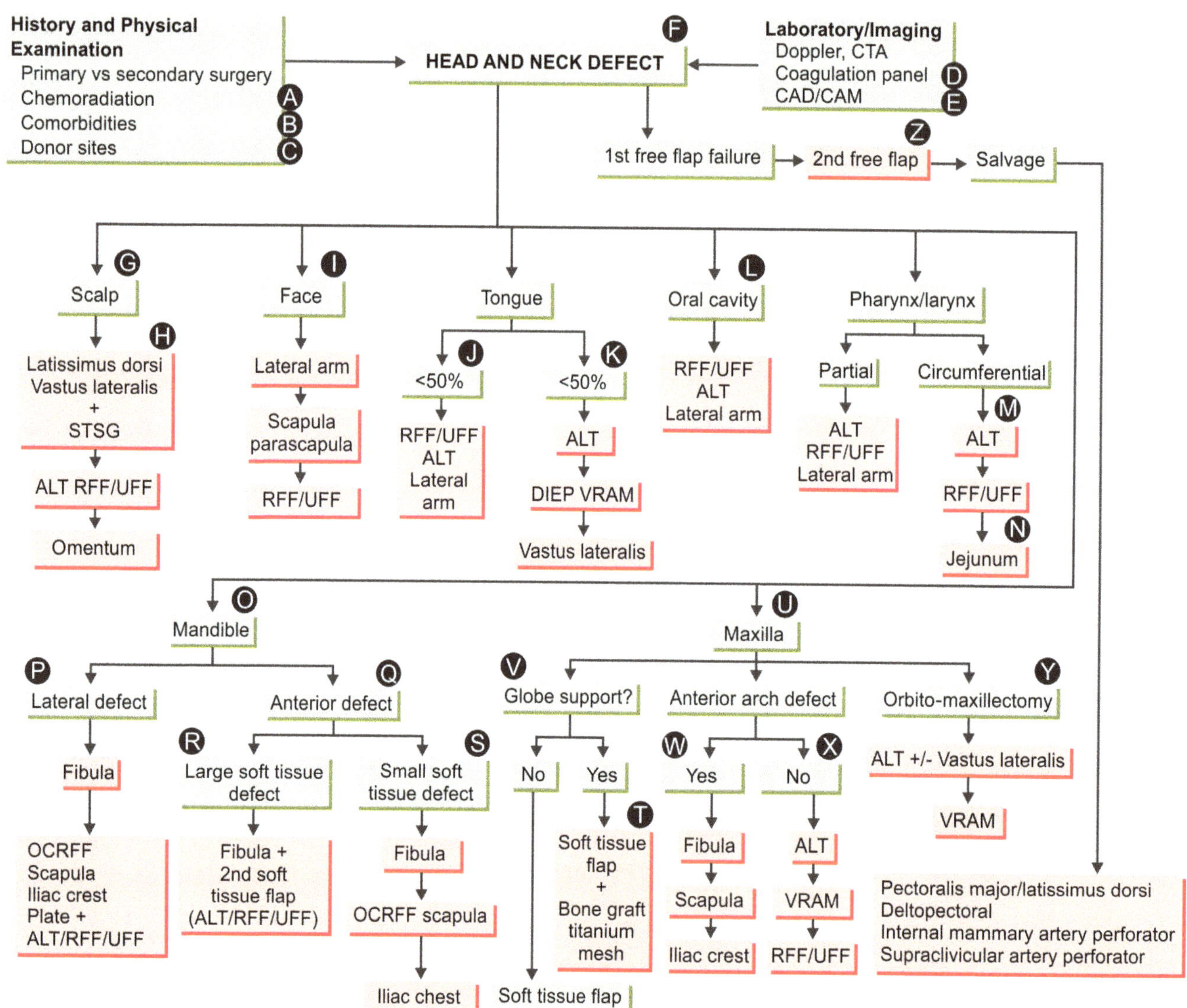

Acquired defects of the head and neck are anatomically multidimensional and may involve multiple tissue types. These defects are functionally morbid and complications such as salivary leak, infection, and fistula can have significant impact on the patient's quality of life. The global goals for reconstruction are to isolate the oropharyngeal cavity from the neck, maximize function, re-establish facial contour, and expedite adjuvant therapy. It is important to address patient expectations and have a close working relationship with the extirpating surgeon for operative planning. This chapter presumes that local tissue options are not reasonable given availability, patient factors, or defect size and complexity, and therefore focuses on free tissue transfer. The majority of defects can be addressed with the following commonly used flaps: anterolateral thigh (ALT), radial or ulnar forearm (RFF/UFF), and fibula or a combination thereof.

A Prior surgical resection, neck dissections, and radiation may all impact treatment choices and determine recipient vessel selection and the need for possible vein grafting.

B Given the length and complexity of these reconstructions, there must be careful consideration of the patients' ability to tolerate surgery in context with the diagnosis. Patients are frequently malnourished and may require prolonged nutritional support requiring a percutaneous endoscopic gastrostomy.

C Likely donor site evaluation must be made with emphasis on evidence of vascular disease such as lack of pulses, skin quality, or chronic wounds and edema, all of which may prompt further objective evaluation of the patient. Allen's test should be performed for forearm-based flaps. Patient-specific donor site characteristics, such as soft tissue thickness and ability to achieve reconstructive goals should ultimately determine flap choice.

D Family or personal history of venous thromboses, multiple spontaneous abortions, or clotting disorders should prompt an evaluation of a possible hypercoagulability state.

E Computer-aided preoperative planning based on three-dimensional computed tomography imaging for bone reconstruction allows for prefabricated guides that can direct mandible osteotomies, individualize reconstruction plates, and guide fibula osteotomies to produce a precise reconstruction with shorter operative time.

F Defining the components of the defect into exposed vital structures, bone support, lining or mucosa, overlying soft tissue or skin, and functional and aesthetic losses will help build a goal-oriented reconstructive plan.

G Goal is brain protection and to cover bone or implant. Large or radiated scalp defects require vascularized tissue typically anastomosed to the superficial temporal vessels. Structural support with synthetic products such as titanium mesh or autologous rib or split calvarium may be needed.

H Muscle only flaps or omentum with split-thickness skin grafts are excellent cover for very large areas as they are easier to design and have good contour as they atrophy.

I Unique to these defects is a consideration for skin with matched quality and color that is best achieved with the lateral arm flap, followed by scapula/parascapular system of flaps.

J Tongue mobility is the primary goal of anterior and smaller tongue defects up to 50% and the best fit is thin, pliable tissue such as the radial forearm.

K The primary goal for posterior or large defects is bulk, as speech and swallow outcomes are improved when the construct is convex. The ALT is the flap of choice. Given many options, muscle only flaps left to mucosalize are not preferred as they are more likely to result in a leak.

L Separating the oral cavity from the major vital structures of the neck while not impacting tongue or jaw mobility is best accomplished with thin pliable fasciocutaneous flaps.

M Fasciocutaneous flaps result in better speech outcomes and are preferred. Advantage of the ALT is a large but pliable flap with the potential for multiple skin paddles or addition of vastus lateralis muscle for more extensive resections. A wider fascial incision also allows for a second layer of closure. Simultaneous extirpation of the cancer and flap harvest is also easier.

N The free jejunum avoids a suture line in circumferential defects but has fallen out of favor due to the need for abdominal surgery, bowel anastomoses and their associated complications. Tolerance for ischemia is also shorter and mucus production may impair the quality of speech.

O Successful reconstruction of the mandible maintains occlusion, facial projection, and range of motion. The fibula remains the standard for mandible reconstruction.

P Soft tissue with or without a reconstruction plate is reasonable in patients who either are not free flap candidates due to comorbidities and poor prognosis, or who will have a difficult recovery after a fibula flap.

Q Bone is required for anterior defects to support the tongue, resuspend the larynx, maintain projection, prevent hardware exposure, and maximize swallowing.

R Consider a second soft tissue free flap such as the ALT or RFF when the soft tissue defect is large and involves significant portions of the tongue.

S The osteocutaneous fibula remains the first choice for the majority of mandible defects but the skin paddle is limited in its mobility or arc of rotation and is best suited for isolated floor of mouth defects or when small portions of the tongue are involved.

T Scapula provides abundant soft tissue but may be bulky and for harvest requires lateral or prone positioning of the patient.

U Midface defects vary widely in their extent and reconstruction may need to support the globe, fill a dead space, separate the oral and nasal cavity, or provide anterior structure and projection. Flaps may need to provide multiple skin paddles or tissue types and the need for bone dictates flap options. Prosthetics such as an obturator should be considered as part of a comprehensive treatment plan and may provide the most functional reconstruction for >50% of the soft palate and a simple option for palatal defects posterior to the canine.

V Support for the globe can be achieved with bone grafts or titanium mesh.

W Projection, support for mastication or prosthetics, and possible dental restoration demand bony reconstruction.

X The ALT is a diverse flap with a long pedicle. Addition of vastus lateralis muscle to the flap provides more bulk and avoids the donor site morbidity of abdominal based flaps.

Y If extensive defects require bone (hard palate resection beyond the ipsilateral canine) over an obturator, consider chimeric flaps with scapula as fibula may not provide sufficient soft tissue.

Z A second free flap is reasonable for salvage if the cause for initial failure is identifiable and can be managed otherwise consider the pectoralis, deltopectoral, latissimus dorsi, and supraclavicular artery flaps.

SUGGESTED READING

Engel H, Huang JJ, Lin CY, et al. A strategic approach for tongue reconstruction to achieve predictable and improved functional and aesthetic outcomes. Plast Reconst Surg. 2010;126:1967-1971.

Hanasano MM, Matros E, Disa JJ. Important aspects of head and neck reconstruction. Plast Reconst Surg. 2014;134:968e-980e.

Tarsitano A, Del Corso G, Ciocca L, et al. Mandibular reconstructions using computer-aided design/computer-aided manufacturing: a systematic review of a defect-based reconstructive algorithm. J Craniomaxillofac Surg. 2015;43:1785-1791.

Yu P, Lewin JS, Reece GP, et al. Comparison of clinical and functional outcomes and hospital costs following pharyngoesophageal reconstruction with the anterolateral thigh free flap versus the jejunal flap. Plast Reconst Surg. 2006;117:968-974.

Reconstruction of Cutaneous Defects of the Head and Neck

John A Zitelli, Gerardo Marrazzo

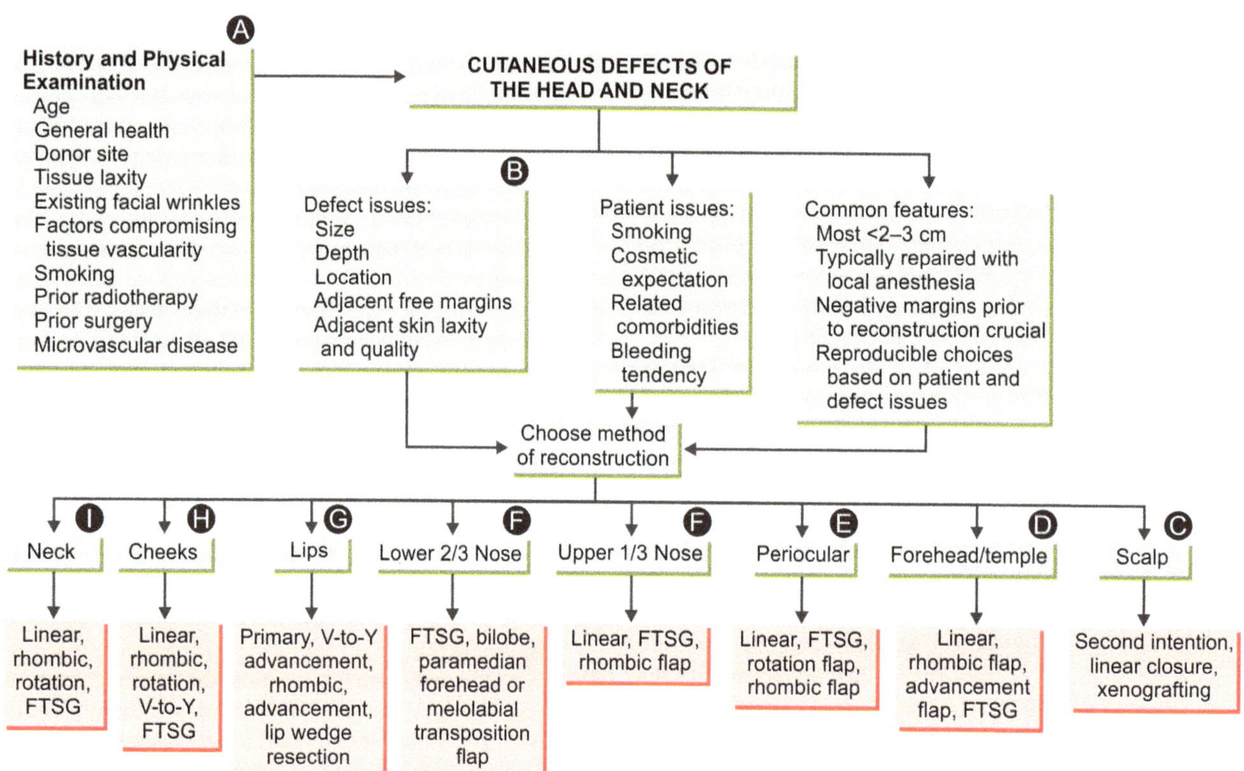

The subtle intricacies of the human face and neck pose a unique and intellectually stimulating challenge to the reconstructive surgeon. When selecting a particular reconstruction on the face, the patient's biologic and psychologic factors, defect characteristics, and defect anatomic location must all be considered. As most defects following excision of cutaneous malignancies measure no greater than 2–3 cm, our discussion will be directed toward wounds of this size.

A When selecting an approach to reconstruction, one must be aware of the patient's clinical and psychologic factors. Tobacco smoking, even if light by a patient's account, significantly hinders the survival of large cutaneous flaps. Importantly, several studies have shown that prescribed anticoagulants should not be discontinued for cutaneous surgery, as the risk of thromboembolic events far outweighs the increased risk of bleeding complications, which are minimal. Additionally, patient expectations must be carefully gauged. The cosmetic appearance of a full-thickness skin graft (FTSG) may be perfectly acceptable to one, and deplorable to another. The patient and his/her defect must be viewed as a whole.

B Once the patient's expectations and tolerances have been analyzed, attention should be turned to the defect itself. The size and depth of the operative wound must be appreciated. Shallow wounds are particularly receptive to healing by secondary intention (best reserved for facial concavities such as the alar crease, melolabial fold, medial canthus, and temple). The location of the defect, and its proximity to free margins such as the eyelid margin, ala, or vermilion lip also influences reconstructive choices. Maintaining normal shape and symmetry is the most important factor. Use of adjacent skin through local flaps is often the best choice because of ideal color and texture match, unless flaps create distortion. Grafts are usually a second choice and are used to prevent distortion, often at the cost of sacrificing color and texture match. Below is a discussion of ideal repairs based on anatomic locations.

C The mobility of the scalp is dependent on a multitude of factors, but is ultimately defined by the galea overlying the calvarium and is significantly variable. Wounds that are exclusively dermal may be left to heal by secondary intention, as the scalp hair bulbs lie within the superficial subcutis and will preserve hair growth. Linear closures are suitable for full-thickness small-to-mid-sized defects. The presence or absence of hair dictates whether a repair must be performed. In wounds that are too large to be closed primarily, second intention healing with or without the assistance of xenografting is often the best choice, particularly in nonhair-bearing scalp.

D Small wounds of the forehead should be closed primarily. Vertical closures better reapproximate static horizontal rhytides of the forehead. Horizontal linear closures, given their elliptical nature, may alter rhytides above and below their widest point. Therefore, more horizontally oriented wounds are closed well with rhombic flaps with horizontally oriented tension vectors and vertically closed donor sites. Defects immediately overlying the eyebrow are well suited for rhombic or bilobe transposition flaps, as well as Burow's advancement flaps (with the Burow's triangle displaced to the medial glabella or lateral canthus so as not to remove the eyebrow with a Burrow's triangle). Defects involving the eyebrow can be closed with an island pedicle (V-to-Y) advancement flap or bilateral advancement flap to preserve the continuity of the brow. Grafts on the forehead are rarely to be used except when necessary to prevent wound contraction and distortion. Second intention healing usually gives a better cosmetic result than a graft. The temple lends itself well to primary closure or rhombic transposition flaps, but can also be managed with second intention healing.

E Periocular lesions can be conceptually divided into medial canthal, eyelid, and eyelid margin defects. Wounds of the eyelid may be closed primarily, with dermal suturing oriented horizontally to avoid tension on the lower eyelid. Eyelid lesions may be repaired with FTSG. Full-thickness lower lid eyelid margin defects can be closed using a wedge resection, with delicate dermal sutures placed to meticulously reapproximate the tarsal plate, or with a Tenzel semicircular flap using a periosteal tacking suture at the lateral canthus to suspend the weight of the flap. Small medial canthal defects can be left to heal by secondary intention or grafted. Flap repair of the medial canthus lends itself to a fullness and protrusion, and should only be considered when bone is exposed (precluding use of FTSG). Primary closure often leads to epicanthal webs and is limited to tiny defects in the medial canthus.

F When reconstructing the nose, tremendous attention to the qualities of the skin and the individual cosmetic units of the nose is required when considering different repair options. The skin of the upper two thirds of the nose is thin and mobile relative to the thick, sebaceous lower third. This transition is highly variable among patients and must be closely studied prior to the design of a repair. Midline defects of the nose are well suited to vertically oriented primary linear closure, with care to extend the Burow's triangles the entire length of the nasal dorsum and nasal tip to avoid a prominent nasal hump at the junction of the nasal bone and upper lateral alar cartilage. Nasal sidewall defects are amenable to rhombic flaps. Repairs of the distal nose must be selected depending on the size and depth of the defect. Shallow defects are amenable to FTSG, with harvest from the conchal bowl providing good color and texture match. Deeper defects roughly ≤1.5 cm are amenable to Zitelli's modification of the bilobe flap, the most commonly used flap of the distal nose. The paramedian forehead flap is often the best selection for larger defects. Defects of the nasal ala are managed well with conchal bowl FTSG. Bilobe flaps, alar rotation flaps,

melolabial interpolation flaps, and paramedian forehead flaps may be used to repair more extensive wounds of the nasal ala, and can be buttressed with a cartilage graft should the inspiratory integrity of the ala be compromised.

G Repair of the lip is highly dependent on the size and location of the wound. Defects of the upper lateral cutaneous lip do especially well with island pedicle (V-to-Y) advancement flaps. This repair, by design, avoids the trap-dooring and hematomas that normally plague repairs in this region. Small wounds can be repaired primarily in a vertical manner with the Burrows triangle extending through the vermilion border and around the lip to the labial mucosa if need be to avoid "bulldozing" or pushing the vermilion border. Larger wounds of the upper cutaneous lip can be closed with advancement or rarely rhombic transposition flaps from the medial cheek, although these repairs obliterate the melolabial fold. Larger wounds up to one third the length of the vermilion lip can be repaired with wedge resections. Healing by secondary intention of small and superficial wounds may give nice results, but large or deep wounds in this area can place the patient at risk of eclabium and should be avoided.

H The cheek is a large and relatively forgiving region for facial reconstruction, given the laxity and tissue reserve most aging faces supply. Even sizable wounds of the cheek can often be closed primarily, with care to orient these closures in a curvilinear manner within relaxed skin tension lines. In the infraorbital region, care should be taken to close the wound with horizontal dermal sutures so as to minimize the risk of ectropion. Rotation flaps can be used in the medial infraorbital region to displace standing cones laterally, but require significant undermining and lead to lengthy scars. Larger wounds of the central cheek lend themselves to closure with rhombic transposition flaps, taking advantage of laxity afforded by the jowls and lateral cheek. Larger defects of the cheek can be repaired by creating sizable Island pedicle (V-to-Y) advancement, bilobe or rotation flaps that extend down into the superior neck. Supraclavicular FTSG can be used to close massive defects of the cheek, but is variable in the final cosmetic outcome.

I The neck can be repaired using the same algorithm applied to the facial defects. Secondary intention healing can be used, but reliably leads to nummular, hypopigmented scar. Linear closures can be used for even sizable neck defects, and flaps need rarely be considered.

SUGGESTED READING

Baker SR. Local Flaps in Facial Reconstruction. Philadelphia, PA: Elsevier; 2014.

Burget GC, Menick FJ. Aesthetic Reconstruction of the Nose. St Louis: Mosby; 1994.

Zitelli JA. Wound healing by secondary intention. J Am Acad Dermatol. 1983;9(3):407-415.

Zitelli JA. The bilobed flap for nasal reconstruction. Arch Dermatol. 1989;125(7):957-959.

Zitelli JA. The nasolabial flap as a single-stage procedure. Arch Dermatol. 1990;126(11):1445-1448.

CHAPTER 166

Maxillofacial Prosthetic Rehabilitation

Matilda Dhima

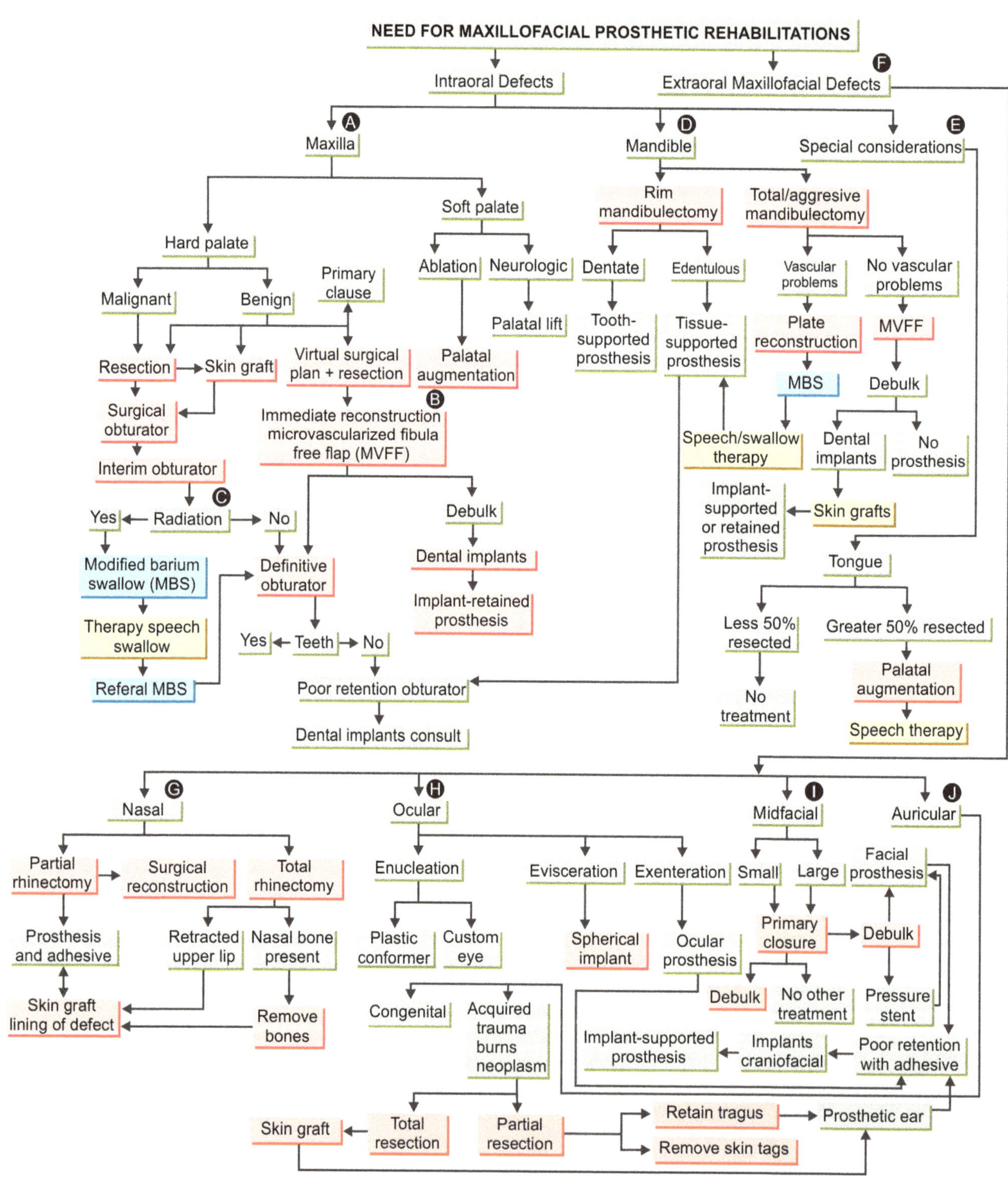

Maxillofacial prosthetic rehabilitation of patients with congenital and acquired defects in the head and neck focuses on improvement of quality of life and management of defects often beginning at the time of surgery or ablation. A thorough examination of the presenting lesion, dentition, and consultation with the patient's surgeon about the nature of the defect, size, location, cause, future planning, and need for immediate dental intervention are important. Preoperative radiographs and photographs, moulages, and in select cases virtual planning are necessary before the main treatment course. Maxillofacial defects can be extraoral or intraoral. In selected patients with extensive defects, a combination of extra- and intraoral defects is present. The quality of life of these patients' can be significantly improved with current advancements in virtual planning, microvascularized fibula free flap reconstruction (MFFR) and dental/craniofacial implant therapy.

For patients who have neoplasms in the head and neck area radiation and chemotherapy sometimes adjuvant to resection or as a primary treatment have helped prolong the patients life. Unfortunately, these treatments may be associated with delayed negative effects on swallow and speech. A multidisciplinary approach with aggressive therapy is key for successful management in this patient population.

A Acquired defects of the soft and hard palate are best treated with an obturator or speech aid regardless of the presence or absence of teeth. In cases of cleft palate, an orthopedic appliance is used to orient the palatal shelves and premaxilla before surgical closure.

B With current advancements in implant therapy and virtual presurgical planning, MFFR for defects in the maxilla and mandible can significantly improve the patient's quality of life. For maxillary defects resulting from resection of benign lesions, concurrent MFFR reconstruction is possible. Even in cases of malignancy where margins are extended beyond those preplanned virtually, the surgical guides can still be used to optimize MFFR. Placement of dental implant has been shown to be more predictable when completed at a second stage. Revision surgery with debulking and often a skin graft is almost always necessary to allow for stable peri-implant tissues when prosthetic reconstruction is complete.

C Adjuvant chemo/radiation therapy requires a careful examination of the dentition and counseling for long/short-term effects of these therapies to head and neck areas. Removal of unsalvageable teeth and daily lifelong fluoride treatment are crucial to the patient's rehabilitation. Speech, swallow, and physical therapy play a major role in minimizing long-term dependency on a PEG tube. It also optimizes the patient's experience with maxillofacial prosthetic rehabilitation.

D Mandibular defects are best treated surgically with the use of a vascularized bone graft to restore the continuity of the mandible and to provide prosthesis-bearing tissue. Use of the bone graft alone, however, will seldom provide an optimum base for a removable prosthesis. Placement of endosseous implants will help anchor a removable prosthesis, minimize bone resorption, and add to the patient's comfort.

E In total glossectomy, a mandibular tongue prosthesis is the treatment of choice. However, if the patient is edentulous or the glossectomy is associated with an unrepaired mandibulectomy, a palatal drop prosthesis is recommended. In partial glossectomy, if <50% of the tongue is removed, no treatment is necessary. When >50% is removed, a lingual or palatal augmentation prosthesis, or a combination, is indicated. Glossectomy patients should be monitored by a Speech Language Pathologist and Nutritionist when necessary.

F Extraoral maxillofacial defects can be congenital (Treacher Collins, Goldenhar, Ectodermal Dysplasia, and cleft lip/palate) or acquired due to trauma or surgical ablation of neoplasms. This includes the nose, orbital region, auricular, midface, and often a combination of such structures.

G Some acquired extraoral defects are small, involve mobile structures such as the nose, eyelid, ear, or lip, or may be present in the cranial vault. In these cases, especially if the margins of the defect are clear of cancer, surgical reconstruction is the treatment of choice.

H Depending on the extent of orbital resection, successful prosthetic reconstruction can be achieved by close collaboration between the surgeon and the maxillofacial prosthodontist.

I The defects affecting the midface are challenging especially when involving the nose and cheek(s). When poor retention or excessive sweating makes it difficult to retain the prosthesis with medical grade adhesive, craniofacial implants have a high success rate and increase retention.

J An immobile bed achieved by skin grafting is key to successful prosthetic replacement of auricular prosthesis. Craniofacial implants with a supporting bar, magnets, and/or clip design are an excellent option to improve retention of prosthesis. A surgical guide designed by the maxillofacial prosthodontist can help the surgeon with proper craniofacial implant placement.

SUGGESTED READING

Akman S, Kalayci A, Ataoğlu H, et al. Complex midfacial reconstruction with an implant-supported framework. J Craniofac Surg. 2011;22(2):724-726.

Claudy MP, Miguens SA Jr, Celeste RK, et al. Time interval after radiotherapy and dental implant failure: systematic review of observational studies and meta-analysis. Clin Implant Dent Relat Res. 2015;17(2):402-411.

Dhima M, Rieck KL, Arce K, et al. Development of stable peri-implant soft tissue and mentolabial sulcus depth with an implant-retained soft tissue conformer after osteocutaneous flap reconstruction. Int J Prosthodont. 2013;26(3):265-267.

Dings JP, Maal TJ, Muradin MS, et al. Extra-oral implants: insertion per- or post-ablation? Oral Oncol. 2011;47(11):1074-1078.

Goyal MK, Goyal S, Dhanasekar B. Modern trends in modeling of extra-oral defects. Indian J Dent Res. 2014;25(1):128-132.

Logemann JA, Kahrilas PJ, Hurst P, et al. Effects of intraoral prosthetics on swallowing in patients with oral cancer. Dysphagia. 1989;4(2):118-120.

Parel SM, Branemark PI, Jansson T. Osseointegration in maxillofacial prosthetics. Part I: Intraoral applications. J Prosthet Dent. 1986;55(4):490-494.

Pauloski BR, Rademaker AW, Logemann JA, et al. Speech and swallowing in irradiated and nonirradiated postsurgical oral cancer patients. Otolaryngol Head Neck Surg. 1998;118(5):616-624.

Zen Filho EV, Tolentino ES, Santos PS. Viability of dental implants in head and neck irradiated patients: a systematic review. Head Neck. 2016;38(Suppl 1):E2229-E2240.

Scar Revision

Vu T Nguyen

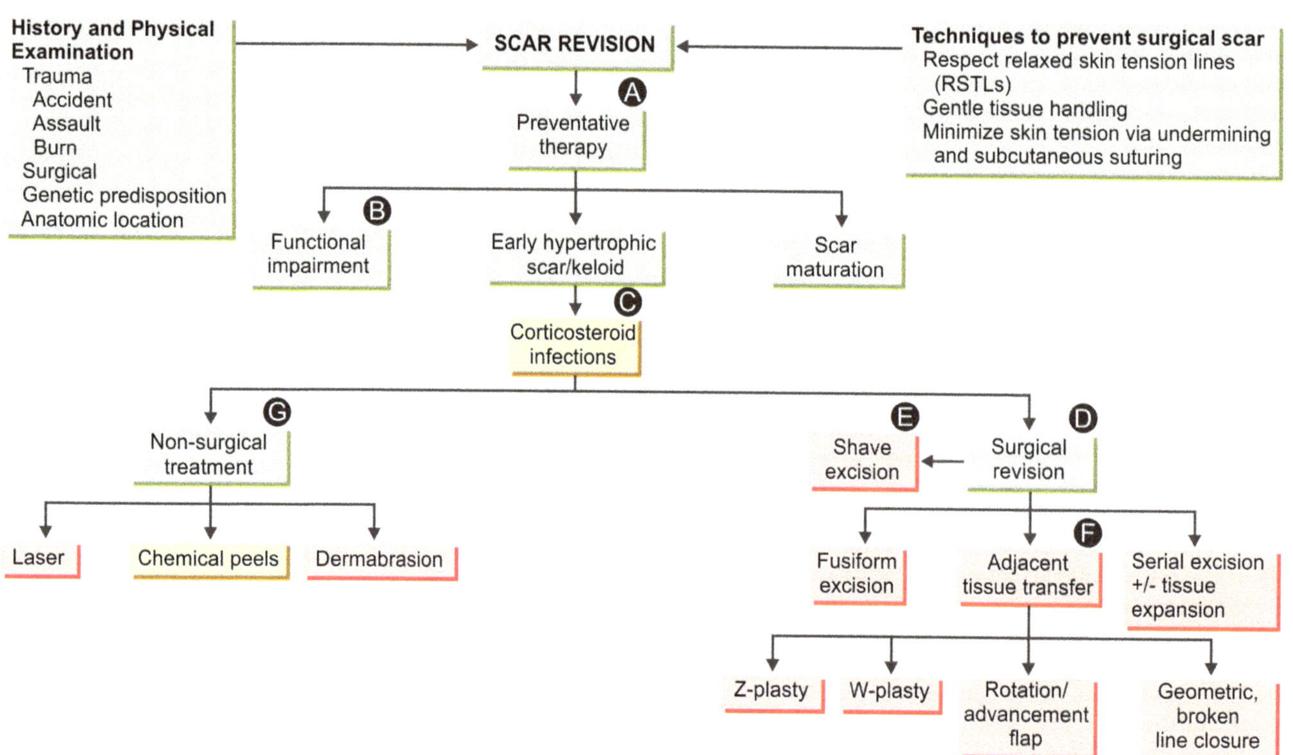

Important aspects regarding scar revision include the origin of the injury (e.g. traumatic versus surgical), a patient's predisposition for pathological scar formation, and the scar's anatomicl location and relationship to surrounding critical structures, including relaxed skin tension lines (RSTLs). Managing patient expectations is also key, recognizing that revision entails an exchange to a more acceptable scar.

Ⓐ Preventative therapy for all scars entails tension relief at the skin margins, hydration/occlusion via silicone therapy, and compression treatment. Additional factors may include avoiding sun exposure and optimizing nutritional status. Silicone therapy in particular has proven efficacy and should be worn a minimum of 12 hours daily, for a period of 3 months.

Ⓑ Functional impairment (e.g. oral/ocular involvement) warrants early intervention at 2–3 months or earlier. Scar maturation, through a process of inflammation, granulation, and remodeling, typically requires a minimum of 9-12 months. Scars however should be evaluated early (4–8 weeks) to assess whether preventative therapy should be discontinued, continued, or intensified.

Ⓒ Early development of hypertrophic scars or keloids may warrant initiation of corticosteroid injection therapy, most commonly in the form of intralesional injection of triamcinolone acetonide 10–40 mg/mL into the papillary dermis every 3–6 weeks, with proven benefit in the majority of patients. Recurrence tends to be high and treatment can be complicated by excessive pain during injection, hypopigmentation, tissue atrophy, and telangiectasias.

Ⓓ Surgical scar revision via fusiform excision may be entertained when scar maturation is complete, other modalities have failed, or when functional impairment exists. Serial excision may also be planned with 3-4 months between procedures. Principles of surgical revision include alignment parallel to RSTLs, gentle techniques for tissue handling, and minimizing skin tension via judicious undermining and/or subcutaneous suturing. When these modalities do not suffice, consideration should be given for methods of adjacent tissue transfer; including Z-plasty, W-plasty, rotation/advancement flap, geometric broken line closure, or serial excision with or without tissue expansion. Regardless of technique, surgical intervention should again be coupled with preventative therapy.

Ⓔ Narrow scars elevated above skin height and scars with irregular levels or sebaceous hypertrophy can be shaved flush to the skin level with a fine scalpel or razor.

F Z-plasty, W-plasty, and geometric broken line closure all reduce the visibility of the scar by converting a noticeable straight-line scar to a less conspicuous camouflaged, irregular scar by creating a series of interposed advancement flaps. Careful planning must be undertaken regarding length, width, and angles when creating these patterns. Similarly, rotation advancement flaps must take into account adjacent areas of soft tissue excess, final location of various scars, and employ techniques of gentle tissue handling and generous soft tissue undermining.

G Less proven therapies for scar revision include nonsurgical treatments, including laser therapy, chemical peels, and dermabrasion, with variable outcomes depending on individual technique and expertise.

SUGGESTED READING

Alster TS, West TB. Treatment of scars: a review. Ann Plast Surg. 1997;39:418-432.

Borges AF. Scar revision. In: Paparella MM, Shumrick DA, Gluckman JL, Meyerhoff WL (Eds). Otolaryngology, 3rd edition, vol 4. Philadelphia, PA: WB Saunders; 1991. p. 2829.

Davidson TM, Webster RC. Scar revision self-instructional package. Am Acad Otolaryngol. 1977.

Gold MH, McGuire M, Mustoe TA, et al. International Advisory Panel on Scar Management. Updated international clinical recommendations on scar management: part 2—algorithms for scar prevention and treatment. Dermatol Surg. 2014;40(8):825-831.

Monstrey S, Middelkoop E, Vranckx JJ, et al. Updated scar management practical guidelines: non-invasive and invasive measures. J Plast Reconstr Aesthet Surg. 2014;67(8):1017-1025.

Rossiter JL. Dermabrasion. Clinical uses in otolaryngology. J Otolaryngol. 1994;23:347-353.

Sykes JM, Byworth PJ. Sutures, needles and techniques for wound closure. In: Baker SR, Swanson NA (Eds). Local Flaps in Facial Reconstruction. St Louis, MO: CV Mosby; 1995. p. 39.

Thomas JR, Frost TW. Scar revision and camouflage. In: Baker SR, Swanson NA (Eds). Local Flaps in Facial Reconstruction. St Louis, MO: CV Mosby; 1995. p. 587.

Urioste SS, Arndt KA, Dover JS. Keloids and hypertrophic scars: Review and treatment strategies. Semin Cutan Med Surg. 1999;18:159-171.

Aging Face and Neck

Grant S Gillman

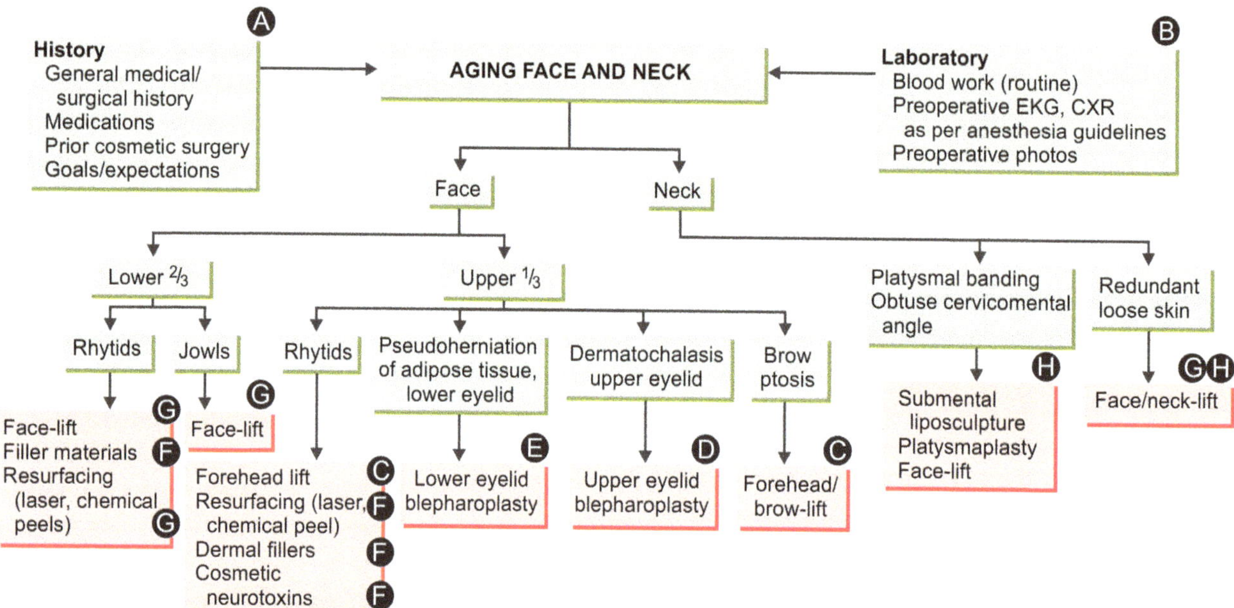

Interest in facial cosmetic procedures continues to grow—with respect to both surgical rejuvenation and nonsurgical treatments (e.g. dermal fillers, superficial peels, and neurotoxin injections). Despite the fact that these procedures are all considered "elective" in nature, the patient's concerns must be evaluated in a systematic and thoughtful way to provide the best and the safest recommendations for ongoing care. Such an approach will generally maximize patient's satisfaction while minimizing complications or the stigmata of "overdone" plastic surgery.

A Management of the patient interested in rejuvenation of the aging face begins with a discussion to define the patient's goals and establish expectations. Unrealistic expectations constitute a relative contraindication to surgery. Other contraindications include patients who are medically or psychologically unstable, heavy smokers, individuals prone to keloid formation, an uncorrectable coagulopathy or serious medical comorbidities (e.g. unstable coronary artery disease, chronic obstructive pulmonary disease, renal failure, and poorly controlled diabetes). Anticoagulant medications must be stopped 1–2 weeks before surgery.

B Required preoperative blood work or testing depends on the patient's age, medical history, and medications. Preoperative photodocumentation is essential.

C There are multiple surgical approaches to a brow lift or forehead lift (direct, mid-forehead, trichophytic, coronal, and endoscopic). Considerations include control of brow position, scar visibility, and hairline position. In general, the closer the incision is to the brow, the greater the control of brow position but with increased risk of visible scarring. Approaches from above the hairline conceal incisional scars but raise the frontal hairline, which is unacceptable to the patient with a high hairline. Individual surgeon's preference will vary.

D An upper eyelid blepharoplasty consists of excision of redundant skin with or without removal of preaponeurotic adipose tissue. If performed simultaneously with a forehead lift, the latter must be done first to minimize the risk of over-resection of eyelid skin and secondary lagophthalmos.

E If skin excision is not required, a transconjunctival blepharoplasty (TCB) approach is preferred. To address a vertical skin excess, a subciliary approach with elevation of a skin–muscle flap or a TCB with skin-pinch excision technique is preferred. In patients with poor lower lid tone preoperatively, a canthopexy, canthoplasty, or lateral orbital rim suspension suture should be done concomitantly to reduce the risk of postoperative ectropion.

F Resurfacing techniques (laser or peels) have a higher risk of complications and should be performed only by those experienced in patient selection and the nuances of each method. Minimally invasive injectable dermal fillers and neurotoxins (botulinum toxin) are very effective and popular owing to their higher safety profiles and negligible downtime. Fillers are used for the camouflage of static wrinkles and cosmetic neurotoxins (e.g. botulinum toxin) are preferred for the treatment of dynamic hyperkinetic lines.

G Many facelift procedures have been described. Preferred techniques all include a subcutaneous flap elevation coupled with suspension (plication or imbrication) of the superficial musculoaponeurotic system. In general, the more extended or deeper the dissection, the greater the risk to the distal branches of the facial nerve. More extensive dissection may better correct difficult areas such as a heavy melolabial fold however. A facelift is often combined with a resurfacing procedure or the use of filler materials to optimize the facial rejuvenation.

H A neck lift will restore a more youthful cervicomental angle and is enhanced by an anterior platysmaplasty (for banding) or submental liposuction for removal of excess adipose tissue when indicated.

SUGGESTED READING

Baker D. Lateral SMASectomy, plication and short scar facelifts: indications and techniques. Clin Plast Surg. 2008;35(4):533-550.

Baker TJ, Gordon HL, Stuzin JM. Surgical Rejuvenation of the Face. St. Louis, MO: CV Mosby; 1996.

Baker TJ, Stuzin JM, Baker TM. Facial Skin Resurfacing. St. Louis, MO: Quality Medical; 1998.

Fagien S. Putterman's Cosmetic Oculoplastic Surgery. Philadelphia, PA: Saunders; 2007.

Hamra ST. The deep-plane rhytidectomy. Plast Reconstr Surg. 1990;86:53-61.

Kontis TC, Lacombe VG. Cosmetic Injection Techniques: A Text and Video Guide to Neurotoxins and Fillers. New York: Thieme; 2013.

Williams EF, Lam SM. Comprehensive Facial Rejuvenation: A Practical and Systematic Guide to Surgical Management of the Aging Face. Philadelphia, PA: Lippincott Williams & Wilkins; 2003.

Cancer of the Skin of the Head and Neck

John A Zitelli, Gerardo Marrazzo

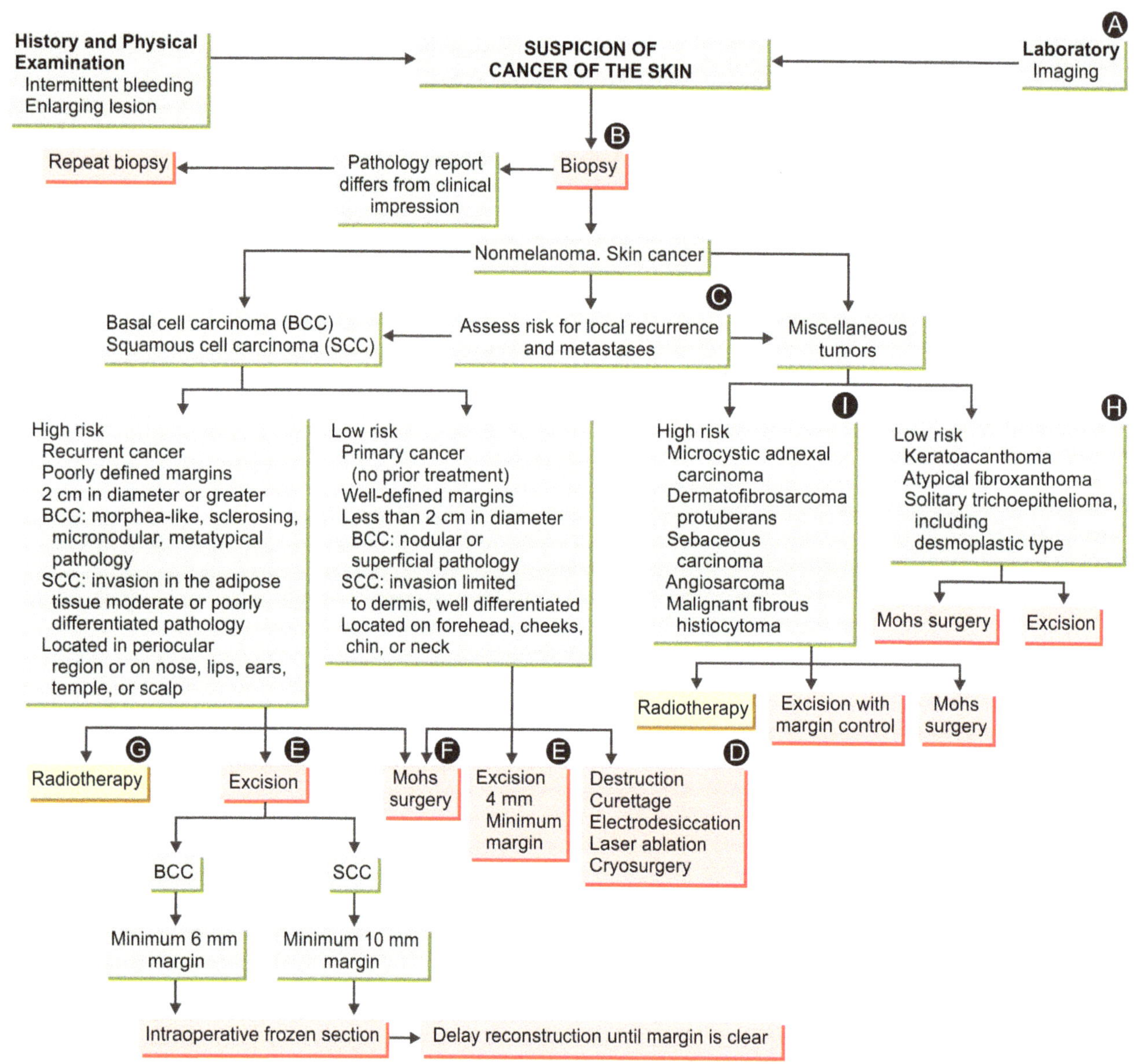

Cutaneous squamous cell carcinoma (SCC) and basal cell carcinoma (BCC), collectively referred to as nonmelanoma skin cancer (NMSC), represent the most common malignancy observed among Caucasians. Estimates of NMSC in 2012 calculated ~5.4 million skin cancers were diagnosed that year. With the burden of disease reaching epidemic levels, it is critical for the surgeon to have a firm grasp of the diagnosis and treatment of NMSC and other less common cutaneous malignancies.

A The most common clinical presentation of skin cancer is a lesion on the skin that bleeds intermittently. Patients often describe cyclical bleeding with perceived healing, or bleeding with minimal trauma. Other presentations include new and enlarging lesions or inexplicable scar-like changes. Squamous cell carcinoma, unlike BCC, may be painful. Other nonmelanoma skin cancers may simulate BCC and are usually diagnosed after biopsy. Patients with a single skin cancer have a 40% risk of a second primary skin cancer within 5 years. Often multiple cancers are diagnosed simultaneously; therefore, a complete cutaneous examination is necessary. The examination should include palpation of draining lymph nodes when high-risk SCCs or other cancers with a high risk for metastases are suspected such as melanoma, Merkel cell carcinoma, or angiosarcoma.

B A biopsy of the skin should include a deep portion of the tumor to provide adequate histologic information to estimate tumor risk. A deep shave or saucerization is preferred. A punch biopsy is adequate; however, if the subcutaneous adipose tissue is entered, curettage cannot be used to treat the tumor following biopsy. The biopsy should not interfere with the ability to determine tumor margins at the time of treatment. For example, some superficial shave biopsies heal quickly without residual markings that allow one to estimate accurate margins. Inflamed scars, suture reactions, and complicated closures of a biopsy may result in overestimation of tumor margins. Therefore, consider the effect of the biopsy procedure on the surgeon's ability to determine clinical margins after the biopsy.

C Once the diagnosis of nonmelanoma skin cancer is made, the options for treatment depend on the risk for local recurrence and metastases. Assessment of these risks depends on the clinical features, type of tumor, and pathology subtypes as well as size, depth, and location. Once these risks are determined, the correct options can be more easily chosen. The goal of surgery for any skin cancer is complete removal with negative histologic margins.

D Destructive techniques include curettage and electro-desiccation, laser ablation, and cryosurgery with liquid nitrogen. All these techniques have a 90–95% cure rate for carefully selected, low-risk tumors but often result in hypopigmented or hypertrophic scars and provide no tissue to assess margins for complete removal. Destructive techniques are not effective for recurrent or high-risk cancers because of much higher recurrence rates.

E Excision begins with a predetermined margin of normal skin surrounding the clinical margins of the tumor that varies depending on tumor type, size, and location. It is important to know that margin assessment for adequacy of excision by traditional bread-loafing of the specimen samples only 0.01% of margin histologically. Reconstruction after excision may minimize scarring. Cure rates range from 90% to 95% for low- to moderate-risk tumors. The cost of excision is greater than that of destruction. The cost of in-office excision is comparable to that for Mohs surgery, but the cost for excision in the hospital or ambulatory surgery section or with frozen-section control exceeds that of in-office surgery.

F Mohs micrographic surgery (MMS) provides extremely high cure rates even for high-risk, recurrent and difficult tumors because it examines 100% of the surgical margin. The more complete margin examination obviates the need for wide surgical margins. The tissue sparing quality of Mohs allows for cosmetically sensitive reconstruction with less morbidity to the patient. The cost of Mohs surgery is greater than that of destruction and similar to that of office-based excision. When available, it is the treatment of choice for most moderate-risk and nearly all high-risk skin cancers.

G Radiation therapy is the most expensive treatment and offers cure rates that are often inferior to that of surgery. Therefore, indications for radiation therapy are usually limited to nonsurgical candidates and infirm patients of advanced age.

H These miscellaneous nonmelanoma skin cancers are at low risk for metastasis or recurrence when completely excised. Keratoacanthomas and atypical fibroxanthomas should be treated with technique similar to well-differentiated SCCs. Solitary trichoepithelioma and desmoplastic trichoepithelioma should be treated by techniques similar to those used to treat low-risk BCC.

I These skin cancers are at high risk for recurrence or metastases. Microcystic adnexal carcinoma should be managed by techniques similar to those for high-risk BCC. Dermatofibrosarcoma protuberans often recurs locally after surgical excision and should be excised by Mohs surgery or with margins of at least 2.5 cm down to and including fascia. Sebaceous carcinoma should be managed similar to a high-risk SCC. Malignant fibrous histiocytoma, Merkel cell carcinoma, and angiosarcoma frequently metastasize and should be either treated with MMS or excised widely; the patient should be monitored closely for local and regional recurrence. Radiation treatment to local and regional areas has been suggested but has not been proved to be of benefit if the cancer is completely excised. Sentinel lymph node biopsy has never been shown to improve survival in any skin cancer.

Reconstruction of the defect with a high-risk cancer should be delayed until permanent pathology sections confirm clear margins.

SUGGESTED READING

Brodland DG, Zitelli JA. Surgical margins for excision of primary cutaneous squamous cell carcinoma. J Am Acad Dermatol. 1992;27:241-248.

Miller SJ. NCCN practice guidelines of care for nonmelanoma skin cancers. Dermatol Surg. 2000;26(3):289-292.

Parker TL, Zitelli JA. Surgical margins for excision of dermatofibrosarcoma protuberans. J Am Acad Dermatol. 1995;32:233-236.

Rogers HW, Weinstock MA, Feldman SR, et al. Incidence Estimate of Nonmelanoma Skin Cancer (Keratinocyte Carcinomas) in the US Population, 2012. JAMA Dermatol. 2015;151(10):1081-1086.

Sladden M, Zagarella S, Popescu C, et al. No survival benefit for patients with melanoma undergoing sentinel lymph node biopsy: critical appraisal of the Multicenter Selective Lymphadenectomy Trial-I Final Report. Br J Dermatol. 2015;172(3):566-571.

Wolf DJ, Zitelli JA. Surgical margins for basal cell carcinoma. Arch Dermatol. 1987;123:340-344.

Malignant Melanoma

Jamie Ahn Ku, Jeffrey N Myers

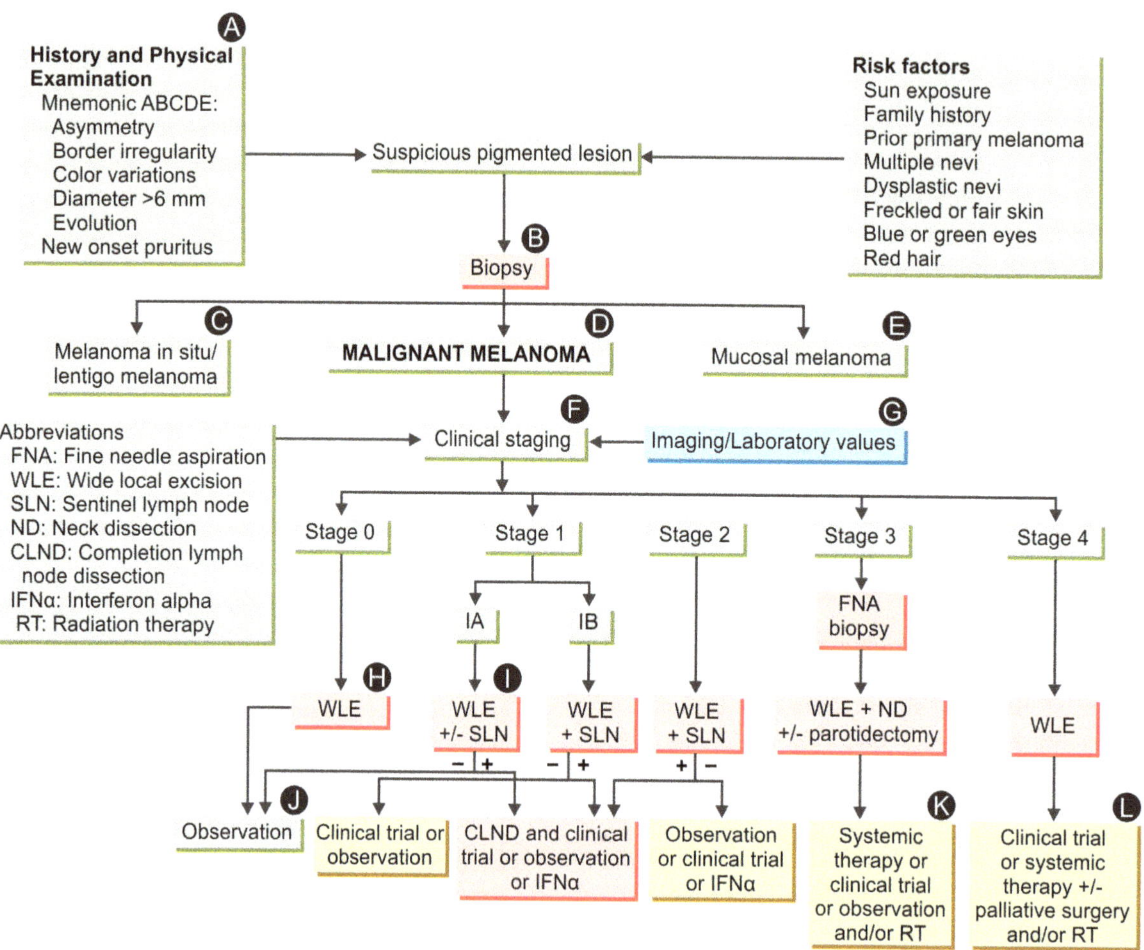

Melanoma comprises only about 5% of all cutaneous malignancies but is responsible for over 75% of skin-cancer-related deaths. Thorough clinical, pathologic, and radiologic evaluation is critical in accurate staging of the disease, and a multidisciplinary approach to treatment is key to improved patient outcome.

A A complete history and physical examination are critical in assessing patients with suspicious pigmented lesions. As most melanomas arise in pre-existing moles, any signs of asymmetry, border irregularity, color variations, diameter of >6 mm, and evolution, or the classic mnemonic "ABCDE," should prompt a biopsy. New onset pruritus is also a notable early clinical symptom. Risk factors for melanoma include sun exposure, family history of melanoma, prior primary melanoma, multiple nevi, dysplastic nevi, freckled or fair skin, blue or green eyes, and red hair.

B Biopsy of a suspicious pigmented lesion may be performed as either an excisional or an incisional biopsy, depending on the location and the size of the lesion. Excisional biopsy is performed with a narrow, 1–3-mm margin of normal-appearing tissue and should include subcutaneous adipose tissue for complete evaluation of depth. Wider margins should be avoided to allow for accurate subsequent lymphatic mapping. If the size or the anatomical location of the lesion precludes excision, incisional or punch biopsies are reasonable alternatives. Fine-needle aspiration, curettage, and shave techniques should not be performed since they do not permit assessment of the depth of invasion if the lesion is invasive melanoma. Excisional biopsy with negative margins is not considered adequate therapy for invasive melanoma. Minimal elements of pathologic evaluation should include Breslow thickness (mm), histologic ulceration, dermal invasion, mitotic rate per mm^2, Clark level, and peripheral and deep margin status.

C Lentigo melanoma (LM) is the most common type of melanoma in situ, and about 5% of LM progress to lentigo maligna melanoma (LMM). Lentigo melanoma lesions are excised with 0.5–1.0-cm margins, although prediction of tumor margins can prove difficult because the lesions are typically ill defined, have subclinical extensive radial growth, may be quite large, and/or located in cosmetically sensitive areas.

D Cutaneous melanomas are categorized into one of the following subtypes: superficial spreading melanoma, nodular melanoma, LMM, acral lentiginous melanoma (ALM), and desmoplastic melanoma. Superficial spreading melanoma is the most common subtype while ALM is more frequently seen in African–American and Hispanic patients. Nodular melanoma is characterized by early vertical growth and is often highly aggressive. Lentigo maligna melanoma typically presents in the head and neck region in the elderly population. Desmoplastic melanoma is rare, accounting for <1% of reported melanoma cases. Up to 75% of cases occur in the head and neck. Desmoplastic melanoma demonstrates tropism for perineural and endoneural tissues, which may account for increased rates of local recurrence in affected patients.

E Primary mucosal melanoma of the head and neck (MMHN) comprises ~1% of all malignant melanoma, and patients with MMHN experience multiple local recurrences and ultimately succumb to a combination of uncontrolled local and distant disease. Complete surgical resection with clear margins remains the primary mode of therapy, and adjuvant radiation therapy may improve locoregional control. The role of systemic therapy, including selective *KIT* inhibitors and immunotherapy, is under investigation.

F Both tumor thickness (Breslow) and level of invasion (Clark) are prognostically important, although thickness alone may be more significant. It has been suggested that traditional tumor thickness divisions of 0.75, 1.50, and 4.0 mm be changed to 1.0, 2.0, and 4.0 mm to simplify stage assignments and improve prognostic grouping. Clinical staging is based on pathologic evaluation of the primary site and on clinical/radiologic evaluation for regional and distant metastases.

G Patients with stage 0–II melanoma, routine imaging, and laboratory tests are not recommended except when evaluating specific signs or symptoms. In patients with stages III–IV, baseline imaging using computed tomography (CT) scan, positron emission tomography/CT, and/or magnetic resonance imaging is recommended as well as obtaining serum lactate dehydrogenase levels.

H Current recommendations for adequate margins include the following (each dependent on anatomic constraints):

Tumor thickness (mm)	Recommended clinical margins (cm)
In situ	0.5–1.0
≤1.00	1.0
1.01–2.00	1.0–2.0
2.01–4.00	2.0
>4.00	2.0

I Sentinel lymph node biopsy (SLNB) is considered standard of care in accurate staging of patients with intermediate thickness and selected thin and thick melanomas. Staging with SLNB identifies patients who may benefit from further therapies, such as a neck dissection or adjuvant therapy. However, no survival benefit has been demonstrated in patients undergoing SLNB. Among patients with a positive SLN, studies have shown additional positive non-SLN in about 18% of patients undergoing completion lymph node dissection (CLND).

J As many as 80% of tumor recurrences will become clinically apparent within 36 months after definitive treatment and within 24 months in patients with regional metastasis. Intervals between follow-up examinations should be every 3–12 months, depending on the initial disease stage. Routine blood tests and radiologic imaging are not recommended unless they are necessary to investigate specific signs or symptoms or to screen for recurrent/metastatic disease in patients with stage IIB–IV disease.

K Systemic therapy may be beneficial in patients with advanced stage, metastatic, or unresectable disease. Options of first-line therapy include immunotherapy (anti PD-1 monotherapy or anti-CTLA4 antibody) and molecularly targeted therapy against tumors carrying *BRAF* mutations. High-dose interleukin 2 and cytotoxic chemotherapy agents can be considered for second-line or subsequent therapies.

L Radiotherapy may improve locoregional control rates in selected patients. For the primary site, adjuvant therapy should be considered in the setting of close or positive margins, extensive perineural invasion, or locally recurrent disease. For the control of regional disease, adjuvant radiation should be considered for patients with nodal stage at least N2 (≥2 lymph nodes), extracapsular extension, ≥3 cm of tumor within a node, and dermal satellite or in-transit disease. Therapy is given in five fractions of 6 Gy each, delivered twice weekly over 2.5 weeks (30 Gy total).

ACKNOWLEDGMENT

We would like to acknowledge the contributions of Dr Andrew Nemechek.

SUGGESTED READING

Ang KK, Peters LJ, Weber RS, et al. Postoperative radiotherapy for cutaneous melanoma of the head and neck region. Int J Radiat Oncol Biol Phys. 1994;30(4):795-798.

Balch CM, Gershenwald JE, Soong SJ, et al. Final version of 2009 AJCC melanoma staging and classification. J Clin Oncol. 2009; 27(36):6199-6206.

Büttner P, Garbe C, Bertz J, et al. Primary cutaneous melanoma. Optimized cutoff points of tumor thickness and importance of Clark's level for prognostic classification. Cancer. 1995;75(10): 2499-2506.

Chen LL, Jaimes N, Barker CA, et al. Desmoplastic melanoma: a review. J Am Acad Dermatol. 2013;68(5):825-833.

Cohen LM. Lentigo maligna and lentigo maligna melanoma. J Am Acad Dermatol. 1995;33(6):923-936.

Erman AB, Collar RM, Griffith KA, et al. Sentinel lymph node biopsy is accurate and prognostic in head and neck melanoma. Cancer. 2012;118(4):1040-1047.

SECTION
7

General

CHAPTER 171

Bleeding Disorders

Winslo K Idicula, Gregory C Allen

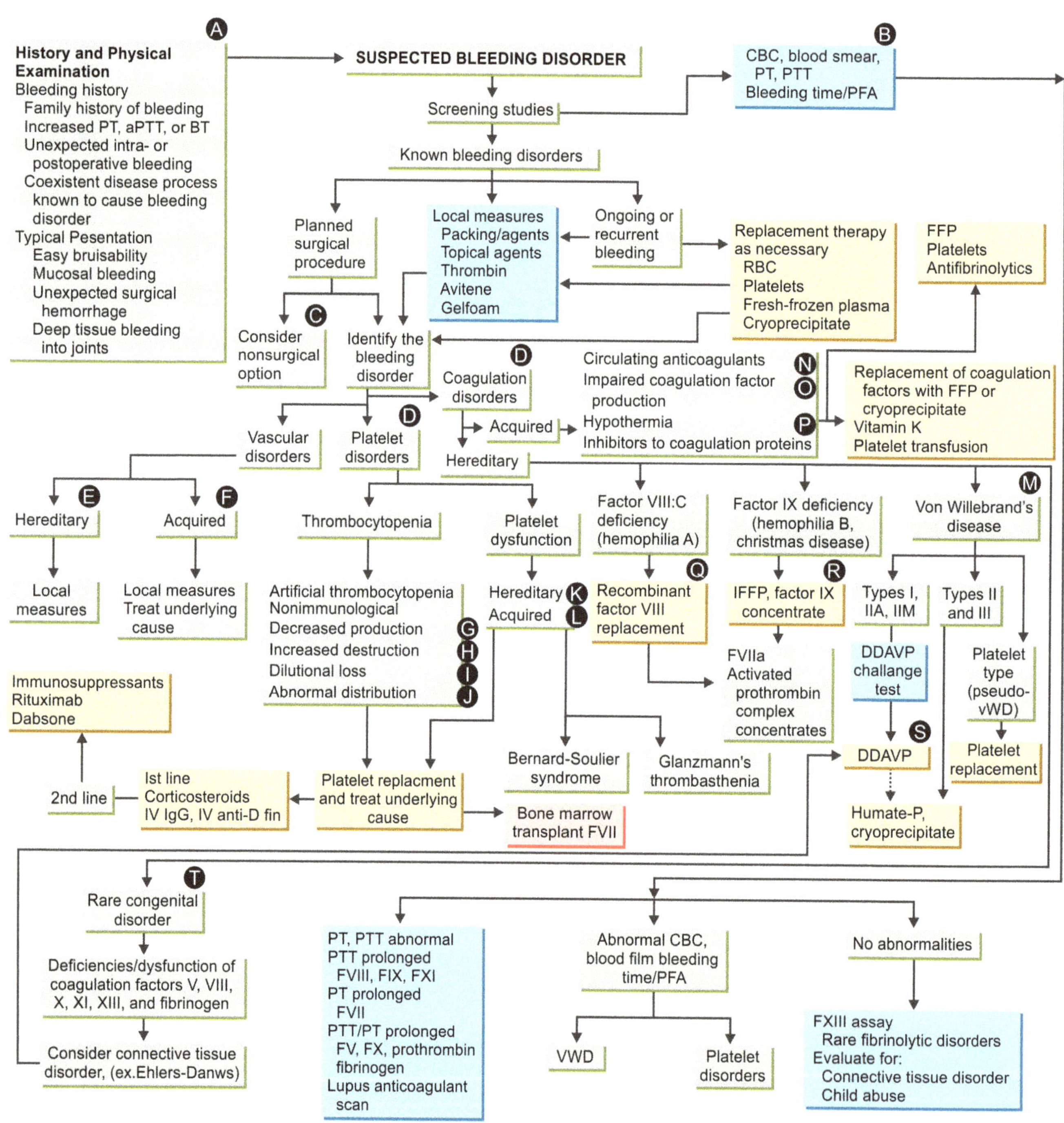

Blood coagulation involves a cascade of activation reactions. Children who have bleeding disorders often present initially to their pediatrician with suspicious signs, abnormal screening from presurgical evaluation, or known family history. Understanding the physiology of coagulation allows the clinician to identify children who have underlying disorders in order to facilitate management and treatment.

A There is general consensus in the literature that a detailed bleeding history and a detailed family history of bleeding disorders are the most sensitive and cost-effective means of evaluating coagulopathies. Bruising in children must be differentiated from extrinsic cause such as child abuse, which is more common than hemophilia. Surgical bleeding in children is associated often with circumcision, tonsillectomy, and dental extractions.

B Screening laboratory testing is reasonable for high-risk procedures in which significant blood loss is anticipated. First-line laboratory screening and second-line specific testing is essential to identify patients with bleeding diatheses. A complete blood count and peripheral blood smear are required as a first step. Bleeding time has low sensitivity and specificity for identifying defects of primary hemostasis. Platelet function assays can guide identification of vWD or platelet function defects. PT measures the extrinsic pathway and the PTT measures the intrinsic/common clotting factors.

C Nonsurgical management is considered when the risk of bleeding is higher than surgical benefit. Bleeding disorders should still be investigated.

D Consider involving a Hematologist at this point.

E Hereditary vascular disorders include hereditary hemorrhagic telangiectasia (Osler-Weber-Rendu disease), Marfan syndrome, Ehlers-Danlos syndrome, osteogenesis imperfecta.

F Acquired vascular disorders include scurvy, senile purpura, steroid-induced purpura, and amyloidosis.

G About 25% of the normal population have thrombocytopenia.

Decreased platelet production can result from bone marrow failure/replacement, selective megakaryocyte depression and hereditary factors.

H Increased platelet destruction can result from immune factors, drugs, and disorders where a large number of platelets are consumed. Nonimmunological causes of thrombocytopenia include thrombotic micro-angioplasties, disseminated intravascular coagulation, thrombotic, thrombocytopenic purpura, hemolytic uremic syndrome, and massive blood transfusions. Immunological causes of thrombocytopenia include neonatal thrombocytopenia, post-transfusion purpura, pregnancy, collagen tissue disorders, lymphoproliferative disorders, and infections.

I Dilutional loss can result from massive transfusion.

J Abnormal distribution can result from splenic/hepatic sequestration or hypothermia.

K Hereditary platelet dysfunctions are abnormalities of platelet number and function. Bernard-Soulier syndrome, defect of platelet glycoprotein complex GPIB/IX/V, presents. Therapeutic approaches include education and aspirin avoidance. Halothane or Dibucaine, anesthetics, compromise platelet reactivity. Desmopressin acetate or 1-deamino-8-D-arginine vasopressin (DDAVP), recombinant FVII, and antifibrinolytic drugs may be beneficial in the treatment of minor bleeding.

Glanzmann's thromblasthenia is a failure of platelets to aggregate when stimulated with adenosine diphosphate. Bone marrow transplant should be considered in patients with recurrent severe bleeding.

L Acquired platelet dysfunction can result from myeloproliferative syndromes, acute myeloblastic leukemia, dysproteinemias, uremia/renal failure, hepatic disease, storage pool deficiency medications cardiac valvular disease, cardiopulmonary bypass, and extracorporeal membrane oxygenation.

M vWD, most common genetic bleeding disorder, presents with different types based on laboratory testing. Type I (70–80% cases) and type III (rare) are characterized by partial and complete deficiency of vWF, respectively. Type II vWD reflects qualitative defect in vWF function.

N Circulating anticoagulants result from drugs (heparin), factor VIII:C inhibitor (develops in 10–15% of patients with factor VIII:C deficiency), factor IX inhibitor (develops in 1–5% of patients with factor IX deficiency), lupus anticoagulant.

O Impaired coagulation factor production results from vitamin K deficiency and hepatic disease.

P Hypothermia results in decreased enzyme activity and potential DIC on rewarming.

Q Generally, recombinant factor VIII is given to increase factor VIII:C activity levels to 100% for major surgical procedures and life-threatening hemorrhage, 50% for other major bleeding, and 30% for lacerations and epistaxis. Patients with antibodies are treated with recombinant FVIIa or activated prothrombin complex concentrates.

R Factor IX activity should be increased to 50% for surgery and maintained at 12–16% postoperatively.

S A DDAVP challenge test should be performed by measuring vWF indices before and after the administrations of DDAVP. DDAVP is administered at a dose of 0.3 μg/kg in 50 mL normal saline over a 30-minute period intravenously and 150–300 mg intranasally. Because of the risk of hyponatremic seizures, DDAVP should be used with caution in children <2 years old. A poor response requires administration of antihemophilic factor VIII or cryoprecipitate. DDAVP is ineffective for Type II and III and require treatment with plasma concentrates and cryopreciptates.

T Rare congenital disorder is typically autosomal recessive with deficiencies or dysfunction of coagulation factors V, VII, X, XI, XII, and fibrinogen. Treatment includes DDAVP with ascorbic acid to assist with crosslinking of collagen.

SUGGESTED READING

Allen GC, Armfield D, BonTempo F, et al. Adenotonsillectomy in children with von Willebrand's disease. Arch Otolaryngol Head Neck Surg. 1999;125:547-551.

Chee YL, Crawford JC, Watson HG, et al. Guidelines on the assessment of bleeding risk prior to surgery or invasive procedure. Br J Haematol. 2008;140:496-504.

Derkay CS, Werner E, Plotnick E. Management of children with von Willebrand's disease undergoing adenotonsillectomy. Am J Otolaryngol. 1996;17:172-177.

Krishnegowda M, Rajashekaraiah V. Platelet disorders: an overview. Blood Coagul Fibrinolysis. 2015;26:479-491.

Sadler JE, Davie EW. Hemophilia A, hemophilia B, and von Willebrand's disease. In: Stamatoyannopoulos G, Majerus PW, Varmus H (Eds). The Molecular Basis of Blood Disease, 2nd edition. Philadelphia, PA: WB Saunders; 1994. p. 675.

Sharathkumar AA, Pipe SW. Bleeding disorders. Pediatr Rev. 2008;29:121-129.

Anesthesia

Gregory L McHugh, Andrew Herlich

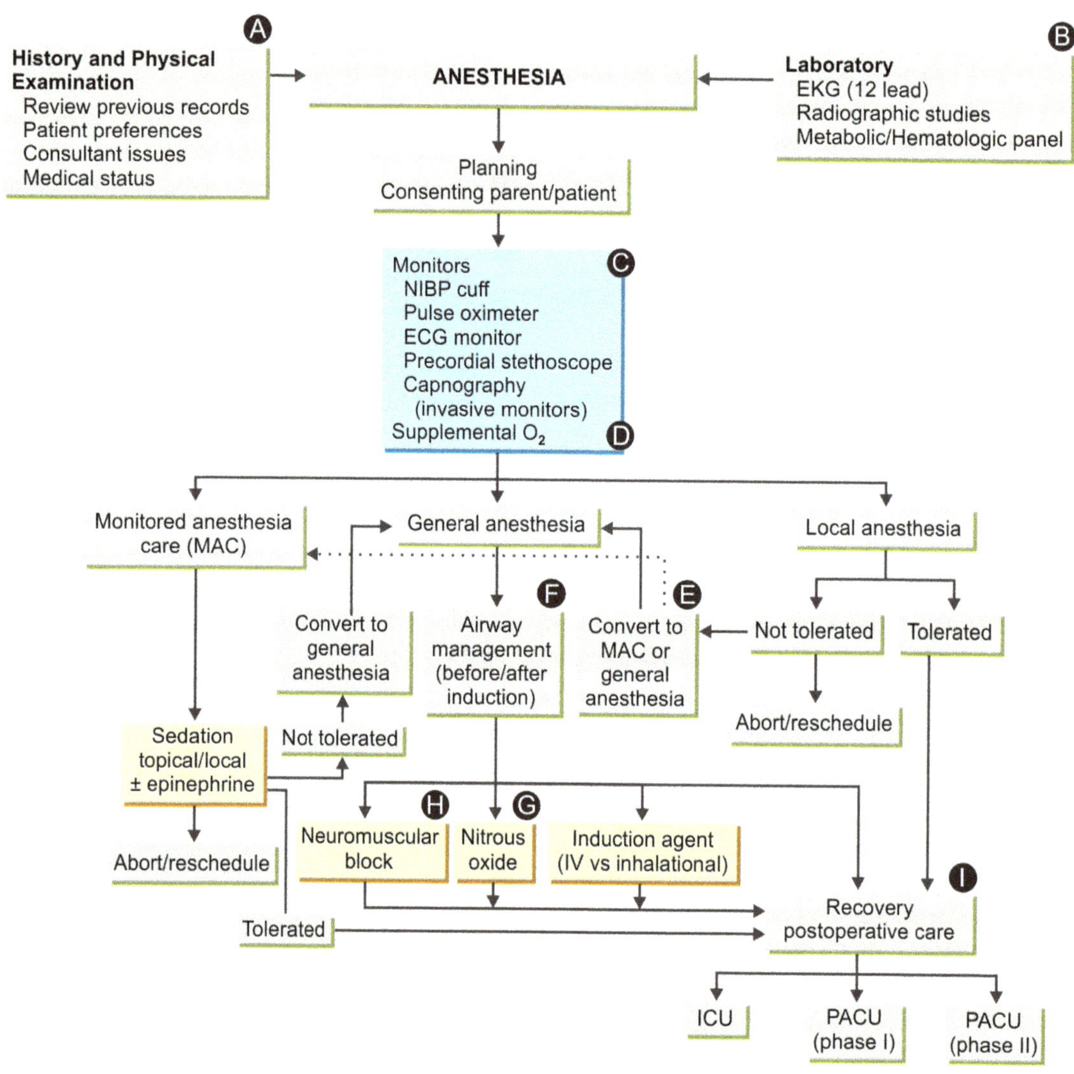

The key to a successful anesthetic plan is to have good communication between the surgeon, anesthesiologist, primary care physician, and operating room staff as far in advance as possible. Otolaryngology patients present unique concerns and potential complications for the anesthesiologist, such as distorted airway anatomy resulting in difficulty with ventilation and/or intubation, managing a "shared" airway with surgical colleagues, and using nonconventional methods of oxygenation and ventilation, such as apneic or intermittent oxygenation and supraglottic or subglottic jet ventilation. For these reasons, communication and collegiality are paramount among all practitioners involved.

A Special equipment, patient position, and prohibition of muscle relaxants need to be communicated before the anesthesia setup. High-risk patients, such as those with pre-existing airway compromise or obstructive sleep apnea and those at the extremes of age, require special attention and planning. Pediatric patients may require preoperative sedation, placement of a functioning intravenous (IV) catheter before induction, and comprehensive discussion with parents before proceeding.

B The primary care physician needs to communicate to the surgical team the patient's optimal medical status considering the disease state. Appropriate specialty consultations should be obtained when warranted. If the surgical procedure needs to be delayed because of the patient's medical status, the risk of delaying surgery versus the risk of proceeding must be weighed among all of the practitioners involved. Preoperative laboratory investigations, including electrocardiography (EKG), radiography, metabolic or hematologic panels, and pulmonary function tests or blood gases, should be determined by patient status and not by age alone. For example, patients with hypertension or coronary disease may benefit from preoperative EKG and metabolic panel if on diuretic medications, asthmatic patients or those with chronic obstructive pulmonary disease may need chest radiography and, if severe, pulmonary function tests (PFTs) and blood gas analysis, those with renal or liver disease should have metabolic, hematologic, and coagulation profiles examined for abnormalities, and diabetic patients should have glucose measurements, EKG, and metabolic panels performed to examine for end organ dysfunction. Healthy patients with no systemic disease, regardless of age, typically do not require preoperative testing. Of particular concern are those patients with morbid obesity and obstructive sleep apnea (OSA), who often require preoperative polysomnography to assess the severity of sleep apnea.

C Regardless of the type of anesthetic care, patients should have minimal monitoring placed before surgery. These include EKG, noninvasive blood pressure monitors, and pulse oximetry. The use of capnography is mandatory intraoperatively. The use of a precordial stethoscope or invasive monitoring should be determined by the nature of the surgery, patient medical status, and the type of anesthesia. It is also important to obtain written informed consent whenever possible.

D The concentration of supplemental oxygen may be necessarily modified by the proximity of electrocautery or laser devices.

E Unless the patient refuses before the initiation of sedation, the patient must understand that monitored anesthesia care (MAC) may become general anesthesia if conditions warrant. The term "MAC" actually includes varying levels of sedation, analgesia, and anxiolysis, but the underlying principle is that the patient remains responsive to verbal, tactile, or painful stimulus. If the patient becomes unresponsive to even painful stimuli, then the anesthetic is considered to be general. Procedures amendable to MAC include laryngeal framework surgery such as thyroplasty, simple vocal cord injections using flexible nasolaryngoscopy, biopsy of superficial lesions, and certain nasal or sinus procedures. Some procedures may be performed with local anesthesia alone, via either field block or specific nerve block, these include excision of superficial masses without known vascular or neural involvement, excision of small soft tissue lesions of the tongue, lip, and buccal mucosa, as well as tracheostomy. Scheduled under local anesthesia, MAC or general anesthesia may become necessary for the patient if he or she is not tolerating the procedure. The surgeon's comfort with an awake or sedated patient and invasive nature of the procedure may also dictate which anesthetic plan is preferable.

F The timing of securing the patient's airway relative to induction of general anesthesia depends on the known difficulties with the patients airway. Awake intubation with topical anesthesia and sedation, awake tracheostomy, or airway management after the induction of anesthesia should be discussed between the surgeon and the anesthesia team.

G Induction of anesthesia may be accomplished by either intravenous technique or spontaneous ventilation using volatile agents with an anesthesia mask. Preoperative sedation is titrated according to the patients needs and physiologic risks, including cardiorespiratory compromise. If the surgeon has any prohibitions against anesthetic agents because of their effect on surgical outcome, such as nitrous oxide for middle ear surgery, they must be conveyed in advance of induction of general anesthesia.

H The requirement for muscle relaxation, as well as its duration and depth, must be discussed with the anesthesia team in advance. Patients in whom the facial nerve will be monitored or may be compromised require modification of anesthetic technique to accommodate surgical needs. The risk of postoperative respiratory compromise due to the use of neuromuscular blocking agents must be weighed against surgical needs for intensity and duration of muscle relaxation.

I The postoperative disposition of the patient, including time to discharge, depends on the immediacy of anesthetic recovery, surgical invasiveness, and the patient's medical status. Phase I postanesthesia care unit (PACU) patients require a standard recovery process from general anesthesia or sedation. Patients who may be transferred directly to phase II PACU are awake, alert, and functional, and have no surgical or airway compromise. Patients requiring immediate intensive care have extensive anesthetic or surgical morbidity requiring such care.

SUGGESTED READING

Brown ACD, Bradford CR. Head and neck Oncologic Surgery. In: Bready LL, Mullins RM, Noorily SH, et al. (Eds). Decision Making in Anesthesiology: An Algorithmic Approach, 3rd edition. St Louis, MO: CV Mosby; 2000. p. 528.

Cavallone LF, Vannucci A.. Extubation of the difficult airway and extubation failure. Anesth Analg. 2013;116:368-383.

Griffin JD, Klein KW. Bronchoscopy. In: Bready LL, Muffins RM, Noorily SH, et al. (Eds). Decision Making in Anesthesiology: An Algorithmic Approach, 3rd edition. St Louis, MO: CV Mosby; 2000. p. 534.

Herlich A. Anesthesia for eye, ear, and throat surgery. In: Reed A (Ed). Clinical Cases in Anesthesia, 2nd edition. New York: Churchill Livingstone; 1995. p. 215.

Mangano DT. Assessment of the patient with cardiac disease. Anesthesiology. 1999;91(5):1521-1526.

Nemeth J, Maghraby N, Kazim S. Emergency airway management: The difficult airway. Emerg Med Clin N Am. 2012;30:401-420.

Management of Syndromic Children

David L Horn

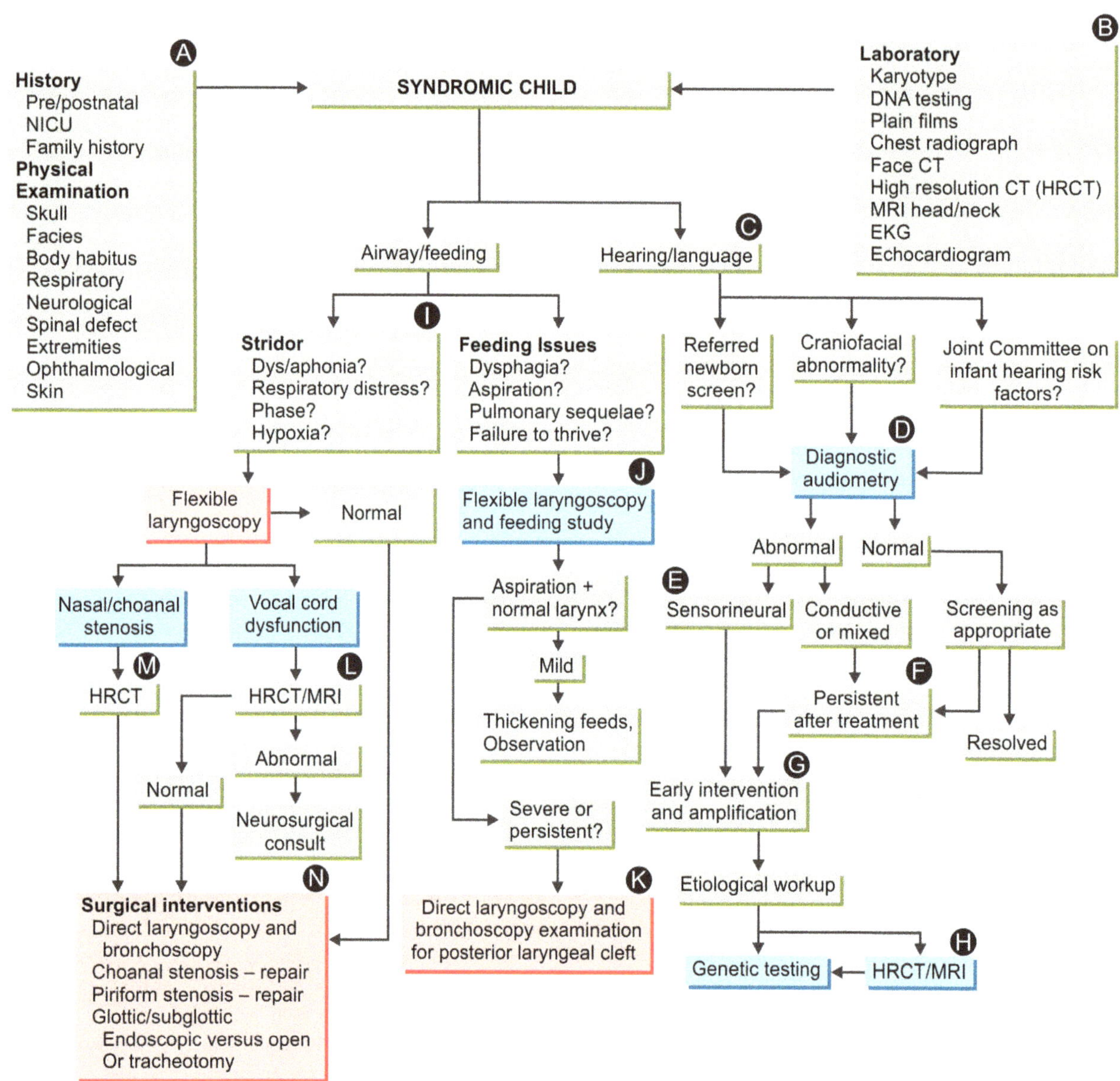

Syndromic children commonly present with otolaryngologic problems including Eustachian tube dysfunction, sensorineural hearing loss, airway obstruction, and dysphagia/aspiration. The following is an algorithm for management of the known or suspected syndromic child in the outpatient clinic setting.

A Children presenting with atypical craniofacial features, hearing problems and/or airway/feeding issues warrant consideration of a syndromic diagnosis. Coloboma, ear anomalies and choanal atresia suggest CHARGE association, while chronic aspiration and tracheoesophageal fistula suggest VATER or VACTERL complex. White forelock, dystopia canthorum, or heterochromia iridis imply Waardenburg

syndrome. Referral to a geneticist can help identify the specific syndrome when not immediately apparent.

B The Otolaryngologist should review any genetic and cardiac records and obtain previous imaging. Chest radiograph may reveal situs inversus associated with Kartagener's syndrome. Facial imaging may reveal craniofacial malformations. Cardiac anomalies can be associated with CHARGE association and 22q11.2 deletion syndrome. Care should be taken in planning anesthetic and surgical management for these patients and preoperative anesthesiology consultation may be warranted.

C Children with known or suspected hearing-loss related syndrome should undergo age-appropriate diagnostic audiometric testing. Children with craniofacial abnormalities or Joint Committee on Infant Hearing (JCIH) risk factors should undergo diagnostic testing by 24–30 months of age regardless of newborn hearing screen status.

D Diagnostic brainstem auditory-evoked response testing should be performed in children who are too young or unable to perform behavioral testing. Children with absent brainstem responses should undergo otoacoustic emissions testing to look for auditory neuropathy/dyssynchrony.

E Syndromes associated with congenital or progressive sensorineural hearing loss include Waardenburg's (white forelock, dystopia canthorum, heterochromia iridis), Usher's syndrome (retinitis pigmentosa and vestibular hypofunction), trisomy 21, Pendred's (mondini, enlarged vestibular aqueduct, and thyroid abnormalities), Branchio-oto-renal (BOR) syndrome, Alport syndrome (glomerulonephritis).

F Hearing loss may be mixed in Pendred's, BOR, and X-linked perilymphatic gusher syndrome or purely conductive as in osteogenesis imperfecta or Turner's syndrome. Children with trisomy 21 commonly have a conductive component to their hearing loss.

G Infants with permanent hearing loss should be enrolled in early intervention and fit with amplification, ideally prior to age 6 months. For children with absent external ear structures, bone-conduction processors can be used. Cochlear-implantation may be an option for children who do not benefit from amplification.

H For patients with sensorineural or mixed hearing loss, computed tomography (CT) scan or magnetic resonance imaging (MRI) can reveal cochleovestibular malformations (as in BOR, Waardenburg's and CHARGE), cochlear nerve or internal auditory canal stenosis, or enlarged vestibular aqueduct (as in Pendred's). Patients with conductive hearing loss should undergo CT to delineate ossicular anomalies. Genetic testing for particular syndromic etiologies can be considered primarily or when imaging is non-diagnostic. Vestibular testing showing bilateral areflexia suggests Usher's syndrome. All children with permanent hearing loss should have a consultation with an Ophthalmologist.

I Neonates and infants with airway compromise present with respiratory distress, noisy breathing, or feeding difficulty. Flexible fiberoptic examination can reveal fixed (piriform aperture stenosis or choanal atresia) and dynamic (laryngomalacia or vocal cord dysfunction) lesions. When airway problems are severe, genetic, intensivist, and pediatric consultation can help evaluate for lethal syndromes and help guide appropriately aggressive interventions. Occasionally, multidisciplinary care and/or ethics committees can help provide guidance when prognosis is poor.

In children with trisomy 21, craniofacial syndromes, or lysosomal storage syndromes, obstructive sleep apnea (OSA) is common. In such patients, polysomnography and evaluation for cor pulmonale should be considered. Tonsillectomy and adenoidectomy may be less effective for these patients than in non-syndromic children.

J A modified barium swallow study (MBSS) or fiberoptic endoscopic evaluation of swallowing (FEES) can be performed to assess for level and severity of dysphagia and to determine what feeding consistencies are safe.

K If aspiration or deep penetration is revealed, without obvious laryngeal abnormalities, the Otolaryngologist should suspect a posterior laryngeal cleft. This diagnosis is made on microdirect laryngoscopy (MDL) in the operating room. Deeper clefts require surgical repair while minor clefts may not require treatment. Test augmentation of the interarytenoid mucosa with absorbable material can be used to guide treatment in the latter case.

L Bilateral vocal cord paralysis may be caused by a central (Arnold-Chiari malformation) or peripheral (post cardiac surgery). MRI of brain can reveal potentially reversible pathology.

M Infants with nasal or choanal stenosis should undergo a CT scan, which can help reveal a specific syndromic diagnosis. Craniofacial synostoses (Apert's or Pfeiffer's syndromes) may be apparent. Mandibular hypoplasia may suggest Treacher Collins or Nager syndrome or Goldenhar syndrome (facial microsomia).

N Syndromic infants who require surgical airway intervention should undergo MDL and bronchoscopy to rule out secondary lesions. Glottic webs can be found in patients with velocardiofacial syndrome and complete tracheal rings can be associated with Pfeiffer's. Tracheomalacia is commonly found in patients with a tracheoesophageal fistula. Children with trisomy 21 may have congenital subglottic stenosis and should be screened preoperatively for atlantoaxial instability. Treatment of nasal/choanal lesions, bilateral vocal cord dysfunction, or infraglottic pathology should proceed as indicated with the caveat that syndromic children are more likely to require tracheotomy than nonsyndromic infants to treat airway obstruction. Preoperative cardiac workup should be considered for patients with choanal atresia (CHARGE), cleft palate (velocardiofacial syndrome), and trisomy 21. Previous uncomplicated anesthesia does not guarantee reliable airway access.

SUGGESTED READING

Joint Committee on Infant Hearing; American Academy of Audiology; American Academy of Pediatrics; American Speech-Language-Hearing Association; Directors of Speech and Hearing Programs in State Health and Welfare Agencies. Year 2000 position statement: principles and guidelines for early hearing detection and intervention programs. Pediatrics. 2000;106(4):798-817.

Rosenfeld RM, Schwartz SR, Pynnonen MA, et al. Clinical practice guideline: tympanostomy tubes in children. Otolaryngol Head Neck Surg. 2013;149(1 Suppl):S1-35.

Sinkueakunkit A, Chowchuen B, Kantanabat C, et al. Outcome of anesthetic management for children with craniofacial deformities. Pediatr Int. 2013;55(3):360-365.

Tan HL, Kheirandish-Gozal L, Abel F, et al. Craniofacial syndromes and sleep-related breathing disorders. Sleep Med Rev. 2015;27:74-88.

Wiley S, Arjmand E, Jareenmeinzen-Derr, et al. Findings from multidisciplinary evaluation of children with permanent hearing loss. Int J Pediatr Otorhinolaryngol. 2011;75(8):1040-1044.

Yoshinaga-Itano C, Sedey AL, Coulter DK, et al. Language of early- and later-identified children with hearing loss. Pediatrics. 1998;102(5):1161-1171.

Radiation Therapy for Head and Neck Cancer

Michael Dohopolski, David A Clump

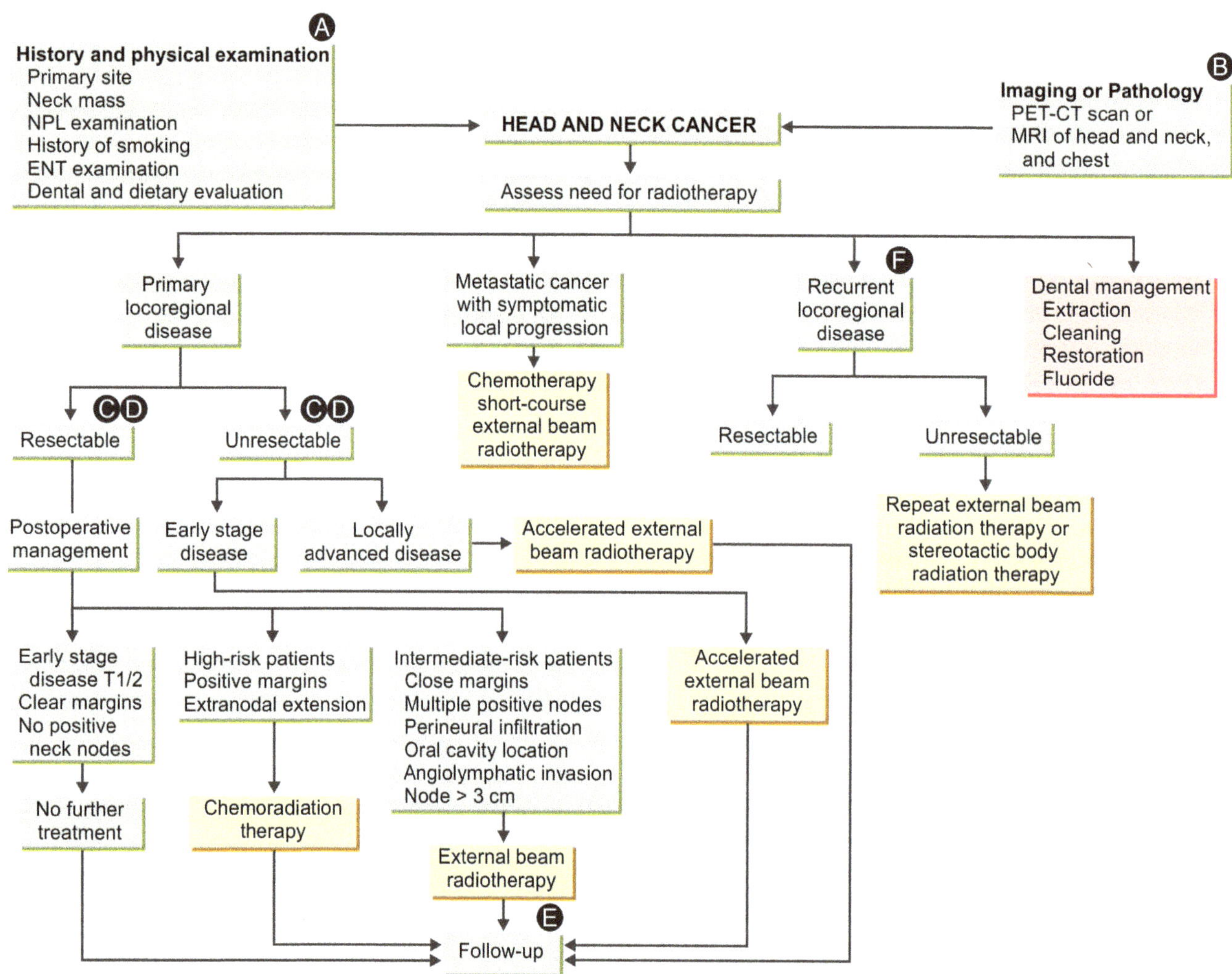

Radiation therapy can be used in definitive management of head and neck (H and N) cancers or in the postoperative setting as an adjuvant treatment to enhance local control. Dose selection and prescription is based on the presence of microscopic versus gross disease, while typical treatment is delivered over 6–7 weeks.

A The history and physical (H&P) including nasopharyngeal laryngoscopy (NPL) examination is central to clinical staging and defining treatment parameters. Historical components including precipitating and exacerbating factors, smoking and alcohol history, and in the case of some H&N malignancies occupational history and birthplace are necessary. Patients should be referred for dental and speech or swallowing evaluation prior to initiating treatment. Identifying the primary tumor, its size and extension into adjacent structures is critical to staging and determining the nodal regions at risk for involvement. Each primary tumor site and its anatomic location in respect to midline influence the potential risk for bilateral hemineck involvement and the subsequent treatment field.

B *Imaging:* CT of the neck and chest including the integration of the fludeoxyglucose-positron emission tomography (FDG-PET) tracer facilitates primary, nodal, and metastatic staging. Additionally, magnetic resonance imaging (MRI) can augment CT in determining primary tumor extension and is especially important in determining skull base involvement and perineural tumor spread.

Pathological assessment: The pathological assessment including both the biopsy as well as final histology is critical. For instance, a low-grade adenoid cystic carcinoma of the parotid gland has minimal-risk for nodal involvement as the primary-pattern of local regional failure is at the primary site and along named nerves. More recently, p16 status assists in the identification of an unknown primary as it is likely to originate from the oropharynx. Most important are the use of the final histology, pathological staging, and risk factors as they influence adjuvant therapies. The high-risk pathological features include positive margins and extracapsular extension while intermediate risk factors include advanced T-stage (T3/4), oral cavity location, perineural invasion (PNI), angiolymphatic invasion (ALI), two or more positive nodes, and lymph nodes measuring greater than 3 cm in size.

C CT-based treatment planning with intravenous (IV) contrast, and preferably PET-CT, in an immobilization mask is necessary for treatment of all H&N malignancies. A 3D-target is identified with assistance of PET and MRI. Here, the primary and nodal gross tumor volume ($GTV_{primary/nodes}$) is identified along with the clinical-target volume ($CTV_{primary/nodes}$) and planning-target volume ($PTV_{primary/nodes}$), an expansion on the CTV(s) to account for motion and set-up uncertainty. $CTV_{primary}$ includes anatomical subsites involved (e.g. entire base of tongue), while CTV_{nodes} includes lymph node stations at risk for microscopic disease involvement. Additionally, normal structures in their entirety should be delineated in order to describe the dose-volume relationship and predict toxicities.

These parameters are combined to create three separate PTVs representing low-risk, intermediate-risk, and high-risk treatment volumes.

(1) PTV1 (low-risk): ($CTV_{primary}$+ CTV_{nodes}) + 0.5 cm;
(2) PTV2 (intermediate-risk): ($CTV_{primary}$ + CTV_{nodes} - involved stations) + 0.5 cm;
(3) PTV3 (high-risk): [($GTV_{primary}$ + 1 cm) + (GTV_{nodes} + 0.5 cm)] + 0.5 cm.

D *Treatment planning:* Intensity-modulated radiation therapy (IMRT) allows for the optimization of tumor coverage while reducing dose to normal surrounding tissues such as the salivary glands, brainstem, and other critical structures. Depending upon the dose and fractionation-regimen selected, a sequential (3-separate plans for PTV1-3) or a dose-painting technique otherwise known as a simultaneous-integrated boost (SIB) plan be created.

Dose selection: PTVs 1-3 are prescribed different doses based upon the extent of disease. Microscopic disease should be prescribed a minimum of 50 Gray while gross disease is typically treated to a total of 70 Gray. For early-stage disease, treated with radiotherapy alone, an accelerated course is preferred while a 7-week regimen is standard for locally-advanced disease that is managed by concurrent chemoradiotherapy. Postoperative radiation therapy consists of a total dose of 50–66 Gray at 2.0 Gray/fraction with the highest dose being delivered to the margin or area of extracapsular spread.

E Patients should be assessed for tumor response and treatment-related toxicities weekly OTVs during the course of therapy. Expected side effects include fatigue, weight loss, taste change, xerostomia, mucositis, odynophagia, and skin erythema. Feeding tube placement is preferred in those with greater than 20% weight loss at presentation and reflexively for those who are unable to maintain weight despite an aggressive speech and swallow regimen. Clinical assessment and restaging with a H&N and lung CT (preferably PET-CT) should be at 8–12 weeks posttreatment and every 3 months for the first year and 4–6 months during the second year. Imaging can be deferred after 2 years except for those with a smoking history and meet criteria for lung cancer screening with a low-dose CT scan. Assessment by the multidisciplinary team for late recurrences as well as toxicities including xerostomia, dental effects, and hypothyroidism should continue in years following treatment.

F Patients with failure within the previously irradiated field are primarily salvaged with surgical management. For those with inoperable cancer and a period of at least 6 months from prior radiation therapy, there is careful consideration for reirradiation. Reirradiation in the form of IMRT can be considered, however, it is associated with significant acute-side effects. For those with limited volume recurrences, a highly conformal form of radiation therapy called stereotactic body radiation therapy (SBRT) can be considered. SBRT is usually limited for those with recurrences less than 100 cc and a total dose of 40–50 Gray delivered in five fractions on nonconsecutive days is utilized.

SUGGESTED READING

Kann BH, Buckstein M, Carpenter TJ, et al. Radiographic extracapsular extension and treatment outcomes in locally advanced oropharyngeal carcinoma. Head Neck. 2014;36:1689-1694.

Kress MA, Sen N, Unger KR, et al. Safety and efficacy of hypofractionated stereotactic body reirradiation in head and neck cancer: Long-term follow-up of a large series. Head Neck. 2015;37(10):1403-1409.

Langer CJ, Harris J, Horwitz EM, et al. Phase II study of low-dose paclitaxel and cisplatin in combination with split-course concomitant twice-daily re-irradiation in recurrent squamous cell carcinoma of the head and neck: results of radiation therapy oncology group protocol 9911. J Clin Oncol. 2007;25:4800-4805.

Lee N, Chan K, Bekelman JE, et al. Salvage reirradiation for recurrent head and neck cancer. Int J Radiat Oncol Biol Phys. 2007;68:731-740.

Leong SC, Javed F, Elliot S, et al. Effectiveness of X-ray and computed tomography screening for assessing pulmonary involvement in patients with head and neck squamous cell carcinoma. J Laryngol Otol. 2008;122:961-966.

National Comprehensive Cancer Network. (2016). NCCN Clinical Practice Guidelines in Oncology (NCCN Guidelines) Head and Neck Cancer. Version 1. [online]. Available from: www.nccn.org/professionals/physician_gls/pdf/head-and-neck.pdf.

Spencer SA, Harris J, Wheeler RH, et al. Final report of RTOG 9610, a multi-institutional trial of re-irradiation and chemotherapy for unresectable recurrent squamous cell carcinoma of the head and neck. Head Neck. 2008;30:281-288.

Sulman EP, Schwartz DL, Le TT, et al. IMRT reirradiation of head and neck cancer-disease control and morbidity outcomes. Int J Radiat Oncol Biol Phys. 2009;73:399-409.

Chemotherapy of Head and Neck Cancer

Jessica L Geiger, Julie E Bauman

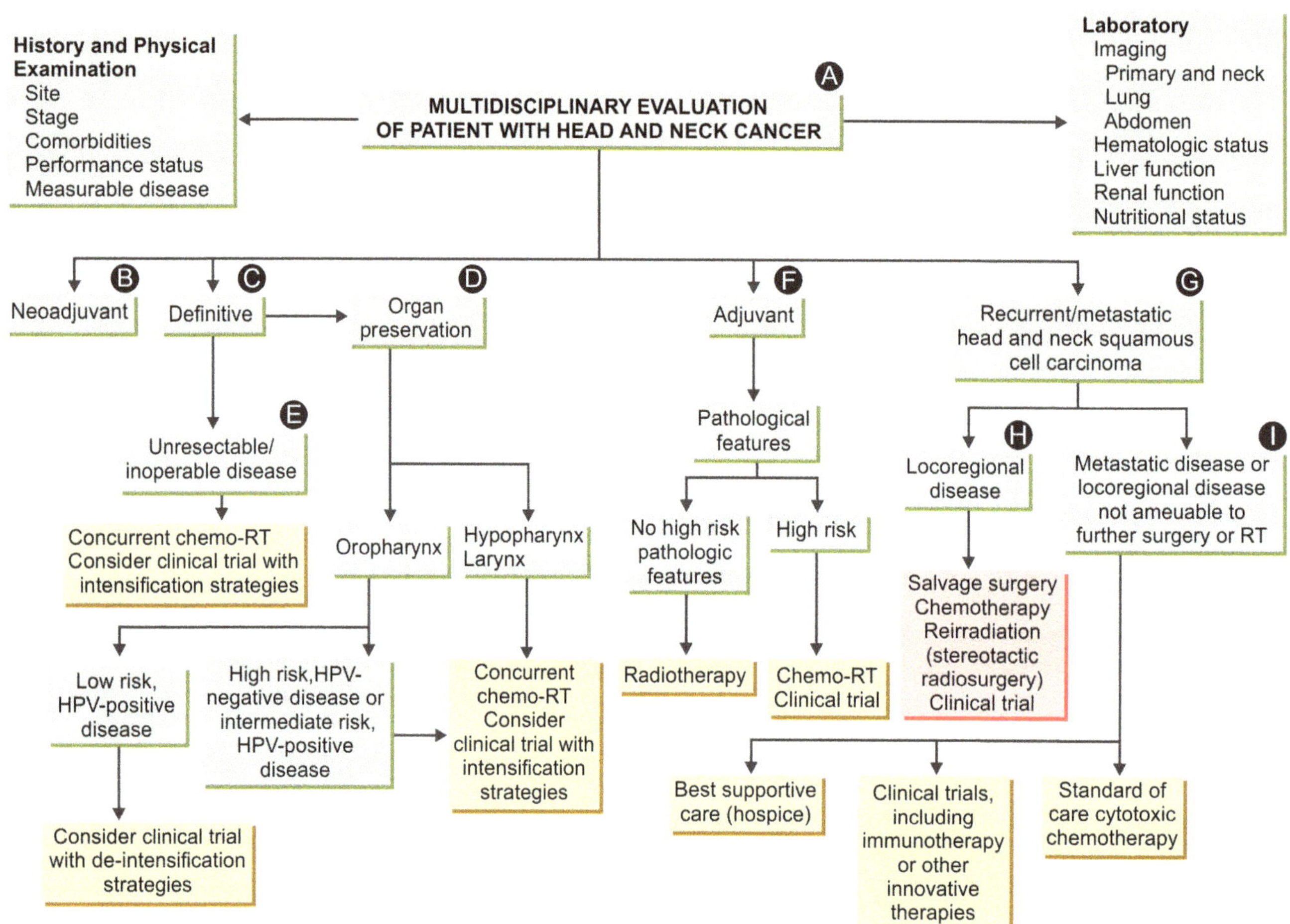

Cancer of the head and neck refers to cancers originating from the epithelial lining of the upper aerodigestive tract and is subdivided by anatomic boundaries: lip and oral cavity, pharynx (including nasopharynx, oropharynx, and hypopharynx), larynx, and nasal cavity and paranasal sinuses. The most common histologic type is squamous cell carcinoma, accounting for 85–95% of all head and neck cancers. Treatment for cancer of the head and neck is multidisciplinary, and long-term treatment-related toxicities demand close follow-up and attention to survivorship issues unique to this patient population.

A Multidisciplinary evaluation at a major medical institution is recommended for all patients with advanced head and neck cancer and should include specialty consultations with Medical Oncology, Radiation Oncology, and Otolaryngologists who specialize in treating head and neck cancer. The multidisciplinary team should also include health care professionals in the areas of nutrition, speech and language pathology, and palliative care

medicine. Concurrent chemoradiotherapy (RT) requires a compliant patient willing to accept 6–7 weeks of aggressive and time-consuming therapy with significant toxicity. Conversely, surgery requires low comorbidity and a patient able to withstand the procedure. Patient preference and the expertise of the treatment team are principal determinants of therapy for all patients with cancer of the head and neck.

B The rationale for the use of neoadjuvant or induction chemotherapy is based on the potential for a greater response to chemotherapy in previously untreated cancers. The role of induction chemotherapy is controversial and used only when followed by surgery or radiation. This approach has not been found superior to surgery and postoperative radiation in randomized trials and is generally reserved for patients with unresectable or inoperable disease. Active chemotherapeutic agents include platinum agents, 5-fluorouracil, taxanes, and cetuximab.

C The standard of care is definitive, concurrent chemotherapy and radiation therapy (chemo-RT) in two situations: (1) when the goal is organ preservation, typically in patients with oropharynx, hypopharynx, or larynx primaries; (2) for patients with a good performance status and very advanced disease in whom surgical resection is not feasible or is likely to lead to excessive morbidity.

D Two landmark trials, one conducted by the Department of Veterans Affairs and one by the European Organization for Research and Treatment of Cancer (EORTC), compared primary surgical management with an organ preservation approach for resectable laryngeal cancer. Overall survival (OS) was comparable in the two groups, and laryngeal preservation was possible in one-half to two-thirds of patients randomized to the nonsurgical arm of both trials. However, the relative contributions of RT and chemotherapy were unclear in both trials. Subsequently, the Intergroup Trial RTOG 9111 concluded that concurrent chemo-RT provided improvement in laryngeal preservation and time to laryngectomy over induction chemotherapy followed by RT and RT alone.

Based on human papillomavirus (HPV) status, pack-years of tobacco use, and nodal stage, patients undergoing definitive chemo-RT can be classified into three groups having low, intermediate, or high risk of death. This classification has framed national clinical trial priorities in head and neck cancer with deintensification strategies being tested in patients with low-risk, HPV-positive disease, whereas intensification strategies are available for patients with high-risk, HPV-negative and intermediate-risk, HPV-positive disease.

E In patients with very advanced, inoperable disease, concurrent chemo-RT is a rational approach to reduce both the rate of locoregional failure and distant metastases. Data from meta-analyses of clinical trials suggest superiority of concurrent chemo-RT over RT alone. Radiotherapy plus cetuximab has also been shown to improve locoregional control and reduce mortality without increased toxicity. Though high-dose cisplatin ($100 \, mg/m^2$ on days 1, 22, and 43) with RT is the preferred regimen, weekly cisplatin ($40 \, mg/m^2$) or cetuximab are also acceptable therapies.

F Chemotherapy given in the postoperative setting as an adjuvant to surgery is administered concurrently with radiation. Postoperative radiation therapy is considered standard for patients with advanced disease at diagnosis (T3 or N1 and higher stage). The addition of chemotherapy is standard in the following situations: (1) close or positive surgical margins, and (2) extracapsular spread in regional lymph nodes, as determined by a combined analysis of the Intergroup Trial RTOG 9501 and EORTC 22931.

G Despite advances in multimodality therapy, 5-year OS of head and neck cancer is 40–60% and has increased only incrementally in the past three decades. Patients with recurrent or metastatic disease have particularly poor prognosis, with median OS of 6–10 months. Responses to standard cytotoxic chemotherapy are of short duration, and there is an unmet need for new agents and innovative approaches for treatment in this area.

H For patients with recurrent cancer not amenable to curative-intent radiation therapy or surgery, the approach to treatment is similar to that for metastatic disease with use of systemic agents. Enrollment in clinical trials is preferred, and there are several studies evaluating reirradiation techniques including stereotactic radiosurgery alone or in combination with chemotherapy or immunotherapy.

I For patients with distant metastatic cancer, systemic therapy is a logical choice with response rates of 15–35%. The addition of cetuximab to cisplatin and 5-fluorouracil (EXTREME regimen) showed improved OS compared to platinum-based chemotherapy plus fluorouracil alone. Six cycles of EXTREME followed by cetuximab maintenance therapy is currently the standard first line in recurrent/metastatic head and neck squamous cell carcinoma. Every effort should be made to enroll patients into clinical trials. Ongoing studies of immunotherapy are well-tolerated with promising preliminary results in overall response rates and stable disease. Palliative care physicians play a crucial role throughout the course of head and neck cancer, and hospice care should be considered in the recurrent/metastatic setting.

SUGGESTED READING

Adelstein DJ, Li Y, Adams GL, et al. An intergroup phase III comparison of standard radiation therapy and two schedules of concurrent chemoradiotherapy in patients with unresectable squamous cell head and neck cancer. J Clin Oncol. 2003;21:92-98.

Ang KK, Harris J, Wheeler R, et al. Human papillomavirus and survival of patients with oropharyngeal cancer. N Engl J Med. 2010;363(1):24-35.

Bernier J, Cooper JS, Pajak TF, et al. Defining risk levels in locally advanced head and neck cancers: a comparative analysis of concurrent postoperative radiation plus chemotherapy trials of the EORTC (#22931) and RTOG (#9501). Head Neck. 2005;27:843-850.

Bonner JA, Harari PM, Giralt J, et al. Radiotherapy plus cetuximab for squamous cell carcinoma of the head and neck. N Engl J Med. 2006;354:567-578.

Forastiere AA, Zhang Q, Weber RS, et al. Long-term results of RTOG 91-11: a comparison of three nonsurgical treatment strategies to preserve the larynx in patients with locally advanced larynx cancer. J Clin Oncol. 2013;31:845-852.

Induction chemotherapy plus radiation compared with surgery plus radiation in patients with advanced laryngeal cancer. The Department of Veterans Affairs Laryngeal Cancer Study Group. N Engl J Med. 1991;324:1685-1690.

Lefebvre JL, Chevalier D, Luboinski B, et al. Larynx preservation in pyriform sinus cancer: preliminary results of a European Organization for Research and Treatment of Cancer phase III trial. EORTC Head and Neck Cancer Cooperative Group. J Natl Cancer Inst. 1996;88:890-899.

Vermorken JB, Mesia R, Rivera F, et al. Platinum-based chemotherapy plus cetuximab in head and neck cancer. N Engl J Med. 2008;359:1116-1127.

Immunotherapy in Head and Neck Cancer

Nicole C Schmitt, Robert L Ferris

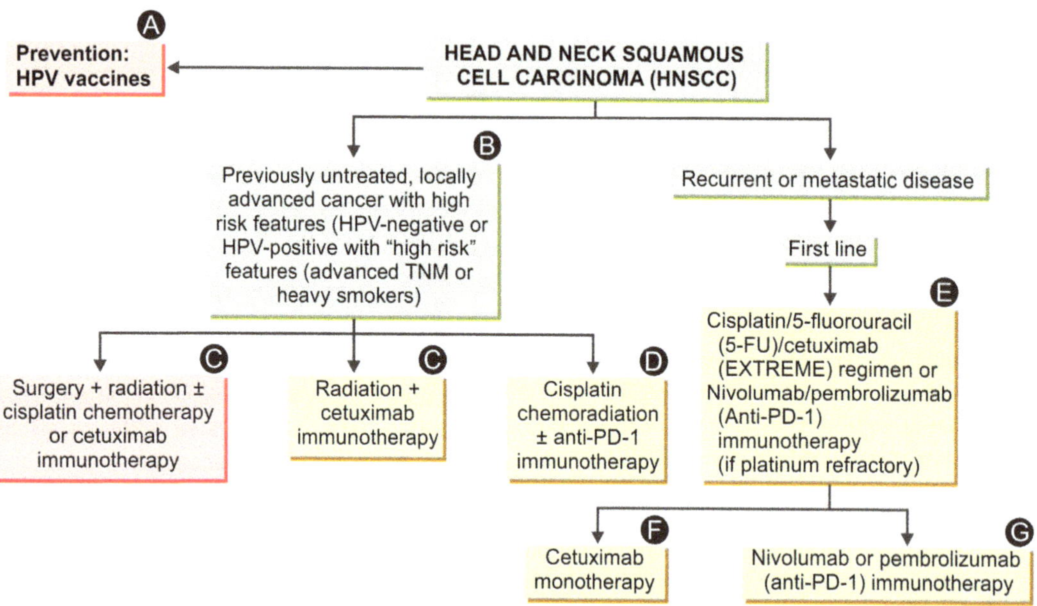

Immunotherapy involves enhancing the antitumor immune response and has been used in addition to standard therapies for head and neck squamous cell carcinoma (HNSCC). Monoclonal antibodies (mAbs) recognize specific tumor proteins, such as epidermal growth factor receptor. Some of these mAbs, such as cetuximab, may enhance antigen-dependent cell-mediated cytotoxicity, antigen presentation, and other mechanisms of antitumor immunity. Immune checkpoint receptors, such as programmed cell death protein 1 (PD-1) and cytotoxic T-lymphocyte-associated protein 4 (CTLA-4), exist to prevent exaggerated immune responses and autoimmunity. Targeting these checkpoint molecules with specific inhibitors has been shown to enhance antitumor immunity for several tumor types, including HNSCC.

A Vaccines to prevent infection with high-risk human papillomavirus (HPV) (Gardasil, Cervarix) have been shown in large studies to prevent HPV-related oropharyngeal and anogenital malignancy.

B Patients with HPV-negative disease or those with HPV-related disease and a smoking history have a relatively poor prognosis, thus they are treated with immunotherapy in addition to standard chemoradiation in attempt to increase survival without disproportionate additional toxicity.

C Cetuximab is approved by the Food and Drug Administration (FDA) approved as an alternative to platinum chemotherapy for previously untreated HNSCC and is often used in patients who cannot tolerate cisplatin.

D Multiple PD-1 inhibitors are under investigation and likely to be approved by the FDA for treatment of locally advanced HNSCC.

E Based on the EXTREME trial, a combination consisting of cisplatin, 5-FU, and cetuximab, is frequently used for recurrent or metastatic HNSCC.

F Cetuximab has been approved by the FDA for use as monotherapy in patients with recurrent or metastatic HNSCC who have been previously treated with cisplatin.

G Anti-PD-1 antibodies (nivolumab and pembrolizumab) have been shown in recent clinical trials in HNSCC to provide sustained responses in a subset of patients with recurrent or metastatic HNSCC. Both PD-1 inhibitors have been approved by the FDA for treatment of recurrent/metastatic, platinum refractory HNSCC in 2016.

SUGGESTED READING

Allen CT, Clavijo PE, Van Waes C, et al. Anti-tumor immunity in head and neck cancer: understanding the evidence, how tumors escape and immunotherapeutic approaches. Cancers. 2015;7: 2397-2414.

Chow LQ, Haddad R, Gupta S, et al. Antitumor activity of pembrolizumab in biomarker-unselected patients with recurrent and/or metastatic head and neck squamous cell carcinoma: results from the phase Ib KEYNOTE-012 expansion cohort. J Clin Oncol. 2016; pii: JCO681478.

Ferris RL. Immunology and immunotherapy of head and neck cancer. J Clin Oncol. 2015;33:3293-3304.

Ferris RL, Blumenschein G Jr, Fayette J, et al. Nivolumab for recurrent squamous-cell carcinoma of the head and neck. N Engl J Med. 2016;375:1856-1867.

Schoppy DW, Sunwoo JB. Immunotherapy for head and neck squamous cell carcinoma. Hematol Oncol Clin North Am. 2015;29: 1033-1043.

Specenier P, Vermorken JB. Cetuximab in the treatment of squamous cell carcinoma of the head and neck. Expert Rev Anticancer Ther. 2011;11:511-524.

Pulmonary Mass in Patients with Head and Neck Cancer

Peter F Ferson

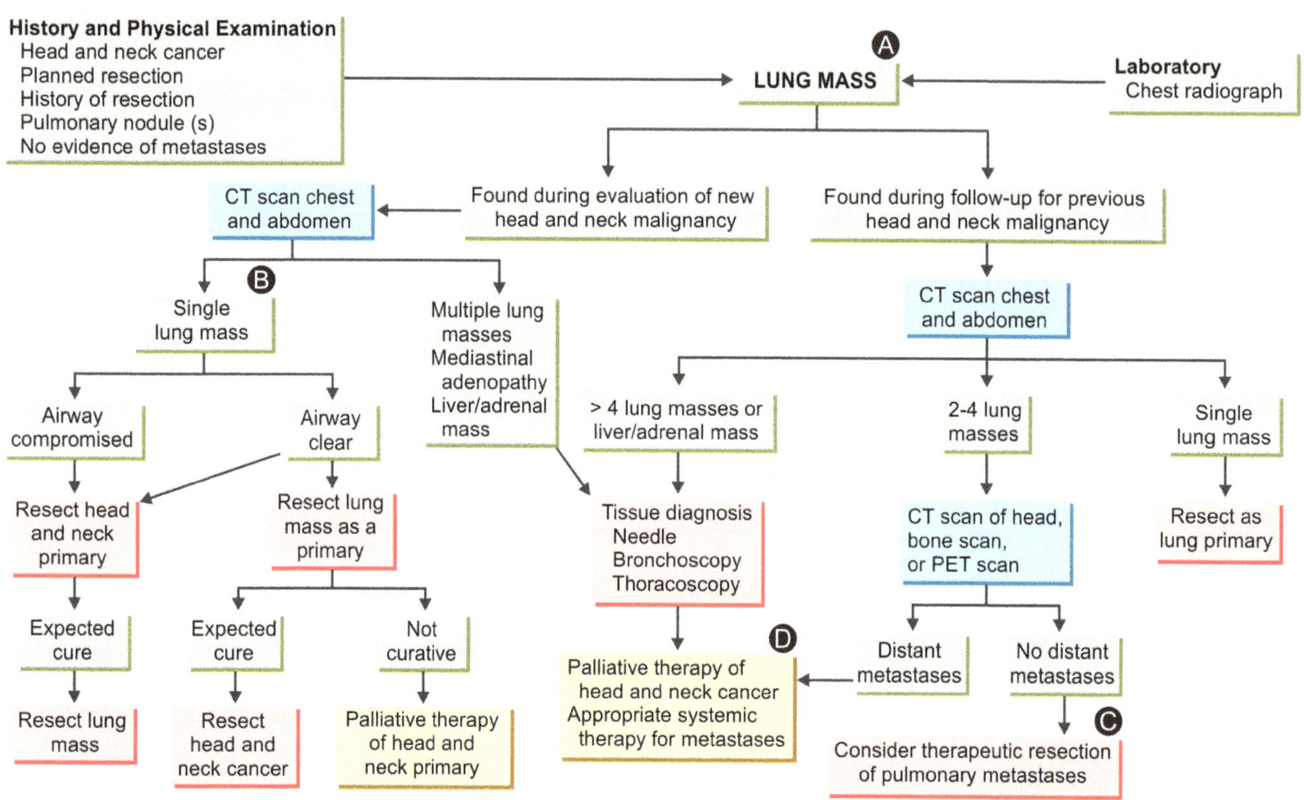

Routine chest radiographs on patients with head and neck cancer will occasionally show unsuspected pulmonary nodules. Diagnostic and therapeutic options for both tumors require careful and thoughtful analysis.

A Because the nasopharynx and the oropharynx are part of the same organ system as the lungs, synchronous or asynchronous masses in both locations can occur. The lung mass or masses may represent metastases from the primary in the head and neck or may be a primary cancer in the lung. Differentiating between the two may be difficult, particularly if there are only one or two nodules. A tissue biopsy may help rule out metastases if the cell types of the lung and the head and neck lesions are different. Often, however, the head and neck tumor is one that is also commonly found as a lung primary, such as adenocarcinoma or squamous cell carcinoma. Similarity in cell types for these cancers does not necessarily imply metastatic disease, but may represent synchronous primaries in different parts of an organ system that have been exposed to the same carcinogens. When the head and neck malignancy is one that is less commonly found in the lung, such as mucoepidermoid carcinoma, adenoid cystic carcinoma, or rhabdomyosarcoma, the diagnosis of metastases may be made with more confidence.

If both cancers are of the same cell type, and if knowledge that the lung mass is a metastasis would alter the approach or intensity of treatment for the head and neck lesion, then deoxyribonucleic acid analysis can be performed on the two biopsies.

B When a potentially resectable lung nodule presents during the initial evaluation for a head and neck primary tumor, a decision must be made concerning the timing of the approach to the two lesions. Simultaneous resections are unwise. If the airway is compromised by the cancer of the head and neck or if maintaining excellent clearance of airway secretions is in question, then the cancer of the head and neck should be resected first. If the airway is stable, however, it is preferable to proceed with the lung resection for two reasons. First, the clinical staging of lung cancer is not uniformly accurate, and findings during lymph node dissection may upgrade a clinically favorable lesion to one that has a poor outcome. The knowledge of a poor prognosis with respect to the lung cancer will obviously have an impact on potential plans for extensive head and neck resections. The second reason relates to airway management during pulmonary resections. Double-lumen endotracheal intubation is commonly used for pulmonary resections, and the insertion of a double-lumen endotracheal tube through an upper airway that is scarred and deformed can be hazardous. Therefore, it is preferable to perform this anesthetic manipulation during the first operation. If a permanent tracheostomy is planned as part of the neck operation, however, subsequent placement of a double-lumen endotracheal tube is quite easy, and the pulmonary operation may safely be delayed as the second operation.

C Resection of pulmonary metastases is appropriate for selected patients. Various criteria for selection of candidates for excision of pulmonary metastases have been proposed. The most commonly accepted criteria require a limited number of metastases (usually four or fewer), ideally a latent period from resection of the primary cancer, no evidence of extrapulmonary metastases, and complete control of the primary cancer.

D Treatment of metastatic cancer requires considerable planning. Palliative therapy for local symptoms from the primary cancer will take precedence and may require major surgical intervention. Distant metastases, verified by scans such as positron emission tomography (PET) may require treatment because of location rather than symptoms, particularly when brain involvement is discovered. Asymptomatic pulmonary metastases may not require immediate intervention.

SUGGESTED READING

Allen MS, Putnum JB. Secondary tumors of the lung. In: Shields T (Ed). General Thoracic Surgery, 7th edition. Philadelphia, PA: Lippincott Williams and Wilkins; 2009. pp. 1619-1646.

Lefor AT, Bredenberg CE, Kellman RM, et al. Multiple malignancies of the lung and head and neck. Second primary tumor or metastases? Arch Surg. 1986;121:265-270.

Massard G, Roeslin N, Jung GM, et al. Bronchogenic cancer associated with head and neck tumors. Survival analysis of 194 patients. J Thorac Cardiovasc Surg. 1992;106(2):218-227.

Massard G, Wihim JM, Ameur S, et al. Association of bronchial and pharyngo-laryngeal malignancies. A reappraisal. Eur J Cardio-thoracic Surg. 1996;10(6):397-402.

Pastorino U, Grunenwald D. Surgical resection of pulmonary metastases. In: Pearson's Thoracic and Esophageal Surgery, 3rd edition. Philadelphia, PA: Churchill Livingston Elsevier; 2008. pp. 851-863.

CHAPTER 178

Follow-Up of Patients with Cancer

Johannes J Fagan

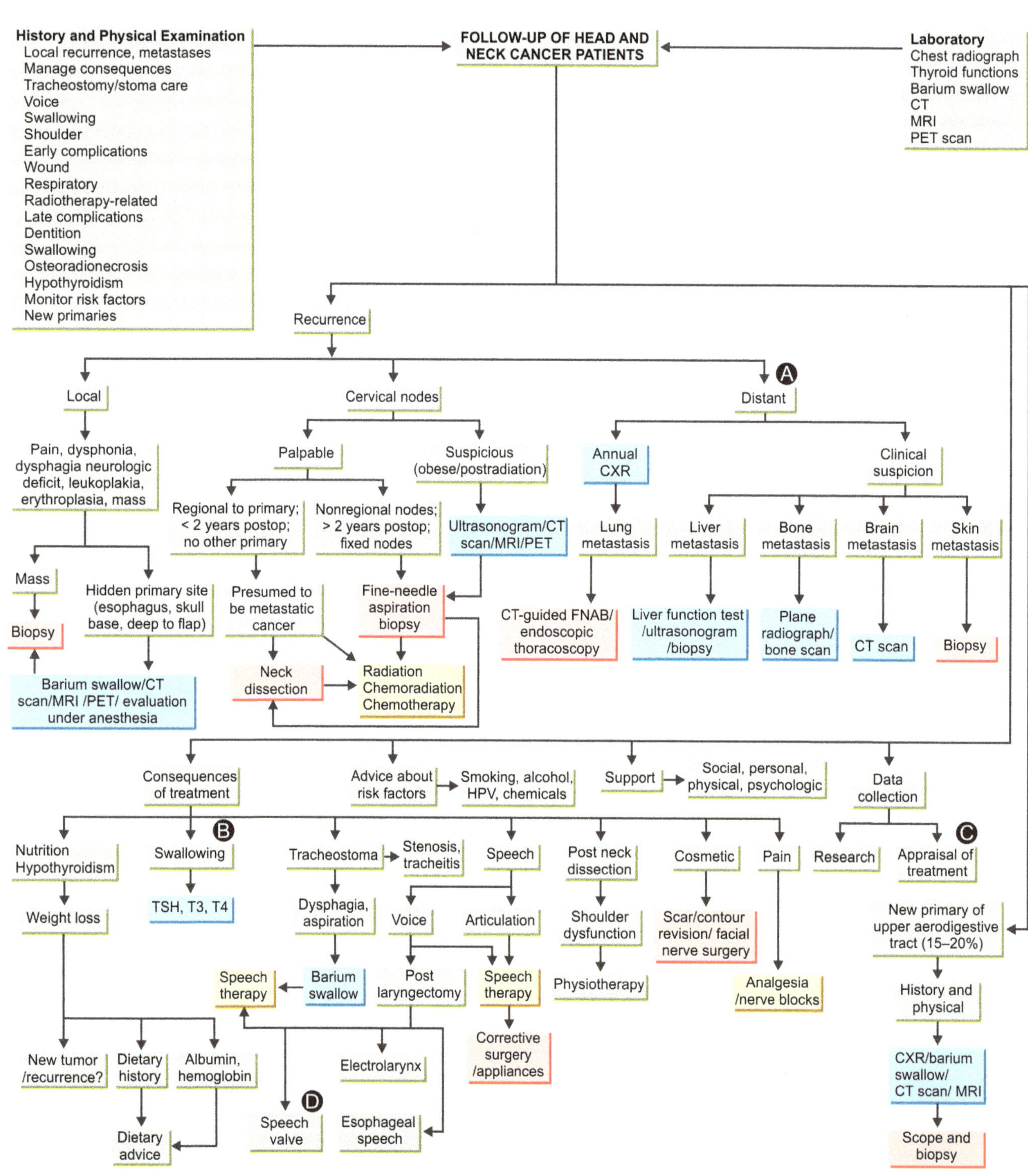

Initial follow-up of patients treated for cancer of the head and neck is directed at detection and management of early complications of treatment. Surgical patients may experience wound complications such as dehiscence, sepsis, flap necrosis, and fistulae or general complications such as pulmonary infection, atelectasis, stridor, deep vein thrombosis, pulmonary embolus, urinary tract infection, and inadequate oral intake. Patients treated with (chemo)radiotherapy may have breakdown of skin and mucosal breakdown and poor oral intake. Patients with a tracheostomy or a laryngectomy stoma are trained in tracheostomy tube and stoma care. Their ability to care for the stoma must be monitored before they are discharged from hospital. Long-term follow-up is directed at detecting new primary cancers, managing the consequences of treatment, monitoring risk factors, and providing emotional support. Data collection for reporting and outcome research is a critical part of any head and neck cancer program and is facilitated by routine follow-up of patients. Time intervals between visits are individualized according to risk of recurrence and other factors. Because~80% of recurrences occur within 2 years, patients are seen 1–3 monthly in the first year, 2–6 monthly in the second year, 4–8 monthly in the third year, and 12 monthly from fifth year onwards.

(A) Treatment of distant metastasis of most cancers of the head and neck is generally palliative. Therefore, despite it being less sensitive than computed tomography (CT) or positron emission tomography (PET)–CT, reliance is generally placed on an annual chest radiograph (CXR; see Chapters 180 and 181).

(B) Hypothyroidism occurs in a significant percentage of patients who have undergone radiation therapy to the neck as well as those who have undergone laryngectomy. It may be subclinical and onset is usually insidious. Patients may present with lethargy, depression, and weight gain. These patients may have a typical puffy appearance on physical examination. Thyroid function tests [thyroid-stimulating hormone (TSH), tri-iodothyronine (T_3), and thyroxine (T_4)] are advisable 6–12 monthly.

(C) Clinical audit permits a critical evaluation of outcomes, and comparison of results of treatment with centers of excellence and may prompt modification of treatment protocols.

(D) Optimal speech results after laryngectomy and tracheoesophageal puncture are facilitated by follow-up with a speech pathologist. Variations in valve selection, such as size and length, indwelling or removable, and duckbill or low pressure, must be individualized. Fungal overgrowth may be treated with oral antifungal preparations. Fungal infection and granulomas at the tracheoesophageal puncture site may require removal and replacement of the valve. Patients who do not achieve speech should undergo videofluoroscopic examination to exclude the presence of spasm or stricture of the pharyngoesophageal segment. These problems are correctable either by surgical means or, in the case of spasm, by injection of botulinum toxin.

SUGGESTED READING

Madana J, Morand GB, Barona-Lleo L, et al. A survey on pulmonary screening practices among otolaryngology—head and neck surgeons across Canada in the post treatment surveillance of head and neck squamous cell carcinoma. J Otolaryngol Head Neck Surg. 2015;44(1):5.

Rønjom MF, Brink C, Bentzen SM, et al. Hypothyroidism after primary radiotherapy for head and neck squamous cell carcinoma: normal tissue complication probability modeling with latent time correction. Radiother Oncol. 2013;109(2):317-322.

Cancer with Distant Metastasis

Julie E Bauman

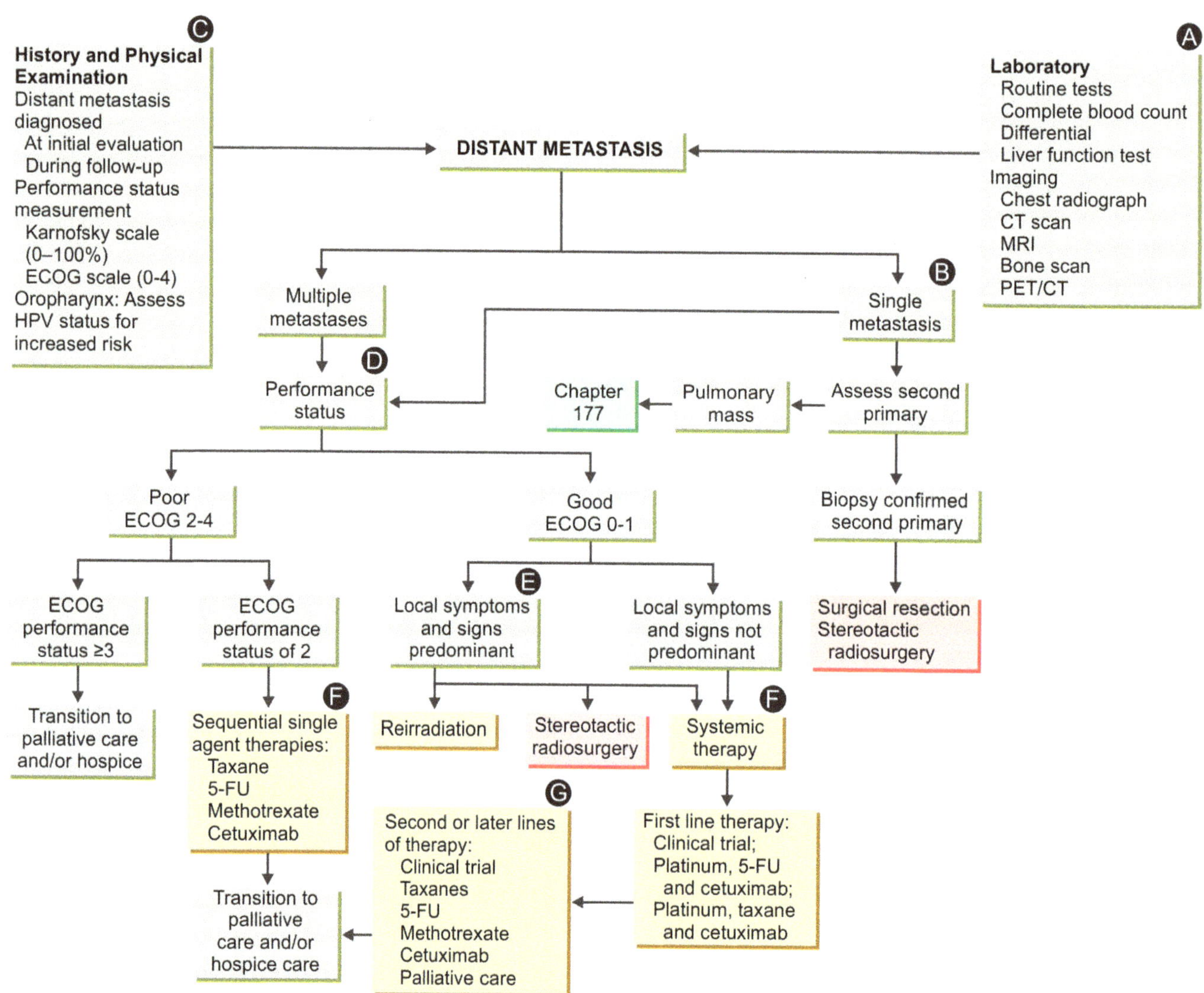

Regional metastases are not uncommon in patients with cancer of the head and neck, and a mass in the neck is often the first sign of the presence of cancer. Management of the neck is a fundamental component of nearly all head and neck cancers, and cure is often possible even with neck metastases. Distant metastases are much less common at initial presentation, and portend a more dire prognosis. Despite this fact, treatment is still possible and many patients benefit from systemic therapy directed against distant disease.

A For patients with clinical stage I–II cancer of the head and neck, cross-sectional locoregional imaging with contrasted computed tomography (CT) or magnetic resonance imaging (MRI) of the neck and chest radiograph is sufficient for radiologic staging; routine cross-sectional thoracic imaging or positron emission tomography (PET)/CT for distant metastases is usually unrewarding and not routinely recommended unless clinical symptoms indicate. Magnetic resonance imaging is superior to CT scans for lesions that may involve the brain or leptomeninges, paranasal sinuses, and/or the skull base. For patients with clinical stage III-IV cancer, comprehensive staging with PET/CT scan, including integrated diagnostic CT of the neck, is preferred. In these cases, the rate of distant metastases and the associated change in clinical management justify the increased cost.

B If an isolated metastasis particularly to the lung is identified in a patient with tobacco-related, human papillomavirus (HPV)-negative disease, consider the possibility that this represents a second primary cancer. Histologic confirmation is essential. Surgical resection or stereotactic radiosurgery may be considered for patients in good overall condition and without significant comorbidities.

C Clinically apparent distant metastases occur in about 11% of patients upon initial diagnosis of squamous cell carcinoma of the head and neck (SCCHN). In patients with HPV-negative disease, the risk increases with Tumor Neck Metastasis (TNM) stage and correlates most closely with nodal stage. In patients with HPV-positive cancer, the risk also increases with TNM stage and is greatest for those with thyroxine (T4) or ≥N2c disease. Irrespective of environmental or viral etiology, the most common site of distant metastases is the lung (52%), and most distant metastases (80%) are diagnosed within 2 years of the primary diagnosis. Autopsy series suggest a much higher incidence of clinically undetected distant metastases (up to 40%) in patients who die of their cancer.

D Performance status is measured either by the Karnofsky (0–100%) or Eastern Cooperative Oncology Group (ECOG) (0–4) scales. Patients who are in poor general condition do not usually benefit from aggressive therapy, and palliation should be the goal. Eligibility for entry into clinical trials is usually restricted to patients with a Karnofsky score >60 and an ECOG score <2.

E Although patients with SCCHN may harbor metastatic cancer, symptoms and morbidity are usually related to the local tumor burden. In certain situations, despite evidence of metastases, effective palliation can be provided by local therapy. Options include conventional (re)irradiation, stereotactic radiosurgery, and surgical debulking or resection. Stereotactic radiosurgery can be combined safely with cetuximab as a radiation sensitizer.

F Palliative systemic therapy is the logical approach to patients with documented metastases, potentially enabling the therapy to reach all tumor sites. In the United States, few systemic agents are approved by the Food and Drug Administration (FDA) for cancer of the head and neck, including methotrexate (1956), fluorouracil (5-FU) (1957), cisplatin (1978), docetaxel (2006), and cetuximab (2006). Because of the dearth of new, effective agents, clinical trials are preferred where available. In patients who have a good performance status (ECOG 0-1), the best evidence supports standard frontline therapy with the combination of platinum, 5-FU, and cetuximab; this combination improved response rate, progression-free and overall survival relative to platinum-5FU in a randomized phase III trial. Due to the impracticality of infusional therapy and the toxicity profile of 5-FU in non-European populations, an alternate frontline combination frequently used in the United States is cisplatin,

taxane, and cetuximab. In patients with an ECOG performance status of 2, single-agent chemotherapy is preferred for frontline management. The choices include single-agent cytotoxic chemotherapy or cetuximab. In patients with an ECOG performance status of ≥3, the toxicities of systemic therapy are very likely to outweigh discernable benefit, and transition to palliative and/or hospice care is recommended.

G When performance status and patient philosophy permit, second or later lines of palliative systemic therapy may be administered. Clinical trials are preferred wherever available. Conventional options include sequential, noncross-resistant, single-agent therapies. For example, in patients who have not been exposed to cetuximab, it is indicated as second-line therapy in platinum-refractory disease. In patients previously exposed to both platinum and cetuximab, single-agent cytotoxics may be considered, such as a taxane, 5-FU, or methotrexate. Given the lack of curative options for patients with distant metastatic disease, the majority of patients will experience a decline in performance status and an increased symptom burden. Early referral to palliative care is encouraged, for comanagement of difficult symptoms and discussions regarding goals of care.

SUGGESTED READING

Agarwal V, Branstetter BF 4th, Johnson JT. Indications for PET/CT in the head and neck. Otolaryngol Clin North Am. 2008;41(1): 23-49.

Fakhry C, Zhang Q, Nguyen-Tan PF, et al. Human papillomavirus and overall survival after progression of oropharyngeal squamous cell carcinoma. J Clin Oncol. 2014;32(30):3365-3373.

O'Sullivan B, Huang SH, Siu LL, et al. Deintensification candidate subgroups in human papillomavirus-related oropharyngeal cancer according to minimal risk of distant metastasis. J Clin Oncol. 2013;31(5):543-550.

Schenker Y, Arnold RM, Bauman JE, et al. An enhanced role for palliative care in the multidisciplinary approach to high-risk head and neck cancer. Cancer. 2016;122(3):340-343.

Vargo JA, Ferris RL, Ohr J, et al. A prospective phase 2 trial of reirradiation with stereotactic body radiation therapy plus cetuximab in patients with previously irradiated recurrent squamous cell carcinoma of the head and neck. Int J Radiat Oncol Biol Phys. 2015;91(3):480-488.

Vermorken JB, Herbst RS, Leon X, et al. Overview of the efficacy of cetuximab in recurrent and/or metastatic squamous cell carcinoma of the head and neck in patients who previously failed platinum-based therapies. Cancer. 2008;112(12):2710-2719.

Vermorken JB, Mesia R, Rivera F, et al. Platinum-based chemotherapy plus cetuximab in head and neck cancer. N Engl J Med. 2008;359(11):1116-1127.

Zbaren P, Lehman W. Frequency and sites of distant metastases in head and neck squamous cell carcinoma: An analysis of 101 cases at autopsy. Arch Otolaryngol Head Neck Surg. 1987;113:762-764.

CHAPTER 180

Management of the Patient with Terminal Cancer

David E Eibling

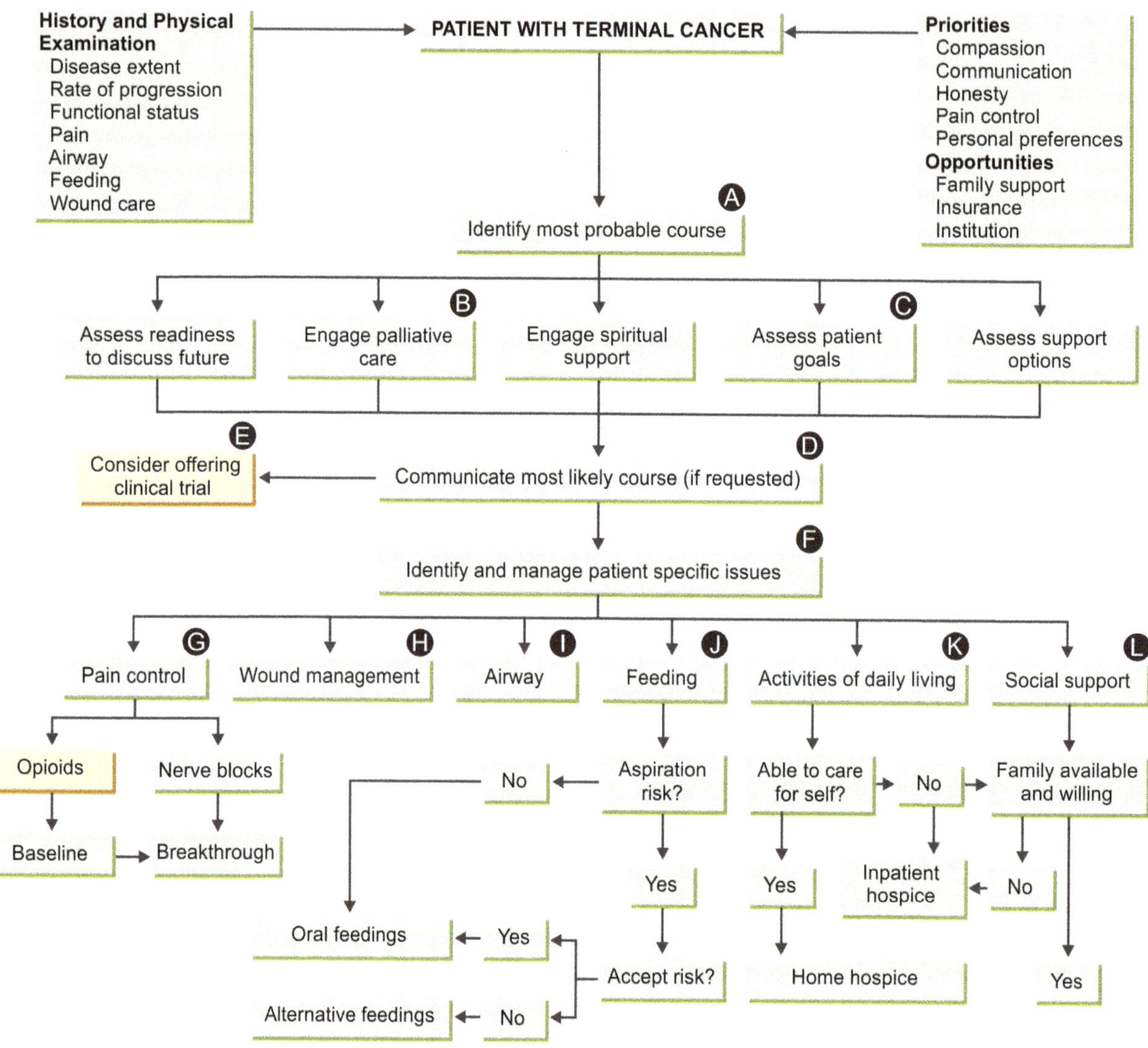

All life is terminal, and all of our patients—and ourselves—will eventually die. Although oncologists are most likely to be called upon to help patients navigate the final chapter of their lives, in reality all physicians will be occasionally called upon to do so. Over the past several years there has developed increasing recognition that most physicians are poorly prepared for this role. In addition to highly developed medical knowledge and specialized communication skills, helping patients and their families' transition this period of their lives requires the highest levels of honesty, candor, empathy, and a willingness to listen to the patient's concerns.

A Perhaps the most difficult part for the physician is to recognize the reality of incurability sufficiently early in the terminal phase of the disease to permit the patient and the family time to accept the inevitability of death. It is natural for physicians to assume that their patient will do better than average. Studies have demonstrated that even when the inevitability of death is understood, the average physician overestimates the chances of cure more than fivefold.

B Early involvement of the Palliative Care Service is invaluable in assisting the treatment team in the required role, and has been shown to improve the quality of life for both the patient and the caregiver(s). Some studies have demonstrated that not only the quality of life, but also the duration of survival is increased by early involvement, probably by reducing the use of morbidity-inducing useless interventions.

At the end of life, one's spiritual life becomes more important, even if it was not important earlier. As such, all patients should be offered pastoral care within the framework of their belief system and culture. Early involvement within the context of a palliative care team is often invaluable to the patient and family, particularly as the end approaches.

C When asked about their goals, patients will naturally state "to be cured". Therefore, a discussion of patient-centered goals must include honest communication of the most likely clinical course (step D). Goal assessment is a conversation that takes time and emotional engagement, not merely asking the question "what do you want us to do?"

D Communication of the likely clinical course is difficult, but necessary in deriving goals and in formulating a management plan. A variety of strategies are taught, and now most medical schools include at least some training in difficult discussions. Communicating the duration of survival is challenging, but necessary for decision making if patients inquire. Most experienced oncologists carefully qualify their predictions with high levels of uncertainty. Studies have demonstrated that patients misinterpret their physicians' statements about prognosis more than half the time. One strategy is to *Ask* (if the patient is ready to hear), *Tell* (as much is known), and *Ask* (did you understand and do you have more questions?).

E Advancing medical knowledge requires that patients be enrolled in clinical trials. Enrolling patients with incurable cancer in Phase 1 or Phase 2 trials is often helpful to advance the science. However, enrolling terminal patients may be harmful as enrollment inevitably implies false hope (even if unstated) and impacts their quality of life through treatment-induced morbidity as well as by reducing the remaining time available to spend doing other things. However, patients who approach such clinical trials with an altruistic intent to help others, with the realization that it is unlikely they will be helped, may benefit by finding some sense of meaning in their life despite their terminal illness.

F All patients with any illness (terminal or not) will have specific issues that vary from patient to patient. Honest assessment based on inquiry is important, and strategies must be based on patient's goals and expectations.

G Fear of pain is often greater than fear of death for the patient with terminal cancer. The assurance that adequate pain control will be provided may be more important than the actual medication itself. Most authorities recommend a graduated baseline level of opioids with additional breakthrough medication available. Addiction is not a concern, and diversion, even though theoretically possible, is not the primary concern.

H Wound management can be challenging, particularly if wounds involve the airway (step I), orocutaneous or pharyngocutaneous fistulae, or major vessels. Competent nursing care is a must, and assessment of the care setting (step L) is necessary. Wounds that present a risk of major bleeding from rupture of a major vessel require specific discussion regarding possibility (step D). Anticipation of the possibility may reduce the emotional trauma on patient and family if such occurs (often as the terminal event).

I Recurrent cancers that involve the airway are problematic, particularly if not able to be easily bypassed with a tracheostomy. Decisions whether to proceed with tracheostomy should be individualized, as, although not intuitive to Otolaryngologists, some patients may elect air hunger rather than prolongation of life with an artificial airway.

J Eating is a fundamental part of the enjoyment of life, and patients with terminal illnesses often elect to continue to eat even when the risk of aspiration pneumonia is high. For others, a palliative gastrostomy may be beneficial, as maintaining fluids and nutrition can improve the quality of life even if it does not prolong survival.

K Assessment of the ability of the patients to care for themselves (activities of daily living) is important and helps drive other conversations. Noting the overall degree of cleanliness may provide some clues. Even if patients are able to care for themselves, home hospice or similar support should be offered early so that meaningful relationships can be built early in the dying process.

L All dying patients will, at some time, need social support. Some patients are fortunate to have nearby family members who participate in care, decision making, as well as provide emotional support. Others are not as fortunate, and these individuals will benefit from placement in an in-patient hospice environment if available.

SUGGESTED READING

Christakis NA, Lamont EB. Extent and determinants of error in physicians' prognoses in terminally ill patients: a prospective cohort study. West J Med. 2000;172:310-313.

Gawande A. Being Mortal: Medicine and What Matters in the End. New York: Metropolitan Books; 2014.

Temel JS, Greer JA, Muzikansky A, et al. Early palliative care for patients with metastatic non-small-cell lung cancer. N Eng J Med. 2010;363:733-742.

Wolf JH, Wolf KS. The Lake Wobegone effect: are all cancer patients above average? Milbank Q. 2013;91(4):690-728.

Approaching Medical Error

David E Eibling

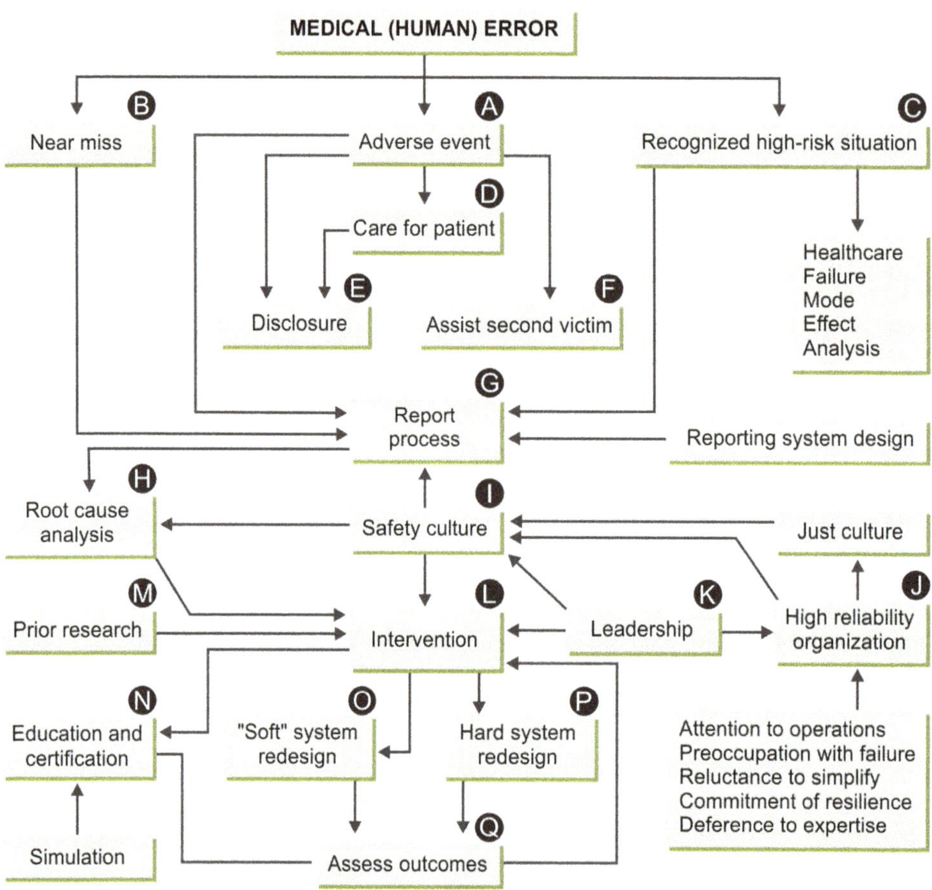

The challenge of medical error burst into the public consciousness with the publication of the seminal Institute of Medicine (IOM) report "To Err is Human" in 1999. The IOM report followed a decade of increasing attention to the issue of medical error, perhaps best summarized by Lucian Leape in 1994. Leape tied the challenge of medical error to pre-existing knowledge of human error in the psychology literature. The very title of the IOM report conveys the fallibility of humans, and the inevitability of error.

Over the past two decades we have come to understand how systems can be improved to reduce the likelihood of error, capture the error before the patient is affected, or mitigate the effects of the error. Accompanying this change is recognition that adverse events long thought to be inevitable, may, in fact, be preventable, and failure of processes to prevent them are considered the errors.

A Recognition that an adverse event was due to human error is often nonintuitive.

B Medical error does not necessarily lead to an adverse outcome for the patient. These so-called "near misses" provide an opportunity for studying and improving systems of care.

C Most healthcare workers recognize risky situations that have the potential for resulting in patient harm. These "nonevents" should be considered a form of human error—in this case, errors in system design. Capturing this "front-line" knowledge permits analysis of the probability of an event occurring and the severity of the event if it should. Formal evaluation using techniques of Healthcare Failure Mode Effect Analysis enables system stakeholders to prioritize interventions.

D Following recognition of an adverse event, the first priority is to provide care for the patient. Often the optimal strategy is to urgently consult ones colleagues, since the practitioner may be unable to make necessary therapeutic decisions when overwhelmed with shame and grief following an event.

E Disclosure of the event to the patient and family, along with authentic expressions of grief and apology, is invaluable to the injured patient and the loved ones. Not only is trust in their physician strengthened by honesty, but knowledge of the event and its sequelae enhance the ability of the patient and family to make what are often difficult decisions. Despite concerns regarding increasing the risk of a tort claim, the reality is that open disclosure and apology reduce the risk, most likely due to abrogating the common perception that there has been a "cover-up". Regardless of legal issues, disclosure is the right thing for the patient and the physician.

F Care for the "second victim" is recognized as a deficiency in US medicine. It falls to all physicians to be aware of the potential for the "second victim" and provide emotional support.

G Lucian Leape pointed out the critical value of reporting as a tool for system improvement. His paper was published nearly two decades after the Aviation Safety Reporting System (ASRS) was established. Two decades later, healthcare is still struggling on how to capture and use the information contained in reports of adverse events. Reporting systems are hampered by multiple factors; however, the biggest impediment remains the culture of the organization (see step "I").

H Analysis of the event, near miss, or high-risk situation is the most challenging aspect of responding to an error. Among the multiple biases that impact the accuracy of the evaluation, the so-called "hindsight bias" is the most difficult to overcome. Reason pointed out that most adverse events occur due to alignment of multiple factors; hence selecting the most salient "root cause" is unlikely to prevent recurrence of the event.

I A safety culture is not a blame-free culture. All high-performing individuals occasionally "bend the rules" to achieve their goal; however, high-reliability organizations do not tolerate reckless behavior. The aviation industry introduced the concept of the "Just Culture" nearly two decades ago and its principles are now making inroads into healthcare systems. The Universal Protocol "Time Out" is one such example. A Just Culture is one in which all employees understand and respect boundaries and are unafraid to report errors. The most critical attribute of a Just Culture is the process whereby boundaries are defined, and who is responsible for doing so.

J Studies of organizations that experience lower-than-expected adverse events, often termed "high-reliability organizations," have identified specific enabling attributes. These include Sensitivity to Operations (what are we doing), Preoccupation with (and attempts to predict) Failure, Reluctance to Simplify, Commitment to Resilience, and Deference to Expertise (wherever it resides).

K Organizational leadership has been repeatedly demonstrated as the most critical factor affecting all of these attributes.

L Rarely is a single intervention likely to be successful in eliminating adverse events. Heimlich has pointed out that although human error cannot be prevented, systems can be designed in such a way to (1) reduce the likelihood of an error, (2) "capture" the error before it reaches the patient, or (3) mitigate the effects on the patient. Resilient systems employ all three strategies. Interventions rarely are successful alone, but require multiple components and implementation in a safety-conscious organization.

M The literature addressing human error is substantial, but most is to be found in the so-called "human factors" research in the engineering and psychology domains. These investigations are based on the understanding that system design affects the probability of human error occurring, as well as the likelihood of resultant injury.

N Deficiencies in knowledge or skills of front-line staff should be considered as a system, not individual human errors. Integrated into effective education is a reliable assessment and certification process. Recently, simulation training has played an ever-increasing role, not only in training, but also in assessment of individual, team, and even system performance.

O Process changes and implementation of policies such as checklists, hand hygiene, and view alerts are "soft" system enhancements in that they can be easily bypassed.

P "Hard" system changes are those that cannot be bypassed, such as unique tubing connectors to prevent accidental misconnection.

Q Assessment of the effectiveness of interventions is often challenging due to the infrequent occurrence of specific adverse events. Centralized reporting, such as the Veterans Administration's National Center for Patient Safety or the Pennsylvania Patient Safety Authority are examples of strategies that facilitate outcome measurement. In reality, most organizations are forced to use process implementation rates rather than actual error rates as surrogate measures.

SUGGESTED READING

Gallagher TH, Studdert D, Levinson W. Disclosing harmful medical errors to patients. N Engl J Med. 2007;356:2713-2719.

Holden R, Ben-Tzion K. A review of medical error reporting system design consideration and a proposed cross-level systems research framework. Hum Factors. 2007;49:257-276.

Lander LI, Connor JA, Shah RK, et al. Otolaryngologists' responses to errors and adverse events. Laryngoscope. 2006;116:1114-1120.

Leape LL. Error in medicine. JAMA. 1994;272:1851-1857.

Marx D. Patient safety and the "Just Culture": a primer for health care executives. Columbia University 2001. [online] Available from: http://www.mers-tm.org/support/Marx_Primer.pdf

Roberson DW, Kentala E, Healy GB. Quality and safety in a complex world: why systems science matters to otolaryngologists. Laryngoscope. 2004;114:1810-1814.

EU GSPR Authorised Reprsentative
Logos Europe, 9 rue Nicolas Poussin
1700, La Rochelle, France
Phone: +33 (0) 6 67 93 73 78
E-mail: contact@logoseurope.eu

www.ingramcontent.com/pod-product-compliance
Ingram Content Group UK Ltd.
Pitfield, Milton Keynes, MK11 3LW, UK
UKHW060047170726
7214IPUK00037B/387